PLANT-BASED NUTRITION IN CLINICAL PRACTICE

PLANT-BASED NUTRITION IN CLINICAL PRACTICE

Edited by
Shireen Kassam MB BS, FRCPATH, PhD, DIPIBLM
Zahra Kassam MB BS, FRCR(UK), FRCPC, MSc, DIPABLM
and
Lisa Simon RD

Foreword by **David JA Jenkins** OC, MD, FRSC, FRCP, FRCPC, PhD, DSc

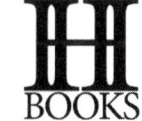

Hammersmith Health Books
London, UK

First published in 2022 by Hammersmith Health Books
– an imprint of Hammersmith Books Limited
4/4A Bloomsbury Square, London WC1A 2RP, UK
www.hammersmithbooks.co.uk

© 2022, Shireen Kassam, Zahra Kassam, Lisa Simon
Reprinted 2022

All rights reserved. No part of this publication may be reproduced, stored in any retrieval system or transmitted in any form or by any means, electronic, mechanical, photocopying, recording or otherwise, without the prior permission of the publishers and copyright holders.

Disclaimer: This book is designed to provide helpful information on the subjects discussed. It is not meant to be used, nor should it be used, to diagnose or treat any medical condition. For diagnosis or treatment of any medical problem, consult your own physician or healthcare provider. The publisher and author are not responsible for any specific health or allergy needs that may require medical supervision and are not liable for any damages or negative consequences from any treatment, action, application or preparation, to any person reading or following the information in this book. References are provided for informational purposes only and do not constitute endorsement of any websites or other sources. Readers should be aware that the websites listed in this book may change. The information and references included are up to date at the time of writing but given that medical evidence progresses, it may not be up to date at the time of reading.

British Library Cataloguing in Publication Data: A CIP record of this book is available from the British Library.

Print ISBN 978-1-78161-198-2
Ebook ISBN 978-1-78161-199-9

Commissioning editor: Georgina Bentliff
Copyedited by: Carolyn White
Designed and typeset by: Julie Bennett of Bespoke Publishing Ltd
Cover design by: Madeline Meckiffe
Cover images by: ©Triff (leaf texture); ©photocell (peas); ©hxdbzxy (broccoli); ©stevemart (apples)
Index by: Dr Laurence Errington
Production: Deborah Wehner of Moatvale Press Ltd
Printed and bound by: TJ Books, Cornwall, UK

Contents

Editor biographies — vii
Author biographies — ix
Acknowledgements — xix
Foreword by David Jenkins — xxi
Preface — xxiii

1. **The impact of plant-based dietary patterns on health and disease** — 1
   Shireen Kassam, Zahra Kassam, Lisa Simon and David Jenkins

2. **Meeting nutritional requirements on a plant-based diet from birth to old age** — 27
   Sandra Hood and Miriam Martinez-Biarge

3. **Plant-based nutrition and cardiovascular disease** — 45
   Nesan Shanmugam

4. **Plant-based nutrition and cancer** — 69
   Aryan Tavakkoli

5. **Plant-based nutrition for respiratory and sleep health** — 89
   Priyumvada Naik

6. **Plant-based nutrition and weight management** — 103
   Sue Kenneally

7. **Plant-based nutrition for the prevention and treatment of diabetes** — 121
   Gemma Newman and Shireen Kassam

8. **Plant-based nutrition and clinical nephrology** — 139
   Leonie Dupuis and Shivam Joshi

9. **Plant-based nutrition and non-alcoholic fatty liver disease** — 149
   Divya Devabhaktuni and Meagan Gray

10. **Plant-based nutrition and gastrointestinal disorders** 163
    Alan Desmond and Rosie Martin

11. **Plant-based nutrition for mental health and wellbeing** 181
    Arvind K Maheru

12. **Plant-based nutrition for male and female health** 197
    Nitu Bajekal and Lisa Simon

13. **Plant-based nutrition and Alzheimer's prevention** 219
    Ayesha Sherzai, Sophia Sherzai, Shireen Kassam and Dean Sherzai

14. **Plant-based nutrition for autoimmunity and chronic inflammation** 229
    Despina Marselou

15. **Plant-based nutrition and bone health** 241
    Rajiv Bajekal and Lisa Simon

16. **Plant-based nutrition and dermatological conditions** 255
    Niyati Sharma

17. **Plant-based nutrition for athletes** 271
    Leila Dehghan-Zaklaki

18. **Barriers and strategies to adopting a plant-based diet** 285
    Trent Grassian and Arvind K Maheru

19. **Lifestyle Medicine in clinical practice** 301
    Laura Freeman

20. **An inclusively responsible food and agriculture system for planetary health** 315
    Laila Kassam and Amir Kassam

Abbreviations 331
Index 333

Editor biographies

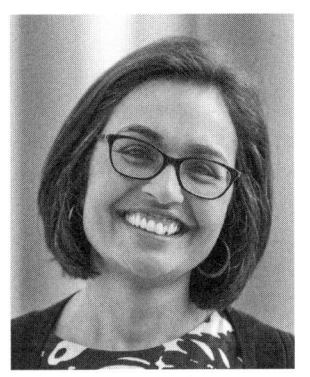

Shireen Kassam MB BS, FRCPATH, PhD, DIPIBLM

Dr Shireen Kassam is a Consultant Haematologist and Honorary Senior Lecturer at King's College Hospital, London, UK with a specialist interest in the treatment of lymphoma. She is also a Visiting Professor at University of Winchester, Hampshire, where she has developed and facilitates the UK's first university-based course on plant-based nutrition.

Shireen is passionate about promoting plant-based nutrition for the prevention and reversal of chronic disease and for maintaining optimal health after treatment for cancer. In 2019 she became certified as a Lifestyle Medicine physician and is also a CHIP facilitator.

Shireen founded Plant-Based Health Professionals UK in 2018, a non-profit, membership organisation whose mission is to provide evidence-based education on whole food plant-based nutrition. In January 2021, she co-founded and launched the UK's first regulated, plant-based, lifestyle medicine healthcare service Plant Based Health Online.

Shireen qualified as a doctor in 2000. During her training, she completed a PhD, which investigated the role of selenium in sensitising cancer cells to chemotherapy. Shireen has published a number of peer-reviewed papers in the field of lymphoma. Her first book, *Eating Plant-Based: Scientific Answers to Your Nutrition Questions*, co-authored with her sister Zahra, was published in January 2022.
(Editor; Chapter 1: The impact of plant-based dietary patterns on health and disease; Chapter 7: Plant-based nutrition for the prevention and treatment of diabetes; Chapter 13: Plant-based nutrition and Alzheimer's prevention)

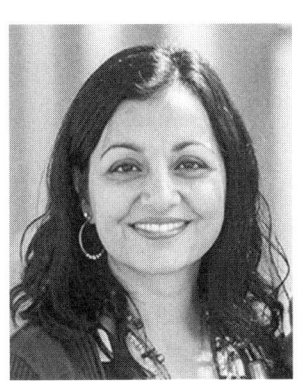

Zahra Kassam MB BS, FRCR(UK), FRCPC, MSc, DIPABLM

Dr Zahra Kassam is a Radiation Oncologist at the Stronach Regional Cancer Centre in Ontario, Canada, and an Assistant Professor in the Department of Radiation Oncology at the University of Toronto. Zahra received her medical degree from the Imperial College of Science, Technology and Medicine in 1995, completed her specialist training in clinical oncology in the UK, followed by three years of clinical and research fellowship training at the Princess Margaret Cancer Centre, Canada, with a Masters in Clinical Epidemiology at the University of Toronto. Her areas of clinical practice are in gastrointestinal and breast cancers. She has published a number of peer-reviewed papers on these malignancies, as well as in education and mentorship.

A few years ago, Zahra discovered the significant body of evidence demonstrating the benefits of nutrition in the prevention and management of chronic diseases, not taught at any stage of her medical training. She is a certified Lifestyle Medicine physician with the American Board of Lifestyle Medicine and has completed the eCornell certification in plant-based nutrition and the Plant-Based Nutrition course at the University of Winchester, UK. Zahra co-founded Plant-Based Canada, a non-profit organisation, in 2019, with the goal of educating the public and health professionals on the evidence-based benefits of plant-based whole food nutrition for individual and planetary health. Their inaugural event was held in 2019, the first Canadian Plant-Based Nutrition conference in Toronto. Her first book, *Eating Plant-Based: Scientific Answers to Your Nutrition Questions*, co-authored with her sister Shireen, was published in January 2022.
(Editor; Chapter 1: The impact of plant-based dietary patterns on health and disease)

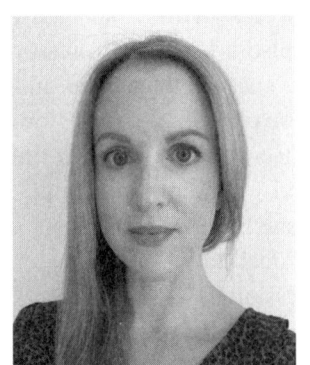

Lisa Simon BSc(HONS), BA(HONS), RD
Lisa Simon, Registered Dietitian, studied Clinical Nutrition and Dietetics at Cardiff Metropolitan University for four years before graduating as a Registered Dietitian with first class Honours in 2014.

She began her career working in Morriston Hospital in Swansea. After a year working with patients with a wide range of clinical conditions, she took up a rotational post at the University Hospital of Wales, where she worked in Neurology, Cardiology and Respiratory Medicine. She then took up a temporary, specialist post in Critical Care in the Royal Gwent Hospital in Newport, before specialising in Gastroenterology in 2016.

Lisa now splits her time working as project lead in the NHS, running outpatient clinics and group workshops, and working at CQC (Care Quality Commission) registered healthcare service, Plant Based Health Online, running individual and group consultations and delivering educational webinars. Her clinical areas of expertise are gastrointestinal conditions, liver and pancreatic disease, and male and female fertility.

Lisa has written a clinical update on diet and fertility for the British Dietetic Association and is writing her first book *The Plant-Based Dietitian's Guide to Fertility: From Pre-Conception to Healthy Birth*, due to be published in 2023.

She is passionate about providing an evidence-based, individualised approach with her patients, using all the pillars of Lifestyle Medicine to enable a holistic and detailed assessment and treatment plan.
(Editor; Chapter 1: The impact of plant-based dietary patterns on health and disease; Chapter 12: 'Plant-based nutrition for male and female health; Chapter 15: Plant-based nutrition and bone health)

Author biographies

Nitu Bajekal MD FRCOG DIPIBLM
Dr Nitu Bajekal is a Senior Consultant Obstetrician and Gynaecologist in the UK with over 35 years of clinical experience in women's health. Her special interests include Lifestyle Medicine, PCOS, endometriosis, period problems, menopause, precancer, complex vulval problems and medical education. She is a keyhole surgeon with experience in laparoscopic procedures including robotics. She is a Fellow of the Royal College and recipient of the Indian President's Gold medal. She is also one of the first board-certified Lifestyle Medicine physicians in the UK. She has written the women's health module for the University of Winchester's plant-based nutrition course.

Dr Bajekal is passionate about educating women, providing reliable medical and lifestyle information for the general public, doctors, workplaces and schools. She is the co-author of *Living PCOS Free*, a book that aims to help people with PCOS to understand their condition better and regain their hormonal health.
(Chapter 12: Plant-based nutrition for male and female health)

Rajiv Bajekal MS FRCS ORTH MCH ORTH DIPIBLM
Mr Rajiv Bajekal is a Consultant Spinal Surgeon practising in London in the National Health Service at the Royal Free Hospital and privately at multiple central and North London hospitals. He is an experienced clinician with a surgical practice mainly in the lumbar spine with a keen interest in managing sciatica, low back pain, spinal stenosis, osteoporotic fractures and infections. He is particularly keen to find simple and often non-surgical solutions for patients in severe pain and practises Lifestyle Medicine to look at problems more holistically rather than just the presenting problem.

Following some personal health issues, he adopted a whole food plant-based diet in 2017 and put his diabetes into remission. He and his wife decided to qualify in Lifestyle Medicine and have been diploma holders from the International Board of Lifestyle Medicine since 2018. As a qualified Lifestyle Medicine practitioner, he now applies the principles to his day-to-day practice and feels he can provide a better service to his patients.

He is a senior examiner for the FRCS Trauma and Orthopaedic Examination and lectures widely nationally and internationally for General Practitioners and is part of a group called Total Orthopaedics which provides high quality patient-focused care.

When not working, he loves walking his dogs, playing golf and cricket and he also cycles. He travels widely with his wife of 35 years who is a Consultant Gynaecologist.
(Chapter 15: Plant-based nutrition and bone health)

Leila Dehghan-Zaklaki MD MSc (NUTR) ANUTR

Dr Leila Dehghan is a doctor turned nutritionist and personal trainer. She received her medical degree from the University of Vienna and completed her internship in the UK. Her debilitating migraines compelled her to quit her medical career.

Although Leila became vegan for ethical reasons, she discovered the power of a whole food plant-based diet and healed her migraines through diet. This experience shifted her professional interests. She pursued a Plant-Based Nutrition Certificate at eCornell, part of Cornell University, and obtained a Master of Science degree in Clinical and Public Health Nutrition from University College London. Her thesis focused on the role of food triggers in migraine.

As an amateur martial artist, she takes a keen interest in sports nutrition and has developed the on-line Plant-Based Sports Nutrition Course for Plant-Based Health Professionals UK and Veganfitness.com. Leila has created a lecture on 'Plant-Based Diets Athletes' for the Plant-Based Nutrition course at the University of Winchester which she also co-facilitates. Leila is passionate about food justice and health equity. Her project 'Food Justice & Race' seeks to introduce a plant-based diet to people of the global majority (a term coined to refer to Black, Indigenous and people of colour).

Leila is a member of the Advisory Board and the education lead for the organisation Plant-based Health Professionals UK and has created the 21 Day Plant-based Health Challenge to invite more people to go plant-based.

(Chapter 17: Plant-based nutrition for athletes)

Alan Desmond MB BCh, BAO, BMEDSc, FRCP

Dr Alan Desmond is a Consultant Gastroenterologist based in Devon. He studied medicine at University College Cork, Ireland and completed his specialist training in Cork, Dublin and Oxford. Having previously published influential work on diagnostic radiation exposure in patients with digestive disorders, he has developed an interest in the dietary management of a range of digestive disorders, particularly Crohn's disease.

Alan takes every opportunity he gets to enjoy the great outdoors, running, biking and rowing. He adheres to, and advocates for, a whole food plant-based diet.

(Chapter 10: Plant-based nutrition and gastrointestinal disorders)

Divya Devabhaktuni MD BSc

Dr Divya Devabhaktuni is a budding hepatologist. She earned her Bachelor of Science in Food Science and Human Nutrition from the University of Florida in Gainesville, FL, US followed by her Doctorate of Medicine from the University of Central Florida College of Medicine. At the time of writing, she is completing her Internal Medicine Residency at the University of Alabama at Birmingham, US, and starts her fellowship in Gastroenterology and Hepatology at the University of Florida in summer 2022. Her areas of research interest are nutritional interventions in patients with chronic liver disease.

(Chapter 9: Plant-based nutrition and non-alcoholic fatty liver disease)

Leonie Dupuis BS

Leonie Dupuis is a medical student at the University of Central Florida College of Medicine (Class of 2023). During medical school, Leonie founded the UCF Lifestyle Medicine Interest Group and helped start up the Healthy Lifestyle Initiative, a volunteer program designed to teach under-served

high schoolers about the pillars of lifestyle medicine. She serves on the Lake Nona Performance Club's Medical Advisory Council where she participates in the development of the Exercise Prescription Program. She looks forward to a career in internal medicine and Lifestyle Medicine.
(Chapter 8: Plant-based nutrition and clinical nephrology)

Laura Freeman MB ChB, MRCGP, DRCOG, CCFP, DipIBLM/BSLM
Dr Laura Freeman obtained her Medical Degree from the University of Edinburgh in 2006. She completed her vocational training in General Practice in 2011. Between May 2012 and May 2019, after attaining full accreditation from the Medical Council of Canada, Dr Freeman ran her own Family Medicine practice in midtown Toronto, taught medical students at the University of Toronto and worked with the Medical Council of Canada as an examiner for international medical graduates.

Both within and outside of her general practice, Dr Freeman has developed a strong interest in plant-based nutrition and optimising health through lifestyle choices. In 2019, Dr Freeman became a diplomat of the International Board for Lifestyle Medicine and a certified CHIP (Complete Health Improvement Program) practitioner.

Dr Laura Freeman is co-founder and medical director of Plant Based Health Online, the UK's first CQC registered online plant-based Lifestyle Medicine healthcare service. She was also one of the first GPs in the UK to bring 'Walk with a Doc' walking groups to her community.
(Chapter 19: Lifestyle Medicine in clinical practice)

Trent Grassian PhD, MPA
Dr Trent Grassian is originally from the US but has been working as a social science researcher in the UK non-profit sector for the past decade, where he has overseen a wide variety of research projects and evaluations across the animal protection, health, education and homelessness sectors. Trent is a passionate social justice advocate and particularly interested in systems thinking approaches and empowering individuals to make changes in their own lifestyles and the world around them. While earning his PhD in Social Policy, Trent conducted research into the impacts of non-profit organisations promoting meat-reduction and veganism, in the largest study of its kind. Trent has given presentations all over the world about the research and his publications include an article in the journal *Appetite* on the process of dietary change and a book chapter on food policy in the foundational volume, *Environmental Nutrition*.
(Chapter 18: Barriers and strategies to adopting a plant-based diet)

Meagan E Gray MD
Dr Meagan Gray is a Transplant Hepatologist in the Division of Gastroenterology and Hepatology at the University of Alabama at Birmingham (UAB), US. She obtained her Bachelor of Science in Biomedical Engineering from Duke University and subsequently her medical degree from the University of Louisville. This was followed by an Internal Medicine residency at the Medical University of South Carolina and fellowships in both Gastroenterology and Transplant Hepatology at the University of Cincinnati. Dr Gray subsequently joined the faculty at UAB where she founded and directs UAB's Non-alcoholic Fatty Liver Disease Clinic. She has been following a plant-based diet for over 10 years and actively promotes this eating pattern to her patients. More recently she has become a Diplomate of the American Board of Obesity Medicine and has also incorporated obesity management into her

practice. Additionally, she is active in clinical research and is the Principal Investigator for multiple actively enrolling NAFLD clinical trials. Her other research interests include plant-based nutrition and healthcare disparities as they relate to NAFLD. When she's not at work, Dr Gray can be found running on one of Alabama's many beautiful trails.
(Chapter 9: Plant-based nutrition and non-alcoholic fatty liver disease)

Sandra Hood RD, BSc(HONS)
Sandra Hood is a Registered Dietitian. She studied at Leeds Metropolitan University where she completed her degree in dietetics. For over 20 years Sandra has worked for the NHS, specialising in various areas, particularly childhood nutrition and diabetes. She has contributed to numerous publications including the *Manual of Dietetic Practice*.
Her experience includes honorary dietitian to the Vegan Society where she was involved in writing the vegan shoppers' guide and liaising with prisons to provide vegan diets.

She worked with Arthur Ling, pioneer of the first plant-based milk in the UK, where she worked on various projects including infant case histories following vegan children from birth to adulthood. This particularly developed her interest in childhood nutrition and led to the publication of her first book in 2005 for the Vegan Society *Feeding Your Vegan Infant – with confidence*. Due to the tremendous shift to plant-based eating over the last few years, Sandra updated her book and last year this was published as *Feeding Your Vegan Child*.

Sandra has been vegan for over 40 years due to her love for animals, and in her spare time enjoys looking after rescued animals, cooking and keeping fit by running, cycling and swimming.
(Chapter 2: Meeting nutritional requirements on a plant-based diet from birth to old age)

David JA Jenkins OC, MD, FRSC, FRCP, FRCPC, PhD, DSc
Dr David JA Jenkins is a University Professor in the Departments of Nutritional Sciences and Medicine, a staff physician in the Division of Endocrinology and Metabolism, the Director of the Clinical Nutrition and Risk Factor Modification Center, and a Scientist in the Li Ka Shing Knowledge Institute, St Michael's Hospital, Toronto, Canada. He was educated at Oxford University, obtaining his DM, DPhil and DSc. He is a fellow of the Royal Colleges of Physicians of London and of Canada. He has served on committees in Canada and the United States that formulated nutritional guidelines for the treatment of diabetes and recommendations for fibre and macronutrient intake under the joint US-Canada DRI system (RDAs) of the National Academy of Sciences. He also served as a member of Agriculture Canada's Science Advisory Board (2004–2009). He has spent much time working with the food industry to develop products for the supermarket shelf, including Kellogg's, Quaker's and Loblaw, Canada's largest supermarket chain. He has written over 300 original publications on the prevention and treatment of hyperlipidaemia and diabetes and related topics. His team was the first to define and explore the concept of the glycaemic index of foods and the blood glucose and cholesterol lowering effects of viscous soluble fibre. His group developed the concept of the cholesterol-lowering dietary portfolio that has entered guidelines in many jurisdictions (e.g., CCS, Heart UK etc). He believes in the therapeutic value of environmentally sustainable plant-based diets.
(Foreword; Chapter 1: The impact of plant-based dietary patterns on health and disease)

Shivam Joshi BSc, MD
Dr Shivam Joshi is an internist, Nephrologist, and plant-based physician practising at NYC Health + Hospitals/Bellevue in New York City, US. He received his Bachelor of Science from Duke University and his medical degree from the University of Miami. He completed his residency at Jackson Memorial Hospital/University of Miami and his nephrology fellowship at the Hospital of the University of Pennsylvania. He is also a Clinical Assistant Professor at the New York University Grossman School of Medicine with research interests in plant-based diets, fad diets and nephrology. He has written numerous scientific articles and speaks nationally on these subjects. He is the youngest nephrologist to receive the NKF's Joel D Kopple award, the highest award in renal nutrition.
(Chapter 8: Plant-based nutrition and clinical nephrology)

Amir Kassam OBE, FRSB, PhD, BSc(Hons), MSc
Prof. Amir Kassam is a Visiting Professor in the School of Agriculture, Policy and Development, University of Reading, UK, Moderator of the Global Platform for Conservation Agriculture Community of Practice (CA-CoP), and Chairman of the International Conservation Agriculture Advisory Panel for Africa (ICAAP-Africa). In 2005, he was awarded an OBE in the Queen's Honours List for services to tropical agriculture and to rural development. He is a Fellow of the Royal Society of Biology (UK), and member of several international advisory committees, boards and panels. He has published widely.

Born in Zanzibar, Tanzania, Prof. Kassam received his BSc (Hons) in Agriculture and PhD in Agroecology from the University of Reading, and MSc in Irrigation from the University of California-Davis. Prof. Kassam's research and development work is focused on sustainable agricultural development and land management to address national and global needs and challenges. During his career, Prof. Kassam has worked with a number of national agricultural research and development institutions internationally, and with several CGIAR centres, UN agencies and NGOs. His former positions include Deputy Director General of WARDA (the Africa Rice Centre); Interim Executive Secretary of the CGIAR Science Council; Chairman of the Aga Khan Foundation (UK); Chairman of the Tropical Agriculture Association, UK; and Chairman of the FOCUS Humanitarian Assistance Europe Foundation.
(Chapter 20: An inclusively responsible food and agriculture system for planetary health)

Laila Kassam PhD, BSc(Hons), MSc
Dr Laila Kassam is a Development Economist and has worked in the international development sector since 2003. She has worked with NGOs, foundations, government ministries and international research and development institutions (including the CGIAR and FAO) focusing on rural development in sub-Saharan Africa and South Asia. Laila is currently based in the UK and is co-founder and Director of Animal Think Tank and co-editor of the book *Rethinking Food and Agriculture: New Ways Forward*. She currently works on issues related to food system transformation, animal freedom and social justice. Laila Kassam has a BSc (Hons) in Economics and Politics (University of Bristol, UK), a MSc in Development Management (London School of Economics and Political Science) and a PhD in Development Economics (School of Oriental and African Studies, University of London). Laila's previous positions include Programme Associate for Rural Development for the Aga Khan Foundation (Geneva); Research Officer for the DFID-funded Coastal Rural Support Programme (Kenya); and Overseas Development Institute (ODI) Fellow at the Ministry of Agriculture (Guyana).
(Chapter 20: An inclusively responsible food and agriculture system for planetary health)

Sue Kenneally MB BS, MRCGP, MSc(ANUTR), DIPBSLM/IBLM

Dr Sue Kenneally is a General Practitioner (GP), Nutritionist and specialist weight management and certified Lifestyle Medicine physician. She enjoys a varied working life in both general practice and as a physician in a NHS specialist weight loss clinic, and also provides private weight loss consultations in various formats that enable her to consult with patients who cannot be referred to her via the NHS.

Regarding her professional roles, she is on the advisory board of Plant Based Health Professionals UK, the obesity lead for the UK GP lifestyle and nutrition committee, a clinical representative in weight loss and nutrition for the Royal College of General Practitioners, a board member of the Welsh Obesity Society, a SCOPE certified member and Wales lead for the Association for the Study of Obesity and a founding member and regional director for the British Society of Lifestyle Medicine where she is involved with the learning academy.

She tutors for the MSc in obesity and weight management via the University of South Wales, teaches the weight loss module for the plant-based nutrition course at University of Winchester, UK, and has worked with the Royal College of General Practitioners, training colleagues to develop expertise in the management of obesity. She has previously written about and spoken on the subject of plant-based diets and weight in many and varied situations and is an international conference speaker. She has eaten a plant-based diet for many years and encourages patients to do likewise as far as is reasonably possible.
(Chapter 6: Plant-based nutrition and weight management)

Arvind Kaur Maheru MB BS, MRCPSYCH, MSc, BSc(Hons), DCH

Dr Arvind Maheru graduated in Medicine from King's College London. She has been a practising medical doctor for over 25 years and a Psychiatrist for over 20 years. She is a member of the Royal College of Psychiatrists, UK. Arvind has worked as a Consultant Psychiatrist in the UK's National Health Service (NHS), with a focus on the areas of general adult, old age and liaison psychiatry. She has a Masters in Psychiatric Research from University College London, UK, and has completed additional training in Motivational Interviewing for health behaviour change.

Arvind and her family adopted a plant-based lifestyle in 2016 due to its multiple health benefits. Since 2016, she has been developing specialist interests in plant-based nutrition, Lifestyle Medicine and preventive medicine. Arvind became a graduate of the AFMCP-UK (Applying Functional Medicine in Clinical Practice) course in 2018. She has completed the eCornell plant-based nutrition certificate and has created the mental health module for the University of Winchester Plant-Based Nutrition course, for which she has been a course tutor since 2019. Arvind is dedicated to educating health professionals, the Indian diaspora, and future generations about the many health advantages of a plant-based lifestyle.
(Chapter 11: Plant-based nutrition for mental health and wellbeing and Chapter 18: Barriers and strategies to adopting a plant-based diet)

Despina Marselou BSc(Hons), MSc(Nutr), RD

Despina Marselou is a Registered Dietitian. She studied at London Metropolitan University in England and her clinical research, 'Thermogenesis, Obesity and the Macro-metabolic Pathways: Relation to Obesity', was published in 2004 in the *Journal of the British Dietetic Association* as one of the best clinical trials among young graduates in the UK. She received a MSc in Clinical Nutrition and Immunology from the University of Surrey in England with an emphasis on dietary support and behaviour modification in patients with immune system disorders, Her professional career as a clinical dietitian at Newcastle upon Tyne and North Tees (NHS) University Hospitals in England enabled her to practise as a senior dietitian in the Centre for Diabetes and Endocrinology. She returned to her native Greece in [year?] where she was introduced as a research associate by the Agricultural University of Athens and was responsible for clinical nutrition seminars for first year and postgraduate students in the period 2007–2009.

She is currently working in her dietetic private practice in Greece with a special interest in evidence-based plant-based diets in supporting the microbiome. She holds a certificate in plant-based nutrition through eCornell University/T Colin Campbell Centre for Nutrition and University of Winchester, UK. She is responsible for the nutritional care of patients with immune disorders, chronic inflammation and neurodegenerative diseases and is passionate about promoting therapeutic nutrition and lifestyle modification protocols.
(Chapter 14: Plant-based nutrition for autoimmunity and chronic inflammation)

Rosemary Martin MSc, BSc, PGDIP, RD
Rosie Martin is a UK-based Registered Dietitian working as Employee Health & Wellness Dietitian for her local NHS trust and as a plant-based specialist through her business Rosemary Nutrition & Dietetics.

As a former zoologist with experience in animal behaviour and welfare, Rosie turned to a fully plant-based diet in 2014 and retrained in nutrition. She has worked with a wide variety of patients within NHS acute and community settings and has specialised in both gastroenterology and oncology. With a diagnosis of coeliac disease in her first year of life, she has lived experience of the dramatic impact of food choices on health and wellbeing.

Having studied and experienced the benefits of Plant-Based nutrition, Rosie now works to support patients and clients to embrace a plant-based diet for disease management and prevention. Rosie is an advisory board member for Plant Based Health Professionals UK, and provides nutrition support for a range of clients, and businesses through her dietetic clinic, talks, workshops and article writing.
(Chapter 10: Plant-based nutrition and gastrointestinal disorders)

Miriam Martinez-Biarge MD PhD
Dr Miriam Martinez-Biarge is a Paediatrician and Neonatologist with a special interest in general and developmental paediatrics, neonatal follow-up and paediatric nutrition, including plant-based nutrition for babies and children. She currently works as an Honorary Consultant Neonatologist & Research Fellow at Imperial College London (Queen Charlotte's and Hammersmith Hospital) and as an Associate Researcher at Bristol University. She also has a private practice in Madrid, Barcelona (Spain) and London (United Kingdom) as a neonatologist and developmental paediatrician. She likes clinical research and works with several research groups in the UK, Spain and other European countries.
(Chapter 2: Meeting nutritional requirements on a plant-based diet from birth to old age)

Priyumvada Naik MD, DIPABLM
Dr Naik is board-certified in Pulmonary Medicine, Critical Care Medicine and Lifestyle Medicine. She has additional training and expertise in lung transplantation, ECMO, interstitial lung disease, genetic lung disease, immunology and nutrition.

She attended Duke University, US, followed by Medical School at The Medical College of Georgia. She did her Internal Medicine residency, and Pulmonary, Critical Care and Lung Transplant fellowship at Emory University. She received additional training in transplant and ECMO in Sydney, Australia before returning to the US to practise as a Transplant Pulmonologist. She has published in the fields of internal medicine, lung transplantation, and organ donor management.

In the intervening years, Dr Naik has founded an Advanced Lung Disease Program, co-founded a Lung Cancer Screening Program, and served as Medical Director for an intensive care unit. She is an adjunct faculty member in the Division of Pulmonary and Critical Care Medicine at Morehouse School of Medicine, Atlanta, US, and is an intensivist for her local Organ Procurement Organization.

Vegan for 11+ years, she has been studying nutrition and lifestyle changes as they relate to chronic disease ever since, and she uses her expertise to help patients and for health coaching clients to prevent, control and even reverse chronic diseases such as diabetes, heart disease, rheumatologic conditions, inflammatory bowel disease, and more.

Her work in Lifestyle Medicine often produces just as dramatic results as her work in critical care and transplantation, and she loves teaching her colleagues how to prescribe plants over pills.
(Chapter 5: Plant-based nutrition for respiratory and sleep health)

Gemma S Newman MB BCh, DFSRH, DRCOG, MRCGP

Dr Gemma Newman is a Medical Doctor and Senior Partner at a family medical practice in West London. She studied at the University of Wales College of Medicine and has worked in many specialties as a doctor before her current specialty of General Practice. She has gained additional qualifications in Gynaecology and Family Planning. She is a founding member and ambassador for Plant-Based Health Professionals UK and a member of BSLM.

Dr Newman has a specialist interest in holistic health, plant-based nutrition and Lifestyle Medicine. She is regularly invited to teach other doctors and the general public via training programmes, podcasts and conferences about the benefits of plant-based nutrition and has authored *The Plant Power Doctor: a simple prescription for a healthier you*, which was a number-one bestseller in popular medicine and green living.

She has also written a chapter for *A Prescription for Healthy Living: a guide to Lifestyle Medicine*, a textbook for clinicians, and contributed content for two books on alcohol-free living: Janey Lee Grace's *Happy Healthy Sober* and Millie Gooch's *The Sober Girl Society Handbook*. She is also host of the popular podcast by Holland and Barratt *The Wellness Edit*. As a broadcaster she has been featured on ITV, Channel 4, Channel 5 and Sky News Sunrise as well as BBC Radio. She has featured in magazines including *Glamour*, *Zest* and *Health* magazine, as well as *The Daily Telegraph*.
(Chapter 7: Plant-based nutrition for the prevention and treatment of diabetes)

Nesan Shanmugam BSc (HONS), MB BS, PGCERTMEDED, MD (RES), FRCP, FHFA

Dr Nesan Shanmugam is a Consultant Cardiologist at St George's University Hospital, London, UK. His specialist interests are in heart failure and cardiac imaging (cardiac magnetic resonance imaging and echocardiography). He also has a particular interest in lifestyle and nutrition in cardiovascular disease (CVD) prevention. He was an integral part of the team that developed and implemented the first national Heart Failure Unit in the UK. The unit opened in 2016, providing specialist nursing, therapist and cardiology care to patients with heart failure.

Dr Shanmugam is an Honorary Senior Lecturer based in the Molecular and Clinical Sciences Research Institute at St George's University of London. He has ongoing research interests in nutrition and CVD, cardiac sarcoidosis and cardiac device therapies in heart failure. He has also obtained a Postgraduate Certificate in Medical Education at University College London and continues to actively teach at an undergraduate and postgraduate level. He is also the South London Clinical Lead for Heart Failure specialist training.

Dr Shanmugam is the Associate Editor of the *European Cardiology Review Journal*. He is a Fellow of the Royal College of Physicians and a Fellow and Education Committee member of the European Heart Failure Association. He is a member of the British Society of Lifestyle Medicine and Plant Based Health Professionals UK.
(Chapter 3: Plant-based nutrition and cardiovascular disease)

Niyati Sharma MB BS, FACD, MPH (NUTRITION)
Raised in Melbourne, Dr Sharma undertook her undergraduate medical degree (MB BS) at Adelaide University before coming back to Melbourne to undertake her internship at Royal Melbourne Hospital. After a few years of working in different parts of Australia, including remote areas, she decided to specialise in dermatology.

As part of her four-year postgraduate training, Dr Sharma spent one year in Singapore at the National Skin Centre learning the nuances of treating Asian skin and its diseases. After finishing her Dermatology fellowship exams (FACD), she undertook a sub-speciality fellowship at Ann & Robert Lurie Children's Hospital in Chicago in paediatric dermatology. This institution is a world leader in treating children's skin diseases.

Dr Sharma has also undertaken her Master of Public Health (MPH), specialising in nutrition, policy and advocacy, at Johns Hopkins University in Baltimore, US. She opened Inside Out Dermatology in April 2020, in Melbourne Australia, to help patients approach their skin diseases in a holistic manner with diet a focus of the consultation.
(Chapter 16: Plant-based nutrition and dermatological conditions)

Ayesha Sherzai MD, MAS
Dr Ayesha Sherzai is a vascular neurologist and a research scientist. After completing her residency, she completed a fellowship in vascular neurology and epidemiology at Columbia University Neurological Institute of New York. She is at the tail end of a Master's degree in public health in lifestyle epidemiology from Loma Linda University. Knowing the importance of empowering her patients, and their communities, she completed an extensive culinary training program in New York and now teaches large populations how to make tasty, easy and healthy meals for their brain health. Ayesha is co-director of Brain Health and Alzheimer's Solution at Loma Linda University. She and her husband are the authors of two best-selling books, *The Alzheimer's Solution* (2017, HarperCollins) and *The 30-day Alzheimer's Solution* (2021, HarperCollins). They are currently leading the largest community-based brain health initiative in the US.
(Chapter 13: Plant-based nutrition and Alzheimer's prevention)

Dean Sherzai MD, PhD, MPH, MAS
Dr Dean Sherzai is a Behavioural Neurologist and Neuroscientist whose entire life has been dedicated

to behavioural change models at the community and population level. He has revolutionised the world of public health nationally (US) and internationally. Dean finished his medical and neurology residencies at Georgetown University, US, with a subsequent fellowship in neurodegenerative diseases at the National Institutes of Health, followed by a second fellowship in Dementia and Geriatrics at the University of California, San Diego. He also holds two Master's Degrees: in advanced sciences at UCSD and in lifestyle epidemiology from Loma Linda University. He has received a PhD in Healthcare Leadership focused on community empowerment from Loma Linda/Andrews University. Finally, he completed the executive leadership program at Harvard Business School. His vision has always been to revolutionise healthcare by empowering communities to take control of their own health.
(Chapter 13: Plant-based nutrition and Alzheimer's prevention)

Sophia Sherzai
Sophia finished high school at age 10 and scored in the 90 percentile on SAT at age 11. Along with her brother, she has published two books, *Walk Like an Elephant* and *SuperMe*, and together they have been on several TV shows and spoken at several conferences and podcasts about healthy living and the power of a plant-based lifestyle. Sophia is currently 15 and a sophomore in college (Cal State LA), majoring in Biomedical Engineering. She is passionate about the environment and science and, along with her brother, has led the online forum 'The Science Kids' since they were young children.
(Chapter 13: Plant-based nutrition and Alzheimer's prevention)

Aryan Tavakkoli MB BS, MRCP, FRACP
Dr Aryan Tavakkoli graduated from the Medical College of St Bartholomew's Hospital, London, UK, in 1991, going on to specialise in Respiratory and General Medicine. She worked as a hospital consultant in Respiratory Medicine for 16 years, before opening her own medical practice.

She is currently the medical director of Quantum Clinic where she provides a progressive approach to adults with cancer, combining her experience in conventional medicine with the benefits of functional medicine and integrative medicine. Her integrative support aims to address root causes of disease using a multi-faceted approach, including whole food plant-based nutrition, modification of lifestyle factors, natural botanicals, micronutrient optimisation, gut microbiome support, oxygenation therapy and mind-body therapy.

Dr Tavakkoli holds additional qualifications in nutrition, functional medicine, phytotherapy (Western herbal medicine), TCM (traditional Chinese medicine) acupuncture, Class 3B laser therapy, oxidative and photonic medicine, HeartMath technology and clinical hypnotherapy. She has written and spoken widely about plant-based nutrition and is regularly invited to speak at conferences about integrative cancer support.

She is a member of the Royal College of Physicians, fellow of the Royal Australasian College of Physicians, member of the British Society for Ecological Medicine, allied member of OncANP (The Oncology Association of Naturopathic Physicians), member of the British Medical Laser Association, member of the British Society of Clinical and Academic Hypnosis, member of Plant-Based Health Professionals UK, and member of the Independent Doctors Federation.
(Chapter 4: Plant-based nutrition and cancer)

Acknowledgements

We would like to acknowledge, and express our appreciation of all those, past and present, who have worked over many decades to further the science of nutrition and lifestyle, and upon whose work this book is based.

We would like to express our deepest gratitude to our authors for the expertise that they put into practice on a daily basis to benefit their patients, for their invaluable contributions to this book to highlight the huge body of evidence supporting plant-based nutrition and Lifestyle Medicine in the medical literature, and for being role models of a new paradigm.

We extend our sincere thanks to our publisher Georgina Bentliff from Hammersmith Health Books for her ongoing support and collaboration, and Carolyn White, our editor, whose efficiency and meticulousness we very much appreciate. Their combined experience in publishing and editing academic books has been invaluable.

Finally, we would like to thank our beloved families and loved ones. Their support and encouragement for this book project and all our endeavors keeps us full of hope, love and gratitude.

Foreword

This textbook was written during the global pandemic caused by the severe acute respiratory syndrome coronavirus 2 (SARS-CoV-2, also referred to as COVID-19 (coronavirus disease 2019)). This has occurred during a time when the world is facing a number of inter-related crises: health, climate and ecological, thus worsening the impact of the pandemic. Our food system and the diets we eat are a central component of these crises. We also have crises of health and ethics whereby more than a billion people remain hungry and at imminent risk of starvation, at a time when the richest nations are facing an obesity epidemic with Western children developing what used to be called maturity-onset diabetes before even entering adulthood.

A global shift to a plant-based food system is considered an essential part of addressing these global issues. Adopting a plant-based diet is the single most impactful change we can make as individuals to improve our health and reduce our impact on the planet, whilst showing kindness to both human and non-human animals with whom we share this planet.

I have spent my career in the field of human nutrition since the early 1980s. I've watched Denis Burkitt bring the dietary fibre concept from Africa to the Western world. This advice was added to the Ancel Keys saturated fat concept that shaped the dietary treatment of cardiovascular disease, with an early emphasis on general advice to eat more plant-based foods. Dietary advice has continued to move in this direction internationally for both human and planetary health. Despite the almost uniform acceptance of this dietary approach to prevent chronic disease, medical education has not been sufficiently influenced and little nutritional education has entered the curriculum of most medical schools.

This textbook fills the current gap in nutrition education in an enlightened way by providing an up-to-date review of the science supporting a healthy plant-based diet for promoting optimal health at all life stages and for preventing and treating chronic illness.

The book starts by providing an overview of plant-based diets and their impact on general health and wellbeing. This is followed by a review of meeting nutritional requirements at all life stages. The book then focuses in on common chronic conditions, with chapters on cardiovascular disease, type 2 diabetes, cancer, mental health and more. Further chapters consider plant-based diet for athletes, overcoming barriers to adopting a plant-based diet, the wider impact of our food system on planetary health, and how plant-based nutrition is incorporated into the newest and fastest growing medical specialty globally, Lifestyle Medicine.

Given the broad and far-reaching impact of diet on health, this book will be a key text for anyone within the medical and healthcare profession. I hope to see it in university and hospital libraries around the world. Its use will not only be for the clinician and dietitian but will provide a major resource for all those who are interested in health while reducing our species' environmental footprint.

David JA Jenkins OC, MD, FRSC, FRCP, FRCPC, PhD, DSc
Director, Clinical Nutrition and Risk Factor Modification Centre, St. Michael's Hospital, Toronto, ON, Canada. Scientist, Li Ka Shing Knowledge Institute, St Michael's Hospital, Toronto, ON, Canada. Staff Physician, Division of Endocrinology, Department of Medicine, St Michael's Hospital, Toronto, ON, Canada

Preface

We are sincerely grateful for the opportunity to edit this academic textbook on *Plant-Based Nutrition in Clinical Practice* as an essential resource for all health professionals. As practising health professionals ourselves, we feel strongly that the evidence presented should be incorporated proactively and urgently into our healthcare systems, given our current and growing pandemic of chronic disease.

Our current medical education, practice and research paradigm is focused on a disease-oriented, 'pathogenic' model of care, using prescription medicines and medical procedures to provide a sticking-plaster approach to dealing with the manifestations of chronic disease, managing symptoms rather than addressing their root causes. Very little of the healthcare budget is allocated to the prevention of chronic disease and 'salutogenesis', which focuses on factors that support human health and wellbeing. The huge progress and ingenuity of modern medicine in treating disease is abundantly clear, but focusing the majority of resources on this approach comes with a huge societal burden in terms of quality of life and economic cost. The current level of chronic disease and its management are simply not sustainable, evidenced by burgeoning healthcare costs both individually and as a society.

Focusing medical practice, education and research more on evidence-based lifestyle measures, of which a plant predominant diet is a key pillar, through all stages of life, can help address these issues, allowing for prevention, management and potential reversal of disease, and a more equitable and sustainable healthcare system.

We now have decades of research on the impact of nutrition on health, yet nutrition education for health professionals needs to catch up with the science. Nutrition has not been consistently taught at medical school or in specialty training. Only recently has it been considered an essential competency in some countries, such as the UK, which now has an established nutrition curriculum. However, implementation will take time, and making time to address diet within clinical practice will take even longer. Education for nutritionists and dietitians also remains grounded in the 'old science' of considering food from animals as essential and desirable and plant-based diets as restrictive and of concern for nutritional deficiencies.

Despite this, we are now seeing an increasing number of committed and passionate health professionals, including our contributing authors, who have independently educated themselves on the huge benefits of nutrition and other lifestyle measures in preventing and managing disease, and who are putting these measures into practice alongside the clinical-guideline-directed medical therapies. This is supported by international consensus, which is becoming apparent in the incorporation of plant-based nutrition into clinical practice guidelines for the prevention and management of chronic disease.

In the medical literature, education has been identified by health professionals as a key barrier to incorporating health promotion into their practice. In the last few years there have been an increasing number of excellent educational opportunities on plant-based nutrition and Lifestyle Medicine, including resources from specialty-specific medical organisations, university-based courses and board certification from the American College of Lifestyle Medicine, the flagship organisation globally for Lifestyle Medicine. In this setting we wished to contribute an academic textbook we have not yet seen, one that is devoted exclusively to plant-based nutrition in clinical practice.

This book contains chapters that cover the abundant evidence for the beneficial impact of plant-based nutrition on the chronic diseases of our time, its impact at all stages of life, the barriers and strategies for behaviour change, and the growth of the evidence-based specialty of Lifestyle Medicine. The book concludes with a chapter on how our food system is in fact a central driver of our current planetary health crises, with root causes that are common to our health crisis, and how a shift to plant-based nutrition can help mitigate them.

We hope this book will be a contribution to educating health professionals so that plant-based nutrition may be added to the toolkit for managing chronic diseases in their patients. More than this, we invite healthcare professionals to consider a more holistic paradigm of health, to focus more on wellness not illness, and where individual health and planetary health are understood to be inextricably linked. Let us educate ourselves so we can be powerful advocates for the wellbeing of our communities and the planet on which we depend.

Chapter 1
The impact of plant-based dietary patterns on health and disease

Shireen Kassam, Zahra Kassam, Lisa Simon and David Jenkins

Introduction

Unhealthy diets are now the single most important risk factor for premature death and chronic illness globally. The Global Burden of Disease Study from 2019 examined dietary consumption between 1990 and 2017 in 195 countries and assessed the contribution to non-communicable diseases and death.[1] The study demonstrated that one in five deaths annually, around 11 million, were caused by an unhealthy diet with most of these deaths due to cardiovascular disease (CVD), followed by cancer and type 2 diabetes.

Unhealthy diets were typically too high in meat and processed foods and deficient in healthy foods such as fruits, vegetables, whole grains, beans, nuts and seeds. This type of diet pattern is typical of the so-called Western-style diet pattern which has been widely adopted in high income, industrialised countries and now exported to middle- and low-income countries.[2] In the UK, Canada and the US for example, more than 50% of calories consumed by children and adults are from ultra-processed foods with consumption of fruits and vegetables at very low levels.[3, 4, 5]

The 2021 Global Nutrition Report paints an even worse picture. It found that diet-related disease and deaths have actually risen, accounting for a quarter (26%) of all adult deaths each year.[6] The proportion of premature deaths attributed to dietary risks is highest in Northern America and Europe (31% each), and lowest but also at notable levels in Africa (17%). No region of the world is meeting recommendations for healthy diets. Fruit and vegetable intake is still about 50% below the recommended level of five servings per day that is considered healthy (60% and 40% respectively), and legume and nut intakes are each more than two thirds below the recommended two servings per day. In contrast, red and processed meat intake is on the rise and almost five times the maximum level of one serving per week, while the consumption of sugary drinks, which are not recommended in any amount, is going up as well.

Over the last few decades, nutrition science has moved away from considering individual nutrients to focusing on healthy foods and diet patterns. This is because studying individual nutrients cannot account for the interactions within foods and the potential synergist effects that are greater than the sum of the individual. In addition, when one food or nutrient is removed from the diet, it is usually replaced by something else, and this substitution effect is very important to consider.

The core components of a healthy diet pattern have been agreed upon for decades and include fruits, vegetables, whole grains, beans, nuts and seeds whilst minimising processed and unprocessed red meat and processed foods, high in salt, sugar and fat. These principles form the basis of most country-based dietary guidelines and healthy eating guidelines from the World Health Organization (WHO).[7] Within this framework there a number of healthy diet patterns that have been widely studied and associated with favourable health outcomes. These includes the Mediterranean, DASH (Dietary Approaches to Stop Hypertension), pescatarian, dietary portfolio, vegetarian, vegan and whole food plant-based dietary pattern, all considered to be either predominantly or exclusively plant-based.[8] Table 1.1 provides definitions of common plant-based dietary patterns. It should not be forgotten that many traditional diet patterns such as the Okinawan, Japanese, Nordic, Indian and African diets are centred around minimally processed plant foods with only small amounts of animal-derived foods included, if any. However, with the corporatisation of our global food system and the transition of people from rural to urban settings, these traditional diets have been eroded, becoming more reliant

Table 1.1: Definitions of plant-based dietary patterns

Diet pattern	Definition
Vegetarian	A general term for a diet pattern that excludes meat, poultry and fish
Lacto-ovo vegetarian	Permits the consumption of dairy and eggs
Lacto-vegetarian	Permits the consumption of dairy but not eggs
Pesco-vegetarian	A diet that incorporates seafood in an otherwise vegetarian dietary pattern
Vegan	Excludes all animal-derived food from the diet, including eggs, dairy and honey
Flexitarian or 'casual vegetarian'	An increasingly popular term used to describe those actively reducing their consumption of meat and dairy, usually to reduce the environmental impact of their diet, but still consuming small amounts of meat, poultry, eggs and dairy
Plant-based	A dietary pattern that is predominately, but not exclusively comprised of plant foods. Although there is no consensus definition, plant-based diets typically include 85–90% plant-derived foods. In the scientific literature, the term 'plant-based' often incorporates all the terms listed above but predominantly vegan and vegetarian dietary patterns
Whole food plant-based	A healthy vegan diet composed of fruits, vegetables, whole grains, legumes, nuts and seeds and minimising/avoiding the consumption of added fat, salt and sugar

on meat, dairy and processed foods.[9] The food industry influence over our food environment, policy decisions, nutrition science and eating habits cannot be underestimated.[10, 11]

The Blue Zones

The term 'Blue Zones' has been coined by the explorer and journalist Dan Buettner, who led a National Geographic expedition to investigate regions of the world where people lived the longest and healthiest lives.[12] He described five Blue Zones where people consistently reach over 100 years of age whilst maintaining an active and vibrant life. The research team identified nine common dietary and lifestyle factors that are shared by people living in these regions. For diet, the common factors are a diet composed predominantly (more than 90%) of minimally processed whole plant-foods, with a particular emphasis on beans and nuts. Meat is eaten infrequently, around five times per month. However, these diets are quite varied. For example, two of the Blue Zones that are in the Mediterranean, Ikaria in Greece and Sardinia, Italy, consume a diet that is relatively high in fat, particularly from extra virgin olive oil. In contrast, Okinawa in Japan has a mainly starch-based diet with 70% or more of calories from the purple or orange sweet potato. Loma Linda in California has a large proportion of citizens who follow a vegetarian or vegan diet. The traditional diet of the Nicoya Peninsula consists of black beans, bananas, plantains, papaya, squash, pejibaje, yams, and homemade corn tortillas. Black beans are eaten daily, often with rice. The diet of these Blue Zones teaches us that the overall quality of the diet is more important than the individual nutrients, with all of these diets centred around minimally processed whole plant foods. The optimal proportion of macronutrients in the diet continues to be a hotly debated topic and that can sometimes take away the focus from the diet quality, which is more important.

Types of nutrition studies

In the last 50 years or so, there has been an exponential rise in the number of studies relating to diet, nutrition and health. Nutrition science relies heavily on epidemiological studies, which are by nature observational. Epidemiology is the study of how often diseases occur in different groups of people and why. Epidemiology measures disease outcomes in a particular population.[13]

Nutrition science is often criticised due to its heavy reliance on epidemiological data rather than data from interventional studies or randomised controlled trials (RCT). The latter are considered to be the gold standard for investigating the effects of pharmaceutical medications, especially if they are randomised, blinded and placebo controlled. One reason for the criticism is that observational studies in of themselves cannot prove causality, only association. However, there are several important examples of how observational data have been instrumental in informing us of the risk of a particular exposure to human health. These include the causal link between cigarette smoking and lung cancer, for which randomised, controlled studies do not exist. Another example would be the adverse effects of industrially produced trans fats on blood lipids and the consequent increased risk of ischaemic heart disease.

The best quality epidemiological study is a prospective cohort study in which participants, who are free of disease at baseline, are followed forward in time, often for decades. Figure 1.1 shows the traditional hierarchy of medical evidence with the strongest evidence at the top of the pyramid.

A further criticism of observational studies is the accuracy of the data collection through the use of dietary questionnaires.[14] Diet and dietary intakes can vary over time and therefore all forms of data collection are prone to error to varying degrees. There are a number of validated

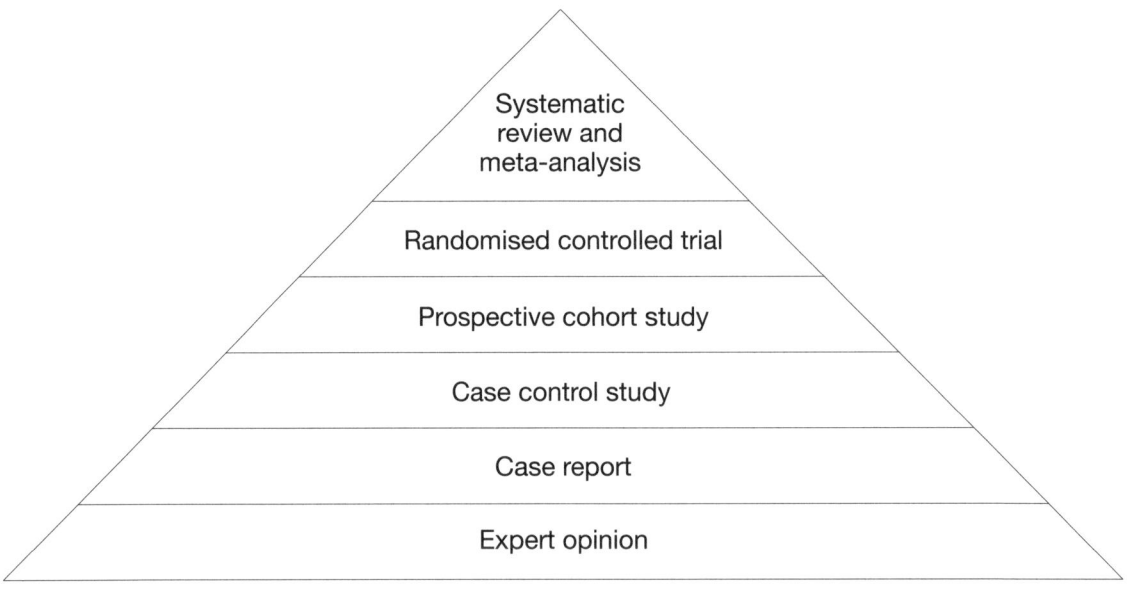

Figure 1.1 Hierarchy of medical evidence

methods for dietary assessment. The most commonly used method for large prospective cohort studies is a food frequency questionnaire, which consists of a structured food list and a frequency response section on which the participant indicates his/her usual frequency of intake of each food over a certain period of time in the past, usually one year. When combined with biological measurements (biomarkers), such as urinary nitrogen for protein intake or 24-hour urinary sodium and potassium excretion, blood lipid and micronutrient measurements, the assessment of nutrient intake can be more objective and therefore can mitigate some of the issues of reporting error.

The medical and scientific community still consider a RCT as the gold standard. This works well when you are only considering one variable, such as whether a particular tablet is taken or not. Nutrition studies do not work in that way. When one component is taken out of the diet, it is replaced by something else, and this may vary between participants. In addition, the length of time required to understand whether a particular diet or intervention is superior for long-term health is just not practical. There are also challenges related to adherence. An example of these challenges is exemplified by the dietary modification component of the Women's Health Initiative study.[15] This is the most expensive human nutrition RCT ever to be conducted, recruiting 48,835 post-menopausal women. The intervention arm was intended to be a low-fat diet group, yet on analysis most of the participants had been unable to reduce their fat intake to the target of 20% of calories. Some of the most successful randomised studies that have been conducted are those that have provided all of the food to the participants in the intervention group, which then of course necessitates a relatively small sample size and short follow-up.

To infer causality from observation studies, the best quality study design is a prospective cohort study. However, this type of study design is still open to confounding. A confounder is a variable that is associated with both the exposure and outcome but is not caused by either and when unaccounted for, introduces bias into the exposure-disease relationship. For example, a study examining the association between body mass index (exposure) and heart disease (outcome) might be confounded by age, diet, smoking status, and a variety of other risk factors that might be unevenly distributed between the groups being compared. So, if people who are of normal weight are also more likely to smoke tobacco, it will appear that being normal weight increases the risk of heart disease when in fact it is the tobacco smoking. To account for this type of bias, potential confounders must be identified and adjusted for in the analysis using statistical methods.

The Hill criteria, published in 1965 by Sir Austin Bradford Hill, are useful in inferring causality from observational data. In his original paper, Hill outlined several key conditions for establishing causality: strength of the data, consistency, temporality (the timing of the exposure is consistent with development of the disease), biological gradient (dose-response – the greater the exposure the higher the risk of disease), plausibility, coherence (makes sense based on knowledge of the natural history and biology of the disease), and experimental evidence.[16] The Hill criteria were used to infer that smoking tobacco causes lung cancer.

The results obtained from prospective, observational studies can be strengthened by data from laboratory studies, mechanistic studies in humans and randomised studies if available. Systematic reviews and meta-analyses of observational data are often considered the best available evidence as they bring together data from a number of studies.[17] However, they are not without issue and the validity of the results are dependent on what data are used in the analysis and how the analysis is conducted. Notable examples of two very misleading systematic reviews and meta-analyses, one published in 2010 and the other in 2014, concluded that saturated fat consumption had no impact on the risk of CVD, leading to headlines such as 'butter is back'.[18, 19] However, these studies failed to consider what nutrient replaced fat in the diet of individuals with lower fat intake i.e., refined carbohydrates and sugar. In addition, most studies included in the meta-analyses did not have participants that were truly consuming a low saturated fat diet, and studies which included those on a vegan or vegetarian diet (thus lower intakes of saturated fat) were given a lower statistical weighting. Thus, what these studies really showed was that substituting fat for refined carbohydrates was equally detrimental for cardiovascular health and that participants didn't differ enough in saturated fat intake to demonstrate a significant difference. Nutrition researchers continue to highlight these very real issues with meta-analyses that can mislead the medical community.[20] Interestingly, a Cochrane systematic review in 2014 concluded that RCTs and observational studies tend to produce similar effect sizes for a range of health outcomes and that disagreements in study conclusions are likely due to other study characteristics such as testing different hypotheses or duration of follow-up rather than the study design alone.[21]

Given the limitations of RCTs for nutrition research and that current approaches for assessing strength of evidence rely heavily on RCTs, a new construct called Hierarchies of Evidence Applied to Lifestyle Medicine (HEALM) has been developed to assess the strength of evidence relevant to the impact of nutrition and other lifestyle behaviours on health outcomes. HEALM incorporates the variety of sources of evidence available and synthesises their contributions into one rating.[22, 23]

Overall, when assessing nutrition data, the entirety of the evidence should be considered. There will always be studies that show unexpected and differing results from the vast majority of the data. These need to be interpreted with knowledge of methodological and statistical considerations. In addition, when considering the impact of a certain food or nutrient on health outcomes, it is essential to know what that food or nutrient is being substituted for.

Healthy, therapeutic diet patterns

The WHO defines a healthy diet as one that emphasises fruits, non-starchy vegetables, whole grains, nuts and seeds; minimises added sugar (less than 10% of total energy intake and salt <5 g per day); limits dietary fat to less than 30% of total energy intake, favouring unsaturated fat (plant sources) over saturated fat (animal sources).[7] Of note, some country-based guidance is more stringent on consumption of foods such as free sugar, including the Scientific Advisory Committee on Nutrition who recommend no more than 5% of daily energy intake from free sugar.[24]

There are several healthy diet patterns that in clinical studies have been shown to reduce the risk of chronic disease, such as heart disease, type 2 diabetes, stroke, hypertension and hyperlipidaemia. They all share in common a focus on whole plant-foods but vary in the amounts of animal-derived foods, including meat and dairy. They all call for minimisation of saturated fat, added sugar and salt and processed foods in general. They encourage the consumption of poultry and fish in place of red and processed meat. The diet patterns that have been studied most extensively include the DASH, Mediterranean, Portfolio, vegetarian, vegan and a low-fat whole food plant-based diet. A systematic review from 2021 evaluated the impact of dietary patterns on all-cause mortality and included 153 articles involving 6,550,664 individuals.[25] The data confirmed that nutrient-dense diet patterns characterised by higher intake of vegetables; legumes; fruit; nuts; either whole grains, cereals or non-refined grains; fish; and unsaturated vegetable oils and by lower or no consumption of animal products (red and processed meat, meat and meat products, and high-fat dairy products); refined grains; and sweets (i.e., higher in added sugars) improve longevity and significantly reduce the risk of death from all causes.

The Dietary Approaches to Stop Hypertension (DASH)

The DASH eating plan or DASH diet was developed by the National Heart, Lung and Blood Institute and based on the vegetarian diet pattern but designed to be more acceptable (as it was thought that recommending a vegetarian diet pattern, proven to be effective at lowering blood pressure, would be unacceptable to most people).[26] It was developed as a therapeutic diet for prevention and treatment of hypertension but has since been shown to benefit other cardiometabolic risk factors.[27] The DASH diet has been further adapted with reduced sodium content and alterations in percentage of fat and protein versus carbohydrate. General principles include eating vegetables, fruits, and whole grains, including fat-free or low-fat dairy products, fish, poultry, beans, nuts, and vegetable oils; limiting foods that are high in saturated fat, such as fatty meats, full-fat dairy products, and tropical oils (coconut, palm kernel and palm oils); limiting sugar-sweetened beverages and sweets.

The Mediterranean diet

There is no one standard Mediterranean diet pattern, given the size of the region. No one component of the diet can account for the health benefits, but as a whole it is associated with a reduced risk of CVD, cancer, dementia, autoimmune disease and type 2 diabetes. The diet pattern has common aspects, including an abundance of whole plant foods, olive oil (usually extra virgin olive oil), limited dairy products, moderate amounts of poultry, fish and wine and low amounts of red and processed meats.[28]

There have been two major randomised studies of a Mediterranean diet in CVD. The Lyon Diet Heart Study was a randomised secondary prevention trial aimed at testing whether a Mediterranean-type diet is associated with a reduced risk of recurrent myocardial infarction *after* a first myocardial infarction. The intervention arm on the Mediterranean diet included eating alpha-linoleic acid (omega-3 fatty acid) and linoleic acid (omega-6 fatty acid) supplemented margarine in place of butter and cream. The study was stopped early due to the benefits in the Mediterranean diet group, which had a significant reduction in recurrent cardiac events and death.[29]

The PREDIMED (the PREvencion con Dieta MEDiterannea) study was a primary prevention study of the Mediterranean diet in people at high risk of cardiovascular disease. It had three study arms; a Mediterranean diet supplemented with extra-virgin olive oil (1 litre per week), a Mediterranean diet supplemented with mixed nuts, or a control diet (advice to reduce dietary fat). Of note, the control diet was not a low-fat diet (as many have suggested) as the control group had a median fat intake of 37% of total energy. The study has also been shrouded in controversy due to errors in the randomisation procedure. However, even after reanalysis and republication, the results continue to show a significant reduction in cardiovascular events in the two Mediterranean diet groups, albeit mainly for reduction in stroke rather than myocardial infarction.[30] There was no reduction in the risk of death from any cause, including CVD. A further analysis of the data showed no difference in rates of heart failure between the three study groups.[31]

In contrast, when the PREDIMED study was analysed using the provegetarian/plant-based diet score, there was significant reduction in the risk of all-cause *and* cardiovascular mortality in those consuming a diet with a high provegetarian score.[32] Of note, the provegetarian score gave positive marks to all plant foods, regardless of quality, and negative marks to all animal-derived foods, including fish and dairy.

In the Greek segment of the European Prospective Investigation into Cancer and Nutrition (EPIC) study, researchers analysed the individual components of the Mediterranean diet and their contribution to a reduction in mortality.[33] The results showed that the components of the diet associated with a mortality benefit were vegetables, legumes, nuts, fruits and unsaturated fatty acids. The foods that did not impact mortality or had an adverse effect on mortality were dairy, fish, meat and alcohol.

Interestingly, researchers have tried to improve upon the traditional Mediterranean diet by adding more plant foods, less meat, green tea, walnuts and Mankai (duckweed) the so-called 'Green Mediterranean diet'. This more plant-based version out-performed the traditional Mediterranean diet for improvements in cardiometabolic risk factors and non-alcoholic fatty liver disease in the randomised studies performed.[34, 35]

It should be noted that although the Mediterranean diet is considered the 'best diet', given the extent of supportive data, this diet pattern is not appropriate for much of the world as it is not relevant to traditional diet patterns such as those consumed in India, Asia and Africa. Thus, we need to be mindful that dietary advice needs to be culturally appropriate and adaptable.

The Portfolio diet

The Portfolio diet or Dietary Portfolio was developed at the University of Toronto and St Michael's Hospital, Toronto. It is a plant-based dietary pattern that was first devised in the early 2000s as a 'portfolio' of four cholesterol-lowering plant foods, each of which has a Food and Drug Administration (FDA), Health Canada, and/or European Food Safety Authority (EFSA) approved health claim for cholesterol-lowering or CVD risk reduction. The four core food components of the Portfolio dietary pattern include (based on a 2000 kcal diet): 42 g nuts (tree nuts or peanuts); 50 g plant protein from soya products or dietary pulses such as beans, peas, chickpeas, and lentils; 20 g viscous soluble fibre from oats, barley, psyllium, eggplant, okra, apples, oranges, or berries; and 2 g plant sterols initially provided in a plant sterol-enriched margarine. An enhanced Portfolio dietary pattern has also been studied in which monounsaturated fat (MUFA) replaces carbohydrate (13% replacement providing 26% energy from MUFA) and is added to the other four components. The studies show benefit for cardiovascular risk factors including reductions in LDL-cholesterol, triglycerides, C-reactive protein and blood pressure.[36] Applying the portfolio dietary pattern to the Women's Health Initiative showed that adherence to the portfolio dietary pattern was associated with a reduced risk of CVD, coronary heart disease and heart failure.[37]

Vegetarian, vegan and whole food plant-based diets

Most of the information we have on the health impacts of a vegetarian or vegan diet comes from the results of prospective cohort studies. There are three main cohorts in which there are significant numbers of vegetarians and vegans. The Adventist Health Studies from North America, the EPIC-Oxford cohort from the UK and The Tzu Chi Health Study from Taiwan.[38] Often, health outcomes for vegetarian and vegan participants are analysed together, so it can be difficult to tease out the impact of eggs and dairy in the diet from these studies.

In general terms, most of these studies, including meta-analyses, have demonstrated significant benefits of eating a vegetarian or vegan diet, especially if the diet is composed of healthy plant foods. A meta-analysis from 2017 showed that vegetarian and vegan diets have a beneficial effect on body mass index, total and LDL-cholesterol, triglycerides and fasting glucose. Vegetarians had a 25% reduction in incidence and mortality from ischaemic heart disease and an 8% reduction in incidence of cancer. Vegans had a 15% reduction in the risk of cancer.[39] An updated meta-analysis specifically assessing the impact of a vegetarian diet on mortality from ischaemic heart disease and all-causes confirmed a 30% reduction in risk of death from ischaemic heart disease, although no impact on cardiovascular or all-cause mortality.[40] Although the studies in this meta-analysis included vegan participants, there was insufficient data to make conclusions on the impact of a vegan diet specifically. Other meta-analyses have confirmed benefits of a vegetarian diet on blood pressure, blood lipid profile and treatment of diabetes with the magnitude of effect often as large as that found with prescribed medication.[41, 42, 43]

The term 'whole food plant-based' (WFPB) diet was coined by Dr T Colin Campbell, Professor Emeritus of Nutritional Biochemistry at Cornell University. He is most well-known for co-authoring the book *The China Study* with his son, Thomas M Campbell. *The China Study* is based on the findings of the China-Cornell-Oxford Project, which was a large observational study conducted in rural China in the 1980s and funded by Cornell and Oxford Universities and the government of China, which involved 6500 participants from 65 different Chinese counties.[44] The findings of the study suggested that Western-style diseases, including CVD and cancer, were associated with diets rich in animal-derived foods, high in animal protein and saturated fat. The opposite was also true. A diet centred around whole plant foods was associated with the lowest incidence of chronic disease.

Since then, a number of researchers have investigated the impact of a whole food plant-based diet as a therapeutic intervention for the reversal of chronic conditions such as obesity, heart disease and type 2 diabetes. A large systematic review including 84 papers investigated the efficacy of vegan, vegetarian and whole food plant-based (exclusively plant-based or minimal animal foods including eggs and dairy) diets in treating obesity, hyperlipidaemia, insulin resistance, glycaemic control, type 2 diabetes, cardiovascular disease and hypertension.[45] Overall, the findings confirmed that all three types of diets reduced body weight to a greater extent than healthy omnivorous diets, including those recommended by the American Heart Association (AHA), American Diabetes Association and the National Cholesterol Education Programme and in some studies performed better than the comparison calorie-restricted diet. The review found that these diet patterns were associated with a greater loss of subcutaneous, visceral and intramuscular fat and all three diets improved glucose control, insulin sensitivity and resulted in reductions in HbA1c in people with diabetes, with the ability to reverse diabetes in some. This has also been shown in the community setting amongst free-living people, such as the BROAD study conducted in New Zealand. Plant-based diets were shown to be very effective at lowering total and LDL-cholesterol but less effective for reducing triglyceride levels and may result in lower HDL-cholesterol levels. Plant-based diets were also found to be effective at lowering blood pressure and markers of inflammation such as high-sensitivity C-reactive protein. Low-fat vegetarian diets have also been shown to have the potential to halt the progression and in some cases even result in regression of atherosclerosis in people with severe coronary artery disease. All of these health outcomes will be discussed in more detail in the relevant chapters.

Overall, the review found that differences between the three categories of plant-based diets were less important than the differences between the conventional comparator diet. Based on the results the authors conclude that recommendations in clinical practice *should* include a plant-based diet comprised mainly of whole plant foods. If animal foods are chosen to be included, then this should be limited to fish and low-fat dairy. White flour products, sugar-sweetened beverages and 'poor-quality' animal foods (factory farmed beef and chicken and processed meat) should be limited/avoided.

Diet quality indices

Several diet quality indices, usually based on established nutrient requirements and dietary guidelines, have been developed to evaluate the healthfulness of individual diets. These scores, reflecting overall diet quality, can help researchers to sort through the nutrient and food-specific findings and provide a measure of diet that incorporates nutrient and food interactions of likely biological importance. The scores are relatively easy for clinicians and dietitians to use for recording people's diet in a clinical setting. The most established scores include the healthy eating index, the alternative healthy eating index, the Mediterranean diet score, the DASH diet score and the provegetarian/plant-based score. Table 1.2 below shows the differences between the DASH and Mediterranean diets and the foods included in the alternative healthy eating index.[46]

The glycaemic index (GI), developed in Oxford and Toronto, is a relative ranking of carbohydrate in foods according to how they affect blood glucose levels. It provides a means of quantifying the effects of carbohydrate-rich foods on blood glucose concentrations. The GI of a food is determined by feeding a portion containing 50 g of carbohydrate to 10 healthy people after an overnight fast. Blood glucose is tested at 15- to 30-minute intervals over the next two hours, and the results are compared with those obtained by feeding a person the same amount of glucose or white bread. A GI below 100 means the food

Table 1.2: Food groups in the DASH, Mediterranean diet and the alternate healthy eating index[46]

Food	Mediterranean diet	DASH	Alternative Healthy Eating Index
Cereals	Included	Whole grains	Whole grains
Vegetables	Included	Included	Included
Fruits	Included	Included	Included
Nuts, legumes	Included	Included	Included
Fish	Included	Encouraged	Encouraged
Meat	Reduced	Lean meat included, red and processed meat limited	Red and processed meat limited
Dairy	Reduced	Low-fat dairy included	Total
Fats	Predominantly olive oil encouraged	Reduction in fats encouraged	Long chain omega-3 and total polyunsaturated fatty acids encouraged
Sweets and sugar-sweetened beverages	Avoided	Avoided	Avoided
Alcohol	Included in moderation		Included in moderation
Sodium		Limited	Limited

has less effect on blood sugar compared with glucose. A higher number means the test food has a greater effect.[47, 48] The lower a food's GI, the slower blood sugar rises after eating that food. In general, the more rapidly digested a food is through cooking or processing, the higher its GI. Also, the glycaemic response can be reduced by added fibre or the presence of protein and fat in a meal. Although the data are not entirely consistent, in general, consuming a low GI diet appears to show benefit in reducing the risk of type 2 diabetes,[49] CVD,[50] some cancers[51] and is beneficial to people living with diabetes.[52] Of course, common sense should be applied when looking at certain low GI foods with high fat content, such as ice cream, as the high saturated fat and sugar content cannot be equated with a reduced risk of chronic disease. Nor should high GI vegetables be avoided as the carbohydrate content (glycaemic load), of, for example, carrots is so small that the GI is irrelevant.

Given that most prospective cohort studies do not include a significant proportion of vegans and vegetarians, researchers have developed the provegetarian score or plant-based diet index (PDI) as a way of scoring data from food frequency questionnaires to assess the health outcomes associated with adherence to a plant-based diet. This plant-based scoring system gives the consumption of plant foods positive marks and the consumption of any animal-derived foods negative marks. Unhealthy plant foods, such as refined grains and sugar and processed foods can also be given negative marks in what is termed the unhealthy plant-based diet index (uPDI) – see Table 1.3. The most frequently asked question about this way of scoring diet quality is why potato consumption is considered as unfavourable. This is mainly because it was Harvard researchers that created this scoring system and they had found in their studies, the Nurses' Health Study and Health Professional follow-up study, that potato consumption has been associated with weight gain,[53] hypertension[54] and type 2 diabetes,[55] regardless of method of preparation. However, it should be noted that these studies are from the USA and in the context of a Western-diet pattern. Cohort studies from other countries have not always confirmed such associations.[56] The impact of potato consumption within the context of a varied and healthy vegan or vegetarian diet is not generally considered unhealthy.

When the PDI scoring system has been applied to dietary data collected from various prospective cohort studies, a healthy plant-based diet has been associated with a significant reduction in the risk of coronary heart disease,[57] stroke,[58] type 2 diabetes,[59] heart failure,[60] renal failure,[61] fatty liver disease,[62] cancer[63] and all-cause mortality[64] with an unhealthy plant-based diet having a neutral or negative impact compared to an omnivorous diet.

These health outcomes are summarised in Table 1.4. In addition, changes towards higher adherence to a plant-based diet over time has also been shown to be beneficial, suggesting that shifting to a plant-based diet can have benefits throughout the life stages for preventing weight gain, type 2 diabetes and cardiovascular disease and all-cause mortality.[65, 66, 67] It should be noted that these studies predominantly include Caucasian participants typically consuming a Western-style diet pattern. Thus, studies going forward should aim to include more diverse populations and communities.

Protein source

The most common concern cited about a plant-based diet, particularly a vegan diet, is the quality of plant protein, which many still consider to be 'inferior' to animal protein. One reason is that animal protein is considered 'complete' i.e., it provides enough of each of the nine essential amino acids to meet human requirements, whereas most plant sources of protein have lower proportions of certain essential amino acids. For example, beans tend to be lower in methionine and whole grains and nuts lower in lysine. In addition, animal-derived protein is more easily digested compared to plant proteins, in which the food matrix (the combination of components present in the food) partly impairs digestibility. However, this is con-

Table 1.3: Plant-based diet index[129]

Healthy plant foods	Unhealthy plant foods	Animal foods
Fruits	Fruit juice	Meat
Vegetables	Refined grains	Fish
Whole grains	Potato	Eggs
Nuts	Sugar-sweetened beverages	Dairy
Tea and coffee	Sweets and desserts	Animal fat
Vegetable oils		

Table 1.4: Health outcomes associated with adherence to a healthy or unhealthy plant-based diet (PDI; plant-based diet index, hPDI; healthy plant-based diet index, uPDI; unhealthy plant-based diet index)

Disease	PDI	hPDI	uPDI
Coronary heart disease[57]	8%↓	25%↓	32%↑
Type 2 diabetes[59]	20%↓	34%↓	16%↑
Total cancer risk[3]	15%↓		
Stroke[58]	Neutral	10%↓	Neutral
Renal failure[61]	6%↓	14%↓	11%↑
Fatty liver[62]	21%↓	24%↓	34%↑
All-cause mortality[64]	5%↓	10%↓	12%↑

sidered an extremely outdated concept.[68]

All plant foods contain all essential amino acids and when eating a variety of whole plant foods throughout the day or even over a few days, when meeting calorie requirements, will mean that protein requirements are easily met without having to worry about specific food combinations. In fact, the lower quantities of certain amino acids such as methionine and branched-chain amino acids (BCAA), leucine, isoleucine and valine, in plant-derived protein may actually be an advantage as they have been implicated in the development of cancer and type 2 diabetes.[69, 70] The lower content of sulphur-containing amino acids in plant foods, such as methionine and cysteine, results in a lower acid load of the diet and thus less burden on the kidneys.[71] There are some 'complete' plant sources of protein, including soya, quinoa, chia seeds and buckwheat. Soya in fact provides protein with a biological value similar to that of animal protein.[72]

More importantly, several lines of evidence demonstrate that obtaining protein from plant sources rather than animal sources is associated with better health outcomes and can reduce the risk of a number of chronic diseases, including cardiovascular disease, type 2 diabetes and certain cancers whilst promoting healthy aging.[73, 74, 75, 76] These studies come from different populations around the world including the USA, Canada, Europe, Japan and China and the results are very consistent.[75, 76, 77, 78] Overall, more is not better when it comes to protein, but the source of protein is key with animal-derived protein adversely affecting health. This is particularly true for animal protein in the form of red and processed meat and poultry, but in some studies even egg protein is found to contribute to ill health.[79] These studies show that just swapping 3% of total energy in the diet from animal protein with plant-derived protein can have a dramatic impact, significantly reducing mortality from several causes with a relative risk reduction in the order of 20–40%.

Processed and unprocessed red meat in particular contribute to harm. In 2015 the World Health Organization determined that processed meat is a major contributor to colorectal cancer, classifying it as a group 1 carcinogen, that is, it causes cancer.[80] Just one hot dog or a few strips of bacon consumed daily increases the risk of colorectal cancer by 18%. At the same time, red meat was classified as a group 2a carcinogen i.e., red meat *probably* causes colorectal cancer. A number of studies have also linked processed and red meat to other cancers including breast, stomach, pancreatic, prostate, and bladder cancers.[81, 82, 83] International cancer guidelines clearly state that processed meat and red meat should be limited or avoided to reduce the risk of developing cancer.[84] According to estimates by the Global Burden of Disease Project, an independent academic research organisation, about 34,000 cancer deaths per year worldwide are attributable to diets high in processed meat, and red meat could be responsible for 50,000 cancer deaths per year worldwide.[1] This will be discussed further in Chapter 4.

Mechanisms by which plant-based diets prevent chronic illness

The main driver of most chronic diseases is inflammation, the body's response to any sort of tissue damage. Usually, inflammation is a protective response against injury. However, when the body becomes overwhelmed, inflammation can lead to damage of normal tissues resulting in chronic disease. Diet and lifestyle choices can either promote or prevent inflammation.[85] Researchers have developed a dietary inflammatory index to provide a summary measure of diet-associated inflammation that could be used in any human population.[86] In general, whole plant foods, tea and coffee are associated with lower levels of inflammation and processed and unprocessed red meat, refined carbohydrates and sources of free sugar are associated with higher levels of inflammation. A number of studies have now confirmed that adherence to a diet with a lower inflammatory potential can reduce the risk of chronic disease.[87] Vegetarian and vegan diets specifically have been shown to lower inflammation.[88, 89]

Causes of inflammation include oxidative stress. Oxidation is a normal process which takes place in the body and refers to a loss of electrons by a molecule, atom or ion. The opposite reaction is called reduction, which is the gain of electrons. These processes are usually in balance and play a crucial role in normal cellular metabolism. An imbalance between oxidation and reduction can give rise to the formation of reactive oxygen species (ROS). ROS are also the by-product of normal cellular metabolism, however, during times of 'stress', ROS levels can rise dramatically resulting in tissue damage through oxidative stress. Oxidative stress can damage proteins, DNA and cell membranes. Stressors that can lead to increased levels of ROS include cigarette smoking, medication, pesticides, radiation and also our diet choices. The body requires antioxidants to counter the effects of these damaging ROS. Studies consistently show that those eating a predominately plant-based diet have higher levels of antioxidants in the body compared to omnivores.[90] Plant foods contain hundreds of antioxidant compounds and have vastly higher antioxidant content than animal-derived foods.[91] These antioxidants come in two broad categories – carotenoids and bioflavonoids. Both are large groups of structurally related compounds that help plants cope with radiation exposure from sunlight. In contrast, some compounds within animal-derived foods, such as haem iron (found in haemoglobin and myoglobin in meat) are pro-oxidants, creating oxidative stress and contributing to cellular damage.[83]

Advanced glycation end products (AGEs) are a group of compounds that induce oxidative stress. They are formed by a spontaneous chemical reaction between an amino acid (protein) and a monosaccharide (glucose). Some AGEs are produced in the body every day. However, diet is the biggest contributor to AGE formation (along with tobacco products). AGEs from food are generated more readily from protein-rich foods, when cooking at high temperatures, for longer and with dry heat cooking (lower AGE formation when there is water/moisture present). Foods that generate the most AGEs are fried and processed foods and also animal-derived foods – meat, dairy, fried eggs. Plant foods such as fruits, vegetables, whole grains and legumes, generate the least amount of AGEs. AGE formation is also increased by altered glucose metabolism – i.e., when there are high blood sugars, insulin resistance and in the presence of diabetes.[92] AGEs accumulate over time and the process for detoxification by the body is slow. AGEs have been shown to result in inflammation, oxidative stress, cellular damage and insulin resistance. AGEs have been implicated in the pathogenesis of a number of chronic diseases, including type 2 diabetes, kidney failure, dementia, cancer and atherosclerosis.[93]

The health of the gut microbiome, the trillions of organisms that live in the gut, plays a key role in determining our overall health. We understand most about the bacteria within our gut, but there are also viruses, fungi and protozoa present too. Dietary choices impact the health of the gut bacteria, which rely predominantly on fibre derived from whole plant foods. Plant-based diets, including vegetarian and vegan diets, increase bacterial diversity and promote the generation of short chain fatty acids (SCFAs), such as butyrate, propionate and acetate.[94] These SCFAs are signalling molecules that are produced by the fermentation of fibre and required for the integrity of the gut lining, maintaining the gut's immune system, reducing colonic pH and protecting against pathogens. One of the largest investigations into the gut microbiome, the American Gut Project, demonstrated that people consuming 30 different plant foods per week had a more diverse and thus healthier gut microbiome than participants consuming less than 10 different plant foods.[95] Diets that are lacking in plant-derived fibre, which is the case for most Western-style diet patterns, are known to result in reduced production of SCFAs, increased production of secondary bile acids (formed by the action of gut bacteria on primary bile acids, which are produced by the liver). Secondary bile acids can damage the gut cells, increase gut permeability and are implicated in the development of cancers of the gastrointestinal tract.[96] Diets high in saturated fat also increase the permeability of the gut lining and allow inflammatory substances, such as bacteria and lipopolysaccharides (bacterial endotoxins), into the circulation, which contributes to inflammation.[97] Diets high in sodium also adversely affect the gut microbiome with salt reduction resulting in increased production of SCFAs.[98] An unhealthy gut microbiome will also result in lower levels of incretin hormones, a group of gut hormones that are released after eating and decrease blood glucose levels, thus promoting the effects of insulin. In people with type 2 diabetes, this incretin effect is reduced or absent.[99]

One mechanism under investigation connecting the gut microbiome with health outcomes is the generation of trimethylamine N-oxide (TMAO) when meat-based diets are consumed. Choline and carnitine, compounds derived mainly from animal foods (red meat, poultry, fish and eggs) are converted by gut microbes to trimethylamine (TMA). TMA is then converted to TMAO by the liver. TMAO is thought to increase the risk of CVD (both heart disease and stroke) by its effects on cholesterol and sterol metabolism, promoting inflammation and by making platelets more reactive thus increasing blood clotting.[100] In addition, higher levels of TMAO have been implicated in the pathogenesis of heart failure, stroke, renal failure and type 2 diabetes.[101] However, there remains uncertainty as to whether TMAO is causal rather than merely a biomarker of underlying chronic illness.[102] What is more certain is that people consuming a plant-based diet have lower levels of TMAO compared to those consuming an omnivorous diet, in part due to the lack of gut microbes responsible for the generation of the metabolite.[103]

A further mechanism by which a plant-based diet low in saturated fat and virtually absent in dietary cholesterol is by preventing dyslipidaemia, specifically high cholesterol.[42] Dyslipidaemia is implicated in causing insulin resistance, atherosclerosis and cognitive decline and is discussed in the relevant disease specific chapters.

International consensus and country based dietary guidelines

There is international consensus on the core components of a healthy diet pattern for prevention of common chronic conditions. These include fruits, vegetables, whole grains, beans, nuts and seeds. In 2016, The American Heart Association and the American College of Cardiology recommended three main dietary patterns for the management of cardiovascular risk factors and prevention of cardiovascular disease.[104] These are the DASH, Mediterranean and vegetarian dietary patterns. The 2019 guideline on the *Primary Prevention of Cardiovascular Disease* published by the American College of Cardiology and the American Heart Association recommends a plant-based or Mediterranean-style diet as optimal, in recognition of the accumulation of evidence supporting plant-based diets for the prevention and treatment of CVD.[105] The updated 2021 guidance from the American Heart Association includes prioritising plant sources of protein and limiting animal sources of fat whilst centring the diet around fruits, vegetables and whole grains.[106]

The 2021 European guidelines for prevention of CVD also recommend 'adopting a more plant- and less animal-based food pattern', specifically recommending the Mediterranean diet given the level of supportive data.[107] In addition to guidelines for CVD prevention, the World Cancer Research Fund recommends a diet pattern centred around fruits, vegetables, whole grains and beans[108] and the American Association of clinical Endocrinologists and American College of Endocrinology have consistently recommended a primarily plant-based meal plan for type 2 diabetes.[109] The American College of Lifestyle Medicine recommends a whole food plant-based diet for the prevention and treatment of chronic disease, including for induction of remission for people with type 2 diabetes.[110] A 100% plant-based diet or vegan is deemed to be nutritionally adequate for all stages of life, with health benefits, by the major dietetic organisations around the world, including in the USA, Canada and UK.[111, 112]

We can no longer consider diet choices without considering the wider impact of our food choices. Our food system is at the centre of the global climate and ecological crises with animal agriculture a key contributor.[113] There is no doubt that a transition to a plant-based food system is required to keep food production within planetary boundaries.[114]

With this in mind, the most up-to-date analysis of what constitutes a healthy diet that is also sustainable for a predicted global population of 10 million by 2050, was conducted by the Eat-Lancet Commission on Food, Planet and Health, which has brought together 37 experts from 16 countries.[115] The work brings together data from several studies on nutrition, health and the environment, whilst considering country-based differences in accessibility to various foods. The recommended reference diet, termed the 'Planetary Health Plate', is one that is composed predominately of whole-plant foods, emphasising fruit, vegetables, whole grains, legumes, nuts and seeds. Animal-derived foods constitute less than 15% of daily calories and there is acceptance that a healthy diet does not need to contain any animal-derived foods at all. Eggs, dairy and poultry are considered optional. In Europe and America this dietary pattern requires a dramatic reduction in the consumption of unhealthy foods, including at least a 90% reduction in the consumption of red meat. At the same time, a more than 100% increase in consumption of whole plant foods is required. It is estimated that the global adoption of this diet pattern could save more than 11 million lives a year, which at the moment are lost due to consequences of an unhealthy diet, whilst keeping the food system within planetary boundaries.

Country-based dietary guidelines are now incorporating aspects of health and environmental sustainability, thus supporting a shift to a plant-based diet. For example, the 2019 Health Canada dietary guideline is mostly plant-based.[116] Three quarters of the diet is recommended to come from fruits, vegetables and whole grains with a quarter from sources of protein, favouring the consumption of beans and nuts in place of animal protein. Dairy has been removed as an essential food group. The 2021 Danish dietary guidelines recommend 'Eat plant-rich, varied and not too much', stating the benefits for health and the climate.[117]

All health professionals have been called to action in the fight to ensure a sustainable future. Supporting patients and clients to adopt a sustainable plant-based diet is one action we can all be a part of. The World Organization of Family Doctors (WONCA) have published a 'Declaration Calling for Family Doctors of the World to Act on Planetary Health'.[118] This includes advising patients to transition to a more plant-based diet in line with the Eat-Lancet planetary health diet. The BDA (the association of UK dietitians) has launched its One Blue Dot campaign, a project aimed at promoting environmentally sustainable diets and providing toolkits for its members to use when advising patients and clients.[119]

Lifestyle medicine and the importance of population-based interventions

In addition to international consensus and the evolution of national dietary guidance towards more plant-based dietary patterns, we are seeing a growing movement of healthcare professionals from different disciplines and specialities, who are recognising the importance of and gaining expertise in the evidence-based field of Lifestyle Medicine and putting the principles into practice. Lifestyle Medicine uses whole food, plant-predominant nutrition, and other important lifestyle measures of optimal sleep, physical activity, avoidance of risky substances such as tobacco, social connection, and stress management, as a primary preventative and treatment modality for chronic disease, where equal focus is placed on Lifestyle Medicine as on medications and procedures.[120] Lifestyle Medicine is now one of the fastest growing healthcare fields globally, recognised in the peer-reviewed literature, with the American College of Lifestyle Medicine as its flagship organisation.[121]

The importance of population-based interventions and community participation is well recognised. Public policy on tobacco consumption is a prime example. An often quoted and inspiring example is the North Karelia Project.[122] In the 1960s it became clear that mortality from coronary heart disease, especially among middle-aged men, was extremely high across Finland especially in North Karelia, the most eastern province of the country, representing the highest rate of coronary disease mortality in the world. This was driven by a diet high in saturated fat, especially heavy in dairy consumption, low consumption of plant-based foods, and tobacco use. In response to this the Finnish government commenced the North Karelia Project in 1972 to carry out a comprehensive community-based prevention program that was subsequently rolled out nationally. Community-based interventions to address risk factors of hypertension, hyperlipidemia and smoking were undertaken. Amongst the range of initiatives, nutrition and education messages were spread through different channels and in connection with different activities in the community, including newspaper articles and distributed leaflets. Hundreds of training seminars were organised for healthcare workers, mass catering personnel, and the general public. Diet was discussed in health education meetings and local associations. Special training meetings were organised to change the diet in mass catering at workplaces, schools, hospitals and restaurants. On a national level, interventions included the publishing of national dietary guidelines in 1981 by the National Nutrition Council, and guidelines on prevention of coronary heart disease in Finland in 1987, together with education contributions by national health authorities and voluntary organisations. The Government made a health policy statement in 1985 where the role of healthy nutrition as an important goal was recognised. Coronary mortality reduced in the middle age population by an incredible 84% from 1972 to 2014, of which about two-thirds of the decline was felt to be due to risk factor changes related to lifestyle. This is a powerful example of how chronic disease burden can be mitigated by purposeful engagement of government and all sectors of the community.

The coronavirus pandemic

As we write this book, the world is dealing with coronavirus disease, COVID-19, caused by severe acute respiratory syndrome coronavirus 2, declared a pandemic on 11th March 2020. It did not take long for healthcare professionals in the front line of the pandemic response to observe that people with underlying chronic health conditions had a greater risk of developing severe COVID-19, requiring hospitalisation, intensive care treatment and ultimately dying. These underlying health conditions were noted to be associated with a number of modifiable risk factors and included overweight and obesity, CVD, cancer, and type 2 diabetes. In the UK, more than 90% of those who died in the first wave of the pandemic had at least one underlying chronic condition.[123] In the USA, 64% of the risk of hospitalisations from COVID-19 was attributable to four underlying health conditions: hypertension, heart failure, type 2 diabetes and obesity.[124] These conditions are intimately related to four modifiable lifestyle factors: tobacco smoking, excessive alcohol consumption, lack of physical activity and unhealthy diets.

Many of these underlying chronic conditions can be prevented and modified by adopting a healthy plant-based diet and lifestyle. It is important to note that there are also risk factors that cannot be modified such as age and male sex, as well as some that cannot easily be modified in the short term but are equally important to address, including socioeconomic status and racial disparities.

Early on in the pandemic general advice on healthy diet and lifestyle was provided to citizens given the known positive impact on immune health.[125] As the pandemic progressed, more specific evidence emerged highlighting the positive impact of a healthy diet, specifically a plant-based diet on reducing COVID-19 severity. Data from China demonstrated that severe disease was associated with specific alterations in the composition of the gut microbiome, including reductions in bacterial species that are known to regulate the immune response. These strains of bacteria thrive on dietary fibre and are important in producing short chain fatty acids. These alterations were more pronounced in patients with a severe disease course and were associated with higher levels of inflammatory markers in the blood.[126]

The first publication to highlight the importance of a healthy plant-based diet pattern reported the results of a case-control study of healthcare workers, mostly physicians, with significant exposure to patients with COVID-19 from six countries.[127] The study included 568 people with COVID-19 and 2316 controls. Those participants who had had COVID-19 were asked to rate the severity based on five options from very mild to critical, requiring intensive care. The results showed that those following a plant-based diet pattern had a 73% reduction in the risk of moderate or severe COVID-19 and those following a pescatarian diet had a 59% reduction in risk. This was independent of body mass index and underlying chronic health conditions. In contrast, participants following a high protein, low carbohydrate diet had a three-fold higher odds of moderate or severe COVID-19 when compared with the plant-based group. Of note, the participants that were classified as plant-based were by no means vegan, vegetarian or whole food plant-based, consuming a median of 3.7 portions of legumes and 9.8 portions of fruits per week and still consuming some animal foods, including similar amounts of dairy and eggs to the non-plant-based group, and similar amounts of refined grains. However, their consumption of legumes, nuts and vegetables was significantly higher and consumption of red/processed meat, sugar-sweetened beverages and alcohol significantly lower than those participants who did not follow a plant-based diet.

The second paper to be published reported more robust data from the Zoe COVID symptom study.[128] This paper analysed diet quality in more than half a million participants from the USA and UK. During the follow-up period, 31,815 COVID-19 cases were documented. The results showed that those participants most adherent to a healthy plant-based diet as defined by the healthy plant-based diet index had a 9% reduction in acquiring COVID-19 infection and a 41% reduction in getting severe disease. The impact of a healthy diet was greatest in those from lower socioeconomic groups and independent of underlying chronic health conditions, body mass index, smoking and physical activity. Based on these results, it was calculated that nearly a third of COVID-19 cases could have been prevented if these differences in diet quality and wealth had not existed. Despite the limitations of the study, these results are fairly remarkable and clearly demonstrate the wide-reaching benefits of a healthy plant-based diet pattern.

Conclusions

There is now ample evidence supporting a plant-based dietary pattern for the prevention and treatment of chronic disease. It is accepted that a healthy diet can be plant-predominant or plant exclusive. A transition to a plant-based food system is also essential for planetary health. This book will discuss the evidence supporting plant-based diets in a variety of chronic conditions, and also includes chapters on barriers and strategies for adopting a plant-based diet, Lifestyle Medicine, and the environmental consequences of our food choices.

References

1. GBD Diet Collaborators. Health effects of dietary risks in 195 countries, 1990–2017: a systematic analysis for the Global Burden of Disease Study 2017. *Lancet* 2019; 393(10184): 1958-1972.
doi.org/10.1016/S0140-6736(19)30041-8

2. Danaei G, Singh GM, Paciorek CJ, Lin JK, Cowan MJ, Finucane MM, et al. The global cardiovascular risk transition: Associations of four metabolic risk factors with national income, urbanization, and western diet in 1980 and 2008. *Circulation* 2013; 127(14): 1493-1502.
doi.org/10.1161/CIRCULATIONAHA.113.001470

3. Rauber F, Louzada MLDC, Martinez Steele E, De Rezende LFM, Millett C, Monteiro CA, et al. Ultra-processed foods and excessive free sugar intake in the UK: A nationally representative cross-sectional study. *BMJ Open* 2019;

4. Nardocci M, Leclerc BS, Louzada ML, Monteiro CA, Batal M, Moubarac JC. Consumption of ultra-processed foods and obesity in Canada. *Can J Public Heal* 2019; 110(1): 4-14. doi: 10.17269/s41997-018-0130-x.
5. Wang L, Martínez Steele E, Du M, Pomeranz JL, O'Connor LE, Herrick KA, et al. Trends in Consumption of Ultraprocessed Foods among US Youths Aged 2-19 Years, 1999-2018. *JAMA* 2021; 326(6): 519-530. doi: 10.1001/jama.2021.10238.
6. The Global Nutrition Report's Independent Expert Group. 2021 Global Nutrition Report [Internet]. 2021. Available from: https://globalnutritionreport.org/reports/2021-global-nutrition-report/
7. World Health Organization. Healthy Diet [Internet]. 2020. Available from: https://www.who.int/news-room/fact-sheets/detail/healthy-diet
8. Cena H, Calder PC. Defining a healthy diet: Evidence for the role of contemporary dietary patterns in health and disease. *Nutrients* 2020: 12(2): 334. doi: 10.3390/nu12020334.
9. Clapp J. The problem with growing corporate concentration and power in the global food system. *Nature Food* 2021; 2: 404-408. doi.org/10.1038/s43016-021-00297-7
10. Nestle M. Corporate funding of food and nutrition research science or marketing? JAMA Internal Medicine 2016; 176(1): 13-14. doi: 10.1001/jamainternmed.2015.6667
11. Barnard ND, Long MB, Ferguson JM, Flores R, Kahleova H. Industry Funding and Cholesterol Research: A Systematic Review. *American Journal of Lifestyle Medicine* 2019; 15(2): 165-172. doi.org/10.1177/1559827619892198
12. Buettner D, Skemp S. Blue Zones: Lessons From the World's Longest Lived. *American Journal of Lifestyle Medicine* 2016; 10(5): 318-321. doi: 10.1177/1559827616637066.
13. Satija A, Yu E, Willett WC, Hu FB. Understanding Nutritional Epidemiology and Its Role in Policy. *Adv Nutr* 2015; 6(1): 5-18. doi: 10.3945/an.114.007492.
14. Shim J-S, Oh K, Kim HC. Dietary assessment methods in epidemiologic studies. Epidemiol Health. 2014; 36: e2014009. doi: 10.4178/epih/e2014009
15. Prentice RL, Howard B V., Van Horn L, Neuhouser ML, Anderson GL, Tinker LF, et al. Nutritional epidemiology and the Women's Health Initiative: a review. American Journal of Clinical Nutrition 2021; 113(5): 1083-1092. doi: 10.1093/ajcn/nqab091.
16. Hill AB. The Environment and Disease: Association or Causation? *Proc R Soc Med* 1965; 58(5): 295-300. PMID: 14283879
17. Askie L, Offringa M. Systematic reviews and meta-analysis. *Seminars in Fetal and Neonatal Medicine* 2015; 20(6): 403-409. doi: 10.1016/j.siny.2015.10.002
18. Siri-Tarino PW, Sun Q, Hu FB, Krauss RM. Meta-analysis of prospective cohort studies evaluating the association of saturated fat with cardiovascular disease. *Am J Clin Nutr* 2010; 91(3): 535-546. doi: 10.3945/ajcn.2009.27725.
19. Willet WC, Stampfer MJ, Sacks FM. Association of dietary, circulating and supplement fatty acids with coronary risk. *Ann Intern Med* 2014; 161(6): 453. doi: 10.7326/L14-5018.
20. Barnard ND, Willet WC, Ding EL. The misuse of meta-analysis in nutrition research. *JAMA* 2017; 318(15): 1435-1436. doi: 10.1001/jama.2017.12083.
21. Anglemyer A, Horvath HT, Bero L. Healthcare outcomes assessed with observational study designs compared with those assessed in randomized trials. *Cochrane Database of Systematic Reviews* 2014; 2014(4): MR000034. doi: 10.1002/14651858.MR000034.pub2.
22. Katz D, Karlsen M, Chung M, Shams-White M, Green L, Fielding J, et al. Hierarchies of Evidence Applied to Lifestyle Medicine (HEALM): Introduction of a Strength-of-evidence Approach Based on a Methodological Systematic Review. *Curr Dev Nutr* 2019; 3: 13.(Supplement_1).
23. Katz DL, Karlsen MC, Chung M, Shams-White MM, Green LW, Fielding J, et al. Hierarchies of evidence applied to lifestyle Medicine (HEALM): Introduction of a strength-of-evidence approach based on a methodological systematic review. *BMC Medical Research*

24. Scientific Advisory Committee on Nutrition. SACN Carbohydrates and Health Report. Public Health England. The Stationery Office 2015. https://assets.publishing.service.gov.uk/government/uploads/system/uploads/attachment_data/file/445503/SACN_Carbohydrates_and_Health.pdf
25. English LK, Ard JD, Bailey RL, Bates M, Bazzano LA, Boushey CJ, et al. Evaluation of Dietary Patterns and All-Cause Mortality: A Systematic Review. *JAMA Network Open* 2021; 4(8): e2122277.
doi: 10.1001/jamanetworkopen.2021.22277
26. Lari A, Sohouli MH, Fatahi S, Cerqueira HS, Santos HO, Pourrajab B, et al. The effects of the Dietary Approaches to Stop Hypertension (DASH) diet on metabolic risk factors in patients with chronic disease: A systematic review and meta-analysis of randomized controlled trials. *Nutr Metab Cardiovasc Dis* 2021; 31(10): 2766-2778. doi: 10.1016/j.numecd.2021.05.030
27. Balasubramaniam J, Hewlings SJ. A Systematic Review of the Efficacy of DASH Diet in Lowering Blood Pressure among Hypertensive Adults. *Topics in Clinical Nutrition* 2021; 36(2): 158-176.
28. Widmer RJ, Flammer AJ, Lerman LO, Lerman A. The Mediterranean diet, its components, and cardiovascular disease. *American Journal of Medicine* 2015; 128(3): 229-238.
doi: 10.1016/j.amjmed.2014.10.014
29. De Lorgeril M, Salen P, Martin JL, Monjaud I, Delaye J, Mamelle N. Mediterranean diet, traditional risk factors, and the rate of cardiovascular complications after myocardial infarction: Final report of the Lyon Diet Heart Study. *Circulation* 1999; 99(6): 1823-1825.
doi: 10.1161/01.cir.99.6.779
30. Estruch R, Ros E, Salas-Salvadó J, Covas M-I, Corella D, Arós F, et al. Primary Prevention of Cardiovascular Disease with a Mediterranean Diet Supplemented with Extra-Virgin Olive Oil or Nuts. *N Engl J Med* 2018; 378(34): e34.
doi: 10.1056/NEJMoa1800389
31. Papadaki A, Martínez-González MÁ, Alonso-Gómez A, Rekondo J, Salas-Salvadó J, Corella D, et al. Mediterranean diet and risk of heart failure: results from the PREDIMED randomized controlled trial. *Eur J Heart Fail* 2017; 19(9): 1179-1185. doi: 10.1002/ejhf.750
32. Martínez-González MA, Sánchez-Tainta A, Corella D, Salas-Salvadó J, Ros E, Arós F, et al. A provegetarian food pattern and reduction in total mortality in the Prevención con Dieta Mediterránea (PREDIMED) study. *American Journal of Clinical Nutrition* 2014; 100(1): 320S-8S. doi: 10.3945/ajcn.113.071431
33. Trichopoulou A, Bamia C, Trichopoulos D. Anatomy of health effects of Mediterranean diet: Greek EPIC prospective cohort study. *BMJ* 2009; 338: b2337. doi: 10.1136/bmj.b2337
34. Tsaban G, Yaskolka Meir A, Rinott E, Zelicha H, Kaplan A, Shalev A, et al. The effect of green Mediterranean diet on cardiometabolic risk; A randomised controlled trial. *Heart* 2020; 2020-317802. doi: 10.1136/heartjnl-2020-317802.
35. Yaskolka Meir A, Rinott E, Tsaban G, Zelicha H, Kaplan A, Rosen P, et al. Effect of green-Mediterranean diet on intrahepatic fat: the DIRECT PLUS randomised controlled trial. *Gut* 2021; 70(11):2085-2095.
doi: 10.1136/gutjnl-2020-323106
36. Chiavaroli L, Nishi SK, Khan TA, Braunstein CR, Glenn AJ, Mejia SB, et al. Portfolio Dietary Pattern and Cardiovascular Disease: A Systematic Review and Meta-analysis of Controlled Trials. *Progress in Cardiovascular Diseases* 2018; 61(1): 43-53.
doi: 10.1016/j.pcad.2018.05.004
37. Glenn AJ, Lo K, Jenkins DJA, Boucher BA, Hanley AJ, Kendall CWC, et al. Relationship between a plant-based dietary portfolio and risk of cardiovascular disease: Findings from the women's health initiative prospective cohort study. *J Am Heart Assoc* 2021; 10(16): e021515.
doi: 10.1161/JAHA.121.021515
38. Orlich MJ, Chiu THT, Dhillon PK, Key TJ, Fraser GE, Shridhar K, et al. Vegetarian Epidemiology: Review and Discussion of Findings from Geographically Diverse Cohorts. *Advances in Nutrition* 2019; 10(4): S284–S295.
doi: 10.1093/advances/nmy109
39. Dinu M, Abbate R, Gensini GF, Casini A, Sofi F. Vegetarian, vegan diets and multiple health

40. Jabri A, Kumar A, Verghese E, Alameh A, Kumar A, Khan MS, et al. Meta-analysis of effect of vegetarian diet on ischemic heart disease and all-cause mortality. *Am J Prev Cardiol* 2021; 7: 100182. doi: 10.1016/j.ajpc.2021.100182

41. Lee KW, Loh HC, Ching SM, Devaraj NK, Hoo FK. Effects of vegetarian diets on blood pressure lowering: A systematic review with meta-analysis and trial sequential analysis. *Nutrients* 2020; 12(6): 1604. doi: 10.3390/nu12061604

42. Yokoyama Y, Levin SM, Barnard ND. Association between plant-based diets and plasma lipids: A systematic review and meta-analysis. *Nutr Rev* 2017; 75(9): 683–698. doi: 10.1093/nutrit/nux030

43. Kahleova H, Levin S, Barnard N. Cardiometabolic benefits of plant-based diets. *Nutrients* 2017; 9(8): 848. doi: 10.3390/nu9080848

44. Campbell TC, Parpia B, Chen J. Diet, lifestyle, and the etiology of coronary artery disease: The Cornell China Study. *American Journal of Cardiology* 1998; 82(10B): 18T-21T. doi: 10.1016/s0002-9149(98)00718-8

45. Remde A, DeTurk SN, Almardini A, Steiner L, Wojda T. Plant-predominant eating patterns – how effective are they for treating obesity and related cardiometabolic health outcomes? – a systematic review. *Nutr Rev* 2021; nuab060. doi: 10.1093/nutrit/nuab060

46. Schulze MB, Martínez-González MA, Fung TT, Lichtenstein AH, Forouhi NG. Food based dietary patterns and chronic disease prevention. *BMJ* 2018; 361: k2396. doi: 10.1136/bmj.k2396

47. Jenkins DJA, Wolever TMS, Taylor RH, Barker H, Fielden H, Baldwin JM, et al. Glycemic index of foods: A physiological basis for carbohydrate exchange. *Am J Clin Nutr* 1981; 34(3): 362-6. doi: 10.1093/ajcn/34.3.362

48. Atkinson FS, Brand-Miller JC, Foster-Powell K, Buyken AE, Goletzke J. International tables of glycemic index and glycemic load values 2021: a systematic review. *Am J Clin Nutr* 2021; 114(5): 1625–1632. doi: 10.1093/acjn/nqab233

49. Livesey G, Taylor R, Livesey HF, Buyken AE, Jenkins DJA, Augustin LSA, et al. Dietary glycemic index and load and the risk of type 2 diabetes: a systematic review and updated meta-analyses of prospective cohort studies. *Nutrients* 2019; 11(6): 1280. doi: 10.3390/nu11061280

50. Jenkins DJA, Dehghan M, Mente A, Bangdiwala SI, Rangarajan S, Srichaikul K, et al. Glycemic Index, Glycemic Load, and Cardiovascular Disease and Mortality. *N Engl J Med* 2021; 384(14):1312-1322. doi: 10.1056/NEJMoa2007123

51. Turati F, Galeone C, Augustin LSA, La Vecchia C. Glycemic index, glycemic load and cancer risk: An updated meta-analysis. *Nutrients* 2019; 11(10): 2342. doi: 10.3390/nu11102342

52. Ojo O, Ojo OO, Adebowale F, Wang XH. The effect of dietary glycaemic index on glycaemia in patients with type 2 diabetes: A systematic review and meta-analysis of randomized controlled trials. *Nutrients* 2018; 10(3): 373. doi: 10.3390/nu10030373

53. Bertoia ML, Mukamal KJ, Cahill LE, Hou T, Ludwig DS, Mozaffarian D, et al. Changes in Intake of Fruits and Vegetables and Weight Change in United States Men and Women Followed for Up to 24 Years: Analysis from Three Prospective Cohort Studies. *PLoS Med* 2015; 12(9): e1001878. doi: 10.1371/journal.pmed.1001878

54. Borgi L, Rimm EB, Willett WC, Forman JP. Potato intake and incidence of hypertension: Results from three prospective US cohort studies. *BMJ* 2016; 353: i2351. doi: 10.1136/bmj.i2351

55. Muraki I, Rimm EB, Willett WC, Manson JE, Hu FB, Sun Q. Potato consumption and risk of type 2 diabetes: Results from three prospective cohort studies. *Diabetes Care* 2016; 39(3): 376-84. doi: 10.2337/dc15-0547

56. Hu EA, Martínez-González MA, Salas-Salvadó J, Corella D, Ros E, Fitó M, et al. Potato consumption does not increase blood pressure or incident hypertension in 2 cohorts of Spanish adults. *J Nutr* 2017; 147(12): 2272-2281. doi: 10.3945/jn.117.252254

57. Satija A, Bhupathiraju SN, Spiegelman D,

Chiuve SE, Manson JAE, Willett W, et al. Healthful and Unhealthful Plant-Based Diets and the Risk of Coronary Heart Disease in U.S. Adults. *J Am Coll Cardiol* 2017; 70(4): 411-422. doi: 10.1016/j.jacc.2017.05.047

58. Baden MY, Shan Z, Wang F, Li Y, Manson JE, Rimm EB, et al. Quality of Plant-Based Diet and Risk of Total, Ischemic, and Hemorrhagic Stroke. *Neurology* 2021; 96(15): e1940-e1953. doi: 10.1212/WNL.0000000000011713

59. Satija A, Bhupathiraju SN, Rimm EB, Spiegelman D, Chiuve SE, Borgi L, et al. Plant-Based Dietary Patterns and Incidence of Type 2 Diabetes in US Men and Women: Results from Three Prospective Cohort Studies. *PLoS Med* 2016; 13(6): e1002039.
doi: 10.1371/journal.pmed.1002039

60. Lara KM, Levitan EB, Gutierrez OM, Shikany JM, Safford MM, Judd SE, et al. Dietary Patterns and Incident Heart Failure in U.S. Adults Without Known Coronary Disease. *J Am Coll Cardiol* 2019; 73(16): 2036-2045. doi: 10.1016/j.jacc.2019.01.067

61. Kim H, Caulfield LE, Garcia-Larsen V, Steffen LM, Grams ME, Coresh J, et al. Plant-based diets and incident CKD and kidney function. Clin J Am Soc Nephrol. 2019;

62. Mazidi M, Kengne A. Higher adherence to plant-based diets are associated with lower likelihood of fatty liver. *Clin Nutr* 2019; 14(5): 682-691. doi: 10.2215/CJN.12391018

63. Kane-Diallo A, Srour B, Sellem L, Deschasaux M, Latino-Martel P, Hercberg S, et al. Association between a pro plant-based dietary score and cancer risk in the prospective NutriNet-santé cohort. *Int J Cancer* 2018; 143(9): 2168-2176. doi: 10.1002/ijc.31593

64. Baden MY, Liu G, Satija A, Li Y, Sun Q, Fung TT, et al. Changes in Plant-Based Diet Quality and Total and Cause-Specific Mortality. *Circulation* 2019; 140(12): 979-991.
doi: 10.1161/CIRCULATIONAHA.119.041014

65. Satija A, Malik V, Rimm EB, Sacks F, Willett W, Hu FB. Changes in intake of plant-based diets and weight change: Results from 3 prospective cohort studies. *American Journal of Clinical Nutrition* 2019; 110(3): 574-582.
doi: 10.1093/ajcn/nqz049

66. Sotos-Prieto M, Bhupathiraju SN, Mattei J, Fung TT, Li Y, Pan A, et al. Association of Changes in Diet Quality and Total and Cause-Specific Mortality. *N Engl J Med* 2017; 377(2): 143-153. doi: 10.1056/NEJMoa1613502

67. Chen Z, Drouin-Chartier JP, Li Y, Baden MY, Manson JAE, Willett WC, et al. Changes in Plant-Based Diet Indices and Subsequent Risk of Type 2 Diabetes in Women and Men: Three U.S. Prospective Cohorts. *Diabetes Care* 2021; 44(3): 663-671. doi: 10.2337/dc20-1636

68. Katz DL, Doughty KN, Geagan K, Jenkins DA, Gardner CD. Perspective: The Public Health Case for Modernizing the Definition of Protein Quality. *Advances in Nutrition* 2019; 10(5): 755-764. doi: 10.1093/advances/nmz023

69. Miousse IR, Tobacyk J, Quick CM, Jamshidi-Parsian A, Skinner CM, Kore R, et al. Modulation of dietary methionine intake elicits potent, yet distinct, anticancer effects on primary versus metastatic tumors. *Carcinogenesis* 2018; 39(9): 1117-1126.
doi: 10.1093/carcin/bgy085

70. Flores-Guerrero J, Osté M, Kieneker L, Gruppen E, Wolak-Dinsmore J, Otvos J, et al. Plasma Branched-Chain Amino Acids and Risk of Incident Type 2 Diabetes: Results from the PREVEND Prospective Cohort Study. *J Clin Med* 2018; 7(12): 513. doi: 10.3390/jcm7120513

71. Rebholz CM, Coresh J, Grams ME, Steffen LM, Anderson CAM, Appel LJ, et al. Dietary Acid Load and Incident Chronic Kidney Disease: Results from the ARIC Study. *Am J Nephrol* 2015; 42(6): 427-35. doi: 10.1159/000443746

72. Young VR. Soy protein in relation to human protein and amino acid nutrition. *Journal of the American Dietetic Association* 1991; 91(7): 828-35.

73. Song M, Fung TT, Hu FB, Willett WC, Longo VD, Chan AT, et al. Association of animal and plant protein intake with all-cause and cause-specific mortality. *JAMA Intern Med* 2016; 176(10): 1453-1463.
doi: 10.1001/jamainternmed.2016.4182

74. Qi XX, Shen P. Associations of dietary protein intake with all-cause, cardiovascular disease, and cancer mortality: A systematic review and meta-analysis of cohort studies. *Nutr Metab*

75. Budhathoki S, Sawada N, Iwasaki M, Yamaji T, Goto A, Kotemori A, et al. Association of Animal and Plant Protein Intake with All-Cause and Cause-Specific Mortality in a Japanese Cohort. *JAMA Intern Med* 2019; 179(11): 1509-1518.
doi: 10.1001/jamainternmed.2019.2806

76. Huang J, Liao LM, Weinstein SJ, Sinha R, Graubard BI, Albanes D. Association between Plant and Animal Protein Intake and Overall and Cause-Specific Mortality. *JAMA Intern Med* 2020; 180(9): 1173-1184.
doi: 10.1001/jamainternmed.2020.2790

77. Zhong VW, Van Horn L, Greenland P, Carnethon MR, Ning H, Wilkins JT, et al. Associations of Processed Meat, Unprocessed Red Meat, Poultry, or Fish Intake with Incident Cardiovascular Disease and All-Cause Mortality. *JAMA Intern Med* 2020; 180(4): 503-512. doi: 10.1001/jamainternmed.2019.6969

78. Naghshi S, Sadeghi O, Willett WC, Esmaillzadeh A. Dietary intake of total, animal, and plant proteins and risk of all cause, cardiovascular, and cancer mortality: Systematic review and dose-response meta-analysis of prospective cohort studies. *BMJ* 2020; 370: m2412.
doi: 10.1136/bmj.m2412

79. Zhong VW, Allen NB, Greenland P, Carnethon MR, Ning H, Wilkins JT, et al. Protein foods from animal sources, incident cardiovascular disease and all-cause mortality: A substitution analysis. *Int J Epidemiol* 2021; 50(1): 223-233.
doi: 10.1093/ije/dyaa205

80. IARC. IARC Monographs evaluate consumption of red meat and processed meat. *World Health Organisation* 2015.

81. Farvid MS, Stern MC, Norat T, Sasazuki S, Vineis P, Weijenberg MP, et al. Consumption of red and processed meat and breast cancer incidence: A systematic review and meta-analysis of prospective studies. *International Journal of Cancer* 2018; 143(11): 2787-2799.
doi: 10.1002/ijc.31848

82. Li F, An S, Hou L, Chen P, Lei C, Tan W. Red and processed meat intake and risk of bladder cancer: A meta-analysis. *Int J Clin Exp Med* 2014; 7(8): 2100-2110.

83. Wolk A. Potential health hazards of eating red meat. *Journal of Internal Medicine* 2017; 281(2): 106-122. doi: 10.1111/joim.12543

84. Clinton SK, Giovannucci EL, Hursting SD. The World Cancer Research Fund/American Institute for Cancer Research Third Expert Report on Diet, Nutrition, Physical Activity, and Cancer: Impact and Future Directions. *Journal of Nutrition* 2020; 150(4): 663-671.
doi: 10.1093/jn/nxz268

85. Furman D, Campisi J, Verdin E, Carrera-Bastos P, Targ S, Franceschi C, et al. Chronic inflammation in the etiology of disease across the life span. *Nat Med* 2019; 25(12): 1822-1832.
doi: 10.1038/s41591-019-0675-0

86. Hébert JR, Shivappa N, Wirth MD, Hussey JR, Hurley TG. Perspective: The Dietary Inflammatory Index (DII) - Lessons Learned, Improvements Made, and Future Directions. *Advances in Nutrition* 2019; 10(2): 185-195.
doi: 10.1093/advances/nmy071

87. Li J, Lee DH, Hu J, Tabung FK, Li Y, Bhupathiraju SN, et al. Dietary Inflammatory Potential and Risk of Cardiovascular Disease Among Men and Women in the U.S. *J Am Coll Cardiol* 2020; 76(19): 2181-2193.
doi: 10.1016/j.jacc.2020.09.535

88. Shah B, Newman JD, Woolf K, Ganguzza L, Guo Y, Allen N, et al. Anti-inflammatory effects of a vegan diet versus the american heart association–recommended diet in coronary artery disease trial. *J Am Heart Assoc* 2018; 7(23): e011367. doi: 10.1161/JAHA.118.011367

89. Craddock JC, Neale EP, Peoples GE, Probst YC. Vegetarian-Based Dietary Patterns and their Relation with Inflammatory and Immune Biomarkers: A Systematic Review and Meta-Analysis. *Advances in Nutrition* 2019; 10(3): 433-451. doi: 10.1093/advances/nmy103

90. Miles FL, Lloren JIC, Haddad E, Jaceldo-Siegl K, Knutsen S, Sabate J, et al. Plasma, urine, and adipose tissue biomarkers of dietary intake differ between vegetarian and non-vegetarian diet groups in the Adventist Health Study-2. *J Nutr* 2019; 149(4): 667-675. doi: 10.1093/jn/nxy292

91. Carlsen MH, Halvorsen BL, Holte K, Bøhn SK, Dragland S, Sampson L, et al. The total

antioxidant content of more than 3100 foods, beverages, spices, herbs and supplements used worldwide. *Nutr J* 2010; 9:3. doi: 10.1186/1475-2891-9-3
92. Uribarri J, Woodruff S, Goodman S, Cai W, Chen X, Pyzik R, et al. Advanced Glycation End Products in Foods and a Practical Guide to Their Reduction in the Diet. *J Am Diet Assoc* 2010; 110(6): 911-16.e12. doi: 10.1016/j.jada.2010.03.018
93. Uribarri J, del Castillo MD, de la Maza MP, Filip R, Gugliucci A, Luevano-Contreras C, et al. Dietary advanced glycation end products and their role in health and disease. *Advances in Nutrition* 2015; 6(4): 461-73. doi: 10.3945/an.115.008433
94. Tomova A, Bukovsky I, Rembert E, Yonas W, Alwarith J, Barnard ND, et al. The Effects of Vegetarian and Vegan Diets on Gut Microbiota. *Frontiers in Nutrition* 2019; 6: 47. doi: 10.3389/fnut.2019.00047
95. McDonald D, Hyde E, Debelius JW, Morton JT, Gonzalez A, Ackermann G, et al. American Gut: an Open Platform for Citizen Science Microbiome Research. *mSystems* 2018; 3:3. doi: 10.1128/mSystems.00031-18
96. Valdes AM, Walter J, Segal E, Spector TD. Role of the gut microbiota in nutrition and health. *BMJ* 2018; 361: k2179. doi: 10.1136/bmj.k2179
97. López-Moreno J, García-Carpintero S, Jimenez-Lucena R, Haro C, Rangel-Zúñiga OA, Blanco-Rojo R, et al. Effect of Dietary Lipids on Endotoxemia Influences Postprandial Inflammatory Response. *J Agric Food Chem* 2017; 65(35): 7756-7763. doi: 10.1021/acs.jafc.7b01909
98. Chen L, He FJ, Dong Y, Huang Y, Wang C, Harshfield GA, et al. Modest Sodium Reduction Increases Circulating Short-Chain Fatty Acids in Untreated Hypertensives. *Hypertension* 2020; 76(1): 73-79. doi: 10.1161/HYPERTENSIONAHA.120.14800
99. Singh RK, Chang HW, Yan D, Lee KM, Ucmak D, Wong K, et al. Influence of diet on the gut microbiome and implications for human health. *Journal of Translational Medicine* 2017; 15(1): 73. doi: 10.1186/s12967-017-1175-y
100. Tang WHW, Wang Z, Levison BS, Koeth RA, Britt EB, Fu X, et al. Intestinal Microbial Metabolism of Phosphatidylcholine and Cardiovascular Risk. *N Engl J Med* 2013; 368(17): 1575-84. doi: 10.1056/NEJMoa1109400
101. Papandreou C, Moré M, Bellamine A. Trimethylamine n-oxide in relation to cardiometabolic health—cause or effect? *Nutrients* 2020; 12(5): 1330. doi: 10.3390/nu12051330
102. Jia J, Dou P, Gao M, Kong X, Li C, Liu Z, et al. Assessment of causal direction between gut microbiota- dependent metabolites and cardiometabolic health: A bidirectional mendelian randomization analysis. *Diabetes*: 2019; 68(9): 1747-1755. doi: 10.2337/db19-0153
103. Heianza Y, Ma W, DiDonato JA, Sun Q, Rimm EB, Hu FB, et al. Long-Term Changes in Gut Microbial Metabolite Trimethylamine N-Oxide and Coronary Heart Disease Risk. *J Am Coll Cardiol* 2020; 75(7): 763-772. doi: 10.1016/j.jacc.2019.11.060
104. Van Horn L, Carson JAS, Appel LJ, Burke LE, Economos C, Karmally W, et al. Recommended Dietary Pattern to Achieve Adherence to the American Heart Association/American College of Cardiology (AHA/ACC) Guidelines: A Scientific Statement from the American Heart Association. *Circulation* 2016; 134(22): e505–e529. doi: 10.1161/CIR.0000000000000462
105. Arnett DK, Blumenthal RS, Albert MA, Buroker AB, Goldberger ZD, Hahn EJ, et al. 2019 ACC/AHA Guideline on the Primary Prevention of Cardiovascular Disease: A Report of the American College of Cardiology/American Heart Association Task Force on Clinical Practice Guidelines. *Circulation* 2019; 140(11): e596-e646. doi: 10.1161/CIR.0000000000000678
106. Lichtenstein AH, Appel LJ, Vadiveloo M, Hu FB et al. 2021 Dietary Guidance to Improve Cardiovascular Health: A Scientific Statement From the American Heart Association. *Circulation* 2021; 144(23): e472-e487. doi: 10.1161/CIR.0000000000001031
107. Visseren FLJ, Mach F, Smulders YM, Carballo D, Koskinas KC, Bäck M, et al. 2021 ESC Guidelines on cardiovascular disease

prevention in clinical practice. *European Heart Journal* 2021; 42(34): 3227-3337. doi: 10.1093/eurheartj/ehab484
108. Rock CL, Thomson C, Gansler T, Gapstur SM, McCullough ML, Patel A V., et al. American Cancer Society guideline for diet and physical activity for cancer prevention. *CA Cancer J Clin* 2020; 70(4): 245-271. doi: 10.3322/caac.21591
109. Garber AJ, Handelsman Y, Grunberger G, Einhorn D, Abrahamson MJ, Barzilay JI, et al. Consensus statement by the American Association of clinical Endocrinologists and American College of Endocrinology on the comprehensive type 2 diabetes management algorithm - 2020 executive summary. *Endocrine Practice* 2020; 26(1): 107-139. doi: 10.4158/CS-2019-0472
110. Kelly J, Karlsen M, Steinke G. Type 2 Diabetes Remission and Lifestyle Medicine: A Position Statement From the American College of Lifestyle Medicine. *American Journal of Lifestyle Medicine* 2020; 14(4): 406-419. doi: 10.1177/1559827620930962
111. BDA. British Dietetic Association confirms well-planned vegan diets can support healthy living in people of all ages. *BDA* 2017. Available from: https://www.bda.uk.com/resource/british-dietetic-association-confirms-well-planned-vegan-diets-can-support-healthy-living-in-people-of-all-ages.html
112. Melina V, Craig W, Levin S. Position of the Academy of Nutrition and Dietetics: Vegetarian Diets. *J Acad Nutr Diet* 2016; 116(12): 1970-1980. doi: 10.1016/j.jand.2016.09.025
113. Poore J, Nemecek T. Reducing food's environmental impacts through producers and consumers. *Science* 2018; 360(6392): 987-992. doi: 10.1126/science.aaq0216
114. Clark MA, Domingo NGG, Colgan K, Thakrar SK, Tilman D, Lynch J, et al. Global food system emissions could preclude achieving the 1.5° and 2°C climate change targets. *Science* 2020; 370(6517): 705-708. doi: 10.1126/science.aba7357
115. Willett W, Rockström J, Loken B, Springmann M, Lang T, Vermeulen S, et al. Food in the Anthropocene: the EAT–Lancet Commission on healthy diets from sustainable food systems. *Lancet* 2019;393(10170): 447-492. doi: 10.1016/S0140-6736(18)31788-4
116. Health Canada. Canada's Dietary Guidelines. *Canada's Food Guide* 2019. Available from: https://food-guide.canada.ca/static/assets/pdf/CDG-EN-2018.pdf
117. Danish dietary guidelines. 2021. Available from: https://altomkost.dk/fileadmin/user_upload/altomkost.dk/Publikationsdatabase/De_officielle_Kostraad_2021/Danish_Official_Dietary_Guidelines_Good_for_Health_and_climate_2021_SCREEN_ENG.pdf
118. WONCA. Declaration calling for family doctors of the world to act on planetary health. 2019. Available from: https://www.globalfamilydoctor.com/site/DefaultSite/filesystem/documents/Groups/Environment/2019 Planetary health.pdf
119. BDA. One Blue Dot: Environmentally Sustainable Diet Toolkit [Internet]. *BDA* 2018. Available from: https://www.bda.uk.com/professional/resources/environmentally_sustainable_diet_toolkit_-_one_blue_dot
120. Bodai B. Lifestyle Medicine: A Brief Review of Its Dramatic Impact on Health and Survival. *Perm J* 2017; 22:17-025. doi: 10.7812/TPP/17-025
121. American College of Lifestyle Medicine. Lifestyle Medicine. *ACLM* 2021. https://lifestylemedicine.org/What-is-Lifestyle-Medicine.
122. Vartiainen E. The North Karelia Project: Cardiovascular disease prevention in Finland. *Glob Cardiol Sci Pract* 2018; 2018(2): 13. doi: 10.21542/gcsp.2018.13
123. Williamson EJ, Walker AJ, Bhaskaran K, Bacon S, Bates C, Morton CE, et al. Factors associated with COVID-19-related death using OpenSAFELY. *Nature* 2020; 584(7821): 430-436. doi: 10.1038/s41586-020-2521-4
124. O'hearn M, Liu J, Cudhea F, Micha R, Mozaffarian D. Coronavirus disease 2019 hospitalizations attributable to cardiometabolic conditions in the united states: A comparative risk assessment analysis. *J Am Heart Assoc* 2021; 10(5): e020859. doi: 10.1161/JAHA.119.020859
125. Calder PC. Nutrition, immunity and

126. Yeoh YK, Zuo T, Lui GCY, Zhang F, Liu Q, Li AYL, et al. Gut microbiota composition reflects disease severity and dysfunctional immune responses in patients with COVID-19. *Gut* 2021; 70(4): 698-706.
doi: 10.1136/gutjnl-2020-323020
127. Kim H, Rebholz CM, Hegde S, Lafiura C, Raghavan M, Lloyd JF, et al. Plant-based diets, pescatarian diets and COVID-19 severity: A population-based case-control study in six countries. *BMJ Nutr Prev Heal* 2021; 4(1).
doi: 10.1136/bmjnph-2021-000272
128. Merino J, Joshi AD, Nguyen LH, Leeming ER, Mazidi M, Drew DA, et al. Diet quality and risk and severity of COVID-19: a prospective cohort study. *Gut* 2021; 70(11): 2096-2104.
doi: 10.1136/gutjnl-2021-325353

Chapter 2
Meeting nutritional requirements on a plant-based diet from birth to old age

Sandra Hood and Miriam Martinez-Biarge

Over time a well-planned vegan diet has been shown to be adequate for all life stages and has the potential to prevent and treat disease and help to slow the ageing process. With appropriate planning it is feasible to meet the requirements for most nutrients from foods on a plant-based diet. Two vitamins, vitamin D and vitamin B12, are not found in plant foods and must be provided in the form of supplements, fortified foods or, in the case of vitamin D, obtained from sun exposure.

Other nutrients, namely iodine, omega-3 fatty acids and selenium, may be in short supply in some plant-based diets, depending on the geographical region, the type of foods included, the way foods are processed and cooked, individual needs and other factors. In plant-based diets, diversity of foods and optimisation of the bioavailability of nutrients are key in order to ensure that nutritional requirements are met.

Contrary to popular belief, protein is not a problem for most people on plant-based diets, as long as energy intake is sufficient, and the diet includes beans and legumes daily. However, suboptimal protein intake can be an issue in the elderly and in other groups with increased needs. On average 85% of plant derived protein foods are digested due to their high fibre and phytochemical content.[1] Accordingly, the protein needs of vegans may be slightly higher than non-vegans to allow for this.

Important nutrients in plant-based diets at all ages

Vitamin B12

Vitamin B12 is not produced by plants or animals, only by bacteria. Small amounts have been occasionally found in sea vegetables, fermented foods or other plants, probably due to bacterial contamination, but no plant food has been proven to be a reliable and significant source of vitamin B12. Many plant milks, cereals, nutritional yeast and other processed foods are fortified, and although absorption from fortified foods is known to be at least as good as from animal foods, for most people it is difficult to reach the recommended daily intake (RDI) with fortified foods alone. Therefore, supplementation is essential at all ages.

The RDIs for vitamin B12 have been derived for the general population, who obtain small amounts of vitamin B12 from multiple animal sources throughout the day. There is no consensus on the best dose and regime of vitamin B12 supplementation for children and adults on plant-based diets, but several studies have shown that oral absorption of both cyanocobalamin and methylcobalamin, the two most common commercially available forms of B12, is good, and that daily or weekly supplementation with different doses can be equally effective to maintain normal blood levels.[2,3]

Vitamin D

Vitamin D has two main forms, D_2 (ergocalciferol) and D_3 (cholecalciferol). Both are equally well absorbed in the intestine, and both need to be hydroxylated twice before becoming the physiologically active form, calcitriol. Vitamin D_3 is more efficiently activated to calcitriol than vitamin D_2.

Mushrooms exposed to sunlight or UV radiation from lamps can generate vitamin D_2 and can be a significant source of vitamin D, providing around 10 mcg/100 g.[4] However, this is not standard commercial practice yet. There are no other plant sources of vitamin D, although many plant-based milks, margarines and other spreads and cereals are fortified with variable amounts.

Vitamin D can be obtained through sunlight exposure, but the time needed to produce the RDI is different in every person and depends on several factors (latitude, altitude, skin type, season, pollution, time of day, amount of skin exposed, duration of exposure, sunscreen use, age), which may be difficult to control and measure.[5] In addition, obesity and other chronic conditions may impair vitamin D production in the skin. Excessive sun exposure is also a strong risk factor for developing skin cancer.[5]

For most people living in Europe, regardless of their diet, taking vitamin D supplements, either in winter or throughout the year, is advisable. Plant-based supplements can be obtained from yeast (ergocalciferol, D_2) or from lichen (cholecalciferol, D_3).

Vitamin A

Plant foods contain only provitamin A carotenoids that the body can convert into vitamin A, but not preformed vitamin A. There are only a few vegetables with adequate amounts of carotenes, and if these foods are not consumed on a daily basis there is the risk of suboptimal vitamin A intake. The best sources of provitamin A are sweet potatoes (not white varieties), carrots, pumpkin, peppers, kale, spinach, Swiss chard and other leafy green vegetables. Heating and the presence of fat in the meal enhance the absorbability of carotenes.[6]

Calcium

Calcium can be found in most plant foods, and as with other micronutrients, the key element to guarantee a good status is to optimise its absorption. The main determinant of calcium absorption is vitamin D. Protein seems to increase absorption, whereas phytate and oxalate are the main inhibitors. Oxalate may reduce calcium absorption in oxalate-rich vegetables (spinach, Swiss chard, sweet potatoes, rhubarb, cocoa) to less than 10%. In contrast, green vegetables low in oxalate (kale, broccoli, pak choi, rocket, lettuce, watercress, spring greens) are one of the best sources of calcium, with absorption rates around 40–60%.[7]

Calcium absorption from other calcium-rich foods like chia seeds, almonds, whole tahini, oranges, figs or beans ranges between 20–40%.[7] Soya products are good sources of calcium, especially calcium-set tofu (up to 400 mg/100 g) and tempeh (110 mg/100 g). Many plant milks and yoghurts are now fortified with calcium, and this can be a very useful source for people with increased needs and for those not able to eat high amounts of green vegetables, like infants and children. Calcium in fortified plant-milks is absorbed at a similar rate as calcium from dairy.[8]

Zinc

The bioavailability of zinc is lower in plant-based diets and people who follow vegetarian and vegan diets consume approximately 10% less zinc and have lower blood levels than non-vegetarians, although there is no evidence of a higher prevalence of clinical zinc deficiency in vegans who live in Western countries.[9]

Phytate, present in cereals, legumes and seeds, impairs iron and zinc absorption. Several household processing methods, such as soaking cereals and legumes in water (followed by decanting the water), germination and fermentation, can reduce the phytate content and facilitate nutrient absorption. Canning and extrusion cooking, malting, milling and hydrothermal treatment are industrial processing practices that can also lower phytate in food.[10]

Seeds (pumpkin, sunflower, and sesame), cashew nuts, grains and legumes are good sources of zinc and provide 1.5–2.5 mg per serving. For people with increased needs, adding one tablespoon a day of nutritional yeast to meals can boost zinc intake.

Iron

Plant foods are rich in iron and the average vegan diet provides more iron than conventional diets, and above the RDI (except for pregnant women). However, absorption of non-haem iron, the form found in plant foods, is less efficient than haem-iron from meat and fish. Studies have consistently shown that vegetarian and vegan adults have lower iron stores and a greater risk of developing deficiency in situations of high demand or when there are other predisposing factors. On the other hand, low ferritin values seem to be protective against type 2 diabetes and metabolic syndrome and could partially explain the lower rates of these conditions found in people following plant-based diets.[11]

Adding iron absorption enhancers to meals (vitamin C and carotenes, other organic acids from fruit and vegetables such as citric, malic, lactic and acetic acids), and reducing phytate content as described before can be the most efficient way of improving iron status.[6, 10]

Iodine

The UK is one of the top 10 iodine-deficient countries in the world.[12] In most countries, the main dietary source of iodine is fortified salt, but in the UK, salt is not iodised, and the only sources of iodine are fish, seaweed and dairy products. Sea vegetables are therefore the only plant food rich in iodine, but the iodine content varies between species and without adequate labelling it is not possible to calculate actual iodine intake. The risk of excessive iodine intake (and subsequent thyroid dysfunction, thyroiditis and thyroid papillary cancer) is real.[12]

Iodine intake in vegans in the UK and many other countries is low and the iodine status of many vegans may be compromised.[13] In the current circumstances the safest and most reliable way to obtain iodine is taking a supplement of potassium iodate that provides 75–100% of the daily RDI (see Table 2.1).

Selenium

The amount of selenium in plant foods is variable and depends on the soil levels, which are low in all Europe including the UK. Several studies have consistently shown suboptimal selenium status in children and adults across Europe.[14] The selenium content in animal products is higher and more stable, partly due to routine feed supplementation; therefore, people on plant-based diets may be at higher risk of selenium deficiency. Vegan women in the UK have been found to have

Table 2.1 RDI for infants, children and adults in the UK (excluding pregnant and breastfeeding women), sources and availability of the main nutrients of interest in plant-based diets

Nutrient	Age (males/females)[45]						
	1–3	4–6	7–10	11–14	15–18	19–64	65+
Protein (g/day)	14.5	19.7	28.3	42.1/41.2	55.2/45.0	55.5/45	53.3/46.5
Vitamin A (mcg/day)	400	400	500	600	700/600	700/600	700/600
Vitamin B12 (mcg/day)	0.5	0.8	1.0	1.2	1.5	1.5	1.5
Vitamin D (mcg/day)	10	10	10	10	10	10	10
Iron (mg/day)	6.9	6.1	8.7	11.3/14.8	11.3/14.8	8.7/8.7-14.8	8.7
Calcium (mg/day)	350	450	550	1000/800	1000/800	700	700
Zinc (mg/day)	5.0	6.5	7.0	9.0	9.5/7.0	9.5/7.0	9.5/7.0
Iodine (mcg/day)	70	100	110	130	140	140	140
Selenium (mcg/day)	15	20	30	45	70/60	75/60	75/60

Best plant sources	Availability	Comments / advice
Beans, peas, legumes, tofu, tempeh, soya mince, seitan, vegan Quorn™, peanuts, nuts, seeds	Increase: milling, dehulling, soaking, boiling, ultra-heating, germination, fermentation	Include one small serving in each meal
Sweet potatoes, carrots, pumpkin, spinach, Swiss chard, pepper, mango	Increase: heat, fat	Include one food from this group every day
Fortified plant milks and yogurts, fortified nutritional yeast and cereals	Good oral absorption from fortified foods and supplements	Supplements can be taken daily or weekly
Sunlight, fortified plant milks and yogurts, fortified spreads and cereals, irradiated mushrooms	Good absorption from fortified foods and supplements. Plant-based D3 from lichen available as supplement	Tolerable upper intake level = 100 mcg/day
Beans, legumes, tofu, tempeh, nuts, seeds, wholegrains, leafy green vegetables, dried fruit	Increase: vitamin C, lysine, organic acids Decrease: phytate, tea, coffee, cocoa	Infants 6–12 months at higher risk of deficiency, consider supplement (1 mg/kg/day)
Cruciferous vegetables, fortified plant milks and yogurts, calcium-set tofu, sesame seeds, almonds, chia seeds, whole-wheat bread, oranges, figs	Increase: vitamin D, dietary protein Decrease: oxalate, phytate	Include 4–5 good sources every day
Pumpkin and sesame seeds, cashew nuts, legumes, whole grains, nutritional yeast	Increase: soaking, fermentation, germination Decrease: phytate	Requirements may be 20–25% higher in high-phytate diets[10]
Sea vegetables (risk of excessive intake), iodised salt		Salt in UK is not iodised
Brazil nuts (1 nut = 80–100 mcg). Small amounts in grains, wheat germ, sunflower seeds, spinach		Tolerable upper intake level (adults) = 400 mcg. Risk of toxicity if excessive intake

significantly lower selenium intakes compared to non-vegan women.[14]

Brazil nuts are the richest source of selenium. One nut (5 g) provides around 100 mcg, which covers 160% and 130% of women and men's daily requirements respectively. Inclusion of 1–2 Brazil nuts once or twice a week is a simple way to guarantee an adequate intake and status. It is better not to eat more than 4–5 nuts at a time, to keep selenium intake below the tolerable upper intake level (400 mcg).

Omega-3 fatty acids

The three most relevant omega-3 fatty acids in human nutrition are alpha-linolenic acid (ALA), eicosapentaenoic acid (EPA), and docosahexaenoic acid (DHA). ALA is considered an essential nutrient that must be obtained from foods and is found in some nuts and seeds (walnuts, chia seeds, linseed, hemp seed), soya products and leafy green vegetables. It can be converted into EPA and then to DHA, but the conversion rate is low. DHA and EPA are produced by microalgae and then consumed by fish, which is the main dietary source in conventional diets. However, it is possible to obtain oil from microalgae and use it as plant-based DHA supplement.

Despite decades of research, the potential benefits of DHA/EPA supplementation in healthy adults and children over two years of age are still controversial.[15, 16] The UK Government and the American Academy of Medicine have not established specific intake recommendations for EPA or DHA, only for ALA. The European Food Safety Authority (EFSA) recommends 100 mg/day for infants 0–2 years, 250 mg for adults and older children and 450 mg/day during pregnancy and breastfeeding.[17]

Planning the diet

The Eatwell Guide was first published in 2016 by Public Health England and summarises government recommendations for a healthy diet.[18] It is applicable to everybody over the age of two years, including people following plant-based diets. The guide shows the proportion of each food group that should be eaten every day. This has been calculated so that the diet provides ≥50% of food energy as carbohydrates, ≤5% as free sugars, ≤35% of food energy as fat; ≤11% as saturated fat; and 15% as protein. The recommended daily intake of fibre is ≥30 g.

Figure 2.1 shows how the national guidelines can be adapted to plant-based diets.

The first two years of life

Exclusive breastfeeding or, if this is not possible, formula feeding, is the recommended way of feeding infants for at least the first four to six months. Small amounts of complementary foods can be introduced from the beginning of the fifth month, but for the first six months infants should be predominantly breast and/or formula fed. Breast or formula milk will still provide most of the energy and nutrient requirements during the second half of the first year.[19]

Between the fifth and the end of the first year, when complementary foods are introduced, infants grow and develop very fast, have high metabolic demands and are most vulnerable to nutritional deficits, especially in relation to energy and iron.

In infants and toddlers the best way to confirm an adequate energy intake is by monitoring growth. Insufficient energy provision can occur when the diet is based on low-energy density, high-volume foods, such as vegetables and fruits. Whereas infants should be offered a wide range of fruits and vegetables and should eat this food group daily, the focus at this age should be high-energy foods, such as the ones shown in Table 2.2. Peanut butter, nut butters, tahini and other seed spreads are very valuable, as fat should constitute

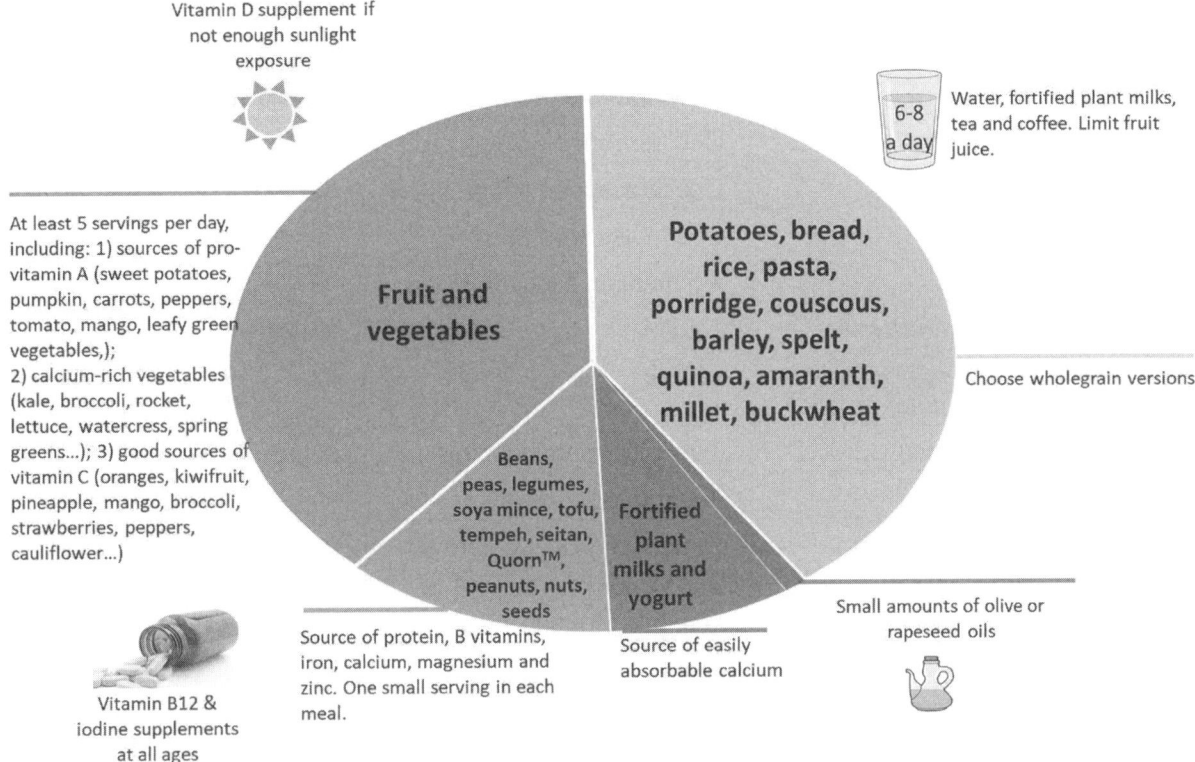

Figure 2.1 Meeting nutritional requirements on plant-based diets from birth to old age

40% of energy intake from 6 to 12 months.

As long as energy requirements are met and the diet has a variety of plant foods from different groups, infants will obtain all the protein and amino acids they need. Milling, dehulling, soaking, boiling, ultra-heating, germination and fermentation have been shown to improve digestibility and bioavailability of plant protein and other nutrients.[20] In infants and young children, processed forms of grains, nuts and pulses (such as bread, rolled oats, pasta, couscous, nut butters, hummus, other bean and pulse spreads) are preferable to intact whole grains and pulses.

Iron requirements are disproportionally high at this age and might be difficult to meet with the diet alone. Breastmilk provides iron in an easily absorbable form. Iron-fortified cereals are often recommended, but many are also high in sugar and many families prefer to use the same cereals that the rest of the family eats. For infants who are not able to eat a good variety of solids, an iron supplement (1 mg/kg/day) can be useful until a diversified diet is well established.

Supplements

The UK Government recommends that all children from six months to five years take a daily supplement containing vitamins A, C and D. Breastfed infants should take a daily supplement containing 400 IU (10 mcg) of vitamin D from birth. In addition, infants on plant-based diets

Table 2.2 High-energy foods for infants and toddlers

Food	Serving size	Energy (kcal)
Peanut butter	One tablespoon (16 g)	95.5
Nut butters	One tablespoon (16 g)	85–100
Tahini	One tablespoon (15 g)	89
Avocado	1/3 medium avocado (50 g)	80
Mature human milk	**100 ml**	**65–70**
SMA® Wysoy® (soya infant formula)	**100 ml**	**67**
Boiled potato	½ medium potato (85 g)	60–65
Hummus	Two tablespoons (28 g)	60
Boiled sweet potato	½ medium sweet potato (75 g)	60
Cooked lentils	Four tablespoons (50 g)	56
Tempeh	30 g	60
Dried fruit	1 dried fig (20 g)	45
Tofu	50 g	40
Banana	½ medium banana (45 g)	40
Wholewheat bread	½ slice	40

Energy requirements in 1-year-old infants are 715 kcal/day (girls), and 765 kcal/day (boys)

should take 2.5 mcg/day or 250 mcg/week of vitamin B12 starting at six months of age.

Iodine is provided during the first year through breast or formula milk. Toddlers 1–2 years who are no longer breastfeeding or taking formula or an iodine-fortified plant-milk will need an iodine supplement.

Key points
- Breast and / or formula milk are the main source of nutrients during the first year. Complementary foods can be introduced from the beginning of the fifth month.
- Infants 6–12 months need high-energy density foods.
- Iron requirements are very high and some infants will need supplements.
- Breastfed infants should take a daily supplement of vitamin D (10 mcg) from the day of birth. From six months they also need a supplement providing vitamins A, C and B12.
- Some infants older than 1 year of age may need an iodine supplement.

Children over two years and adolescents

The distribution of food groups should be very similar to the adult diet. Energy requirements vary with age, sex, physical activity and other individual factors, and general recommendations should be used as an approximation.

Table 2.3 shows the number of servings per each food group that are recommended at each age. Children with higher levels of physical activity will require more servings, as well as male adolescents compared to females.

Vegan 'meat alternatives' are not necessary but are enjoyed by many children and adolescents and can be a useful addition to the diet two to three times a week. They can replace one serving of legumes or tofu. These numbers of servings have been calculated so that the diet provides at least 90% of the RDI of energy, protein, iron, zinc, calcium, and ALA.[21] Supplementation with vitamin B12, vitamin D, and iodine is recommended in all cases.

Table 2.3 Recommended number of daily portions for children and adolescents

Food group	Portion size	2–3 years	4–10 years	11–17 years
Whole grains and potatoes	Two slices of bread (60 g), ½ cup of oats / other breakfast cereals, one medium potato / sweet potato, one cup of cooked rice, quinoa, spelt, 80 g of cooked pasta	3–4	4–5	6–9
Beans and legumes, including tofu, tempeh, textured soya protein	One small bowl of cooked lentils, chickpeas or beans; (or 4 tbsp); 80–100 g of hummus (5 tbsp); 80 g of firm tofu, 60 g of tempeh, 30 g of texturised soya protein (dried)	1–2	2–3	2–4
Vegan 'meat alternatives'	One medium vegan burger, two small tofu sausages, four 'meat' balls	0–1	0–1	0–2
Fortified soya or other plant-milks	1 glass (200–250 ml), 150 ml of soya yoghurt	1–2	1–2	2
Fruit	One medium piece or two small ones, 10–12 grapes or berries, 30 g (one handful) of dried fruit	2	2–3	3–5
Vegetables	One small bowl of cooked vegetables or salad	2	3	4–5
Nuts and seeds	30 g (one handful) or 2 tbsp of nut spread/butter	1	1–2	2–3

Adapted from: Menal-Puey S, Martinez-Biarge M, Marques-Lopes I. Developing a Food Exchange System for Meal Planning in Vegan Children and Adolescents. *Nutrients*. 2018;11:43.[21]

> **Key points**
> - The distribution of food groups should be the same as in adults.
> - When energy requirements are met, and the distribution of food groups is adequate the diet provides the RDIs for all the main nutrients.
> - Supplementation with vitamins D, B12 and iodine is recommended.

Pregnancy and lactation

General nutritional recommendations of particular relevance during this period include those for vitamin D, folic acid and calcium, and for vegans, vitamin B12 and iodine. Other nutrients that often raise concern specifically for those following a plant-based diet include protein, iron and omega-3 fatty acids. However, with careful planning these can be accommodated by a varied, mixed plant-based diet and are all addressed below.

Current evidence encourages eating a wide variety of foods and not avoiding anything unless there is a known intolerance or allergy.[22] Care needs to be taken with vegetables and salads which should be washed carefully. This is in case they have been in contact with soil contaminated with the parasite toxoplasma gondii, which can cause toxoplasmosis. This is usually harmless but in pregnant women there is a small risk that the infection could cause miscarriage or birth defects.

Folate (folic acid)

Folate is a B vitamin of crucial importance in early pregnancy, directly involved in DNA and RNA synthesis. A deficiency can cause neural tube defects such as spina bifida. Plant-based diets are usually rich in this B vitamin and studies have shown vegans typically have higher intakes than non-vegans.[23] Plant sources include green leafy vegetables, beans, pulses, nuts and oranges. Nevertheless, it is prudent for all women planning a pregnancy to take a daily folic acid supplement of 400 mcg continuing up to the 12th week of pregnancy. There is an increased requirement for women with diabetes or epilepsy, or with a family history of neural tube defects and these women should receive personalised advice from their doctor.

Vitamin B12

Adequate supplementation of vitamin B12 is essential during pregnancy and breastfeeding, as the B12 stores of infants at birth are dependent upon the levels of this vitamin circulating in the mother's bloodstream during pregnancy. Healthy newborns have been found to have twice their mothers' levels of B12.[24] Therefore, it is important to ensure a minimum daily intake of at least 3 mcg from fortified foods or a supplement containing a minimum of 10 mcg daily, or at least 2000 mcg weekly. Although the body has the ability to store and recycle this vitamin in the liver, pregnant women should not rely on their reserves. This is because there is some uncertainty about the impact of vitamin B12 stores on the vitamin B12 status of the foetus.

It is also particularly important that the mother's B12 levels are sufficient so that breast milk levels of this vitamin meet the infant's needs. Vegan women who take B12 supplements have similar B12 content in their milk compared to non-vegan women.[25]

Vitamin D and calcium

Demands for vitamin D increase during pregnancy and lactation, due to the need for extra calcium to form the foetus's bones and to produce milk. Infants rely on stored vitamin D obtained prior to birth because human breast milk has low vitamin D levels. Therefore, the UK Department of Health recommends that all pregnant women take a supplement of 10 mcg per day and continue through breast feeding.

During pregnancy there is no need to consume more calcium as the efficiency of calcium absorption increases at this time.[26] Nevertheless, it is sensible to ensure a good calcium intake. Intakes in women have been shown to be below the current recommendations of 700 mg per day with a significant percentage not meeting the LRNI (the lower recommended nutrient intake) to meet requirements.[27] This understandably raises concerns but with careful planning recommendations can be met.

For breastfeeding an extra 550 mg per day is required and this can be met by adding extra calcium-rich snacks through the day. For example:
- a bowl of cereal with 150 ml of fortified plant milk would provide at least 200 mg
- two slices of wholemeal bread and small tin of baked beans would provide at least 150 mg
- a handful (30 g) of almonds and a large orange would provide at least 120 mg
- a portion (50 g) of scrambled calcium-set tofu with 50 g of steamed spinach would provide at least 320 mg.

Iodine

This mineral is essential for foetal growth and brain development, and requirements increase from 150 mcg to 200 mcg daily during pregnancy, and breastfeeding. However, approximately 60% of pregnant women do not meet the recommended intake.[12] As explained previously, vegan women may be at even higher risk of low iodine intake.

Due to the critical nature of getting iodine intake right, it may be prudent to take a supplement. This should contain up to 150 mcg in the form of potassium iodine or potassium iodate and the remainder requirement can be met by the diet.

Iron

There is an extra demand for iron during pregnancy for the developing foetus and to form haemoglobin. However, with the cessation of periods more iron is available and in addition there is increased absorption during this time. The RDI for the latter half of pregnancy increased from 14.8 to 27 mg.[28]

Iron deficiency anaemia rates are no different in vegans and anaemia can be a problem during any pregnancy, regardless of the diet.[23] All pregnant women need to eat foods rich in iron together with adequate vitamin C to aid iron absorption. Iron supplements are only necessary if there is a deficiency and can interfere with other minerals' absorption. They can also lead to constipation.

Omega-3 fatty acids

The long chain omega-3 fatty acids EPA and DHA are important for the development of the foetus and newborn's brain and visual system[29] and understandably there has been a lot of discussion as to whether vegans need to consume a direct source of these fatty acids. A recent meta-analysis found that maternal supplementation was significantly associated with a reduced risk of preterm birth and low birthweight in the foetus.[30] It seems prudent that pregnant and breastfeeding women take a supplement that provides 400–550 mg of a combination of DHA and EPA. Limiting sources of linoleic acid (LA) e.g. oils of sunflower, corn and sesame and increasing intake of foods rich in alpha ALA foods e.g. walnuts, ground linseed (flaxseed), shelled hemp seeds, chia seeds and vegetable (rapeseed) oil in cooking will optimise conversion of ALA to EPA and DHA.

Protein

Protein requirements increase by 6 g a day in the third trimester and by 11 g a day when breastfeeding. This increased requirement can easily be met if a variety of plant foods are eaten, and calorie requirements are met. For example by ensuring a good source of protein at every meal and adding in one or two extra protein-rich snacks.

> **Key points**
> - Daily requirements of protein and iron increase in the second half of pregnancy, whereas extra calcium is needed during breastfeeding. These extra requirements can be met with careful planning.
> - Daily supplementation with 400 mcg of folic acid is recommended for all women, including vegan women, starting before pregnancy and continuing up to the 12th week of pregnancy.
> - Pregnant women on plant-based diets are advised to continue taking their vitamin D, B12 and iodine supplementation.
> - A daily supplement providing 400–550 mg of DHA-EPA is also recommended.

Nutrition in elderly vegans

There is no definitive age at which someone becomes elderly, but it is usually considered to be a person over 65 years of age. With life expectancy rising to 82.9 years for women and 79.3 for men in the UK (Office for National Statistics 2016–2018) it is more important than ever to ensure healthy ageing. Unfortunately, there have been no studies looking at the nutritional needs of elderly vegans. What we do know is that a vegan diet may offer some protection against many chronic conditions such as cardiovascular disease,[31] diabetes,[32] and certain cancers.[33] Indeed, it has been suggested that physicians should consider recommending a plant-based diet for those with health conditions such as hypertension, diabetes, cardiovascular disease and obesity.[34, 35]

Therefore, it is supposed that elderly vegans should have a lower risk for the various diseases that afflict conventional eaters. Surveys suggest that typical older vegetarians have a more nutrient-dense diet than meat eaters,[36] benefit from being leaner than omnivores, and have good bowel regularity due to a high fibre diet.[37] In short a plant-based diet offers potential health benefits that can help to slow the ageing process.

Nevertheless, with increasing age comes the inevitable challenge of physical and mental changes, reduction in lean body mass and bone tissue. These issues need to be addressed.

It is recognised that the nutritional requirements of older adults differ from younger adults.[27] Calorie requirements decrease and maintaining a nutrient dense, varied and balanced diet can be difficult. The risk of malnutrition can be high and whether the situation is any different for vegans is unclear.

Age-related issues include:
- increased risk for the development of non-communicable diseases such as osteoporosis, cardiovascular disease, diabetes and cancer
- dementia
- loss of taste, sight and hearing
- dental problems
- loss of ability to shop or cook
- reduced appetite
- malnutrition including weight loss and weight gain.

Bone status (see Chapter 16) is of particular concern after a recent study found that vegans had higher risks of fractures compared with meat eaters and vegetarians.[38] It was suggested that these risks were likely partly due to lower BMI and possibly lower intakes of calcium and protein. Therefore, careful consideration should be given to ensuring adequate intake of protein and calcium, along with vitamin B12, vitamin D, folate and fluids, as well as maintaining a healthy body weight. These issues are addressed below together with other nutrients that often raise concern for vegans.

Protein

Protein requirements for the elderly was previously recommended at 0.8 g per kg per day. This has now been increased to a minimum of 1 g per kg per day in combination with varied daily activity to help preserve lean body mass and prevent its loss throughout ageing.[39] Therefore recommendations are that 1.0–1.2 g protein per kg of body weight per day should be used and for those with complex medical conditions. During illness the European Society for Clinical Nutrition and Metabolism (ESPEN) and the Parenteral and Enteral Nutrition Group (PENG) recommend 1.5–2.0 g per kg per day.[39] Since vegans may have higher protein requirements than non-vegans due to the reduced digestibility of protein from whole foods it is important to ensure that the diet includes good protein sources. Some choices that provide a relatively high amount of protein in a small amount include firm tofu, tempeh, soya mince, seitan and vegan Quorn™. Other good quality sources are beans, pulses, nuts, seeds and protein-rich grains such as quinoa, millet and buckwheat.

Calcium and vitamin D

Ensuring a good intake of calcium and vitamin D to aid absorption is essential. Frailty and illnesses such as gastrointestinal (GI) disorders may affect the absorption rate of various nutrients. If there are any concerns with meeting calcium requirements, a calcium supplement is recommended. In addition, due to the declining synthesis of vitamin D with increasing age, the British Dietetic Association (BDA) recommends a supplement of 10 mcg per day for those over 65 years of age regardless of dietary preference.

Vitamin B12

It is recognised that the capacity to absorb vitamin B12 may decrease with aging due to digestive changes.[40] However, there is currently no recommended increment for older people and vegans should continue taking the same supplementation regime.

Folate

This B vitamin plays a role in helping prevent heart disease and low levels are linked to osteoporosis. Deficiency is also associated with depression and dementia and an increased risk of Alzheimer's disease and vascular dementia.[41] Vegans generally have higher intakes of folic acid than omnivores but nevertheless it is important to ensure a good intake with concentrated sources such as oranges, lentils, greens and avocados.

Fluid

Adequate fluid intake is important to keep the urinary tract and kidneys healthy. The elderly can be more vulnerable to dehydration due to a number of factors including loss of thirst, reduced renal function, swallowing difficulties or a reluctance to drink to prevent visits to the toilet. Dehydration can lead to low blood pressure and increased risk of falls, urinary tract infections, poor healing and reduced mental ability, as well as being one of the most common causes of constipation. However, fluid requirements in the elderly is estimated to be slightly less at 30 ml/kg/day than an adult's requirements of 35 ml/kg/day.[42]

Fibre

Maintaining an adequate fibre intake has been shown to be problematic for meat eaters, with many struggling to meet the minimum requirement of 30 g a day leading to a high prevalence of gastrointestinal (GI) disorders such as diverticular disease, diarrhoea and constipation. Vegans generally have more robust digestive systems and have been shown to consume significantly more fibre than omnivores, with numerous beneficial health effects including weight management and healthy aging.[43, 44]

However, too much fibre can result in a low energy intake and, as with children, the elderly can feel full before they have met their energy requirements. Therefore, if weight is low and there is difficulty in meeting calorie requirements, a shift towards a higher fat intake can be encouraged. Many plant-based sources are rich in unsaturated, heart-healthy fats such as avocado, nuts and seeds. Other energy dense foods include dried fruit, cakes and biscuits which can be included as part of a balanced vegan diet.

Omega-3 long chain fatty acids

There is limited evidence for the benefit of taking omega-3 supplements for protecting cognitive health.[16] Nevertheless, ensuring a good intake of ALA to generate adequate EPA and DHA is important. Micro algae supplements containing EPA and DHA are available but whether these are necessary or of benefit is unclear.

Body weight

Appetite can decrease with ageing due to a number of reasons and can cause weight loss. Vegans tend to have a lower BMI than their peers and maintaining a healthy weight in later life is important. Being underweight can increase the risk of health problems as much as being overweight. Weight loss can reduce muscle strength, impact on the immune system, lead to frailty and increase the risk of falls. Ensuring an energy dense diet, eating regular meals and including nutritious snacks will ensure adequate calories. If taste acuity is a problem, meals can be perked up with herbs and spices for added flavour.

Physical activity

Sufficient exercise is important in protecting mental and physical health. Older people are encouraged to do some type of physical activity every day. This should include activities that improve strength, balance and flexibility on at least two days a week.[46] There are now many opportunities for group activities for the older person and local health centres and libraries can provide further information.

> **Key points**
> - Physical and mental changes associated with increased age may hinder adequate nutrition.
> - Energy requirements decrease, whereas the need for protein increase and absorption of other nutrients may be compromised.
> - Ensuring enough fluid intake and good hydration status is essential for the health and wellbeing of the elderly.
> - Supplementation with vitamin B12, vitamin D and iodine is recommended for all vegans over 65 years.
> - Regular physical activity can protect mental and physical health and should be promoted.

References

1. Lonnie M, Hooker E, Brunstrom JM et al. Protein for Life: Review of Optimal Protein Intake, Sustainable Dietary Sources and the Effect on Appetite in Ageing Adults. *Nutrients* 2018; 10(3): 360. doi: 10.3390/nu10030360
2. Obeid R, Fedosov SN, Nexo E. Cobalamin coenzyme forms are not likely to be superior to cyano- and hydroxyl-cobalamin in prevention or

treatment of cobalamin deficiency. *Mol Nutr Food Res* 2015; 59(7): 1364-1372. doi: 10.1002/mnfr.201500019.

3. Del Bo' C, Riso P, Gardana C et al. Effect of two different sublingual dosages of vitamin B12 on cobalamin nutritional status in vegans and vegetarians with a marginal deficiency: A randomized controlled trial. *Clin Nutr* 2019; 38(2): 575-583. doi: 10.1016/j.clnu.2018.02.008

4. Cardwell G, Bornman JF, James AP, Black LJ. A Review of Mushrooms as a Potential Source of Dietary Vitamin D. *Nutrients* 2018; 10(10): 1498. doi: 10.3390/nu10101498

5. Wacker M, Holick MF. Sunlight and Vitamin D: A global perspective for health. *Dermatoendocrinol* 2013; 5(1): 51-108. doi: 10.4161/derm.24494

6. Platel K, Srinivasan K. Bioavailability of Micronutrients from Plant Foods: An Update. *Crit Rev Food Sci Nutr* 2016; 56(10): 1608-1619. doi: 10.1080/10408398.2013.781011

7. Weaver CM, Proulx WR, Heaney R. Choices for achieving adequate dietary calcium with a vegetarian diet. *Am J Clin Nutr* 1999; 70(3 Suppl): 543S-548S. doi: 10.1093/ajcn/70.3.543s

8. Tang AL, Walker KZ, Wilcox G, Strauss BJ, Ashton JF, Stojanovska L. Calcium absorption in Australian osteopenic post-menopausal women: an acute comparative study of fortified soymilk to cows' milk. *Asia Pac J Clin Nutr* 2010; 19(2): 243-249.

9. Foster M, Chu A, Petocz P, Samman S. Effect of vegetarian diets on zinc status: a systematic review and meta-analysis of studies in humans. *J Sci Food Agric* 2013; 93(10): 2362-2371. doi: 10.1002/jsfa.6179

10. Gibson RS, Raboy V, King JC. Implications of phytate in plant-based foods for iron and zinc bioavailability, setting dietary requirements, and formulating programs and policies. *Nutr Rev* 2018; 76(11): 793-804. doi: 10.1093/nutrit/nuy028

11. Haider LM, Schwingshackl L, Hoffmann G, Ekmekcioglu C. The effect of vegetarian diets on iron status in adults: A systematic review and meta-analysis. *Crit Rev Food Sci Nutr* 2018; 58: 1359-1374. doi: 10.1080/10408398.2016.1259210

12. Bouga M, Lean MEJ, Combet E. Contemporary challenges to iodine status and nutrition: the role of foods, dietary recommendations, fortification and supplementation. *Proc Nutr Soc* 2018; 77(3): 302-313. doi: 10.1017/S0029665118000137

13. Eveleigh ER, Coneyworth LJ, Avery A, Welham SJM. Vegans, Vegetarians, and Omnivores: How Does Dietary Choice Influence Iodine Intake? A Systematic Review. *Nutrients* 2020; 12(6): 1606. doi: 10.3390/nu12061606

14. Stoffaneller R, Morse NL. A review of dietary selenium intake and selenium status in Europe and the Middle East. *Nutrients* 2015; 7(3): 1494-1537. doi: 10.3390/nu7031494

15. Abdelhamid AS, Brown TJ, Brainard JS et al. Summerbell CD, Worthington HV, Song F, Hooper L. Omega-3 fatty acids for the primary and secondary prevention of cardiovascular disease. *Cochrane Database Syst Rev* 2020; 3(2): CD003177. doi: 10.1002/14651858.CD003177.pub3

16. Deane KHO, Jimoh OF, Biswas P, et al. Omega-3 and polyunsaturated fat for prevention of depression and anxiety symptoms: systematic review and meta-analysis of randomised trials. *Br J Psychiatry* 2021; 218(3): 135-142. doi: 10.1192/bjp.2019.234

17. EFSA Panel on Dietetic Products, Nutrition, and Allergies (NDA); Scientific Opinion on Dietary Reference Values for fats, including saturated fatty acids, polyunsaturated fatty acids, monounsaturated fatty acids, trans fatty acids, and cholesterol. *EFSA Journal* 2010; 8(3): 1461. doi: 10.2903/j.efsa.2010.1461

18. Public Health England. From Plate to Guide: What, why and how for the eatwell mode. [Published Nov 2016]. https://assets.publishing.service.gov.uk/government/uploads/system/uploads/attachment_data/file/579388/eatwell_model_guide_report.pdfl

19. Fewtrell M, Bronsky J, Campoy C et al. Complementary Feeding: A Position Paper by the European Society for Paediatric Gastroenterology, Hepatology, and Nutrition (ESPGHAN) Committee on Nutrition. *J Pediatr Gastroenterol Nutr* 2017; 64(1): 119-132. doi: 10.1097/MPG.0000000000001454

20. Sá AGA, Moreno YMF, Carciofi BAM. Food processing for the improvement of plant proteins digestibility. *Crit Rev Food Sci Nutr* 2020; 60(20): 3367-3386. doi: 10.1080/10408398.2019.1688249

21. Menal-Puey S, Martinez-Biarge M, Marques-Lopes I. Developing a Food Exchange System for Meal Planning in Vegan Children and Adolescents. *Nutrients* 2018; 11: 43. doi: 10.3390/nu11010043
22. Greer FR, Sicherer SH, Burks AW. The effects of early nutritional interventions on the development of atopic disease in infants and children: The role of maternal dietary restriction, breastfeeding, hydrolysed formulas and timing of introduction of allergenic complementary foods. *Pediatrics* 2019; 143(4): e20190281. doi: 10.1542/peds.2019-0281
23. Sebastiani G, Herranz Barbero A, Borrás-Novell C, et al. The Effects of Vegetarian and Vegan Diet during Pregnancy on the Health of Mothers and Offspring. *Nutrients* 2019; 11(3): 557. doi: 10.3390/nu11030557
24. Frery N Huel G Leroy M et al. Vitamin B12 among parturients and their newborns and its relationship with birthweight. *Eur J Obstet Gynecol Reprod Biol* 1992; 45(3): 155-163. doi: 10.1016/0028-2243(92)90076-b
25. Karcz K, Królak-Olejnik B. Vegan or vegetarian diet and breast milk composition - a systematic review. *Crit Rev Food Sci Nutr* 2021; 61(7): 1081-1098. doi: 10.1080/10408398.2020.1753650
26. Kovacs CS. Maternal Mineral and Bone Metabolism During Pregnancy, Lactation, and Post-Weaning Recovery. *Physiol Rev* 2016; 96(2): 449-547. doi: 10.1152/physrev.00027.2015
27. SACN (Scientific Advisory Committee on Nutrition) Statement on nutrition and older adults living in the community, January 2021. www.gov.uk/government/publications/sacn-statement-on-nutrition-and-older-adults
28. Pavord S, Daru J, Prasannan N et al. BSH Committee. UK guidelines on the management of iron deficiency in pregnancy. *Br J Haematol.* 2020; 188(6): 819-830. doi: 10.1111/bjh.16221
29. Shulkin M, Pimpin, L, Bellinger et al. n-3 Fatty Acid Supplementation in Mothers, Preterm Infants, and Term Infants and Childhood Psychomotor and Visual Development: A Systematic Review and Meta-Analysis. *J Nutr* 2018; 148(3): 409-418. doi: 10.1093/jn/nxx031
30. Middleton P, Gomersall JC, Gould JF, Shepherd E, Olsen SF, Makrides M. Omega-3 fatty acid addition during pregnancy. Cochrane Database of Systematic Reviews 2018, 11. doi: 10.1002/14651858.CD003402.pub3
31. Craig WJ. Health effects of vegan diets. *Am J Clin Nutr* 2009; 89(5): 1627S-1633S. doi: 10.3945/ajcn.2009.26736N
32. Papier K, Appleby PN, Fensom GK et al. Vegetarian diets and risk of hospitalisation or death with diabetes in British adults: results from the EPIC-Oxford study. *Nutr Diabetes* 2019; 9(1): 7. doi: 10.1038/s41387-019-0074-0
33. Key TJ, Appleby PN, Spencer EA et al. Cancer incidence in British vegetarians. *Br J Cancer* 2009; 101(1): 192-197. doi: 10.1038/sj.bjc.6605098
34. Tuso PJ, Ismail MH, Ha BP, Bartolotto C. Nutritional update for physicians: plant-based diets. *Perm J* 2013; 17(2): 61-66. doi: 10.7812/TPP/12-085
35. Farmer B, Larson BT, Fulgoni VL 3rd, Rainville AJ, Liepa GU. A vegetarian dietary pattern as a nutrient-dense approach to weight management: an analysis of the national health and nutrition examination survey 1999-2004. *J Am Diet Assoc* 2011; 111(6): 819-827. doi: 10.1016/j.jada.2011.03.012
36. Dwyer JT. Nutritional consequences of vegetarianism. *Annu Rev Nutr* 1991; 11: 61-91. doi: 10.1146/annurev.nu.11.070191.000425
37. Bingham SA. Diet and colorectal cancer prevention. *Biochem Soc Trans* 2000; 28(2): 12-16. doi: 10.1042/bst0280012
38. Tong TYN, et al. Vegetarian and vegan diets and risks of total and site-specific fractures: results from the prospective EPIC-Oxford study. *BMC Med 2020* 18(1): 353. doi: 10.1186/s12916-020-01815-3
39. Volkert D, Beck AM, Cederholm T, et al. ESPEN guideline on clinical nutrition and hydration in geriatrics. *Clin Nutr* 2019; 38(1): 10-47. doi: 10.1016/j.clnu.2018.05.024
40. Stover PJ. Vitamin B12 and older adults. *Curr Opin Clin Nutr Metab Care* 2010; 13(1): 24-7. doi: 10.1097/MCO.0b013e328333d157
41. Reynolds EH. Folic acid, ageing, depression and dementia. *BMJ* 2002; 324(7352): 1512-1515. doi: 10.1136/bmj.324.7352.1512
42. National Institute for Health and Care Excellence. Intravenous fluid therapy in adults in hospital.

Clinical guideline. Published: 10 December 2013. Last updated: May 2017. www.nice.org.uk/guidance/cg174
43. Davies GJ, Crowder M, Dickerson JW. Dietary fibre intakes of individuals with different eating patterns. *Hum Nutr Appl Nutr* 1985; 39(2): 139-148.
44. Dreher ML. Whole Fruits and Fruit Fiber Emerging Health Effects. *Nutrients* 2018; 10(12): 1833. doi: 10.3390/nu10121833
45. Nutrition Science Team, Public Health England 2016. Government Dietary Recommendations. https://assets.publishing.service.gov.uk/government/uploads/system/uploads/attachment_data/file/618167/government_dietary_recommendations.pdf [Accessed 21st March 2022].
46. NHS. Exercise. www.nhs.uk/live-well/exercise/?msclkid=a83bf920a93311ec90811bf4aff92150 [Accessed 21st March 2022].

Chapter 3
Plant-based nutrition and cardiovascular disease

Nesan Shanmugam

Introduction

Cardiovascular disease (CVD) is an umbrella term that encompasses several conditions including coronary heart disease (CHD), heart failure (HF), stroke and vascular dementia. The largest contributor to CVD, and a leading cause of death worldwide, is CHD.[1]

The last century has seen a steady decline in cardiovascular deaths, driven by advances in therapeutics and increased access to healthcare. Death from heart disease has declined 70% over the past four decades. However, these figures have plateaued and the gains are projected to decline, likely a result of diet and lifestyle factors.[2]

Epidemiological studies have provided important information on cardiovascular (CV) risk factors, such as hypercholesterolaemia, hypertension, obesity and diabetes in predicting CV events, thereby leading to the development of primary and secondary prevention strategies.[3] The data suggest that addressing unhealthy diets, physical inactivity and obesity may prevent up to 80% of CVD with interventions earlier in the life course yielding optimal benefits.[4] Diet represents an important modifiable risk factor and thus it is imperative that clinicians are familiar with the scientific evidence underpinning cardiovascular dietary recommendations. The chapter will focus specifically on the prevention and management of CHD, HF, stroke and CVD risk factors including hypertension and hypercholesterolaemia.

Coronary heart disease: what constitutes a heart healthy dietary pattern?

Tsimane case study

In this fascinating study, 705 members of the indigenous Bolivian Tsimane tribe underwent CT coronary artery calcium (CAC) score assessment, a reliable predictor of myocardial infarction (MI) and cardiovascular events.[5] The tribe live a subsistence lifestyle of hunter gathering and horticultural farming, with 6–7 hours of physical labour per day. Approximately half of subjects displayed high inflammatory burden, as measured by high-sensitivity CRP (hsCRP), secondary to parasitic pathogens exposure. However, they are observed to possess optimal cardiovascular risk factors, including low-density lipoprotein cholesterol (LDL-C) levels and the majority being non-diabetic and normotensive. The Tsimane are reported to have the lowest prevalence of atherosclerosis compared with any other populations with an 80-year-old Tsimane having the same arterial age as an American in their mid-50s.[6] The Tsimane consume an atheroprotective diet: high in unrefined, unprocessed high fibre carbohydrates (plantain, rice, wild nuts and fruit), as well as low in refined sugar and saturated fat. This dietary pattern is approximately 80% plant predominant with 20% sourced from fish and wild game.

The Tsimane case study highlights the importance of focusing on healthy dietary patterns rather than nutritional recommendations advocating specific macronutrient combinations.

'Heart healthy' dietary patterns are commonly:
- high in plants, fruit and grains
- low in saturated fats i.e., animal foods
- free of trans fatty acids
- low in refined carbohydrates
- minimally processed food content.

The 2015 World Heart Federation concluded that: 'on the basis of current evidence the traditional Mediterranean diet including plant foods and emphasis on plant proteins provides a well-tested healthy dietary pattern to reduce CVD'.[7] The Dietary Approaches to Stop Hypertension (DASH) diet and plant-based diets as heart healthy dietary patterns were also referenced. Similar recommendations have been published by the European Society of Cardiology (ESC)[8] and American College of Cardiology and American Heart Association (ACC/AHA).[9] The most consistent benefits to have been reported with vegetarian and vegan diet patterns is a significant reduction in ischaemic heart disease, in the order of 25–30% reduction in incidence and mortality, in part due to the association of these diets with a significant reduction in cardiovascular risk factors.[10] It is also important to consider dietary patterns that are harmful in CVD (see Table 3.1).

Atherosclerosis

At the core of CVD is atherosclerotic plaque formation, a process that may develop as early as infancy.[14] It is recognised that atherosclerosis is influenced by oxidative damage resulting in inflammation, initially caused by oxidised LDL-C penetrating the vascular endothelium. The progression of atherosclerosis correlates with loss of endothelial function further exacerbated by cardiovascular risk factors such as smoking, diabetes and hypertension.

The endothelium is involved in the production of nitric oxide (NO) via the precursor amino acid l-arginine and endothelial NO synthase (eNOS), which leads to the regulation of blood pressure, immunity and clotting function, as well as inhibition of plaque formation. Also, the glycocalyx, a protective gel-like layer of the vascular endothelium, maintains vascular endothelial function. Reductions in glycocalyx depth or barrier function predispose to the oxidised atherogenic LDL-C entering the intima layer triggering a cascade of maladaptive inflammatory and oxidative stress pathways. Adhesive molecules are expressed by damaged endothelial cells, which in turn, trigger accumulation of monocytes. Monocytes penetrate the sub-endothelial intima and differentiate into macrophages, which envelop modified oxidised LDL-C particles that form foam cells (fatty streak) and lead to the development of plaques. Activated macrophages also release pro-inflammatory cytokines, inducing vascular smooth muscle cell migration and formation of a fibrous cap over the cholesterol-rich necrotic plaque. Thick atherosclerotic caps ensure plaque stability, however, thinned capped plaques are vulnerable to rupture (exposing the necrotic core), leading to thrombosis and arterial occlusion and subsequent myocardial infarction (MI).[15, 16]

Table 3.1: Harmful dietary patterns in cardiovascular disease

Southern United States dietary pattern	Characterised by processed foods high in saturated fats, refined carbohydrates and animal products. The Reasons for Geographic and Racial Differences in Stroke (REGARDS) study demonstrated a significant 56% increase in cardiac events over a median 5.8 years follow-up associated with the Southern United States dietary pattern.[11]
Low carbohydrate dietary pattern (ketogenic, Atkins, and paleo diets)	These dietary patterns focus on high animal fat and protein intakes. Despite short-term weight loss and improvements in glucose metabolism, concerns remain about elevation of LDL-cholesterol and associations with increased all-cause mortality when adopted over longer durations.[12]
Unhealthy plant-based diet	Plant-based diets that emphasise consumption of foods such as fruit juices, sugar-sweetened beverages, refined grains (white pasta, rice, and processed breads and cereals) and potatoes (French fries and potato chips), while reducing the intake of unprocessed plant foods has been shown to adversely affect CVD outcomes, similar to following an animal-based dietary patterns.[13]

Lipids

The key stage in atherosclerosis development is cholesterol infiltration of the arterial wall. Lipids are non-soluble and therefore circulate within lipoproteins. Seven classes of lipoproteins exist and are classified according to their size and density (see Table 3.2). The external shell of lipoproteins consists of phospholipid and cholesterol, combined with apolipoproteins, which define the type, function and destination of the lipoprotein. Apoprotein B (ApoB) is specifically associated with atherosclerosis and acts as a binding point on LDL receptors throughout the body. Hydrophobic triglycerides and cholesterol esters form the inner lipoprotein core.

Lipoprotein size and density determines atherogenic capacity. Lipoproteins with diameters of >75 nm exceed arterial penetrability; thus, chylomicrons and large VLDL particles are not atherogenic. Conversely, smaller particles, namely small VLDL, IDL, LDL, and Lp(a), are pro-atherogenic ApoB lipoproteins. Smaller, low-density HDL is also capable of penetrating arteries; however, it has the capacity to exit arterial adventitia therefore evading arterial accumulation.

Individual CVD risk is not solely dependent on magnitude of elevated LDL-C alone, but also duration of exposure. Thus, the role of LDL-C in driving atherosclerosis is cumulative over the lifespan. Furthermore, differing densities of the same lipoprotein subtypes exist, thereby altering atherogenic risk. Small, dense LDL-C is most associated with CVD risk. The number of LDL particles also influences risk. The same amount of cholesterol can be carried by a high number of small LDL particles or a small number of large particles. The quantity of LDL particles may be estimated by measuring ApoB levels. Atherosclerosis results from arterial infiltration of ApoB containing lipoproteins, therefore quantifying circulating ApoB is a better predictor of heart disease than LDL-C.[18]

Table 3.2: Major lipoprotein classes

Lipoprotein	Density (g/ml)	Size (nm)	Major ApoLipo-protein
Chylomicrons	0.93	75–1200	ApoB-48
Chylomicron remnants	0.93–1.006	30–80	ApoB-48
VLDL	0.93–1.006	30–80	ApoB-100
IDL	1.006–1.019	25–35	ApoB-100
LDL	1.019–1.063	18–25	ApoB-100
HDL	1.063–1.210	5–12	ApoA-1
Lp(a)	1.050–1.120	25	ApoB-100

Abbreviations: very-low density lipoprotein (VLDL); intermediate density lipoprotein (IDL); low density lipoprotein (LDL); high density lipoprotein (HDL); lipoprotein A (Lp(a)).

Adapted from: Chapter 31 Disorders of lipoprotein metabolism. In: Loscalzo J *Harrison's Cardiovascular Medicine*. 2nd ed.[17]

Lipid heart hypothesis

The seminal Framingham Study demonstrated a strong exponential association with high total cholesterol (TC) and CHD development.[3] These results have been replicated in numerous populations. The Seven Countries Study, involving 12,763 men in seven countries demonstrated, at population and individual levels, that CHD mortality was strongly correlated with dietary saturated fatty acids (SFA) intake and elevated blood cholesterol levels.[19] Furthermore, migrant studies indicate the importance of dietary modulation following adoption of new dietary lifestyles in populations with the same genetic background. In the Japanese Ni-Hon San Study, Japanese Americans in Hawaii and California were observed to have significantly higher total serum cholesterol levels and higher CHD risk relative to the men in Japan, despite greater smoking numbers in Japan.[20]

In the 1960s Finnish men had the highest CHD mortality in the world. Their diet was high in saturated fat (19–24% of total energy), predominantly from dairy products, with high salt intakes and smoking was also prevalent. A population-based intervention initiated in North Karelia, and later nationally, aimed to reduce four major risk factors: TC, hypertension, body mass index (BMI) and smoking. During 35 years of follow-up, a remarkable 80% reduction in coronary mortality was observed, with TC reductions of 67%, despite little change in smoking rates and increased BMI. Importantly, this correlated with a significant decline in total SFA intake from 22% of energy intake to 13%.[21]

The 2020 Cochrane review on SFA consumption and CVD included 15 randomised controlled trials (RCT) and demonstrated that reducing SFA intake over two years reduced CVD events by 21% with greater benefits achieved with greater reductions in SFA.[22] Population-based metabolic studies have also demonstrated that CVD reductions are mediated via reductions in atherogenic lipoproteins.[23] Data from meta-regression analysis of LDL-C reduction approaches (non-statins and statins) indicate that for every 1mmol LDL-C reduction there is a 23% risk reduction in major vascular events.[24]

When adopting cardioprotective strategies to reduce SFA consumption, careful consideration must be made about the macronutrient substituting SFA. A meta-analysis of randomised controlled trials (RCTs) showed that polyunsaturated fatty acid (PUFA) replacement for SFA reduced CHD events by 19%.[25] Similarly, replacement of 5% energy of SFA with monounsaturated fatty acids (MUFA) was associated with 15% CHD risk reduction[26] with significantly lower CHD risk when SFAs were replaced with plant versus animal derived MUFA.[27]

However, these substitution effects are dependent on the quality of carbohydrates also consumed. Substitution of 5% energy from SFA with complex carbohydrates from whole grains was associated with an 11% reduction in risk for CHD, compared to refined carbohydrates or trans fats, which had significantly worse outcomes.[26]

SFA is predominantly animal derived, however, it is important to appreciate that plant sources like coconut (90% SFA) and palm oils (50% SFA) should also be minimised. In a meta-analysis of 16 trials, coconut oil consumption significantly increased LDL-C concentrations compared with non-tropical vegetable oils. The authors extrapolated that the 0.3 mmol/l (10.47 mg/dL) increase in LDL-C resulting from the replacement of non-tropical vegetable oils with coconut oil may translate to 6% increased risk of major vascular events and a 5.4% increase in CHD mortality.[28]

Primary prevention CHD dietary studies

The most widely studied dietary pattern in relation to CVD health is the Mediterranean diet. The Prevention With Mediterranean Diet study (PREDIMED) was the first large landmark primary cardiovascular prevention RCT demonstrating the CV benefits of the Mediterranean diet.[29] A total of 7447 participants deemed at high CVD risk were randomised to one of three dietary options: 1) Mediterranean diet supplemented with extra virgin olive oil (EVOO); 2) Mediterranean diet supplemented with mixed nuts; or 3) low-fat American Heart Association (AHA)-recommended control diet. Of note, the low-fat group had poor adherence and did not significantly change their fat intake compared to baseline.

Over a mean follow-up period of 4.8 years, a 30% reduction in the primary end point of MI, stroke, or death from cardiovascular causes was observed when compared to the AHA low-fat diet, but without an advantage for overall mortality. However, when the data were analysed using the pro-vegetarian diet score, a higher consumption of plant-derived foods was associated with reduced risk of all-cause and CV mortality.[30] The ability of a healthy plant-based diet as defined by the plant-based dietary index to reduce the risk of cardiovascular events and mortality has subsequently been shown in large prospective cohort studies.[31,32]

The only randomised comparison of the PREDIMED diet with a healthy low-fat vegan diet (100% plant-based) is a 16-week crossover trial in 62 overweight adults. The results showed that the vegan group achieved an average 6 kg weight loss, with significant reductions in total and visceral fat, and improvements in TC and LDL-C levels, blood pressure (BP) and insulin sensitivity. No weight reduction or cardiometabolic benefits other than BP improvements were achieved in the Mediterranean group.[33]

Secondary prevention CHD dietary studies

Patients with established CVD or diabetes are at increased risk of further CVD events. Therefore, it is imperative that patients remain on disease-modifying therapies, such antiplatelet agents, statins, angiotensin modulators, and beta-blockers, as each alone can reduce CVD event risk by almost 25%.[34] However, despite these therapies, there remains a sizeable residual risk. Therefore, adherence to healthy lifestyle factors such as diet confers additional significant benefits.

The Lyon Diet Heart Study was a secondary prevention RCT involving 605 patients who had experienced a first MI.[35] Patients were randomised to a Mediterranean-style diet or a 'prudent' low-fat diet, with statins not routinely prescribed. The trial was stopped early at 27 months when participants on the Mediterranean diet showed a remarkable 73% reduction in CHD event rates and cardiovascular mortality.

In a cohort of patients investigated before and after their MI, the Alternative Healthy Eating Index 2010 (AHEI2010), which mostly scores plant-derived foods favourably, was examined.[36] Greater adherence to the AHEI2010 score was associated with a 29% reduction in all-cause mortality and 40% cardiovascular mortality reduction. Higher consumption of refined grains, high fat dairy, French fries, sweets and red or processed meats were associated with worse CV outcomes. The Mediterranean diet resembles the AHEI2010 dietary pattern, except for higher intakes of EVOO and red wine.

In individuals with stable CHD, the Stabilization of Atherosclerotic Plaque by Initiation of Darapladib Therapy (STABILITY) trial also confirmed the CV benefits of plant-predominant Mediterranean diet.[37] The study included 15,828 participants across 39 countries, followed for a median of 3.7 years, and showed that adherence to a more plant-predominant Mediterranean dietary pattern was associated with a lower risk of CVD, MI, stroke and all-cause death.

Diet and atherosclerotic plaque burden

A meta-regression analysis of lipid treatment trials using intravascular ultrasound (IVUS) of coronary arteries in over 6,000 patients showed that a 1% reduction in atheroma volume is associated with an approximately 20% reduction of incurring a major cardiovascular event.[38] Mechanistically, this could explain some of the clinical benefits seen in the dietary prevention studies previously discussed. The adoption of a plant-predominant diet is hypothesised to reduce atherosclerotic plaque burden, leading to plaque progression cessation or possibly plaque regression. Interruption of plaque progression is observed at LDL-C levels of <1.8 mmol/l with potential plaque regression at LDL-C levels <1.4 mmol/l.[39]

A seminal study investigating dietary approaches is the Ornish Lifestyle Heart RCT, which examined effects of a comprehensive lifestyle program involving 48 patients with angiographically documented CHD.[40] The intervention arm included a low-fat vegetarian diet (10% of calories as fat and 5 mg or less cholesterol per day), stress management training, moderate exercise, smoking cessation and weekly psychosocial support. After one year, LDL-C significantly decreased from 3.92 mmol/L (151 mg/dL), at baseline, to 2.46 mmol/L (95 mg/dL), as well as substantial ApoB reductions in the intervention group compared to the control group.

At five years, there was reported 3.1% plaque regression compared to baseline.[41] This modest regression of coronary artery stenoses also translated to reduced size and severity of perfusion abnormalities on functional dipyridamole positron emission tomography (PET) imaging, and 2.5 times fewer cardiac event rates.[42] Greater adherence to lifestyle intervention translated to greater percentage change in arterial stenosis. Furthermore, this correlated with significant improvements in functional status, with a 91%

reduction in anginal symptoms at one year, in comparison to a 165% increase in the control-group. Although small and underpowered, the study highlights the significance of a multidisciplinary lifestyle approach in halting atherosclerosis, although differentiating the specific effect of diet from the other lifestyle interventions is difficult.

The St Thomas' Atheroma Regression Study (STARS) specifically examined a plant-predominant diet on image analysis of quantitative coronary angiograms in 90 hypercholesterolaemic men with established ischaemic heart disease (IHD).[43] This was compared to an intervention group receiving diet and cholestyramine (a bile acid sequestrant drug inhibiting intestinal cholesterol uptake) and a usual care control group. Coronary angiography was performed at baseline and at 39 months. Compared to the low-fat Ornish Study, total fat intake was 27% of dietary energy, with SFA content set at 8–10% of dietary energy and dietary cholesterol to 100 mg/1000 kcal. Both interventions considerably reduced the frequency of cardiovascular events. Dietary change alone retarded overall progression and increased overall regression of coronary artery disease (CAD), and diet plus cholestyramine was additionally associated with a net increase in coronary lumen diameter. The overall net regression seen in the diet-only and diet/lipid lowering group correlated with a reduction in LDL-C of 16% and 36% respectively. No significant LDL-C change was seen in the usual care group.

Esselstyn et al. have reported outcomes in 198 patients with angiography-documented CAD.[44] Patients followed a low-fat (less than 10% calories from fat) whole food plant-based diet along with cholesterol-lowering therapies if required, to achieve target total cholesterol levels <3.88 mmol/L (<150 mg/dL), thus arrest or reverse CAD progression, as measured by coronary angiography. A 10% event rate was seen in those adherent to the intervention, compared to a 62% event rate in the non-adherent group over a mean 3.7 year follow-up period. However, the absence of a control arm and confounding effects of cholesterol lowering medications were significant limitations, impacting the ability to establish specific dietary intervention causality.

Similar inferences were noted in the Mount Abu Open Heart Trial involving patients with moderate to severe CHD who underwent an Ornish-style lifestyle program, including a high fibre, low-fat, plant-centred diet.[45] However, the study was unblinded and did not include a control group. The angiographic mean percent diameter stenosis decreased by 6.1% after two years, and patients with the highest adherence exhibited a significant 18.23% regression compared to 10.56% in those least adherent.

Recent studies have questioned the reliability of quantitative invasive angiography as an imaging tool to accurately detect plaque progression and regression.[46] Notwithstanding these criticisms, outcome data from the PREDIMED, LYON Heart Study and large prospective cohort studies have established the important benefits of plant-based dietary patterns on CVD. Further mechanistic dietary RCTs utilising more advanced coronary imaging modalities such as IVUS are required to clarify the debate surrounding plaque reversal.

Mechanisms underpinning a heart healthy dietary pattern

The common nutritional constituents and mechanisms underpinning heart healthy dietary patterns are shown in Table 3.3.[47]

Anti-inflammatory

Chronic inflammation is widely implicated in chronic diseases, including CVD. In a meta-analysis of 14 studies using the dietary inflammatory index, a pro-inflammatory diet is associated with an increased risk CVD incidence and mortality. Anti-inflammatory foods include vegetables, fruit, fibre, whole grains, spices and seasonings, rich in phytochemicals and micronutrients.[48] Healthy dietary patterns reduce inflammatory markers, for example a healthy vegan diet was shown to reduce hsCRP by 32% after eight weeks in those with CHD, when compared to the AHA diet. Although the study was not powered to assess cardiovascular outcomes, it is well established that lower hsCRP levels reduce cardiovascular risk.[49]

Endothelial function

Dietary nitrates, found predominantly in green leafy vegetables elevate systemic nitrite through an entero-salivary pathway. Nitrites are reduced to NO, with consistent data showing improved BP and arterial stiffness. In a study of 53,150 participants followed up over 23 years, a moderate vegetable nitrate intake (one cup of green leafy vegetables) was associated with 15% lower CVD risk and 12%, 15%, 17% and 26% lower risk of CHD, HF, stroke and peripheral artery disease hospitalisations, respectively.[50] Daily ingestion of leafy green vegetables has also been shown to favour increased circulating endothelial progenitor cells (EPCs),[51] which critically maintain vasculature integrity, with lower EPCs associated with poorer CVD outcomes.[52]

Vegetarian diets are also associated with improved atherosclerotic biomarkers. Compared to omnivores, vegetarians are shown to have lower myeloperoxidase (MPOs) and metalloproteinases (MMPs).[53] MPOs are pro-oxidant enzymes which generates reactive oxygen species (ROS) and are implicated in endothelial dysfunction. MMPs, are a family of proteases that degrade the atheromatous fibrous plaque cap.

Haem iron-rich meat and N-nitroso compounds generated from nitrates and nitrites in processed meats, may also generate ROS, resulting in oxidative stress and endothelial dysfunction.[54]

Advanced glycated end products (AGEs) are a heterogeneous group of compounds originating from spontaneous reactions of reducing sugars with amino acids. AGEs form continuously through a variety of reactions, which markedly

Table 3.3: Cardiovascular benefits of a healthy plant-based diet

Healthy attributes	Benefits
Low energy density	Maintaining a healthy weight
High fibre	Promoting insulin sensitivity and glucose regulation
High in unsaturated fats	Healthy blood lipids
High in antioxidants	Healthy blood pressure
Low in harmful dietary components i.e. haem iron, saturated fats	Optimal vascular health
High in healthy micronutrients i.e. vitamins, potassium, magnesium	Reduction in inflammation
	Healthy gut microbiome

Adapted from Satija A, Hu FB. Plant-based diets and cardiovascular health. *Trends Cardiovasc Med* 2018; 28(7): 437–441. doi: 10.1016/j.tcm.2018.02.004.[56]

increase with hyperglycaemia, insulin resistance or elevated oxidative stress. They are also generated in foods via high-temperature cooking processes, with animal products having the highest concentrations of pre-formed AGEs. AGEs negatively impact endothelial function through oxidative and inflammatory pathways and reduced NO production.[55]

Gut microbiome

Fibre remains a significant component of the heart healthy plant-predominant diet, with a dose response between higher fibre intake (>30 g/day), and lower mortality and CHD incidence.[56] These observed benefits are linked to the relationship between adequate fibre and a healthy gut microbiota.

A novel biochemical pathway has been elucidated describing the association between gut microbiota and atherosclerosis. Choline and carnitine – compounds derived mainly from animal foods – are converted by gut microbes to trimethylamine (TMA), which is absorbed and metabolised in the liver to trimethylamine N-oxide (TMAO). TMAO increases CVD in a dose-dependent way via effects on cholesterol and sterol metabolism and increasing inflammation and platelet reactivity.[57] Whether the link between TMAO is association or causative is still being investigated.[58] Data from the Nurses' Health Study cohort show that the highest levels of TMAO were associated with a 58–79% higher risk of CHD compared to those with the lowest TMAO levels and attenuated with a plant-centric diet.[59] The higher prevalence of specific gut bacteria when consuming a vegetarian diet can positively influence the change in pro-atherogenic oxidised LDL-C, thus further impacting cardiovascular risk.[60] SFA's from animal-derived foods can damage the epithelial lining of the gut and allow endotoxins, including lipopolysaccharides (from the bacterial contamination of meat) into the blood, resulting in inflammation within arteries.[61]

Antioxidants

A plant-predominant diet is rich in antioxidants, such as vitamins C and E, beta-carotene and polyphenols. Polyphenols significantly contribute to cardiovascular health, via scavenging and neutralising ROS, limiting LDL oxidation, modulating endothelial function through NO production, inhibiting platelet aggregation, and ultimately, reducing inflammation.[62]

Epigenetics

Epigenetics refers to the process by which genes can be switched on and off by environmental triggers like lifestyle. Recent analysis across four studies involving over 55,000 participants showed that among those at high CV genetic risk, a favourable lifestyle (no smoking or obesity, regular physical activity and a healthy diet) attenuated the relative risk of developing CAD by 50%, compared to unfavourable lifestyles.[63] Intensive lifestyle interventions may modulate gene expression by favourably altering the expression of genes involved in immune function, lipid metabolism, BP regulation, inflammation and oxidative stress. Several epidemiologic surveys have also observed an association of short telomere length with CVD development. Critically, short telomeres lead to cellular dysfunction contributing to atherogenesis. CHD risk factors such as smoking, and hypertension may accelerate telomere shortening through inflammation or increased oxidative stress. Conversely, disease protective factors, such as exercise and healthy diet, can activate telomerase activity, thus maintaining telomere length. In a sample of healthy individuals, analyses revealed that the relation between having shorter telomeres and the presence of CT CAC was attenuated in the presence of low meat, high fruit and vegetable diets.[64]

Cardiovascular risk factors

In this section, we focus on the role of nutrition in the management of hypertension and hypercholesterolemia, both important modifiable cardiovascular risk factors. Data from the UK Biobank has shown a 1 mmol/L reduction in LDL-C and a 10 mmHg lowering in BP is associated with 80% lower risk of CV disease.[4]

Hypertension

Hypertension is defined as systolic BP (SBP) ≥130 mmHg or diastolic BP ≥80 mmHg. The condition is identified as the number one risk factor worldwide for deaths and disability-adjusted life years, with just over 40% of CV deaths related to hypertension.[73]

In line with international hypertension guidelines, lifestyle and non-pharmacologic interventions are pivotal in hypertension prevention and reduction.[65] In addition to physical exercise, recommended non-pharmacological interventions include:
1. Decreased dietary sodium consumption.
2. Increased dietary potassium consumption.
3. Weight loss.
4. Adoption of heart-healthy dietary patterns (DASH, plant-based).
5. Alcohol reduction/avoidance.

Hypertension healthy dietary patterns

There are important pathological interplays between high sodium and low potassium intakes, leading to vascular smooth muscle cell contraction, increased peripheral vascular resistance and subsequent hypertension. Heart healthy plant-predominant dietary patterns have lower sodium and higher potassium, thereby improving BP, independent of weight loss and exercise.

The DASH diet initially promoted to control hypertension was inspired by the BP lowering effects of vegetarian diets, with later introduction of low-fat dairy foods. The standard DASH diet in combination with 2300 mg sodium restriction is associated with an 11 mmHg reduction in SBP in those with baseline SBP of 150 mm Hg or greater and a reduction of 4 mmHg in those with baseline SBP of 130 mm Hg or less.[66] A 1500 mg daily sodium DASH variant was associated with further BP reductions[67] with additional weight reduction resulting in superior SBP reductions than the DASH diet alone.[68]

Vegetarian and vegan diets have been shown to be effective at maintaining a normal BP, especially if low in salt. In the large Adventist Health Study-2[69] and EPIC-Oxford cohort[70] vegetarians and vegans had the lowest risk of hypertension (up to 60% reduced risk compared to omnivores). A large meta-analysis of RCTs found that vegetarian diets lower BP compared with omnivorous diets independent of weight loss. Importantly, a reduction in SBP by 5 mmHg correlates with a 7% reduction in all-cause mortality, and a 9% and 14% reduced mortality due to CHD and stroke respectively.[71]

Emerging evidence indicates that plant-predominant diets rich in fruits, vegetables, whole grains and nuts contain components with specific anti-hypertensive properties.[72,73,74]

In addition to higher potassium content, plant-predominant diets rich in leafy green vegetables and beetroot are nitrate rich, possessing vasodilatory benefits, with evidence indicating that beetroot consumption can lead to equivalent SBP reductions as medication.[75] Regular consumption of flaxseeds (30 g/day) and blueberries (1 cup per day) has also been shown to significantly lower BP in randomised studies.[76,77]

Hypercholesterolaemia

International primary and secondary CV guidelines recommend significant serum cholesterol reductions with lifestyle and therapeutic interventions guided by risk stratification tools.[78] The principles of dietary lipid reduction are summarised below.

Reduction in saturated fat

SFA consumption, predominantly from animal sources, results in a direct, linear increase in blood cholesterol levels and is the single most important factor driving atherosclerosis. There is evidence that replacement of 1% daily energy intake from SFAs by equivalent energy from PUFA, whole grains or plant proteins is associated with a 6–8% reduction in CVD risk. Individual SFA also confer differential effects on lipid profiles, with lauric, myristic, and palmitic acids raising LDL-C concentrations, and stearic acid having a neutral effect.[79]

Reduction in trans fatty acids

Industrial hydrogenation converts the *cis* forms of PUFA to the *trans* configurations, forming trans fatty acids (TFA), thereby increasing the shelf life of vegetable oils and ability to convert oils into semi-solid fats like margarines. Considerable data now shows that TFA detrimentally increases serum lipids to the same extent as SFA and are linked with worse CVD outcomes.[80] Consequently, current guidelines recommend TFA limitation to 1% of total dietary energy. Unfortunately, these recommendations are not universally adopted, thus foods labelled as containing partially hydrogenated oils should be avoided.

Reduction in dietary cholesterol

Dietary cholesterol in Western diets derives from animal products and regardless of which animal protein sources are consumed, LDL-C, ApoB, HDL, and small and medium LDL-C, are all similarly increased.[81] Dietary cholesterol is less potent than SFA in elevating blood cholesterol concentrations, however, its ability to increase total and LDL-C is well established.[82] Eggs, especially the yolk, are significant contributors to dietary cholesterol, confirmed by several large meta-analyses that indicate higher consumption of dietary cholesterol or eggs significantly raise LDL-C in a dose-dependent manner and is associated with increased CVD and all-cause mortality.[83] It should be noted that 60% of studies evaluating the effect of eggs on blood cholesterol were industry funded, resulting in conclusions that downplay the association. In fact, more than 85% of research studies, regardless of funding sources, showed that eggs have unfavourable effects on blood cholesterol.[84]

The effect of dietary cholesterol on LDL-C should also be analysed in the context of baseline dietary patterns. Additional dietary cholesterol in the context of a pre-existing cholesterol-rich diet has been found not to significantly increase LDL-C as levels tend to plateau.[85]

Increase in dietary fibre

Dietary fibre, especially soluble fibre in fruits, vegetables, legumes and whole grain cereals has been shown to lower cholesterol. Multiple mechanisms have been proposed including substitution effect with SFA, its effect on bile acid secretion, reduction in liver cholesterol concentrations and upregulation of LDL receptors.

An experimental diet based on increasing fibre consumption was created in a study by Jenkins et al.[86] The diet contained 63 servings of fruit and vegetables a day (50 g fibre/1000 kcal). A 33% reduction in LDL-C was seen in only two weeks. Interestingly, when compared to a starch-based diet (similar to the Mediterranean diet) consisting of 19 g/1000 kcal fibre, significant reduction in serum lipids remained but were of smaller magnitude. No significant improvements in lipid profile were observed with a low-fat therapeutic diet, with a dietary fibre intake identical to current recommendations of 25–30 g daily fibre; indicating that much greater fibre intake is required to reduce serum lipids than currently recommended.

Increase in plant phytosterols

Studies have demonstrated that plant sterols present in vegetable oils, vegetables, fruits, nuts and grains can reduce cholesterol absorption with 2 g of plant sterols daily reducing LDL-C by 15%.[87]

Lipid lowering dietary patterns

Combined with moderate physical activity and weight reduction, plant-predominant dietary patterns possess many lipid-lowering properties, including being extremely low in SFA, devoid of dietary cholesterol, and rich in soluble fibre and polyphenols. This may explain why vegetarians and healthy vegan diets improve blood lipid levels when compared with conventional omnivore dietary patterns.[88] The Portfolio dietary pattern includes a range of cholesterol-lowering foods (2 g plant sterols, 50 g nuts, 10–20 g soluble fibre from a variety of plant foods, and 50 g soya protein as a replacement to animal-based products), and was studied in a 351 participant RCT, comparing the portfolio dietary pattern to a low SFA control group. A 13–14% LDL-C reduction was observed with the portfolio diet compared to a 3% reduction in the control group.[87]

Triglyceride reduction

High blood triglycerides (TG) levels also increase CVD risk as elevated TGs are atherogenic, particularly with concurrent elevated ApoB related cholesterol levels.[89] In contrast, isolated high TGs with low ApoB levels is not atherogenic, as the cholesterol is transported in larger chylomicrons and VLDL. Several lifestyle factors cause TG elevation, including calorie overconsumption, increased alcohol intake, physical inactivity and weight gain. A Mediterranean diet may improve TG levels better than vegetarian diet patterns as shown in the CARDIVEG study as well as, avoiding refined carbohydrates, which may elevate hepatic TG synthesis via de novo lipogenesis.[90]

Specific foods

Dairy

Dairy foods have differing nutritional composition (e.g., low-fat and full-fat whole milk, butter, and fermented dairy such as yogurt and cheese) with low-fat and fermented dairy often incorporated within heart healthy dietary patterns. However, the increased SFA content of dairy (approximately 65%) and subsequent LDL-C elevation requires consideration, particularly with butter and whole fat milk, as evidenced from the pioneering Finnish public health intervention where 50% saturated fat (predominantly butter) reduction led to 80% CVD mortality reduction.[21] However, data from meta-analysis of prospective cohort studies of dairy (low-fat or full-fat) and its association with CVD and all-cause mortality remain equivocal or neutral.[91] These findings may be related to different forms of dairy, which are often categorised as one entity when studied.

The association of dairy with the risk of CVD will also depend on what food you are comparing with. Data from the Nurses' Health and Health Professionals Follow-up studies demonstrated that adults who consumed the most dairy, compared with the least, had the highest risk for total mortality, cardiovascular and cancer mortality.[92] The study also found that when replacing dairy with legumes, whole grains, or nuts, mortality rates were reduced. However, replacing dairy with red and processed meat increased this risk.

Olive oil

The Blue Zones observational longevity data suggests that regions with diets high in olive oil (Ikaria and Sardinia) are associated with improved long-term survival.[93] Furthermore, results from the Mediterranean lifestyle studies with preponderance to increased olive oil consumption demonstrate improved cardiovascular outcomes.[29, 35] The quality of olive oil is important. Cold-pressed, unripened olives contain higher levels of antioxidants such as tocopherols, polyphenols (including oleocanthal) and phytosterols. These have multiple pleiotropic benefits including anti-inflammatory, enhancement of endothelial function, inhibition of platelet aggregation, reduction in LDL-C and improved HDL functionality. The substitution of SFA and refined carbohydrates with plant-derived MUFA will also improve cardiovascular outcomes.[94]

Small studies linking oil consumption with endothelial dysfunction and negative cardiovascular outcomes forms the basis for some to advocate a low/no oil approach for atherosclerosis protection.[95] However, the entirety of the data more consistently shows a beneficial impact on endothelial function and cardiovascular risk factors,[96, 97] in addition to the benefits shown in clinical outcomes including cardiovascular events.[29, 35] The ACC Prevention of Cardiovascular Disease Council consensus statement in 2017 recommends extra virgin olive oil use in moderation, as part of a heart healthy dietary pattern.[98]

Omega-3 PUFAs

The omega-3 PUFA family has long been the subject of scrutiny, specifically the omega-3 long chain-PUFAs, docosahexaenoic acid (DHA), eicosapentaenoic acid (EPA) and docosapentaenoic acid (DPA). Mechanistically, these omega-3 fatty acids reduce triglycerides, have anti-inflammatory, antihypertensive, and antiplatelet effects, with higher circulating levels of EPA and DHA associated with a lower risk of CV death.[99] Fish consumption (high in EPA and DHA) has also consistently been associated with significant reductions in cardiovascular disease and mortality.[100]

Evidence for long-chain omega-3 supplementation remains controversial due to conflicting data from clinical trials.[101, 102]

EPA versus DHA

Recent clinical trials using high dose EPA supplements show significant cardiovascular event reductions, leading some to postulate that the EPA component of omega-3 supplements confers the cardioprotective benefits.[103] A meta-analysis assessing the impact of DHA and EPA supplementation separately found a greater impact associated with EPA.[104]

Extrapolating from the available evidence, supplementation with omega-3 PUFA at a dose of 800–1000 mg per day may confer added cardiovascular benefits, especially if there is variable compliance in the consumption of ALA-rich plant foods. It is important to note that algae oil-based omega-3 supplements have been shown to be as effective as fish oil equivalents, in increasing levels of DHA and EPA.[105] Plant-based diets that exclude fish consumption, such as vegetarian and vegan diets, have been shown to benefit cardiovascular health, but whether further benefits could be derived from the addition of an algae-based supplement is currently not known.

Heart failure (HF)

HF affects over 26 million individuals worldwide with a rising global burden due to an ageing population and increased survival from acute cardiac events, such as MIs.[106] Despite advances in HF therapeutics mortality remains high.

Prevention and treatment of CHD, the leading cause of HF, is pivotal in HF prevention. Recent HF guidelines also emphasise the importance of targeting the preclinical stages of HF and targeting modifiable risk factors.[107] Emerging data highlights the increasing importance of diet and lifestyle on HF prevention and management.

Heart failure healthy dietary patterns

The DASH dietary pattern has the most evidence base for HF and has been adopted by the ACC/AHA CVD Risk Prevention Guidelines and is viewed the most optimal dietary plan for symptomatic HF.[108] Multiple observational studies show the DASH diet's association with reduced HF incidence.[109] Moreover, greater adherence with a DASH diet is associated with improvements of surrogate markers of both systolic and diastolic heart function whilst improving exercise capacity and quality of life.[110]

Large prospective studies also report the Mediterranean diet's association with reduced HF incidence with a meta-analysis involving 10,950 participants demonstrating a 70% risk reduction in HF with greater adherence conferring a dose-dependent benefit.[111]

When comparing the DASH versus Mediterranean diet, a follow-up of 3215 hospitalised women with HF over a median 4.6 years revealed that participants with higher DASH diet scores were associated with significantly lower mortality rates compared with a nonsignificant trend towards a decrease in mortality with the Mediterranean diet scores.[112]

Specific plant predominant dietary patterns

The recommendations of specific components of a HF 'healthy' dietary pattern from the ACC's Nutrition and Lifestyle Committee for the Prevention of Cardiovascular Disease Council[124] include:
- plant-based
- low sodium/high potassium content
- antioxidant rich
- inorganic nitrates rich.

A large prospective study of interest including 30,000 Americans followed for a median of 8.7 years demonstrated that adherence to a 'plant-based' diet had the lowest risk of HF (41% reduced risk) compared to other diets, even after adjusting for other known risk factors.[113]

An extensive review of the data on diet and heart failure found certain foods and nutrients associated with a reduced risk (vegetables, fruit, soya protein, whole grains, legumes, extra virgin olive oil, fibre, MUFAs, PUFAs, dietary nitrate, antioxidants and potassium), certain foods and nutrients associated with an increased risk (meat, salty snacks, fried foods, eggs, fried fish, sugar-sweetened beverages, SFAs, TFAs, dietary cholesterol and sodium) and some foods with inconsistent or no reported association (nuts, poultry, dairy, oily and white fish).[114]

Sodium restriction is beneficial for HF prevention, although its role in established HF is less clear. Data on most dietary supplements and HF is conflicting and not recommended with only limited supportive data for coenzyme Q10, functioning as an antioxidant.[114]

Future studies in patients with HF are needed to evaluate the impact of nutrition on cardiac function with hard clinical end points. Healthful eating patterns, particularly those that are based on consumption of foods derived predominantly from plants, such as the DASH and the Mediterranean diet should be advocated in all stages of HF. This should be incorporated into an overall lifestyle intervention, including regular exercise and mindfulness interventions.

Stroke

Ischaemic strokes comprise the greatest proportion of strokes (87% ischaemic versus 13% haemorrhagic),[115] although both share common cardiovascular risk factors. Stroke represents a huge burden of disease globally with a stroke risk of approximately 25% among both men and women.[116]

The data supporting dietary patterns for stroke prevention and management is not as robust as for CHD, partly related to less research in this area. Nevertheless, broad observations can be made in that those eating greater fruits and vegetables and reduced meat have a lower incidence of ischaemic stroke.[117]

Dietary patterns emphasising more whole plant foods and minimising animal-derived foods, DASH[118] and Mediterranean diets,[119] have been associated with a lower stroke risk. The PREDIMED study showed a reduction in cardiovascular events, predominately related to reduced stroke risk.[29]

Prospective cohort studies examining vegetarian and vegan diets, have shown variable results on the risk of stroke. The EPIC-Oxford study demonstrated an increased risk of haemorrhagic stroke in an analysis that combined both vegetarian and vegan diets.[120] This may be related to lower LDL-C levels, although the overall benefit of lower cholesterol for prevention of ischaemic heart disease far exceeds any potential risk. Interestingly, a reduced risk of both ischaemic and haemorrhagic stroke was demonstrated with a vegetarian diet pattern in the Tzu-Chi cohort, where diets are higher in soya foods and participants don't consume alcohol.[121] A meta-analysis and systematic review of prospective cohort studies did not show an impact of a vegetarian diet pattern on the risk of stroke – neither positive nor negative – when compared to non-vegetarian diet patterns.[122] When diet quality was assessed, higher adherence to a healthy plant-based diet was shown to reduce the risk of total stroke by 10%.[123]

Conclusion

Adoption of a fibre-rich, low-saturated fat, whole food plant-predominant dietary pattern with minimal refined carbohydrate and ultra-processed foods has proven pleiotropic benefits for primary and secondary CVD prevention, including modulation of cardiovascular risk factors. The totality of evidence for this dietary approach, in combination with other lifestyle interventions, has been shown to reduce symptoms and crucially improve clinically relevant cardiovascular endpoints.

References

1. Abbafati C, Abbas KM, Abbasi-Kangevari M, Abd-Allah F, Abdelalim A, Abdollahi M, et al. Global burden of 369 diseases and injuries in 204 countries and territories, 1990–2019: a systematic analysis for the Global Burden of Disease Study 2019. *Lancet* 2020; 396(10258): 1204-1222.
doi: 10.1016/S0140-6736(20)30925-9
2. Nabel EG, Braunwald E. A Tale of Coronary Artery Disease and Myocardial Infarction. *N Engl J Med* 2012; 366(1): 54-63.
doi: 10.1056/NEJMra1112570
3. Dawber TR, Moore FE, Mann G V. Coronary heart disease in the Framingham study. *Int J Epidemiol* 2015; 44(6): 4-24.
doi: 10.2105/ajph.47.4_pt_2.4
4. Ference BA, Bhatt DL, Catapano AL, Packard CJ, Graham I, Kaptoge S, et al. Association of Genetic Variants Related to Combined Exposure to Lower Low-Density Lipoproteins and Lower Systolic Blood Pressure with Lifetime Risk of Cardiovascular Disease. *JAMA* 2019; 322(14):

1381-1391. doi: 10.1001/jama.2019.14120
5. Kaplan H, Thompson RC, Trumble BC, Wann LS, Allam AH, Beheim B, et al. Coronary atherosclerosis in indigenous South American Tsimane: a cross-sectional cohort study. *Lancet* 2017; 389(10080): 1730-1739.
doi: 10.1016/S0140-6736(17)30752-3
6. Tota-Maharaj R, Blaha MJ, Blankstein R, Silverman MG, Eng J, Shaw LJ, et al. Association of coronary artery calcium and coronary heart disease events in young and elderly participants in the multi-ethnic study of atherosclerosis: A secondary analysis of a prospective, population-based cohort. *Mayo Clin Proc* 2014; 89(10): 1350-9. doi: 10.1016/j.mayocp.2014.05.017
7. Anand SS, Hawkes C, de Souza RJ, Mente A, Dehghan M, Nugent R, et al. Food Consumption and its Impact on Cardiovascular Disease: Importance of Solutions Focused on the Globalized Food System. *J Am Coll Cardiol* 2015; 66(14): 1590-1614.
doi: 10.1016/j.jacc.2015.07.050
8. Piepoli MF, Hoes AW, Agewall S, Albus C, Brotons C, Catapano AL, et al. 2016 European Guidelines on cardiovascular disease prevention in clinical practice. *European Heart Journal* 2016; 37(29): 2315-2381.
doi: 10.1093/eurheartj/ehw106
9. Arnett DK, Blumenthal RS, Albert MA, Buroker AB, Goldberger ZD, Hahn EJ, et al. 2019 ACC/AHA Guideline on the Primary Prevention of Cardiovascular Disease: A Report of the American College of Cardiology/American Heart Association Task Force on Clinical Practice Guidelines. *Circulation* 2019; 140(11): e596-e646. doi: 10.1161/CIR.0000000000000678
10. Jabri A, Kumar A, Verghese E, Alameh A, Kumar A, Khan MS, et al. Meta-analysis of effect of vegetarian diet on ischemic heart disease and all-cause mortality. *Am J Prev Cardiol* 2021; 7: 100182. doi: 10.1016/j.ajpc.2021.100182
11. Shikany JM, Safford MM, Newby PK, Durant RW, Brown TM, Judd SE. Southern dietary pattern is associated with hazard of acute coronary heart disease in the reasons for geographic and Racial Differences in Stroke (REGARDS) study. *Circulation* 2015; 132(9): 804-14.
doi: 10.1161/CIRCULATIONAHA.114.014421
12. Mazidi M, Katsiki N, Mikhailidis DP, Sattar N, Banach M. Lower carbohydrate diets and all-cause and cause-specific mortality: A population-based cohort study and pooling of prospective studies. *Eur Heart J* 2019; 40: 2870-2879.
13. Satija A, Bhupathiraju SN, Spiegelman D, Chiuve SE, Manson JAE, Willett W, et al. Healthful and Unhealthful Plant-Based Diets and the Risk of Coronary Heart Disease in U.S. Adults. *J Am Coll Cardiol* 2017; 70(4): 411-422.
doi: 10.1016/j.jacc.2017.05.047
14. Tanaka K, Masuda J, Imamura T, Sueishi K, Nakashima T, Sakurai I, et al. A nation-wide study of atherosclerosis in infants, children and young adults in Japan. *Atherosclerosis* 1988; 72(2–3): 143-56.
doi: 10.1016/0021-9150(88)90075-5
15. Kim YH, Nijst P, Kiefer K, Tang WHW. Endothelial Glycocalyx as Biomarker for Cardiovascular Diseases: Mechanistic and Clinical Implications. *Current Heart Failure Reports* 2017; 14(2): 117-126.
doi: 10.1007/s11897-017-0320-5
16. Huang A, Patel S, McAlpine CS, Werstuck GH. The role of endoplasmic reticulum stress-glycogen synthase kinase-3 signaling in atherogenesis. *International Journal of Molecular Sciences* 2018; 19(6): 1607. doi: 10.3990/ijms19061607
17. Loscalzo J. Harrison's Cardiovascular Medicine. *Mcgraw-Hill Publ.Comp* 2010.
18. Pencina MJ, D'Agostino RB, Zdrojewski T, Williams K, Thanassoulis G, Furberg CD, et al. Apolipoprotein B improves risk assessment of future coronary heart disease in the Framingham heart study beyond LDL-C and non-HDL-C. *Eur J Prev Cardiol* 2015; 22(10). doi: 10.1177/2047487315569411
19. Kromhout D, Menotti A, Bloemberg B, Aravanis C, Blackburn H, Buzina R, et al. Dietary saturated and transfatty acids and cholesterol and 25-year mortality from coronary heart disease: The seven countries study. *Prev Med (Baltim)* 1995; 24(3): 308-315.
20. Worth RM, Kato H, Rhoads GG, Kagan A, Syme SL. Epidemiologic studies of coronary heart disease and stroke in Japanese men living in Japan, Hawaii and California: Mortality. *Am J*

21. Vartiainen E, Laatikainen T, Peltonen M, Juolevi A, Männistö S, Sundvall J, et al. Thirty-five-year trends in cardiovascular risk factors in Finland. *Int J Epidemiol* 2010; 39(2): 504-18. doi: 10.1093/ije/dyp330

22. Hooper L, Martin N, Jimoh OF, Kirk C, Foster E, Abdelhamid AS. Reduction in saturated fat intake for cardiovascular disease. *Cochrane Database of Systematic Reviews* 2020; (6): CD011737. doi: 10.1002/14651858.CD011737

23. Borén J, John Chapman M, Krauss RM, Packard CJ, Bentzon JF, Binder CJ, et al. Low-density lipoproteins cause atherosclerotic cardiovascular disease: Pathophysiological, genetic, and therapeutic insights: A consensus statement from the European Atherosclerosis Society Consensus Panel. *European Heart Journal* 2020; 41(24): 2313-2330. doi: 10.1093/eurheartj/ehz962

24. Silverman MG, Ference BA, Im K, Wiviott SD, Giugliano RP, Grundy SM, et al. Association between lowering LDL-C and cardiovascular risk reduction among different therapeutic interventions: A systematic review and meta-analysis. *JAMA* 2016; 316(12): 1289-97. doi: 10.1001/jama.2016.13985

25. Mozaffarian D, Micha R, Wallace S. Effects on coronary heart disease of increasing polyunsaturated fat in place of saturated fat: A systematic review and meta-analysis of randomized controlled trials. *PLoS Med* 2010; 7(3): e1000252. doi: 10.1371/journal.pmed.1000252

26. Li Y, Hruby A, Bernstein AM, Ley SH, Wang DD, Chiuve SE, et al. Saturated Fats Compared with Unsaturated Fats and Sources of Carbohydrates in Relation to Risk of Coronary Heart Disease A Prospective Cohort Study. *J Am Coll Cardiol* 2015; 66(14): 1538-1548. doi: 10.1016/j.jacc.2015.07.055

27. Zong G, Li Y, Sampson L, Dougherty LW, Willett WC, Wanders AJ, et al. Monounsaturated fats from plant and animal sources in relation to risk of coronary heart disease among US men and women. *Am J Clin Nutr* 2018; 107(3): 445-453. doi: 10.1093/ajcn/nqx004

28. Neelakantan N, Seah JYH, Van Dam RM. The Effect of Coconut Oil Consumption on Cardiovascular Risk Factors: A Systematic Review and Meta-Analysis of Clinical Trials. *Circulation* 2020; 141(10): 803-814. doi: 10.1161/CIRCULATIONAHA.119.043052

29. Estruch R, Ros E, Salas-Salvadó J, Covas M-I, Corella D, Arós F, et al. Primary Prevention of Cardiovascular Disease with a Mediterranean Diet Supplemented with Extra-Virgin Olive Oil or Nuts. *N Engl J Med* 2018; 378(25): e34. doi: 10.1056/NEJMoa1800389

30. Martínez-González MA, Sánchez-Tainta A, Corella D, Salas-Salvadó J, Ros E, Arós F, et al. A provegetarian food pattern and reduction in total mortality in the Prevención con Dieta Mediterránea (PREDIMED) study. *American Journal of Clinical Nutrition* 2014; 100(1): 320S-8S. doi: 10.3945/ajcn.113.071431

31. Satija A, Bhupathiraju SN, Spiegelman D, Chiuve SE, Manson JAE, Willett W, et al. Healthful and Unhealthful Plant-Based Diets and the Risk of Coronary Heart Disease in U.S. Adults. *J Am Coll Cardiol* 2017; 70(4): 411-422. doi: 10.1016/j.jacc.2017.05.047

32. Kim H, Caulfield LE, Garcia-Larsen V, Steffen LM, Coresh J, Rebholz CM. Plant-Based Diets Are Associated With a Lower Risk of Incident Cardiovascular Disease, Cardiovascular Disease Mortality, and All-Cause Mortality in a General Population of Middle-Aged Adults. *J Am Heart Assoc* 2019; 8: e012865. doi: 10.1161/JAHA.119.01286

33. Barnard ND, Alwarith J, Rembert E, Brandon L, Nguyen M, Goergen A, et al. A Mediterranean Diet and Low-Fat Vegan Diet to Improve Body Weight and Cardiometabolic Risk Factors: A Randomized, Cross-over Trial. *J Am Coll Nutr* 2021; 1-13. doi: 10.1080/07315724.2020.1869625

34. Yusuf S. Two decades of progress in preventing vascular disease. *Lancet* 2002; 360(9326): 2-3. doi: 10.1016/S0140-6736(02)09358-3

35. De Lorgeril M, Salen P, Martin JL, Monjaud I, Delaye J, Mamelle N. Mediterranean diet, traditional risk factors, and the rate of cardiovascular complications after myocardial infarction: Final report of the Lyon Diet Heart Study. *Circulation* 1999; 99(6): 779-785. doi: 10.1161/01.cir.99.6.779

36. Li S, Chiuve SE, Flint A, Pai JK, Forman JP, Hu

FB, et al. Better diet quality and decreased mortality among myocardial infarction survivors. *JAMA Intern Med* 2013; 173(19): 1808-1818. doi: 10.1001/jamainternmed.2013.9768
37. Stewart RAH, Wallentin L, Benatar J, Danchin N, Hagström E, Held C, et al. Dietary patterns and the risk of major adverse cardiovascular events in a global study of high-risk patients with stable coronary heart disease. *Eur Heart J* 2016; 37(25): 1993-2001.
doi: 10.1093/eurheartj/ehw125
38. Bhindi R, Guan M, Zhao Y, Humphries KH, Mancini GBJ. Coronary atheroma regression and adverse cardiac events: A systematic review and meta-regression analysis. *Atherosclerosis* 2019; 284: 194-201.
doi: 10.1016/j.atherosclerosis.2019.03.005
39. Ahmadi A, Argulian E, Leipsic J, Newby DE, Narula J. From Subclinical Atherosclerosis to Plaque Progression and Acute Coronary Events: JACC State-of-the-Art Review. *Journal of the American College of Cardiology* 2019; 74(12): 1608-1617. doi: 10.1016/j.jacc.2019.08.012
40. Ornish D, Brown SE, Billings JH, Scherwitz LW, Armstrong WT, Ports TA, et al. Can lifestyle changes reverse coronary heart disease? The Lifestyle Heart Trial. *Lancet* 1990; 336(8708): 129-33. doi: 10.1016/0140-6736(90)91656-u
41. Ornish D, Scherwitz LW, Billings JH, Lance Gould K, Merritt TA, Sparler S, et al. Intensive lifestyle changes for reversal of coronary heart disease. *J Am Med Assoc* 1998; 280(23): 2001-7. doi: 10.1001/jama.280.23.2001
42. Gould KL, Ornish D, Scherwitz L, Brown S, Edens RP, Hess MJ, et al. Changes in Myocardial Perfusion Abnormalities by Positron Emission Tomography After Long-term, Intense Risk Factor Modification. *JAMA* 1995; 274(11): 894-901. doi: 10.1001/jama.1995.03530110056036
43. Watts GF, Lewis B, Lewis ES, Coltart DJ, Smith LDR, Swan A V., et al. Effects on coronary artery disease of lipid-lowering diet, or diet plus cholestyramine, in the St Thomas' Atherosclerosis Regression Study (STARS). *Lancet* 1992; 339(8793): 563-569.
doi: 10.1016/0140-6736(92)90863-x
44. Esselstyn CB, Gendy G, Doyle J, Golubic M, Roizen MF. A way to reverse CAD? *J Fam Pract* 2014; 63(7): 356-364b.
45. Gupta SK, Sawhney RC, Rai L, Chavan VD, Dani S, Arora RC. Regression of Coronary Atherosclerosis through Healthy Lifestyle in Coronary Artery Disease Patients - Mount Abu Open Heart Trial. *Indian Heart J* 2011; 63: 461–9.
46. Berry C, L'Allier PL, Grégoire J, Lespérance J, Levesque S, Ibrahim R, et al. Comparison of intravascular ultrasound and quantitative coronary angiography for the assessment of coronary artery disease progression. *Circulation* 2007; 115(14): 1851-1857.
doi: 10.1161/CIRCULATIONAHA.106.655654
47. Satija A, Hu FB. Plant-based diets and cardiovascular health. *Trends in Cardiovascular Medicine* 2018; 28(7): 437-441.
doi: 10.1016/j.tcm.2018.02.004
48. Shivappa N, Godos J, Hébert JR, Wirth MD, Piuri G, Speciani AF, et al. Dietary inflammatory index and cardiovascular risk and mortality—a meta-analysis. *Nutrients* 2018; 10(2): 200.
doi: 10.3390/nu10020200
49. Shah B, Newman JD, Woolf K, Ganguzza L, Guo Y, Allen N, et al. Anti-inflammatory effects of a vegan diet versus the american heart association–recommended diet in coronary artery disease trial. *J Am Heart Assoc* 2018; 7(23): e011367.
doi: 10.1161/JAHA.118.011367
50. Bondonno CP, Dalgaard F, Blekkenhorst LC, Murray K, Lewis JR, Croft KD, et al. Vegetable nitrate intake, blood pressure and incident cardiovascular disease: Danish Diet, Cancer, and Health Study. *Eur J Epidemiol* 2021; 36(8): 813-825.
doi: 10.1007/s10654-021-00747-3
51. Mano R, Ishida A, Ohya Y, Todoriki H, Takishita S. Dietary intervention with Okinawan vegetables increased circulating endothelial progenitor cells in healthy young women. *Atherosclerosis* 2009; 204(2): 544-8.
doi: 10.1016/j.atherosclerosis.2008.09.035
52. Werner N, Kosiol S, Schiegl T, Ahlers P, Walenta K, Link A, et al. Circulating Endothelial Progenitor Cells and Cardiovascular Outcomes. *N Engl J Med* 2005; 353(10): 999-1007.
doi: 10.1056/NEJMoa043814

53. Navarro JA, de Gouveia LA, Rocha-Penha L, Cinegaglia N, Belo V, Castro MM de, et al. Reduced levels of potential circulating biomarkers of cardiovascular diseases in apparently healthy vegetarian men. *Clin Chim Acta* 2016; 461: 110-3. doi: 10.1016/j.cca.2016.08.002
54. Wolk A. Potential health hazards of eating red meat. *Journal of Internal Medicine* 2017; 281(2): 106-122. doi: 10.1111/joim.12543
55. Ren X, Ren L, Wei Q, Shao H, Chen L, Liu N. Advanced glycation end-products decreases expression of endothelial nitric oxide synthase through oxidative stress in human coronary artery endothelial cells. *Cardiovasc Diabetol* 2017; 16(1): 52. doi: 10.1186/s12933-017-0531-9
56. Threapleton DE, Greenwood DC, Evans CEL, Cleghorn CL, Nykjaer C, Woodhead C, et al. Dietary fibre intake and risk of cardiovascular disease: Systematic review and meta-analysis. *BMJ* 2013; 347: f6879. doi: 10.1136/bmj.f6879
57. Tang WHW, Wang Z, Levison BS, Koeth RA, Britt EB, Fu X, et al. Intestinal Microbial Metabolism of Phosphatidylcholine and Cardiovascular Risk. *N Engl J Med* 2013; 368(17): 1575-1584.
doi: 10.1056/NEJMoa1109400
58. Jia J, Dou P, Gao M, Kong X, Li C, Liu Z, et al. Assessment of causal direction between gut microbiota- dependent metabolites and cardiometabolic health: A bidirectional mendelian randomization analysis. *Diabetes* 2019; 68(9): 1747-1755. doi: 10.2337/db19-0153
59. Heianza Y, Ma W, DiDonato JA, Sun Q, Rimm EB, Hu FB, et al. Long-Term Changes in Gut Microbial Metabolite Trimethylamine N-Oxide and Coronary Heart Disease Risk. *J Am Coll Cardiol* 2020; 75(7): 763-772.
doi: 10.1016/j.jacc.2019.11.060
60. Djekic D, Shi L, Brolin H, Carlsson F, Särnqvist C, Savolainen O, et al. Effects of a Vegetarian Diet on Cardiometabolic Risk Factors, Gut Microbiota, and Plasma Metabolome in Subjects With Ischemic Heart Disease: A Randomized, Crossover Study. *J Am Heart Assoc* 2020; 9(18): e016518. doi: 10.1161/JAHA.120.016518
61. López-Moreno J, García-Carpintero S, Jimenez-Lucena R, Haro C, Rangel-Zúñiga OA, Blanco-Rojo R, et al. Effect of Dietary Lipids on Endotoxemia Influences Postprandial Inflammatory Response. *J Agric Food Chem* 2017; 65(35): 7756-7763.
doi: 10.1021/acs.jafc.7b01909
62. Tangney CC, Rasmussen HE. Polyphenols, inflammation, and cardiovascular disease. *Curr Atheroscler Rep* 2013; 15(5): 324.
doi: 10.1007/s11883-013-0324-x
63. Genetic Risk, Lifestyle, and Coronary Artery Disease. *N Engl J Med* 2017; 376(12): 1192-1195. doi: 10.1056/NEJMc1700362
64. Diaz VA, Mainous AG, Everett CJ, Schoepf UJ, Codd V, Samanii NJ. Effect of healthy lifestyle behaviors on the association between leukocyte telomere length and coronary artery calcium. *Am J Cardiol* 2010; 106(5): 659-663.
doi: 10.1016/j.amjcard.2010.04.018
65. Whelton PK, Carey RM, Aronow WS, Ovbiagele B, Casey DE, Smith SC, et al. 2017 Guideline for the Prevention, Detection, Evaluation, and Management of High Blood Pressure in Adults A Report of the American College of Cardiology/The American Heart Association. *Journal of American College of Cardiology* 2017; 23976. doi: 10.1016/j.jacc.2017.07.745
66. Appel LJ, Moore TJ, Obarzanek E, Vollmer WM, Svetkey LP, Sacks FM, et al. A clinical trial of the effects of dietary patterns on blood pressure. DASH Collaborative Research Group. *N Engl J Med* 1997; 336(16): 1117-24.
doi: 10.1056/NEJM199704173361601
67. Sacks F, Svetkey LP, Vollmer WM, Appel LJ, Bray GA, Harsha D, et al. Effects on blood pressure of reduced dietary sodium and the Dietary Approaches to Stop Hypertension (DASH) diet. DASH-Sodium Collaborative Research Group. *New Engl J Med* 2001; 344(1): 3-10.
doi: 10.1056/NEJM200101043440101
68. Blumenthal JA, Babyak MA, Hinderliter A, Watkins LL, Craighead L, Lin PH, et al. Effects of the DASH diet alone and in combination with exercise and weight loss on blood pressure and cardiovascular biomarkers in men and women with high blood pressure: The ENCORE study. *Arch Intern Med* 2010; 170(2): 126-135.
doi: 10.1001/archinternmed.2009.470
69. Pettersen BJ, Anousheh R, Fan J, Jaceldo-Siegl K, Fraser GE. Vegetarian diets and blood

pressure among white subjects: Results from the Adventist Health Study-2 (AHS-2). *Public Health Nutr* 2012; 15(10): 1909-1916. doi: 10.1017/S1368980011003454
70. Appleby PN, Davey GK, Key TJ. Hypertension and blood pressure among meat eaters, fish eaters, vegetarians and vegans in EPIC–Oxford. *Public Health Nutr* 2002; 5(5): 645-654. doi: 10.1079/PHN2002332
71. Yokoyama Y, Nishimura K, Barnard ND, Takegami M, Watanabe M, Sekikawa A, et al. Vegetarian diets and blood pressure ameta-analysis. *JAMA Intern Med* 2014; 174(4): 577-587. doi: 10.1001/jamainternmed.2013.14547
72. Wang L, Manson JE, Gaziano JM, Buring JE, Sesso HD. Fruit and vegetable intake and the risk of hypertension in middle-aged and older women. *Am J Hypertens* 2012; 25(2): 180-189. doi: 10.1038/ajh.2011.186
73. Tighe P, Duthie G, Vaughan N, Brittenden J, Simpson WG, Duthie S, et al. Effect of increased consumption of whole-grain foods on blood pressure and other cardiovascular risk markers in healthy middle-aged persons: A randomized controlled trial. *Am J Clin Nutr* 2010; 92(4): 733-740. doi: 10.3945/ajcn.2010.29417
74. Mohammadifard N, Salehi-Abargouei A, Salas-Salvadó J, Guasch-Ferré M, Humphries K, Sarrafzadegan N. The effect of tree nut, peanut, and soy nut consumption on blood pressure: A systematic review and meta-analysis of randomized controlled clinical trials. Am J Clin Nutr 2015; 101(5): 966-982. doi: 10.3945/ajcn.114.091595
75. Coles LT, Clifton PM. Effect of beetroot juice on lowering blood pressure in free-living, disease-free adults: A randomized, placebo-controlled trial. *Nutr J* 2012; 11(1): 106. doi: 10.1186/1475-2891-11-106
76. Johnson SA, Feresin RG, Navaei N, Figueroa A, Elam ML, Akhavan NS, et al. Effects of daily blueberry consumption on circulating biomarkers of oxidative stress, inflammation, and antioxidant defense in postmenopausal women with pre- and stage 1-hypertension: A randomized controlled trial. *Food and Function* 2017; 8: 372-380. doi: 10.1039/C6FO01216G
77. Khalesi S, Irwin C, Schubert M. Flaxseed consumption may reduce blood pressure: A systematic review and meta-analysis of controlled trials. *J Nutr* 2015; 145(4); 758-765. doi: 10.3945/jn.114.205302
78. Mach F, Baigent C, Catapano AL, Koskinas KC, Casula M, Badimon L, et al. 2019 esc/eas guidelines for the management of dyslipidaemias: Lipid modification to reduce cardiovascular risk. *Eur Heart J* 2020; 41(1): 111-188. doi: 10.1093/eurheartj/ehz45510.1093/eurheartj/ehz455
79. Zong G, Li Y, Wanders AJ, Alssema M, Zock PL, Willett WC, et al. Intake of individual saturated fatty acids and risk of coronary heart disease in US men and women: Two prospective longitudinal cohort studies. *BMJ* 2016; 355: i5796. doi: 10.1136/bmj.i5796
80. Nishida C, Uauy R. Who scientific update on health consequences of trans fatty acids: Introduction. *European Journal of Clinical Nutrition* 2009; 63 Suppl 2: S1-4. doi: 10.1038/ejcn.2009.13
81. Bergeron N, Chiu S, Williams PT, M King S, Krauss RM. Effects of red meat, white meat, and nonmeat protein sources on atherogenic lipoprotein measures in the context of low compared with high saturated fat intake: a randomized controlled trial. *Am J Clin Nutr* 2019; 110(1): 24-33. doi: 10.1093/ajcn/nqz035
82. Vincent MJ, Allen B, Palacios OM, Haber LT, Maki KC. Meta-regression analysis of the effects of dietary cholesterol intake on LDL and HDL cholesterol. *Am J Clin Nutr* 2019; 109(1): 7-16. doi: 10.1093/ajcn/nqy273
83. Khalighi Sikaroudi M, Soltani S, Kolahdouz-Mohammadi R, Clayton ZS, Fernandez ML, Varse F, et al. The responses of different dosages of egg consumption on blood lipid profile: An updated systematic review and meta-analysis of randomized clinical trials. *J Food Biochem* 2020; 44(8): e13263. doi: 10.1111/jfbc.13263
84. Barnard ND, Long MB, Ferguson JM, Flores R, Kahleova H. Industry Funding and Cholesterol Research: A Systematic Review. *American Journal of Lifestyle Medicine* 2019; 15(2): 165-172. doi: 10.1177/1559827619892198
85. Hopkins PN. Effects of dietary cholesterol on serum cholesterol: A meta-analysis and review. *American Journal of Clinical Nutrition* 1992;

55(6): 1060-1070. doi: 10.1093/ajcn/55.6.1060
86. Jenkins DJA, Kendall CWC, Popovich DG, Vidgen E, Mehling CC, Vuksan V, et al. Effect of a very-high-fiber vegetable, fruit, and nut diet on serum lipids and colonic function. *Metabolism* 2001; 50(4): 494-503.
doi: 10.1053/meta.2001.21037
87. Chiavaroli L, Nishi SK, Khan TA, Braunstein CR, Glenn AJ, Mejia SB, et al. Portfolio Dietary Pattern and Cardiovascular Disease: A Systematic Review and Meta-analysis of Controlled Trials. *Progress in Cardiovascular Diseases* 2018; 61(1): 43-53.
doi: 10.1016/j.pcad.2018.05.004
88. Wang F, Zheng J, Yang B, Jiang J, Fu Y, Li D. Effects of vegetarian diets on blood lipids: A systematic review and meta-analysis of randomized controlled trials. *J Am Heart Assoc* 2015; 4(10): e002408. doi: 10.1161/JAHA.115.002408
89. Sarwar N, Danesh J, Eiriksdottir G, Sigurdsson G, Wareham N, Bingham S, et al. Triglycerides and the risk of coronary heart disease: 10 158 Incident cases among 262 525 participants in 29 Western prospective studies. *Circulation* 2007; 115(4): 450-458.
doi: 10.1161/CIRCULATIONAHA
90. Sofi F, Dinu M, Pagliai G, Cesari F, Gori AM, Sereni A, et al. Low-calorie vegetarian versus mediterranean diets for reducing body weight and improving cardiovascular risk profile. *Circulation* 2018; 137(11): 1103-1113.
doi: 10.1161/CIRCULATIONAHA.117.030088
91. Guo J, Astrup A, Lovegrove JA, Gijsbers L, Givens DI, Soedamah-Muthu SS. Milk and dairy consumption and risk of cardiovascular diseases and all-cause mortality: dose–response meta-analysis of prospective cohort studies. *Eur J Epidemiol* 2017; 32(4): 269-287.
doi: 10.1007/s10654-017-0243-1
92. Ding M, Li J, Qi L, Ellervik C, Zhang X, Manson JE, et al. Associations of dairy intake with risk of mortality in women and men: Three prospective cohort studies. *BMJ* 2019; 367: l6204.
doi: 10.1136/bmj.l6204
93. Buettner D, Skemp S. Blue Zones: Lessons From the World's Longest Lived. *American Journal of Lifestyle Medicine* 2016; 10(5): 318-321.
doi: 10.1177/1559827616637066
94. Nocella C, Cammisotto V, Fianchini L, D'Amico A, Novo M, Castellani V, et al. Extra Virgin Olive Oil and Cardiovascular Diseases: Benefits for Human Health. *Endocrine, Metab Immune Disord - Drug Targets* 2017; 18(1): 4-13.
doi: 10.2174/1871530317666171114121533
95. Vogel RA, Corretti MC, Plotnick GD. The postprandial effect of components of the Mediterranean diet on endothelial function. *J Am Coll Cardiol* 2000; 36(5): 1455-1460.
doi: 10.1016/s0735-1097(00)00896-2
96. Schwingshackl L, Christoph M, Hoffmann G. Effects of olive oil on markers of inflammation and endothelial function—A systematic review and meta-analysis. *Nutrients* 2015; 7(9): 7651-7675. doi: 10.3390/nu7095356
97. Schwingshackl L, Krause M, Schmucker C, Hoffmann G, Rücker G, Meerpohl JJ. Impact of different types of olive oil on cardiovascular risk factors: A systematic review and network meta-analysis. *Nutr Metab Cardiovasc Dis* 2019; 29(10): 1030-1039.
doi: 10.1016/j.numecd.2019.07.001
98. Freeman AM, Morris PB, Barnard N, Esselstyn CB, Ros E, Agatston A, et al. Trending Cardiovascular Nutrition Controversies. *Journal of the American College of Cardiology* 2017; 69(9): 1172-1187. doi: 10.1016/j.jacc.2016.10.086
99. Harris WS, Tintle NL, Imamura F, Qian F, Korat AVA, Marklund M, et al. Blood n-3 fatty acid levels and total and cause-specific mortality from 17 prospective studies. *Nat Commun* 2021; 12(1): 2329. doi: 10.1038/s41467-021-22370-2
100. Jayedi A, Shab-Bidar S. Fish Consumption and the Risk of Chronic Disease: An Umbrella Review of Meta-Analyses of Prospective Cohort Studies. *Advances in Nutrition* 2020; 11(5): 1123-1133. doi: 10.1093/advances/nmaa029
101. Abdelhamid AS, Brown TJ, Brainard JS, Biswas P, Thorpe GC, Moore HJ, et al. Omega-3 fatty acids for the primary and secondary prevention of cardiovascular disease. *Cochrane Database of Systematic Reviews* 2020; 7(7): CD003177.
doi: 10.1002/14651858.CD003177.pub3
102. Manson JE, Cook NR, Lee I-M, Christen W, Bassuk SS, Mora S, et al. Marine n−3 Fatty Acids and Prevention of Cardiovascular Disease and Cancer. *N Engl J Med* 2019; 380(1): 23-32.

doi: 10.1056/NEJMoa1811403

103. Bhatt DL, Steg PG, Miller M, Brinton EA, Jacobson TA, Ketchum SB, et al. Cardiovascular Risk Reduction with Icosapent Ethyl for Hypertriglyceridemia. *N Engl J Med* 2019; 380(1): 11-22. doi: 10.1056/NEJMoa1812792

104. Khan SU, Lone AN, Khan MS, Virani SS, Blumenthal RS, Nasir K, et al. Effect of omega-3 fatty acids on cardiovascular outcomes: A systematic review and meta-analysis. *EClinicalMedicine* 2021; 38: 100997. doi: 10.1016/j.eclinm.2021.100997

105. Kagan ML, West AL, Zante C, Calder PC. Acute appearance of fatty acids in human plasma - A comparative study between polar-lipid rich oil from the microalgae Nannochloropsis oculata and krill oil in healthy young males. *Lipids Health Dis* 2013; 12(1): 102. doi: 10.1186/1476-511X-12-102

106. Savarese G, Lund LH. Global Public Health Burden of Heart Failure. *CRF J* 2017; 3(1): 7-11. doi: 10.15420/cfr.2016:25:2

107. Schocken DD, Benjamin EJ, Fonarow GC, Krumholz HM, Levy D, Mensah GA, et al. Prevention of heart failure: A scientific statement from the American Heart Association Councils on epidemiology and prevention, clinical cardiology, cardiovascular nursing, and high blood pressure research; Quality of Care and Outcomes Research Interdisciplinary Working Group; and Functional Genomics and Translational Biology Interdisciplinary Working Group. *Circulation* 2008; 117(19): 2544-65. doi: 10.1161/CIRCULATIONAHA.107.188965

108. Eckel RH, Jakicic JM, Ard JD, De Jesus JM, Houston Miller N, Hubbard VS, et al. 2013 AHA/ACC guideline on lifestyle management to reduce cardiovascular risk: A report of the American College of cardiology/American Heart Association task force on practice guidelines. *Circulation* 2014; 129(25 Suppl 2): S76-99. doi: 10.1161/01.cir.0000437740.48606.d1

109. Salehi-Abargouei A, Maghsoudi Z, Shirani F, Azadbakht L. Effects of Dietary Approaches to Stop Hypertension (DASH)-style diet on fatal or nonfatal cardiovascular diseases-Incidence: A systematic review and meta-analysis on observational prospective studies. *Nutrition* 2013; 29(4): 611-618. doi: 10.1016/j.nut.2012.12.018

110. Rifai L, Pisano C, Hayden J, Sulo S, Silver MA. Impact of the Dash Diet on Endothelial Function, Exercise Capacity, and Quality of Life in Patients with Heart Failure. *Baylor Univ Med Cent Proc* 2015; 28(2): 151-156. doi: 10.1080/08998280.2015.11929216

111. Liyanage T, Ninomiya T, Wang A, Neal B, Jun M, Wong MG, et al. Effects of the mediterranean diet on cardiovascular outcomes-a systematic review and meta-analysis. *PLoS ONE* 2016; 11(8): e0159252. doi: 10.1371/journal.pone.0159252

112. Levitan EB, Lewis CE, Tinker LF, Eaton CB, Ahmed A, Manson JE, et al. Mediterranean and DASH diet scores and mortality in women with heart failure the women s health initiative. *Circ Hear Fail* 2013; 6(6): 1116-1123. doi: 10.1161/CIRCHEARTFAILURE.113.000495

113. Lara KM, Levitan EB, Gutierrez OM, Shikany JM, Safford MM, Judd SE, et al. Dietary Patterns and Incident Heart Failure in U.S. Adults Without Known Coronary Disease. *J Am Coll Cardiol* 2019; 73(16): 20136-20145. doi: 10.1016/j.jacc.2019.01.067

114. Kerley CP. A Review of Plant-based Diets to Prevent and Treat Heart Failure. *Card Fail Rev* 2018; 4(1): 54–61. doi: 10.15420/cfr.2018:1:1

115. Benjamin EJ, Virani SS, Callaway CW, Chamberlain AM, Chang AR, Cheng S, et al. Heart Disease and Stroke Statistics-2018 Update: A Report From the American Heart Association. *Circulation* 2018; 137(12): e67-e492. doi: 10.1161/CIR.0000000000000558

116. GBD 2016 Lifetime Risk of Stroke Collaborators, Feigin VL, Nguyen G, Cercy K, Johnson CO, Alam T, Parmar PG, et al. Global, Regional, and Country-Specific Lifetime Risks of Stroke, 1990 and 2016. *N Engl J Med* 2018; 379(25): 2429-2437. doi: 10.1056/NEJMoa1804492

117. Campbell T. A plant-based diet and stroke. *Journal of Geriatric Cardiology* 2017; 14(5): 321–326. doi: 10.11909/j.issn.1671-5411.2017.05.010

118. Feng Q, Fan S, Wu Y, Zhou D, Zhao R, Liu M, et al. Adherence to the dietary approaches to stop hypertension diet and risk of stroke: A meta-analysis of prospective studies. *Med (United States)* 2018; .

119. Saulle R, Lia L, De Giusti M, La Torre G. A systematic overview of the scientific literature on the association between Mediterranean Diet and the Stroke prevention. *Clin Ter* 2019; 170(5): e396-e408. doi: 10.7417/CT.2019.2166
120. Tong TYN, Appleby PN, Bradbury KE, Perez-Cornago A, Travis RC, Clarke R, et al. Risks of ischaemic heart disease and stroke in meat eaters, fish eaters, and vegetarians over 18 years of follow-up: Results from the prospective EPIC-Oxford study. 97(38): e12450*BMJ* 2019; 366: l4897. doi: 10.1136/bmj.l4897
121. Chiu THT, Chang H-R, Wang L-Y, Chang C-C, Lin M-N, Lin C-L. Vegetarian diet and incidence of total, ischemic, and hemorrhagic stroke in 2 cohorts in Taiwan. *Neurology* 2020; 94(11): e1112-e1121.
wdoi: 10.1212/WNL.0000000000009093
122. Glenn AJ, Viguiliouk E, Seider M, Boucher BA, Khan TA, Blanco Mejia S, et al. Relation of vegetarian dietary patterns with major cardiovascular outcomes: A systematic review and meta-analysis of prospective cohort studies. *Frontiers in Nutrition* 2019; 6: 80. doi: 10.3389/fnut.2019.00080
123. Baden MY, Shan Z, Wang F, Li Y, Manson JE, Rimm EB, et al. Quality of Plant-Based Diet and Risk of Total, Ischemic, and Hemorrhagic Stroke. *Neurology* 2021; 96(15): e1940-e1953. doi: 10.1212/WNL.0000000000011713
124. Aggarwal M, Bozkurt B, Panjrath G, Aggarwal B, Ostfeld RJ, Barnard N, et al. American College of Cardiology's Nutrition and Lifestyle Committee of the Prevention of Cardiovascular Disease Council. Lifestyle Modifications for Preventing and Treating Heart Failure. *J Am Coll Cardiol* 2018;72(19): 2391-2405. doi: 10.1016/j.jacc.2018.08.2160

Chapter 4
Plant-based nutrition and cancer

Aryan Tavakkoli

Introduction

Worldwide, cancer is the second leading cause of death, accounting for about 17 million new cases, and 10 million deaths, per year.[1]

In the UK, over 360,000 people are diagnosed with cancer annually. For people born after 1960, an estimated 50% have a lifetime risk of being diagnosed with cancer, with cancers of the breast, prostate, lung and bowel being the most common.[2]

Current medical practice focuses on eradicating tumour cells using a combination of surgery, radiotherapy, chemotherapy and targeted medical treatments, but very few oncologists currently advise their patients regarding the role of nutrition and lifestyle factors in the prevention, or recurrence, of cancer and the potential for improving outcomes after a diagnosis of cancer.

The understanding that the genes we are born with contribute to the development of cancer in only 5–10% of cases, and that environmental factors, including modifiable lifestyle behaviours, play a major role in cancer development, accounting for 90–95% of cancers, emphasises further the need for doctors to better understand the importance of advising their patients on lifestyle factors, especially nutrition. Most oncologists provide no dietary advice at all to their patients at any stage, or, if advice is provided, it is often incomplete, inconsistent or inaccurate.[3] With up to 35% of all cancer potentially linked to diet[4] the lack of knowledge in the area of nutrition is an area that requires significant improvement within the oncology field.

In every phase of cancer, from reducing risk factors, to curbing early development and DNA damage, to decreasing inflammation and oxidative stress, and reducing risk of recurrence after treatment, nutrition plays a significant role and has the potential not only for improving outcomes but also for improving energy levels, wellbeing, patients' tolerance to aggressive treatments and accelerated recovery following treatment.[5]

Pathophysiological mechanisms of cancer development

The metabolic landscape of cancer is extremely complex. Cancer cells are able to use many different pathways in order to access fuel, to direct information to one another, to grow new blood vessels, proliferate and metastasise. Although we are developing a greater understanding of the multiplicity of biological mechanisms involved in cancer development and progression, there is still much to be discovered in this field.

Through ongoing research, a number of characteristic features of cancer cells have been identified, termed the 'hallmarks of cancer'.[6] These comprise:
- sustained proliferative signalling
- resisting cell death
- activating invasion and metastasis
- inducing angiogenesis
- evading growth suppressors
- enabling replicative immortality
- avoiding immune destruction
- deregulating cellular energetics
- enabling characteristic: genomic instability and mutation
- enabling characteristic: tumour-promoting inflammation.

Phytochemicals within whole plant foods can play a major role in the prevention, progression and treatment of cancer, alongside standard treatment measures, through the modulation of each of these hallmarks.[7]

In most cancers, there is epigenetic silencing of genes that control cell growth. The phytochemicals in plant foods bind to multiple receptors to modulate cellular behaviour and impact the expression of numerous tumour suppressor genes and oncogenes to modulate abnormal cell growth by affecting the production of substances such as protein kinases, growth factors, inflammatory cytokines and inflammatory enzymes[8] (see Table 4.1).

Table 4.1 Anti-cancer activity of phytonutrients
NB This is not an exhaustive list

Some sources	Bioactive compound	Chemical structure	Examples of anti-cancer activity
Turmeric	Curcumin		Induces apoptosis, suppresses glutaminolysis, IGF-1, aerobic glycolysis, mTOR and NF-kB
Red grapes, pistachios, blueberries, dark chocolate	Resveratrol		Suppresses NF-kB, COX-1 and COX-2 signalling pathways, suppresses VEGF
Green tea	Epigallocatechin-3-gallate (EGCG)		Suppresses wnt signalling pathway, suppresses multiple metalloproteinases
Soya beans	Genistein		Activates p53 tumour suppressor gene, suppresses Hedgehog signalling pathway

Cruciferous vegetables	Sulphoraphane		Suppresses the Notch signalling pathway, inhibits angiogenesis, activates transcription factor nrf-2
Parsley, celery, oregano	Apigenin		Triggers apoptosis, induces cell cycle arrest, inhibits hypoxia inducible factor (HIF-1)
Tomatoes	Lycopene		Inhibits IGF-1, inhibits angiogenesis
Ginger	Gingerol		Inhibits NF-kB, COX-2 signalling pathways
Citrus fruit peel	D-limonene		Suppresses mTOR signalling pathway, induces apoptosis
Cruciferous vegetables	Indole-3-carbinol		Modulates e-cadherin and BRCA1
Apples, onions, leafy vegetables	Quercetin		Induces apoptosis, suppresses IGF-1, Notch and wnt signalling pathways
Peppermint, rosemary, sage, thyme	Rosmarinic acid		Inhibits ERK and COX-2 signalling pathways
Raspberries, blackberries, chestnuts, walnuts	Ellagic acid		Inhibits platelet-derived growth factor (PDGF), induces apoptosis
Black cumin seeds	Thymoquinone		Induces apoptosis and cell cycle arrest, modulates NF-kB, inhibits angiogenesis
Cranberries, apples	Ursolic acid		Inhibits glutaminolysis, inhibits STAT3 signalling pathway
Peppers, celery	Luteolin		Inhibits aerobic glycolysis, inhibits Notch signalling pathway

Inflammation

The presence of chronic, low-grade inflammation increases the risk of cancer development and progression.[9] A high level of inflammation is closely associated with cancer-associated symptoms such as fatigue, depression and weight loss, as well as lower survival rates.[10, 11, 12, 13]

The possible causes of chronic inflammation are diverse and include:
- a pro-inflammatory diet (for example, high in saturated fat and processed foods)
- a gut microbiome that is imbalanced, or lacks diversity (intestinal dysbiosis)
- insulin resistance and metabolic syndrome
- oxidative stress
- exposure to carcinogens and environmental toxins
- hormone dysregulation.

Cancer cells themselves secrete inflammatory cytokines, such as IL-6, resulting in an inflamed microenvironment around tumours that facilitates further tumour growth, angiogenesis and metastasis.

NFκB

Nuclear Factor kappa-B, or NFκB, is a transcription factor that possesses several pro-tumourigenic actions, such as upregulating telomerase activity in order to enable immortality; stimulating the release of inflammatory cytokines and prostaglandins such as TNFα, IL-1, IL-8 and COX2; stimulating angiogenesis via the release of vascular endothelial growth factor (VEGF); and inhibiting apoptosis via the modulation of several apoptosis genes such as Bcl-x.

When activated, NFκB triggers multiple inflammatory pathways. Consequently, any intervention that regulates this transcription factor can curtail downstream inflammatory pathways.

Many phytochemicals have been shown to reduce NFκB activation,[4] including indole-3-carbinol from the brassica family; lycopene from tomatoes; apigenin from celery and parsley; curcumin; quercetin; resveratrol; sulphoraphane and zingiber (see Table 4.2). The myriad of phytochemicals present in whole plant foods explain the anti-inflammatory nature of whole food plant-based nutrition that is observed in practice.

Table 4.2 NFκB inhibition by phytonutrients
NB This is not an exhaustive list

NFκB suppression	Curcumin
	Berberine
	Resveratrol
	Sulphoraphane
	Quercetin
	Astragalus
	Boswellic acid
	Xanthohumol
	Honokiol
	Ginger
	Thymoquinone
	Lycopene
	Genistein
	Capsaicin
	Silybinin
	EGCG
	Luteolin
	Kaempferol
	Naringenin
	Mangiferin
	Caffeic acid
	Carnosic acid
	Artemisinin

Other ways in which inflammation can be modulated are via the gut microbiota and by weight control. The phytonutrients in whole plant foods impact both of these important areas.

Gut microbiome

The high amount of fibre in whole plant foods acts as a prebiotic for beneficial gut flora such as *Bifidobacterium* and *Lactobacillus* species, enabling them to perform their physiological functions including the production of short chain fatty acids, which are anti-inflammatory and protective to the gut mucosa.

Compared with animal proteins that possess a high saturated fat content and can stimulate inflammatory pathways, plant proteins (such as legumes, nuts, seeds, vegetable proteins) protect the gut barrier and reduce inflammation[14] whilst encouraging a more favourable gut microbiome.

Maintaining a healthy weight

Obesity is a major risk factor for cancer, accounting for 20% all cancer diagnoses in women and 14% all cancer diagnoses in men. Obesity is identified as a cause in at least 13 types of cancer.[15]

In the UK, maintaining a healthy weight is the second biggest preventable cause of cancer after tobacco smoking.

A number of mechanisms have been proposed to explain the higher incidence of cancer with obesity as listed below.
- Excess weight contributes to inflammation, which in itself increases the risk of cancer.
- Insulin resistance as a metabolic adaptation to the increased circulation of free fatty acids released from adipose tissue, results in increased insulin secretion, which again is a risk factor for cancer development.
- Increased circulating levels of oestrogen (synthesised by adipose tissues) and altered sex hormone metabolism.
- The storage of more fat-soluble toxins in adipose tissue.
- Increased availability of IGF-1, a growth factor implicated in the growth of many cancers.[16]

As well as posing an increased risk for cancer development, obesity is also associated with a poorer prognosis and higher risk of recurrence after a cancer diagnosis, along with reduced effectiveness of systemic therapies in some cancers.[15]

In comparison with animal-based foods that tend to possess a high calorie density, the low-calorie and high nutrient-density of whole plant foods facilitates healthy weight maintenance whilst reducing the development of conditions that promote further inflammation, such as insulin resistance, type 2 diabetes mellitus and cardiovascular disease.

Specific diet related carcinogens and associated factors

In 2015, The International Agency for Research on Cancer (IARC), the specialised cancer agency of the World Health Organisation, determined that convincing evidence exists that eating processed meat causes colorectal cancer, and that, at the time of convening, there was strong mechanistic evidence from epidemiological studies showing a positive association between eating red meat and developing colorectal cancer.

The IARC graded processed meat as a group 1, that is, definitely carcinogenic to humans, and red meat as group 2a, that is, probably carcinogenic to humans.

In keeping with this direction, UK data[17] from half a million individuals established that every 25 g/day increment in processed-meat intake (equivalent to about one rasher of bacon or one slice of ham) is associated with a 19% increase in risk for colorectal cancer, and every 50 g/day increment of red meat intake (equivalent to one thick slice of roast beef, or one lamb cutlet) is associated with an 18% increased risk of colorectal cancer.

A number of studies have also linked processed and red meat to other cancers including breast, stomach, pancreatic, prostate, and bladder cancer.[18, 19, 20] International cancer guidelines clearly state processed meat and red meat should be limited or avoided to reduce the risk of developing cancer.

Animal-based foods are not only devoid of beneficial anti-cancer nutrients such as fibre, phytochemicals, antioxidants and most vitamins, but also contain certain compounds that are known to trigger inflammatory pathways and induce oxidative stress and DNA damage.

The following potentially carcinogenic compounds derived from meat and other animal products have been the subjects of numerous studies, and some of the potential mechanisms of carcinogenicity identified.

Nitrates, nitrites and N-nitroso compounds

Nitrates are natural compounds found in many foods. Celery, beetroots, leafy greens such as spinach and arugula are examples of nitrate-rich plant foods. Nitrates are converted to nitrites by salivary organisms in the oral microbiome, using the enzyme nitrate reductase. Nitrites can be metabolised to produced nitric oxide, which is known for its beneficial effects on blood pressure, and other cardiovascular disease risk factors.

However, when nitrites are consumed in the absence of phytonutrients, carcinogenic compounds called N-nitroso compounds (NOC), such as nitrosamines, are formed. Nitrites are also artificially added to processed meat in the form of preservatives, leading to the formation of NOCs in meat.

The connection between NOCs in processed meats such as sausages, bacon, ham and deli meats is now well established, accounting for the IARC's position in categorising these processed meats as definite carcinogens to humans.[21]

Alkylating signature associated with processed and red meat consumption in colorectal cancer

In 2021, Gurjao et al. reported on a study that undertook whole-exome sequencing data from 900 colorectal cancer cases that had occurred in three US-wide prospective studies, the Nurses' Health Studies and Health Professionals Follow-up Study.[22] The data showed a previously undescribed alkylating signature that was associated with high intakes of processed and unprocessed red meat prior to diagnosis, providing molecular evidence of this dietary factor's mutagenic impact. Higher alkylating damage was found in tumours harbouring cancer driver mutations KRAS p.G12D, p.G13D and PIK3CA p.E545K. In addition, higher levels of alkylating damage were associated with a 47% greater risk of dying from colorectal cancer compared to patients with lower levels of damage. These results link for the first time a colorectal mutational signature to a component of diet and further implicate the role of red meat in colorectal cancer initiation and progression.

Trimethylamine N-oxide (TMAO)

TMAO is a highly inflammatory molecule produced in the liver via the oxidation of trimethylamine (TMA), which is generated by the gut bacteria through the process of metabolising choline and L-carnitine. The highest concentration of choline is found in red meat, poultry, fish, dairy and eggs. L-carnitine is almost exclusively found in these animal products.

High blood levels of TMAO have been linked to colorectal cancer, cardiovascular disease, diabetes and early death from all causes. People found to have higher blood levels of TMAO also have a four-fold greater risk of premature death from any cause.[23, 24]

Consuming whole plant foods, especially increased vegetable consumption, alters the gut microbiota and the enzymes necessary for converting TMA into TMAO, leading to reduced TMAO levels.

Haem iron

Dietary iron occurs in two forms – haem iron and non-haem iron. Non-haem iron is derived from plant foods such as legumes, whole grains, vegetables, fruits, nuts and seeds. Haem iron is derived from animal foods, predominantly red and processed meat, in the form of haemoglobin and myoglobin. Haem iron is also present in white meat, fish and other seafood.

Whilst iron is an essential mineral in the body, at high levels it acts as a pro-oxidant and can induce oxidative stress and DNA damage through free radical formation.

There are several ways in which haem iron may lead to an increased risk of malignancy:
- Haem iron that cannot be fully degraded in the small intestine, accumulates in the large intestine, exerting cytotoxic damage to the cells of the intestinal mucosa. This results in the proliferation and hyperplasia of crypt cells, which is an early change that is often observed to precede colorectal cancer.
- Free haem iron accumulation results in the production of reactive oxygen species, that induce DNA damage and gene mutations.[25]
- Haem iron is involved in the formation of carcinogenic N-nitroso compounds and cytotoxic, DNA-damaging aldehydes via lipoperoxidation.[26]

Haem iron is also associated with numerous inflammatory conditions such as metabolic syndrome and coronary heart disease, which are covered elsewhere in this book.

With regard to its role in cancer development, in numerous systematic reviews and meta-analyses, haem iron specifically has been found to be linked to an increased risk of developing cancer.[27]

A higher intake of haem iron is associated with a higher risk of colorectal cancer,[26] breast cancer,[28] and oesophageal cancer.[29]

No significant association has been found with endometrial cancer or adult glioma, and mixed results have been found with lung cancer, with some meta-analyses showing a positive association between meat consumption and lung cancer.[27, 30, 31]

One systematic review[32] found no link between haem iron and colorectal cancer, however this review included only experimental studies of animal models and cell cultures, using 'semi-purified diets designed to mimic the nutrient loads in current westernised diets'. This type of study design is typical in attempting to generate confusion with experimental study designs that carry little relevance to human anatomy, when the close relationship of red meat consumption and colorectal cancer has already been elucidated with large population studies and prospective cohort studies.

Heterocyclic amines and polycyclic aromatic hydrocarbons (HCAs and PAHs)

HCAs and PAHs are two groups of potentially carcinogenic chemical compounds formed during the cooking of meat.

HCAs are formed mainly in muscle tissue (red meat, poultry) cooked at high temperatures (such as frying, grilling and barbecuing). They are also formed in fish, eggs and cheese.

PAHs are formed when meat is exposed to smoke, such as over an open fire, under a grill, or in certain food production processes such as smoking meats.

Considerable evidence in the medical literature points to the positive association between meat consumption and cancer risk via the production of these mutagenic compounds.[33]

One HCA, 2-amino-1-methyl-6-phenylimidazo[4,5-b]pyridine (PhIP), formed in very well done meat, has been shown to activate oestrogenic signalling and the mitogen-activated protein kinase (MAPK) pathway, both being signalling pathways used in the progression of cancer, with implications for numerous cancers that involve oestrogen signalling.[34]

Eating cruciferous vegetables may reduce the absorption and subsequent oxidative-induced DNA damage from HCAs.[35]

Insulin-like growth factor-1 (IGF-1)

IGF-1 is a growth hormone that is mainly secreted by the liver but also by many other tissues. The highest rate of production occurs around puberty, and levels reduce once the natural growth period is completed. At this point, high levels of IGF-1 are no longer necessary and if present, can stimulate cell signalling, leading to cellular proliferation and an increased risk of developing cancer.

Once cancer has developed, IGF-1 is a potent stimulator of progression.[36] Possible mechanisms by which IGF-1 may lead to cancer progression include its interactions with oncogenes and tumour suppressors, and interactions with the sex hormones.[37]

Serum IGF-1 levels are strongly influenced by diet. Plant-based diets and short-term fasting both lower IGF-1 levels.[38, 39]

Dairy

A number of systematic reviews and meta-analyses have implicated dairy, especially whole milk intake, as a risk factor for developing prostate cancer.[40]

Possible reasons for this may include: the intake of exogenous hormones naturally present in cow's milk, such as oestrogen and bovine growth hormone; the intake of IGF-1; the intake of potentially carcinogenic proteins in dairy, such as casein;[41] the intake of saturated fat, which is associated with aggressiveness of prostate cancer;[42] the intake of carcinogenic pesticides from non-organic products.

A recent study funded by the National Cancer Institute, the National Institutes of Health, and the World Cancer Research Fund, found that in a large cohort of over 52,000 American women, a significantly increased risk of developing breast cancer occurred with higher intakes of dairy calories and especially dairy milk, with one cup per day increasing the risk by 50%, and two to three cups per day increasing the risk up to 80%.[43]

It is worth mentioning that studies have shown a reduced risk of colorectal cancer with dairy consumption.[44] This is considered predominantly because of the calcium content of dairy which acts to neutralise the negative impact of secondary bile acids in the gut, compounds that are more readily formed when eating the standard Western-style diet. Calcium can of course be obtained from healthier plant-based sources.

At the current time, studies on dairy as a risk factor for cancers (other than prostate cancer) show differing results although it is possible that some results may be skewed due to an element of bias arising from industry-funded research.

The reader should be alerted to studies sponsored by profit-driven industries that may be designed to produce desired outcomes that conflict with the substantial weight of evidence to the contrary. An example is a 2011 study funded by the National Cattlemen's Beef Association (USA) which found no association between red meat consumption and colorectal cancer.

International guidelines on dairy intake and its relation to cancer prevention will likely evolve as data grows in this area.

Microplastics

Recent years have seen the world's oceans become vastly polluted with toxic waste from industrial and agricultural processes. Microplastics are now universally found throughout the world's oceans, accumulating in the flesh of fish and other aquatic species that mistake small plastic fragments for food. Eighty percent of European anchovies are contaminated with microplastics, along with a significant proportion of other small, oily fish.[45] Over 70% of wild-caught Atlantic fish that have previously been considered to be pure and toxin-free, are now contaminated with microplastics.[46]

Microplastics are highly toxic to the immune system. They are known endocrine disruptors that mimic endogenous hormones such as oestrogen and have been implicated in hormone-driven cancers.[47]

Consuming docosahexaenoic acid (DHA) and eicosapentaenoic acid (EPA) from marine algae would provide a safer source of these long chain fatty acids, given that the manufacturing process usually involves organic cultivation of marine algae that are uncontaminated with pollutants such as microplastics.

Pesticides and persistent organic pollutants

Ocean and land contamination with industrial and agricultural pollutants, collectively known as persistent organic pollutants (POPs), is a global issue, with POPs found in fish in all of the world's oceans and land farmed animals.[48]

These environmental toxins are also present in virtually all non-organic foods and are associated with an increase in the risk of various cancers including thyroid cancer,[49] prostate cancer,[50] lung cancer,[51] colorectal cancer, and increasing the risk of metastasis in breast cancer.[52]

In 2015, the International Agency for Research on Cancer (IARC) classified certain chemicals used in farming, including malathion, glyphosate and diazinon, as group 2 carcinogens.[53] Two large population studies have also shown a potential association between consuming organically produced animal and plant foods and cancer. The Million Women study reported a 21% lower risk of non-Hodgkin lymphoma but not other cancers.[54] The French NutriNet Santé Study demonstrated a significantly lower level of cancer with a 25% reduction in those consuming the most organic foods, mainly due to a 76% reduction in risk for lymphoma and 34% reduction in the risk of post-menopausal breast cancer.[55]

The current guideline for cancer prevention from the American Cancer Society acknowledges the possible link between chemicals used in farming and the development of cancer, although prioritises fruit and vegetable intake in general rather than choosing organic produce, where cost can be prohibitive.

Co-morbidities in cancer development and outcomes

The presence of chronic disease, such as cardiovascular disease, diabetes and kidney disease significantly increases both the risk of developing cancer and the risk of death from cancer, not surprising when we consider that these diseases share common underlying mechanisms including inflammation, insulin resistance, dyslipidaemia and dysbiosis.

Lifestyle factors that are known to increase the risk of comorbidities and chronic disease, such as smoking, being overweight, lack of physical exercise, and high alcohol intake, all contribute to a higher risk of developing and dying from cancer. Conversely, avoiding these risk factors, whilst consuming a diet consisting of a high intake of vegetables, fruits, whole grains, unsaturated fats, and omega-3 fats, and a low intake of red and processed meat, salt, sugar-sweetened beverages, and trans-fats, results in a significantly reduced risk of death from cancer.[56]

One study from Taiwan following more than 400,000 participants for nearly nine years found that around a third of the risk of dying from cancer was due to underlying chronic health conditions, with a further third from unhealthy lifestyle habits.[57] As well as healthy nutrition, physical activity is notably one of the most effective forms of reducing cancer risk, and has been shown to attenuate cancer incidence by 48% and cancer mortality by 27%, in people with underlying chronic disease.

Another study, with data from the Nurses' Health Study and the Health Professionals Follow-up Study from the US followed almost 200,000 participants over 30 years.[58] Participants with a new diagnosis of type 2 diabetes during the follow-up period had a significantly increased risk of developing cancer, particularly, colorectal, lung, pancreas, oesophageal, liver, thyroid, breast, and endometrial cancers. This risk was increased in the first eight years following diagnosis of type 2 diabetes but not after this. Data from the study suggested that high insulin levels may be the contributing factor. Overall, there was a 21% increased risk of total cancer, 28% increased risk of obesity-related cancer, and 25% increased risk of diabetes-related cancer comparing participants with and without diabetes.

Unfortunately the risk of a second primary cancer is also increased by already having a diagnosis of cancer, with potential contributing factors including genetic predisposition, having the same ongoing lifestyle related risk factors, and secondary effects of cancer treatment.[59]

Role of plant-based nutrition for prevention of cancer

The main preventable lifestyle factors that increase the risk of cancer development are tobacco smoking, unhealthy diet, alcohol, lack of physical activity, and unsafe sun exposure, accounting for 40 to 50% of all cancers overall.[4, 56] Although estimates vary, as well as by cancer subtype, the evidence suggests that diet can be the underlying driver in up to 35% of cancer deaths.

Healthy nutrition is one of the cornerstones of cancer prevention advice provided by major international organisations, with a focus on increasing whole plant foods such as vegetables, fruits, whole grains and legumes, and reducing animal products and ultra-processed foods.

These recommendations are based on convincing evidence from epidemiological studies and large prospective cohort studies.

Studies showing reduced risk of cancer with plant-based diets

The Adventist Health Study[60] followed a cohort of over 34,000 Seventh-day Adventists. Cancers of the colon and prostate were significantly more likely in nonvegetarians compared with vegetarians, and higher consumption of fruit was associated with lower risks of lung, prostate, and pancreatic cancers.

The Adventist Health Study II which involved over 73,000 participants, identified a 16% reduced risk of cancer in those consuming a vegan diet, and an 8% reduced risk of cancer in those eating a vegetarian diet, compared to non-vegetarians.[61]

Pooled results from the EPIC-Oxford Study[62] and the Oxford Vegetarian Study[63] reported that that vegetarians (including vegans) had a lower risk than did nonvegetarians for all cancers combined, as well as a lower risk of cancers of the stomach, bladder, and cancers of the lymphatic and haematopoietic tissue, but a higher risk of cervical cancer. The increased risk of cervical cancer in vegetarians in this study was a non-significant finding, having been observed in only 50 cases overall and reported by the researchers as possibly being related to non-dietary factors, or having occurred by chance. The total cancer incidence was 19% lower in vegans compared with meat eaters.[64]

The reduced risk of developing cancer in vegans and vegetarians compared with meat eaters has been consistently reproduced, as evidenced by the above large prospective cohort studies and a recent systematic review and meta-analysis of cross-sectional and prospective cohort studies that showed a 15% reduced risk of cancer in those consuming a vegan diet.[65]

Ultraprocessed foods

Ultraprocessed foods are usually packaged foods that contain added ingredients such as preservatives and colourings, or that are cooked in ways that are known to generate carcinogens. They comprise a significant percentage of food, and about 50% of total calories, bought from UK supermarkets.

In a large population-based cohort study involving over 100,000 individuals, a 10% increase in the proportion of ultra-processed foods in the diet was associated with a 12% increased risk of overall cancer.[66]

Alcohol

Globally, an estimated 749,300 cases, accounting for 4·1% of all new cases of cancer in 2020 were attributable to alcohol consumption. Cancers of the oesophagus, liver, and breast contributed the most cases.[67]

There are various possible mechanisms by which alcohol may induce malignant change.[68] Ethanol is oxidised to acetaldehyde by alcohol dehydrogenase enzymes. Acetaldehyde, categorised by the IARC as a group 2B carcinogen (i.e. possibly carcinogenic to humans), may contribute to oxidative stress by binding to DNA and stimulating several pathways including lipid peroxidation, resulting in the release of oxygen free radicals.

Excessive alcohol induces the CYP2E1 pathway which enhances the catabolism of retinoic acid. This can impact several signalling pathways, including oestrogen signalling, which may enhance malignant transformation of pre-cancerous cells.

Chronic alcohol intake can also lead to an increase in the types of immune cells that hinder immunosurveillance against malignant cells, such as regulatory T cells.

It is generally agreed that there is no safe limit for alcohol consumption in cancer prevention, and therefore international guidelines concur that alcohol should be minimised, if not removed completely, for cancer prevention.

International recommendations for cancer prevention

The most recent dietary recommendations for the prevention of cancer by the World Cancer Research Fund (WCRF) and American Institute of Cancer Research comprise the following:[69]
- keeping weight within the healthy range throughout life (BMI of 18.5–24.9)
- undertaking moderate physical activity
- eating a diet that is high in all types of plant foods including at least five portions or servings of a variety of non-starchy vegetables and fruit every day, at least 30 g per day of fibre, and that contains wholegrains, non-starchy vegetables, fruit and pulses (legumes) such as beans and lentils in most meals
- limiting consumption of processed foods such as burgers, chips, sugary drinks and products made from white flour

- limiting red meat to no more than three portions per week, and consuming very little, if any, processed meat
- avoiding drinks sweetened with sugar
- avoiding the use of high-dose dietary supplements for cancer prevention, instead aiming to meet nutritional needs through diet
- for mothers, breastfeeding the baby to protect against breast cancer
- continuing to follow this guidance following a cancer diagnosis.

Very similar nutrition guidance is advised by the American Cancer Society,[70] again with a focus on nutrient-dense plant foods including vegetables and fruits of different colours, whole grains and legumes. The American Cancer Society guidelines are more explicit in stating that a healthy diet limits *or does not include* red and processed meats.

Benefits of whole plant foods for cancer prevention

Fibre
Dietary fibre is a complex carbohydrate that is inversely associated with colorectal cancer.[71]

Possible mechanisms include improving gut transit time and bowel frequency, thus potentially reducing the amount of time carcinogens in food spend in close contact with the gut mucosa. Insoluble fibre in particular, such as that found in nuts, beans and wholegrains, increases stool size, partly through higher water retention, thus diluting potential carcinogens and secondary bile acids, a mechanism that may protect against the development of colorectal cancer.

Fibre also acts as a prebiotic for gut microbiota, enabling the production of anti-inflammatory short chain fatty acids such as butyrate, which protects the colorectal mucosa from oxidative stress and malignant change.

Both soluble and insoluble fibre intake helps to maintain a healthy weight, an important factor in preventing cancer.

Dietary fibre is present only in whole plant foods such as fruits, vegetables and legumes, with a recommended daily intake of fibre of 30g a day at the time of printing.

Whole grains
Wholegrains are the seeds of cereal plants, with preservation of their bran (fibre-rich outer layer), germ (nutrient-rich inner layer) and endosperm (starchy core). The bran and germ layers are removed during processing methods, resulting in the typical white appearance of refined grains.

Dietary intake of whole grains, such as brown rice, oats, quinoa, whole wheat, buckwheat and millet, is associated with a lower cancer mortality, with every 90 g/day intake of whole grains associated with a 15% lower risk of cancer death.[72]

Fruits and vegetables
Fruits and vegetables contain a plethora of antioxidants and nutrients known to reduce cancer risk via a variety of mechanisms. A low intake of fruits and vegetables is associated with deficiency of vital nutrients such as folate, dietary fibre and the antioxidant vitamins, A, C and E, leading to DNA instability, increased oxidative stress and inflammation and reduced capacity for initiating programmed cell death, or apoptosis.

Most current authorities recommend a minimum of five portions of fruits and vegetables a day, although a recent meta-analysis of prospective studies estimated that about 7.8 million premature deaths could be prevented every year by increasing fruit and vegetable consumption to about ten portions a day.[73]

Legumes
Legumes are a rich source of fibre, protein, B vitamins and minerals. Meta-analyses reveal that higher legume consumption is associated with a reduced risk of colorectal[74] and prostate cancer.[75]

Higher legume and lentil consumption is associated with between 37–49% lower risk of cancer mortality.[76]

Soya

A meta-analysis of 23 prospective studies involving over 330,000 individuals identified an inverse relationship of soya and cancer mortality, with a 10 mg per day intake of soya associated with 7% decreased mortality from all cancers, and each 5 g per day associated with a 12% reduction in breast cancer deaths.[77] Another large analysis of all the human data on soya consumption, which includes 114 meta-analyses and systematic reviews reported a significant reduction in the risk of a number of cancers, including ovarian (48% reduction), gastric (37%), prostate (29%), breast (13%), colorectal (24%), endometrial (19%) and lung (17%).[78]

Role of plant-based nutrition during cancer treatment

The optimum diet whilst undergoing treatment for cancer is an area of ongoing research. Current international guidelines for nutrition during cancer treatment, are similar to those for cancer prevention, with recommendations to aim for a low saturated fat and high-fibre diet by eating more plant-based foods and avoiding or limiting the intake of processed and red meats, processed foods, and alcohol.[79]

There is growing evidence that a healthy gut microbiome is associated with improved outcomes with certain treatments, especially immunotherapies but also chemotherapy and some targeted therapies.[80]

The gut microbiota interacts closely with the immune system and can impact treatment efficiency through various measures including: modulating drug metabolism; overcoming drug resistance; promoting the maturation of immune cells such as dendritic cells and natural killer cells; mediating toxicity; and anti-inflammatory cytokine production, amongst other proposed mechanisms.[81]

Lifestyle factors such as adequate sleep, physical exercise and stress are all important factors in influencing the gut microbiota. Nutrition also plays a leading role, with plant foods providing fibre to feed and enhance the diversity of beneficial microbiota.[14]

Fasting

Cancer cells are dependent on a continuous supply of nutrients, and vulnerable when this supply is interrupted. Mounting evidence from pre-clinical studies supports the role of short term fasting during cancer treatments, with data showing that short-term fasting generates a differential stress resistance between healthy cells and tumour cells, essentially increasing the resilience of healthy cells to treatment toxicity, whilst augmenting the sensitivity of tumour cells to the same treatment.

The mechanisms for inducing differential stress resistance are still being explored but one of the likely regulators is the growth factor IGF-1, levels of which are reduced following short-term fasting. Nutrient-sensing pathways are also modulated in the presence of nutrient scarcity, and re-directed to enhance cellular repair, rather than cellular growth.[38]

Pre-clinical studies show that short-term fasting, or calorie restriction of 48 hours is safe and may reduce chemotherapy-related side effects and improve treatment efficacy.[38]

In 2020, de Groot et al. reported the findings of the first randomised study of fasting, using the fasting mimicking diet (FMD), in patients with cancer.[82] The FMD is a five-day plant-based low calorie diet (800–1,100 calories/day) developed by Dr Valter Longo and designed to mimic the effects of water fasting. The study was based on

131 patients with breast cancer requiring chemotherapy and randomised to either FMD for three days pre chemotherapy and on the day of chemotherapy or to continue their usual diet. The results showed that the response to chemotherapy was better in the FMD group, with potentially less treatment toxicity. Unfortunately, there was a high dropout rate in the FMD group due to tolerability of the fasting regimen, and in the control group, five people fasted even though they were not meant to.

The data so far on fasting as a therapeutic modality are preliminary only. More information is required on the optimal composition and acceptability of the fasting diet, the mechanisms, and its efficacy in different cancer subtype and treatment settings. Fasting is not recommended in patients who are underweight, and caution must be used for those with underlying medical conditions such as diabetes. In these circumstances fasting should be undertaken only under medical supervision.

Role of plant-based nutrition after a cancer diagnosis

Following a diagnosis of cancer, there is evidence that altering the diet to include more whole plant foods and reduce the intake of saturated fats may improve several parameters including survival.[83]

In men diagnosed with early-stage prostate cancer, intervention with whole food plant-based nutrition, regular physical exercise and stress relieving activities, resulted in a drop in prostate specific antigen (PSA) levels and a reduced need for conventional treatment.[84]

In a large randomised controlled study by the Women's Health Initiative, of 48,835 postmenopausal women, with 19.6 years median follow up, mortality rates, including a 21% reduced risk of dying of breast cancer, dropped significantly in those who consumed a low-fat, mainly plant-based diet following a diagnosis of breast cancer, compared to those who did not.[85]

In colorectal-cancer, those who consume a prudent diet (mainly plant-based and low saturated fat diet with high intakes of fruit, vegetables and whole grains) have improved overall survival and reduced rates of colorectal cancer recurrence, compared to those who consume a Western-type diet (high saturated fat intake, higher meat and high fat dairy products, refined grains, and desserts).[86]

Maintaining a healthy body weight is important following a cancer diagnosis, as patients with a raised BMI have a higher risk of recurrence and mortality.[87]

International guidelines recommend similar dietary guidance, both for cancer prevention and following a cancer diagnosis.[69]

Conclusion

Ample data point to the fact that the adoption of whole food plant-based nutrition, providing high-fibre, antioxidant-rich, phytochemical-rich, nutrient-dense plant foods, is one of the most effective measures that can be taken both to reduce the risk of cancer development and to improve outcomes following a diagnosis of cancer.

The inclusion of appropriate dietary advice is a vital aspect of a physician's armamentarium in treating cancer. Education on nutrition should be incorporated into training programmes for oncologists and all health professionals involved in cancer care and should be viewed as an integral part of routine oncology appointments.

References

1. WHO. Cancer. Key Facts. World Health Organization. www.who.int/news-room/fact-sheets/detail/cancer [accessed 3 April 2021]

2. Smittenaar CR, Petersen KA, Stewart K, Moitt N. Cancer incidence and mortality projections in the UK until 2035. *Br J Cancer* 2016; 115(9): 1147-1155. doi:10.1038/bjc.2016.304
3. Champ CE, Mishra MV, Showalter TN et al. Dietary recommendations during and after cancer treatment: consistently inconsistent? *Nutr Cancer* 2013; 65(3): 430-439.
doi: 10.1080/01635581.2013.757629
4. Anand P, Kunnumakkara AB, Sundaram C et al. Cancer is a preventable disease that requires major lifestyle changes. *Pharm Res* 2008; 25(9): 2097-2116. doi: 10.1007/s11095-008-9661-9
5. Ravasco P. Nutrition in Cancer Patients. *J Clin Med* 2019; 8(8): 1211. doi: 10.3390/jcm8081211
6. Hanahan D, Weinberg RA. Hallmarks of cancer: the next generation. *Cell* 2011; 144(5): 646-674. doi: 10.1016/j.cell.2011.02.013
7. Lachance JC, Radhakrishnan S, Madiwale G et al. Targeting hallmarks of cancer with a food-system-based approach. *Nutrition* 2020; 69: 110563. doi: 10.1016/j.nut.2019.110563
8. Chirumbolo S, Bjørklund G, Lysiuk R et al. Targeting Cancer with Phytochemicals via Their Fine Tuning of the Cell Survival Signaling Pathways. *Int J Mol Sci* 2018; 19(11): 3568. doi: 10.3390/ijms19113568
9. Grivennikov SI, Greten FR, Karin M. Immunity, inflammation, and cancer. *Cell* 2010; 140(6): 883-899. doi: 10.1016/j.cell.2010.01.025
10. Bower JE, Lamkin DM. Inflammation and cancer-related fatigue: mechanisms, contributing factors, and treatment implications. *Brain Behav Immun* 2013; 30 Suppl(0): S48-S57.
doi: 10.1016/j.bbi.2012.06.011
11. Lanser L, Kink P, Egger EM et al. Inflammation-Induced Tryptophan Breakdown is Related With Anemia, Fatigue, and Depression in Cancer. *Front Immunol* 2020; 11: 249.
doi: 10.3389/fimmu.2020.00249
12. Webster JM, Kempen LJAP, Hardy RS, Langen RCJ. Inflammation and Skeletal Muscle Wasting During Cachexia. *Front Physiol* 2020; 11: 597675. doi: 10.3389/fphys.2020.597675
13. Proctor MJ, McMillan DC, Horgan PG, Fletcher CD, Talwar D, Morrison DS. Systemic inflammation predicts all-cause mortality: a glasgow inflammation outcome study. *PLoS One* 2015; 10(3): e0116206.
doi: 10.1371/journal.pone.0116206
14. Singh RK, Chang HW, Yan D, Lee KM, Ucmak D, Wong K, Abrouk M, Farahnik B, Nakamura M, Zhu TH, Bhutani T, Liao W. Influence of diet on the gut microbiome and implications for human health. *J Transl Med* 2017; 15(1): 73.
doi: 10.1186/s12967-017-1175-y
15. De Pergola G, Silvestris F. Obesity as a major risk factor for cancer. *J Obes* 2013; 2013: 291546. doi:10.1155/2013/291546
16. Renehan AG, Zwahlen M, Egger M. Adiposity and cancer risk: new mechanistic insights from epidemiology. *Nat Rev Cancer* 2015; 15(8): 484-98. doi: 10.1038/nrc3967
17. Bradbury KE, Murphy N, Key TJ. Diet and colorectal cancer in UK Biobank: a prospective study. *Int J Epidemiol* 2020; 49(1): 246-258.
doi: 10.1093/ije/dyz064
18. Farvid, MS, Stern MC, Norat T, et al. Consumption of red and processed meat and breast cancer incidence: A systematic review and meta-analysis of prospective studies. *International Journal of Cancer* 2018; 143(11): 2787-2799.
doi: 10.1002/ijc.31848
19. Li F, An S, Hou L, Chen P, Lei C, Tan W. Red and processed meat intake and risk of bladder cancer: a meta-analysis. *Int J Clin Exp Med* 2014; 7(8): 2100-2110.
20. Wolk, A. Potential health hazards of eating red meat. Journal of Internal Medicine 2017; 281(2): 106-122. doi:10.1111/joim.12543
21. Hughes R, Cross AJ, Pollock JR, Bingham S. Dose-dependent effect of dietary meat on endogenous colonic N-nitrosation. Carcinogenesis 2001; 22(1): 199-202. doi: 10.1093/carcin/22.1.199
22. Gurjao C, Zhong R, Haruki K, et al. Discovery and Features of an Alkylating Signature in Colorectal Cancer. *Cancer Discov* 2021; 11(10): 2446-2455. doi:10.1158/2159-8290.CD-20-1656
23. Janeiro MH, Ramírez MJ, Milagro FI et al. Implication of Trimethylamine N-Oxide (TMAO) in Disease: Potential Biomarker or New Therapeutic Target. *Nutrients* 2018; 10(10): 1398. doi: 10.3390/nu10101398
24. Guertin KA, Li XS, Graubard BI et al. Serum Trimethylamine N-oxide, Carnitine, Choline, and Betaine in Relation to Colorectal Cancer Risk

in the Alpha Tocopherol, Beta Carotene Cancer Prevention Study. *Cancer Epidemiol Biomarkers Prev* 2017; 26(6): 945-952. doi: 10.1158/1055-9965
25. Fiorito V, Chiabrando D, Petrillo S et al. The Multifaceted Role of Heme in Cancer. Front Oncol 2020; 9: 1540. doi: 10.3389/fonc.2019.01540
26. Bastide NM, Pierre FH, Corpet DE. Heme iron from meat and risk of colorectal cancer: a meta-analysis and a review of the mechanisms involved. Cancer Prev Res (Phila) 2011; 4(2): 177-184. doi: 10.1158/1940-6207.CAPR-10-0113
27. Fonseca-Nunes A, Jakszyn P, Agudo A. Iron and cancer risk--a systematic review and meta-analysis of the epidemiological evidence. *Cancer Epidemiol Biomarkers Prev* 2014; 23(1): 12-31. doi: 10.1158/1055-9965
28. Chang VC, Cotterchio M, Khoo E. Iron intake, body iron status, and risk of breast cancer: a systematic review and meta-analysis. *BMC Cancer* 2019; 19(1): 543. doi: 10.1186/s12885-019-5642-0
29. Ma J, Li Q, Fang X et al. Increased total iron and zinc intake and lower heme iron intake reduce the risk of esophageal cancer: A dose-response meta-analysis. *Nutr Res* 2018; 59: 16-28. doi: 10.1016/j.nutres.2018.07.007
30. Ward HA, Whitman J, Muller DC et al. Haem iron intake and risk of lung cancer in the European Prospective Investigation into Cancer and Nutrition (EPIC) cohort. *Eur J Clin Nutr* 2019; 73(8): 1122-1132. doi: 10.1038/s41430-018-0271-2
31. Gnagnarella P, Caini S, Maisonneuve P, Gandini S. Carcinogenicity of High Consumption of Meat and Lung Cancer Risk Among Non-Smokers: A Comprehensive Meta-Analysis. *Nutr Cancer* 2018; 70(1): 1-13. doi: 10.1080/01635581.2017.1374420
32. Turner ND, Lloyd SK. Association between red meat consumption and colon cancer: A systematic review of experimental results. *Exp Biol Med* 2017; 242(8): 813-839. doi: 10.1177/1535370217693117
33. Chiavarini M, Bertarelli G, Minelli L, Fabiani R. Dietary Intake of Meat Cooking-Related Mutagens (HCAs) and Risk of Colorectal Adenoma and Cancer: A Systematic Review and Meta-Analysis. *Nutrients* 2017; 9(5): 514. doi: 10.3390/nu9050514
34. Gooderham NJ, Creton S, Lauber SN, Zhu H. Mechanisms of action of the carcinogenic heterocyclic amine PhIP. *Toxicol Lett* 2007; 168(3): 269-277. doi: 10.1016/j.toxlet.2006.10.022
35. Murray S, Lake BG, Gray S et al. Effect of cruciferous vegetable consumption on heterocyclic aromatic amine metabolism in man. *Carcinogenesis* 2001; 22(9): 1413-1420. doi: 10.1093/carcin/22.9.1413
36. Bowers LW, Rossi EL, O'Flanagan CH et al. The Role of the Insulin/IGF System in Cancer: Lessons Learned from Clinical Trials and the Energy Balance-Cancer Link. *Front Endocrinol* 2015; 6: 77. doi: 10.3389/fendo.2015.00077.
37. Grimberg A. Mechanisms by which IGF-I may promote cancer. *Cancer Biol Ther* 2003; 2(6): 630-635.
38. de Groot S, Pijl H, van der Hoeven JJM, Kroep JR. Effects of short-term fasting on cancer treatment. *J Exp Clin Cancer Res* 2019; 38(1): 209. doi: 10.1186/s13046-019-1189-9
39. Allen NE, Appleby PN, Davey GK et al. The associations of diet with serum insulin-like growth factor I and its main binding proteins in 292 women meat-eaters, vegetarians, and vegans. *Cancer Epidemiol Biomarkers Prev* 2002; 11(11): 1441-1448.
40. Aune D, Navarro Rosenblatt DA, Chan DS et al. Dairy products, calcium, and prostate cancer risk: a systematic review and meta-analysis of cohort studies. *Am J Clin Nutr* 2015; 101(1): 87-117. doi: 10.3945/ajcn.113.067157
41. Park SW, Kim JY, Kim YS et al. A milk protein, casein, as a proliferation promoting factor in prostate cancer cells. *World J Mens Health* 2014; 32(2): 76-82. doi: 10.5534/wjmh.2014.32.2.76
42. Allott EH, Arab L, Su LJ et al. Saturated fat intake and prostate cancer aggressiveness: results from the population-based North Carolina-Louisiana Prostate Cancer Project. *Prostate Cancer Prostatic Dis* 2017; 20(1): 48-54. doi: 10.1038/pcan.2016.39
43. Fraser GE, Jaceldo-Siegl K, Orlich M, Mashchak A, Sirirat R, Knutsen S. Dairy, soy, and risk of breast cancer: those confounded milks. *Int J Epidemiol* 2020; 49(5): 1526-1537. doi: 10.1093/ije/dyaa007
44. Aune D, Lau R, Chan DSM, et al. Dairy products

and colorectal cancer risk: A systematic review and meta-analysis of cohort studies. *Annals of Oncology* 2012; 23(1): 37-45 doi:10.1093/annonc/mdr269

45. Collard F, Gilbert B, Compère P et al. Microplastics in livers of European anchovies (Engraulis encrasicolus, L.). *Environ Pollut* 2017; 229: 1000-1005. doi: 10.1016/j.envpol.2017.07.089

46. Wieczorek AM, Morrison L, Croot PL et al. Frequency of Microplastics in Mesopelagic Fishes from the Northwest Atlantic. *Frontiers in Marine Science* 2018; 5: 39. doi: 10.3389/fmars.2018.00039

47. Campanale C, Massarelli C, Savino I et al. A Detailed Review Study on Potential Effects of Microplastics and Additives of Concern on Human Health. *Int J Environ Res Public Health* 2020; 17(4): 1212. doi: 10.3390/ijerph17041212

48. Bonito LT, Hamdoun A, Sandin SA. Evaluation of the global impacts of mitigation on persistent, bioaccumulative and toxic pollutants in marine fish. *PeerJ* 2016; 4: e1573. doi: 10.7717/peerj.1573

49. Han MA, Kim JH, Song HS. Persistent organic pollutants, pesticides, and the risk of thyroid cancer: systematic review and meta-analysis. *Eur J Cancer Prev* 2019; 28(4): 344-349. doi: 10.1097/CEJ.0000000000000481

50. Lim JE, Park SH, Jee SH, Park H. Body concentrations of persistent organic pollutants and prostate cancer: a meta-analysis. *Environ Sci Pollut Res Int* 2015; 22(15): 11275-11284. doi: 10.1007/s11356-015-4315-z

51. Park EY, Park E, Kim J, Oh JK, Kim B, Hong YC, Lim MK. Impact of environmental exposure to persistent organic pollutants on lung cancer risk. *Environ Int* 2020; 143: 105925. doi: 10.1016/j.envint.2020.105925

52. Koual M, Cano-Sancho G, Bats AS, et al. Associations between persistent organic pollutants and risk of breast cancer metastasis. *Environ Int* 2019; 132: 105028. doi: 10.1016/j.envint.2019.105028

53. Guyton KZ, Loomis D, Grosse Y, et al. Carcinogenicity of tetrachlorvinphos, parathion, malathion, diazinon, and glyphosate. *Lancet Oncol* 2015; 16(5): 490-491. doi:10.1016/S1470-2045(15)70134-8

54. Bradbury KE, Balkwill A, Spencer EA, et al. Organic food consumption and the incidence of cancer in a large prospective study of women in the United Kingdom. *Br J Cancer* 2014; 110(9): 2321-2326. doi:10.1038/bjc.2014.148

55. Baudry J, Assmann KE, Touvier M, et al. Association of Frequency of Organic Food Consumption with Cancer Risk: Findings from the NutriNet-Santé Prospective Cohort Study. *JAMA Internal Medicine* 2018; 178(12): 1597-1606.

56. Li Y, Pan A, Wang DD et al. Impact of Healthy Lifestyle Factors on Life Expectancies in the US Population. *Circulation* 2018; 138(4): 345-355. doi: 10.1161/CIRCULATIONAHA.117.032047

57. Tu H, Wen CP, Tsai SP et al. Cancer risk associated with chronic diseases and disease markers: prospective cohort study. *BMJ* 2018; 360: k134. doi: 10.1136/bmj.k134

58. Hu Y, Zhang X, Ma Y, et al. Incident Type 2 Diabetes Duration and Cancer Risk: A Prospective Study in Two US Cohorts. *JNCI: Journal of the National Cancer Institute* 2021; 113(4): 381-389. doi: 10.1093/jnci/djaa141

59. Sung H, Hyun N, Leach CR, Yabroff KR, Jemal A. Association of First Primary Cancer With Risk of Subsequent Primary Cancer Among Survivors of Adult-Onset Cancers in the United States. *JAMA* 2020; 324(24): 2521–2535. doi:10.1001/jama.2020.23130

60. Fraser GE. Associations between diet and cancer, ischemic heart disease, and all-cause mortality in non-Hispanic white California Seventh-day Adventists. *Am J Clin Nutr* 1999; 70(3 Suppl): 532S-538S. doi: 10.1093/ajcn/70.3.532s

61. Segovia-Siapco G, Sabaté J. Health and sustainability outcomes of vegetarian dietary patterns: a revisit of the EPIC-Oxford and the Adventist Health Study-2 cohorts. *Eur J Clin Nutr* 2019; 72(Suppl 1): 60-70. doi: 10.1038/s41430-018-0310-z

62. Davey GK, Spencer EA, Appleby PN, Allen NE, Knox KH, Key TJ. EPIC-Oxford: lifestyle characteristics and nutrient intakes in a cohort of 33 883 meat-eaters and 31 546 non meat-eaters in the UK. *Public Health Nutr* 2003; 6(3): 259-69. doi: 10.1079/PHN2002430

63. Appleby PN, Thorogood M, Mann JI, Key TJ. The Oxford Vegetarian Study: an overview. *Am J Clin*

Nutr 1999; 70(3 Suppl): 525S-531S. doi: 10.1093/ajcn/70.3.525s

64. Key TJ, Appleby PN, Crowe FL et al. Cancer in British vegetarians: updated analyses of 4998 incident cancers in a cohort of 32,491 meat eaters, 8612 fish eaters, 18,298 vegetarians, and 2246 vegans. *Am J Clin Nutr* 2014; 1(1): 378S-85S. doi: 10.3945/ajcn.113.071266

65. Dinu M, Abbate R, Gensini GF, Casini A, Sofi F. Vegetarian, vegan diets and multiple health outcomes: A systematic review with meta-analysis of observational studies. *Crit Rev Food Sci Nutr* 2017; 57(17): 3640-3649. doi: 10.1080/10408398.2016.1138447

66. Fiolet T, Srour B, Sellem L et al. Consumption of ultra-processed foods and cancer risk: results from NutriNet-Santé prospective cohort. *BMJ* 2018; 360: k322. doi: 10.1136/bmj.k322

67. Rumgay H, Shield K, Charvat H, Ferrari P, Sornpaisarn B, Obot I, Islami F, Lemmens VEPP, Rehm J, Soerjomataram I. Global burden of cancer in 2020 attributable to alcohol consumption: a population-based study. *Lancet Oncol* 2021; 22(8): 1071-1080. doi: 10.1016/S1470-2045(21)00279-5

68. Ratna A, Mandrekar P. Alcohol and Cancer: Mechanisms and Therapies. *Biomolecules* 2017; 7(3): 61. doi: 10.3390/biom7030061

69. World Cancer Research Fund. Cancer Prevention Recommendations. www.wcrf.org/dietandcancer/cancer-prevention-recommendations [Accessed 30th March 2021]

70. Rock CL, Thomson C, Gansler T et al. American Cancer Society guideline for diet and physical activity for cancer prevention. *CA Cancer J Clin* 2020; 70(4): 245-271. doi: 10.3322/caac.21591

71. Murphy N, Norat T, Ferrari P et al. Dietary fibre intake and risks of cancers of the colon and rectum in the European prospective investigation into cancer and nutrition (EPIC). *PLoS One* 2012; 7(6): e39361. doi: 10.1371/journal.pone.0039361

72. Aune D, Keum N, Giovannucci E et al. Whole grain consumption and risk of cardiovascular disease, cancer, and all cause and cause specific mortality: systematic review and dose-response meta-analysis of prospective studies. *BMJ* 2016; 353: i2716. doi: 10.1136/bmj.i2716

73. Aune D, Giovannucci E, Boffetta P et al. Fruit and vegetable intake and the risk of cardiovascular disease, total cancer and all-cause mortality-a systematic review and dose-response meta-analysis of prospective studies. *Int J Epidemiol* 2017; 46(3): 1029-1056. doi: 10.1093/ije/dyw319

74. Zhu B, Sun Y, Qi L, Zhong R, Miao X. Dietary legume consumption reduces risk of colorectal cancer: evidence from a meta-analysis of cohort studies. *Sci Rep* 2015; 5: 8797. doi: 10.1038/srep08797

75. Li J, Mao QQ. Legume intake and risk of prostate cancer: a meta-analysis of prospective cohort studies. *Oncotarget* 2017; 8(27): 44776-44784. doi: 10.18632/oncotarget.16794

76. Papandreou C, Becerra-Tomás N, Bulló M et al. Legume consumption and risk of all-cause, cardiovascular, and cancer mortality in the PREDIMED study. *Clin Nutr* 2019; 38(1): 348-356. doi: 10.1016/j.clnu.2017.12.019

77. Nachvak SM, Moradi S, Anjom-Shoae J et al. Soy, Soy Isoflavones, and Protein Intake in Relation to Mortality from All Causes, Cancers, and Cardiovascular Diseases: A Systematic Review and Dose-Response Meta-Analysis of Prospective Cohort Studies. *J Acad Nutr Diet* 2019; 119(9): 1483-1500.e17. doi: 10.1016/j.jand.2019.04.011

78. Li N, Wu X, Zhuang W, Xia L, Chen Y, Zhao R, Yi M, Wan Q, Du L, Zhou Y. Soy and Isoflavone Consumption and Multiple Health Outcomes: Umbrella Review of Systematic Reviews and Meta-Analyses of Observational Studies and Randomized Trials in Humans. *Mol Nutr Food Res* 2020; 64(4): e1900751. doi: 10.1002/mnfr.201900751

79. American Cancer Society. Nutrition and Physical Activity During and After Cancer Treatment: Answers to Common Questions. www.cancer.org/treatment/survivorship-during-and-after-treatment/staying-active/nutrition-and-physical-activity-during-and-after-cancer-treatment.html [Accessed 3 April 2021]

80. Ma W, Mao Q, Xia W, Dong G, Yu C, Jiang F. Gut Microbiota Shapes the Efficiency of Cancer Therapy. *Front Microbiol* 2019; 10: 1050. doi: 10.3389/fmicb.2019.01050

81. Gopalakrishnan V, Helmink BA, Spencer CN, Reuben A, Wargo JA. The Influence of the Gut Microbiome on Cancer, Immunity, and Cancer Immunotherapy. *Cancer Cell* 2018; 33(4):

570-580. doi: 10.1016/j.ccell.2018.03.015

82. de Groot S, Lugtenberg RT, Cohen D, et al. Dutch Breast Cancer Research Group (BOOG). Fasting mimicking diet as an adjunct to neoadjuvant chemotherapy for breast cancer in the multicentre randomized phase 2 DIRECT trial. *Nat Commun* 2020; 11(1): 3083.
doi: 10.1038/s41467-020-16138-3

83. Li H, Zeng X, Wang Y, Zhang Z, Zhu Y, Li X, Hu A, Zhao Q, Yang W. A prospective study of healthful and unhealthful plant-based diet and risk of overall and cause-specific mortality. *Eur J Nutr* 2021; 61(1): 387-398.
doi: 10.1007/s00394-021-02660-7

84. Ornish D, Weidner G, Fair WR et al. Intensive lifestyle changes may affect the progression of prostate cancer. *J Urol* 2005; 174(3): 1065-1069. doi: 10.1097/01.ju.0000169487.49018.73

85. Chlebowski RT, Aragaki AK, Anderson GL et al. Women's Health Initiative. Dietary Modification and Breast Cancer Mortality: Long-Term Follow-Up of the Women's Health Initiative Randomized Trial. *J Clin Oncol* 2020; 38(13): 1419-1428. doi: 10.1200/JCO.19.00435

86. Meyerhardt JA, Niedzwiecki D, Hollis D, Saltz LB, Hu FB, Mayer RJ, Nelson H, Whittom R, Hantel A, Thomas J, Fuchs CS. Association of dietary patterns with cancer recurrence and survival in patients with stage III colon cancer. *JAMA* 2007; 298(7): 754-764. doi: 10.1001/jama.298.7.754

87. Calle EE, Rodriguez C, Walker-Thurmond K, Thun MJ. Overweight, obesity, and mortality from cancer in a prospectively studied cohort of U.S. adults. *N Engl J Med* 2003; 348(17): 1625-1638. doi: 10.1056/NEJMoa021423

Chapter 5
Plant-based nutrition for respiratory and sleep health

Priyumvada Naik

Introduction

The scientific literature examining the effects of animal foods and lung health largely focuses on the environmental effects of living near or working in large animal farms; and to some extent the global environmental health effects caused by climate change (in large part driven by of our dependence on animal industries). Any examination of the impacts of animal foods on lung health must be conducted with the understanding that occupational and other exposures to animals are not generally considered by physicians. As the focus of this text is the impacts of diets which incorporate animal-based foods, occupational and environmental exposures will not be addressed here, but the author encourages healthcare professionals to study this essential influence on human health.

There is a dearth of existing literature and ongoing studies examining the potential relationship between purely plant-based diets (PBDs) – diets devoid of any animal products whatsoever – and lung health. Most dietary studies looking at healthfulness of diets and association with diseases involve 'plant forward' diets, such as the Mediterranean diet. Despite this potential limitation, there are sufficient data suggesting an association between low fruit and vegetable, fibre, and antioxidant intake, and decline in lung function. Herein, we present the available data examining PBDs (or diets that emphasise plant-based foods) and lung diseases.

Weight and respiratory health

No examination of respiratory health is complete without addressing the importance of maintaining a healthy weight. Multiple disease processes managed by the general and specialist clinician are impacted by excess body weight, and this is particularly critical for chronic lung diseases. Extra pulmonary restriction (reduction of functional lung volume unrelated to lung parenchymal disease), decreased exercise tolerance, sleep disordered breathing, decreased respiratory muscle strength, and dysfunctional respiratory and diaphragm mechanics with decreased respiratory system compliance and increased pulmonary resistance have been documented in the setting of excess weight. Even gas exchange and bronchial hyperresponsiveness can be impacted. Many of these changes are due to the mechanical aspects of holding excess weight, particularly if the distribution of adipose tissue is in the thorax or abdomen[1] but adipose tissue itself is associated with production of many proinflammatory markers, all of which can have profound effects on airways and lung parenchyma.[2]

Plant-based diets may modulate these effects through decreased inflammatory burden and decreased adiposity. The potential anti-inflammatory effects of PBDs are discussed in later sections.

Multiple groups have reported that plant-based diets result in significant weight loss.[3] In fact, a 2006 review of 87 studies by Berkow and Barnard concluded that a vegan or vegetarian diet is effective for weight loss independent of activity level, with an average loss of one pound per week. The group found in both this review and a more recent study that a vegan diet caused more calories to be burned after meals, in contrast to non-vegan diets; they hypothesise that a non-vegan diet may result in fewer calories being burned because food is being stored as fat.[4] Furthermore, in an analysis of national data from the National Health and Nutrition Examination Survey (NHANES) (1999–2004), Wang and Beysoun found a positive association between meat consumption and obesity.[5]

Most studies group vegan and vegetarian diets together or include the Mediterranean diet as a 'plant forward' diet, though the latter two eating patterns do include animal products to varying degrees. Furthermore, much of the data comes from observational trials. Interestingly, a recent study in the Journal of the American College of Nutrition did a head-to-head comparison of a purely plant-based diet with the Mediterranean diet (following the PREDIMED protocol[6]). They found that the purely PBD group had an average weight loss of 6 kg in 16 weeks (no mean change in the PREDIMED group) and lost more overall fat mass as well as visceral fat. They further had improvements in lipid concentrations and insulin sensitivity.[7]

Importantly, multiple large-scale studies indicate that PBDs are an excellent weight loss and weight maintenance strategy. Both the EPIC[8] and Adventist[9] cohorts amongst others[4] have reported lower BMIs on average amongst vegans when compared to meat eaters. With this in mind, it is clear that a PBD can and should be an important tool in the prevention and treatment of many chronic respiratory diseases, particularly those influenced by weight.

For a more in-depth discussion of plant-based nutrition and overweight and obesity, please see Chapter 6.

Chronic obstructive pulmonary disease (COPD)

COPD is the third leading cause of death worldwide, and the fourth leading cause of death in lower-middle-income countries[10] (see Figures 5.1 and 5.2). In 2019, this translated to 3.23 million deaths, over 80% of which occurred in low- and middle-income countries.[11]

COPD is an umbrella term for multiple, progressive respiratory illnesses, including emphysema, chronic bronchitis, and small airways obstruction. The hallmark of all of these disorders is chronic inflammation of the airways and lung parenchyma which result in irreversible airflow limitation.[12] Clinically, patients may experience dyspnoea, cough with or without sputum, and bronchospasm (wheezing, chest tightness), though there is some variability in symptoms.[13] Radiographically, COPD can vary based on type of disease, but may include hyper-inflated lungs with flattened diaphragms, decreased peripheral bronchovascular markings, increased lung lucency, and prominent hilar vessels on chest radiographs.[14]

Smoking is, of course, the major cause of COPD, but not all smokers develop the disease.[15] Meanwhile, between 25 and 45% of patients have no history of smoking.[16] Besides genetic factors

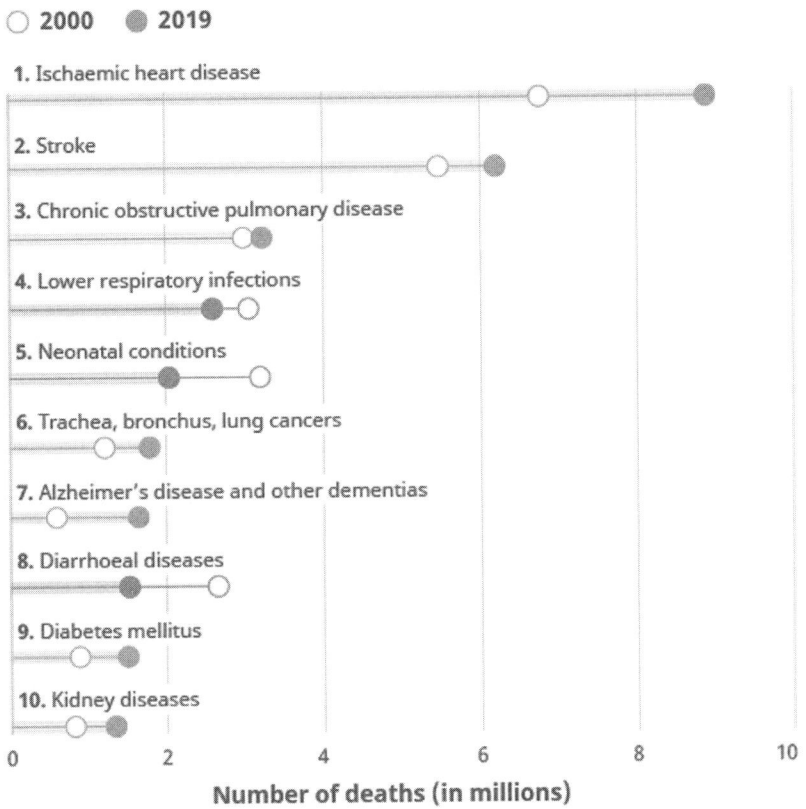

Figure 5.1 WHO factsheet: Leading causes of death globally

Reproduced from WHO. WHO Newsroom Factsheet. Top 10 Causes of Death.[10]

such as alpha 1 anti-trypsin deficiency (which only accounts for up to 3% of cases[17]), candidate genes have been identified which amplify smoking induced lung damage.[18] Additionally, studies link environmental exposures such as biomass smoke, air pollution, and fumes and dust exposures to increased risk of COPD development, particularly globally.[19]

There is compelling data indicating that a plant forward dietary plan can protect lung health. Whilst there are no studies examining a diet completely devoid of all animal products, many studies point to the importance of the nutrients that are most plentiful in healthy whole food, plant-based diets. For example, a recent systematic review and meta-analysis has shown an increased risk of COPD with 'unhealthy/Western-style' dietary pattern and a decreased risk with healthier eating patterns.[20]

Given the role of oxidative stress in the pathogenesis of lung injury and airway remodelling, including COPD,[21] it is conceivable that certain nutrients found in plant foods, such antioxidants, may explain this benefit. In a cross-sectional study, Strachan and colleagues reported that amongst both smokers and non-smokers with no history of chronic pulmonary disease, lack of fresh fruit and fruit juice intake was associated with a mean adjusted lower forced expiratory volume in one second (FEV1) of 78 mL.[22] In a follow

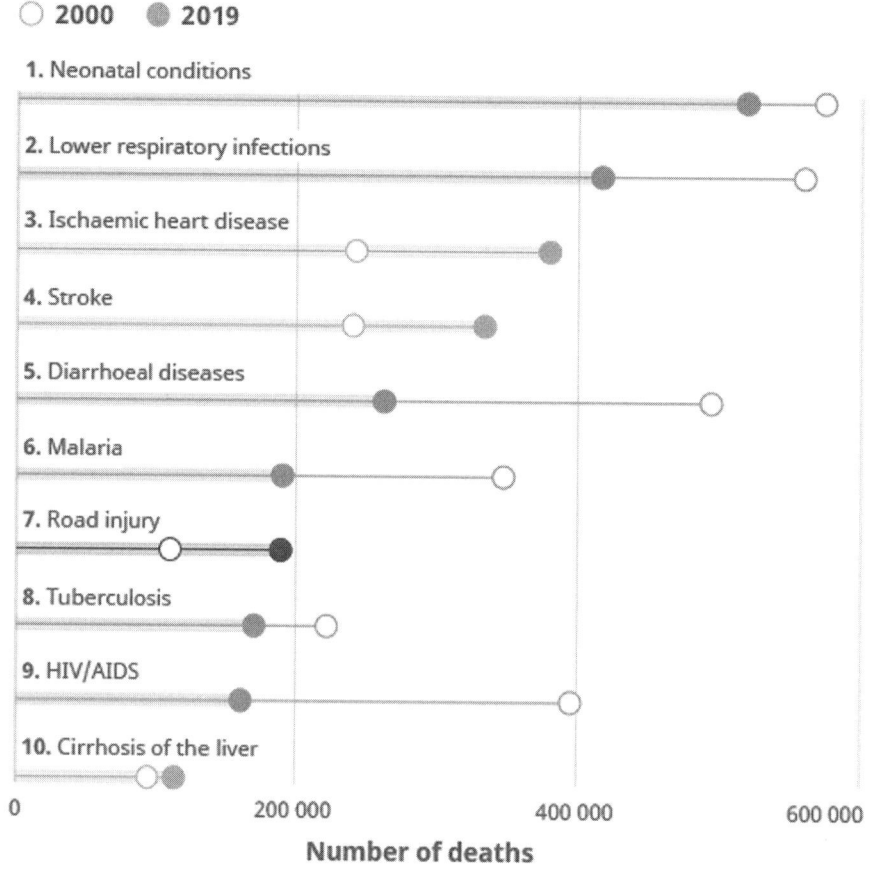

Figure 5.2 WHO factsheet: Leading causes of death in low-income countries
Reproduced from WHO. WHO Newsroom Factsheet. Chronic obstructive pulmonary disease (COPD).[11]

up larger cross-sectional study conducted seven years later, they noted that decreases in fresh fruit consumption were associated with decreased FEV1. Specifically, for those who reduced their consumption to the greatest degree, the fall in FEV1 was an average of 107 mL, whilst there was no similar drop seen for those with consistent levels of fruit intake.[23]

The authors hypothesise that one particular antioxidant, vitamin C, is a key factor to explain these changes. In fact, some studies have established that low serum levels or low intake of vitamin C are associated with smoking-related obstructive airway disease (OAD),[24, 25] or lower lung function independent of smoking or lung disease history.[26] For example, an increase of 20 mmol/L in plasma vitamin C was associated with a 13% lower risk of OAD,[24] and a 50 mmol/L difference was associated with a 0.22 litre difference in FEV1.[26]

Other oxidant-antioxidant imbalances that have been suggested to play a role in severity of COPD include malondialdehyde (MDA), superoxide dismutase (SOD), glutathione peroxidase (GPx), and glutathione.[27, 28] Despite this, antioxidant and vitamin supplementation as a preventative or treatment for COPD is not well established. A randomised placebo control trial of 64 patients admitted for inpatient pulmonary rehabilitation (PR) examined supplementation with vitamins C and E, zinc, and selenium. Eighty-one per cent showed at least one antioxidant deficiency, and whilst supplementation failed to show benefit for muscle endurance, muscle strength was increased.[29]

It is conceivable that the benefits seen with fruit and vegetable in these, and other studies, are related not only to antioxidant intake, but to fibre intake as well. The association between fibre and lung function is well documented.[30, 31, 32, 33] Studies comparing a 'prudent' diet (ample fruit, vegetables, whole grains and fish) was associated with decreased risk (by as much as 50%) of a new diagnosis of COPD whilst a 'Western' diet (high intake of cured and red meat, desserts, refined grains etc) was associated with as much as 4.5 times increased risk of COPD.[31, 32] Cured meats have specifically been linked to increased risk of COPD, but not asthma, suggesting the risk may be related to smoking-related OAD in particular.[34, 35]

Though many of the studies showing benefits to adequate fibre intake have been conducted in North America or Europe, similar results have been seen in Asian studies as well. A retrospective study comparing spirometry between 2012 and 2017 and validated dietary intake questionnaires during the same time period in 1,439 subjects in Seoul, Korea showed an OR of 2.7 for new airflow limitation (compared with normal spirometry in 2012) for every 10% decrease in the daily recommended allowance of vitamin C, folic acid and fibre[25] (see Figure 5.3).

On a macronutrient level, this data seems to compare with studies showing that, to the authors' own surprise, a diet rich in fat was associated with more dyspnoea in COPD than a carbohydrate-rich diet, despite the lower respiratory quotient and lower CO_2 production associated with fat.

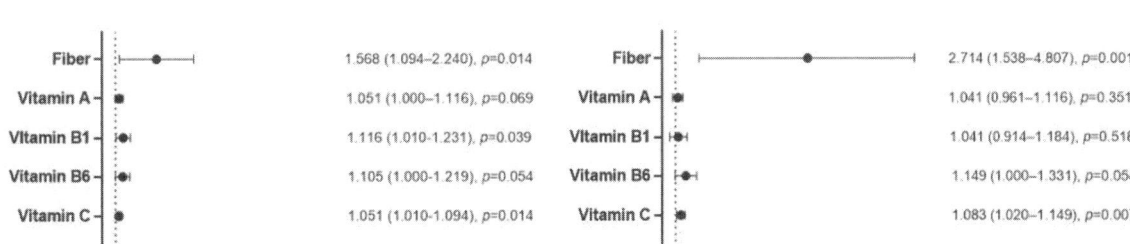

Figure 5.3 Unadjusted and adjusted OR for the development of airflow limitation on spirometry by dietary nutrient

Association between new airflow limitation onset and nutrient intake differences between the baseline and 5-year follow-up. Adjusted for gender, age, smoking history, and FEV1/FVC at baseline (2012). (A) Unadjusted OR (B) Adjusted ORs. All values are expressed with a 95% confidence interval. OR, odds ratio. Source: Jung et al.[25]

Glucose is more rapidly available and oxidised in COPD patients, who have lower oxidative capacity as discussed earlier, which may explain these findings.[36]

Though healthcare professionals may attend to nutrition as a prevention or treatment for COPD, the mainstay therapies are pharmacological therapies and pulmonary rehabilitation. Patients with COPD are at risk of malnutrition, with some studies placing risk as high as 45% of outpatients and 60% of inpatients.[37] Multiple studies have shown that nutritional status is a key factor in disease progression or stability.[22,23,38] For many patients with COPD, weight loss represents an ominous finding. As mentioned, malnutrition is an issue, but often for patients with COPD, cachexia and muscle wasting, rather than obesity, present a problem, with low BMI being a significant predictor of mortality.[39] The prevalence of obesity in COPD is not well known, and may be related to differences in obesity rates from country to country, or COPD phenotypes (e.g., 'pink puffers' or emphysema vs 'blue bloaters' or chronic bronchitis).[40] Because COPD has a heterogeneous pathophysiology, the effects of obesity on lung function are harder to determine, though studies indicate greater dyspnoea with earlier physical and mechanical limitations resulting in lower exercise tolerance.[40] Complicating matters is the well described 'obesity paradox' in which mortality seems decreased in overweight and obese patients with COPD in Global Initiative for Chronic Obstructive Lung Disease (GOLD) stage 3-4, while it is increased in those with GOLD stage 1-2 disease with (pre)obesity.[41] Thus, whilst the issue of excess adiposity is not settled in regards to COPD, the evidence for the benefits of a diet rich in antioxidants and fibre seems clearer.

And yet, despite a large body of evidence supporting the benefits of an antioxidant and fibre rich diet in the prevention and stabilisation of COPD, there is a lack of literature examining strict PBDs. Diets heavily focused on plant foods (and occasional dairy and fish) have been shown to be protective. However, purely plant-based diets are generally lower in fat content and higher in carbohydrates and fibre,[42] suggesting this diet may confer even larger benefits for prevention and stabilisation of COPD. More studies are needed in this area, particularly studies comparing a purely plant-based diet to a similarly healthful diet such as the Mediterranean diet in relation to COPD.

Asthma

Asthma is a heterogeneous respiratory disease marked by variable, usually reversible, airflow limitation and characterised by chronic airway inflammation and airway narrowing. Common symptoms include wheezing, chest tightness, shortness of breath, and cough. Though there are recognisable clusters of symptoms (called 'asthma phenotypes'), these don't have consistent pathological correlates and may not respond to similar treatment plans. Like COPD, the diagnosis involves history, physical examination, and spirometry. In asthma, airflow limitation is reversible after bronchodilator administration.[43]

As with COPD, there is a growing body of evidence that diet influences the development of asthma, as well as progression and severity. However, definitive answers for strict PBDs are similarly difficult to find. Mediterranean diets, with an emphasis on fruits, vegetables, and whole grains and which tend to be lower in saturated fat protect against the development of asthma or asthma symptoms, but 'Western' diets (deficient in fruits, vegetables, and whole grains, and high in refined grains and saturated fat) increase the risk of asthma.[44,45] Patients with severe asthma have decreased plasma levels of multiple antioxidants,[46] but replacing vitamins A, E, and C have not been shown in large systematic reviews to have sufficient benefit to make recommendations, partly due to the heterogeneity of dosing, exacerbation definitions, and more.[47] In a recent case-control study of adults, a 'Western diet' with a high 'dietary inflammatory index' was associated with asthma, reduced lung function and increased plasma levels of the inflammatory cytokine interleukin-6 (IL-6). The asthmatics in this study ate notably more pro-inflammatory foods. Higher serum levels of inflammatory markers such as IL-6, TNFα, CRP were found in those who ingested high fat meals, whilst foods high in n-3 polyunsaturated fats, fibre, vitamin E, vitamin C, and β-carotene have been associated with lower levels of systemic inflammation.[48]

Similar findings have been reported in children. Forastiere and colleagues reported an association between intake of citrus or kiwi fruit and odds ratio (OR) of wheeze, with the most pronounced protective effect occurring in those with asthma, and those who ate fruit 5–7 times per week.[49] In a cross-sectional school based survey of children aged 8–11, children who never ate fresh fruit had an estimated FEV1 of 79 mL (4.3%) lower that those who ate fresh fruit more than once a day. This persisted even after adjustment for socioeconomic status and passive smoking exposure. Interestingly, in this group, plasma vitamin C levels did not correlate with FEV1.[50]

Another mechanism by which dietary oxidative stress occurs is via the highly inflammatory compound advanced glycation end products (AGEs), and their corresponding receptors (RAGEs). RAGE is highly expressed in the lungs, and dysregulation of the AGE-RAGE interaction plays a role in lung cancer, fibrosis, and even graft dysfunction post lung transplantation.[51] Wang and colleagues noted in a large review of National Health and Nutrition Examination Survey (NHANES) data that meat consumption was associated with increased odds of wheezing at baseline, during sleep, and with exercise, including wheezing requiring medications.[52]

AGEs are found in many foods, particularly animal derived foods. Furthermore, cooking processes can promote AGEs. Restriction of dietary AGEs (dAGEs) has been shown to prevent and reduce vascular and kidney dysfunction, accelerate wound healing, improve insulin sensitivity and reduce markers of oxidative stress.[53] Uribarri and colleagues' database of high and low dAGEs foods shows that animal derived foods, particularly high fat animal derived foods (beef, cheeses, poultry, pork, fish, eggs) were naturally high in dAGEs, and even lean meats and poultry contained high dAGEs when cooked under dry heat (Maillard reaction). Conversely, carbohydrate rich foods (grains, legumes, breads made without significant sources of fat, fruits, vegetables and low-fat milks) had far lower levels of dAGEs either naturally or through cooking.[53]

As discussed earlier, weight is a significant influencing factor on the severity of asthma. The incidence of asthma is nearly 1.5 times higher in obese individuals, and large cohort studies have shown that a higher BMI is associated with worsened control of asthma. Whilst it may seem intuitive that this worsened control is related to the respiratory mechanics of carrying excess adipose tissue (e.g., extra pulmonary restriction), in fact, studies have shown that the overall higher inflammatory milieu of excess adiposity likely contributes.[2] Bates describes two distinct phenotypes related to asthma in obese patients: an early onset form with an allergic component that is worsened by obesity, and a non-allergic form that is later in onset and exclusively occurs in the presence of obesity.[54]

Asthma is a complex disease influenced by many factors. Whilst more studies are needed to examine the effects of a plant-based diet on asthma development, progression, and stabilisation or remission, based on current data it is relevant to the clinician, whether a generalist or specialist, to add nutrition counselling as a therapeutic tool in the armamentarium currently available to treat asthma. A lower inflammatory burden, through the direct pathway of ingesting anti-inflammatory foods against a background of maintaining a healthier weight and therefore lower baseline inflammatory environment, should be part of any discussion on risk mitigation strategies in the same manner one would discuss allergen avoidance and adherence to medication regimens.

Pulmonary hypertension

Pulmonary hypertension (PH) is a disease of the pulmonary vessels characterised by increased pulmonary vascular resistance and results in elevated pulmonary pressures. The specific pathogenesis of the various subsets of pulmonary hypertension are wide-ranging, and beyond the scope of this discussion. Very little data exists on the benefits of a plant-based diet and pulmonary hypertension. There is one case report of a subject with idiopathic pulmonary arterial hypertension (not specified in the report but based on description group 5) who began eating a whole foods PBD and had some reduction in her mean pulmonary arterial pressures. The authors note this is only a hypothesis-generating case, and postulate that (based on animal models) dietary nitrites seem to reduce PH.[55]

Diffuse lung diseases

Diffuse lung diseases (DLD), colloquially known as scarring lung diseases, include lung parenchymal diseases such as sarcoidosis, pulmonary fibrosis (idiopathic and other), hypersensitivity pneumonitis, cystic fibrosis, and more. There is no data available on plant-based diets and DLD. For diseases such as idiopathic pulmonary fibrosis (IPF) and sarcoidosis, maintaining a healthy weight is paramount (particularly for end stage disease where lung transplantation may be a consideration), so a PBD may be an excellent opportunity for these patients to lose weight or maintain a healthy weight.

Obstructive sleep apnoea

Obstructive sleep apnoea (OSA) is characterised by repeated episodes of extra thoracic upper airway obstruction or reductions in breath amplitude; the resultant intra-arterial hypoxaemia and hypercapnia lead to transient arousals from sleep, which then lead to fragmented sleep.[56]

Estimating prevalence of OSA is challenging due to methodological variability in studies. One systematic review suggested that at ≥5 events/h apnoea-hypopnea index (AHI) (mild OSA), the overall population prevalence ranged from 9% to 38% and was higher in men. It increased with increasing age and, in some elderly groups, was as high as 90% in men and 78% in women. At ≥15 events/h AHI, the prevalence in the general adult population ranged from 6% to 17%, being as high as 49% in the advanced ages. OSA prevalence was also greater in obese men and women.[57] Moreover, OSA is increasingly being recognised as a cause of cardiovascular mortality.[58]

Whilst positive airway pressure (PAP) is the mainstay for many who suffer from OSA, weight loss is also a critical adjunctive therapy.[59] As discussed earlier, PBDs are an excellent tool for patients to maintain a healthy weight or lose excess weight.

Anecdotally, many patients endorse an improvement in sleep quality and duration after transitioning to a PBD. Often, this is the first health benefit they notice. Clearly, this would not be attributable to significant weight loss. While there are no formal studies looking at this on a larger scale, there are theoretical mechanisms of action. Smaller studies have shown that higher percentages of plant-based protein intake trended towards a positive association with sleep duration, better sleep quality and lower insomnia.[60] Some possible mechanisms of action include the known association between higher soya isoflavone intake and less daytime sleepiness in women as well as an overall inverse association between isoflavone intake and sleep duration, with higher daily isoflavone intake associated with better sleep duration and quality.[61, 62]

Another possible mechanism includes the relatively high amount of tryptophan in plant-based proteins, in light of the fact that tryptophan is a precursor to neurotransmitters such as melatonin and serotonin, both involved in sleep regulation. Since animal proteins can also be high in tryptophan, without head-to-head studies, this mechanism is speculative.[60]

Obesity hypoventilation syndrome

Obesity hypoventilation syndrome (OHS) is characterised by the combination of obesity (body mass index [BMI] ≥ 30 kg/m2), sleep-disordered breathing, and awake daytime hypercapnia (awake resting $PaCO2 \geq 45$ mm Hg at sea level), after excluding other causes for hypoventilation.[63, 64] OHS is the most severe form of obesity-induced respiratory compromise and is linked to

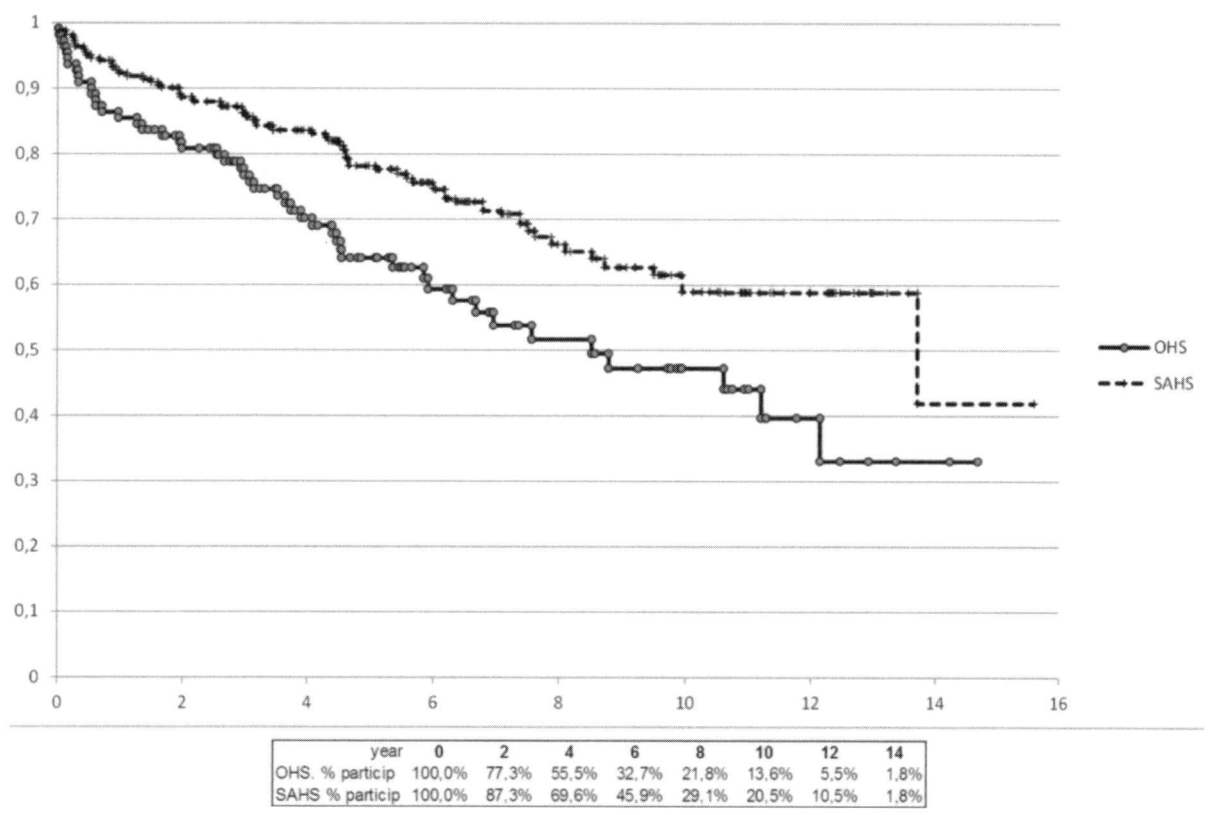

Figure 5.4 Kaplan-Meier curves for time to first cardiovascular event
OHS=Obesity Hypoventilation Syndrome; SAHS=Sleep Apnoea-Hypopnoea Syndrome
Source: Castro-Añón et al.[65]

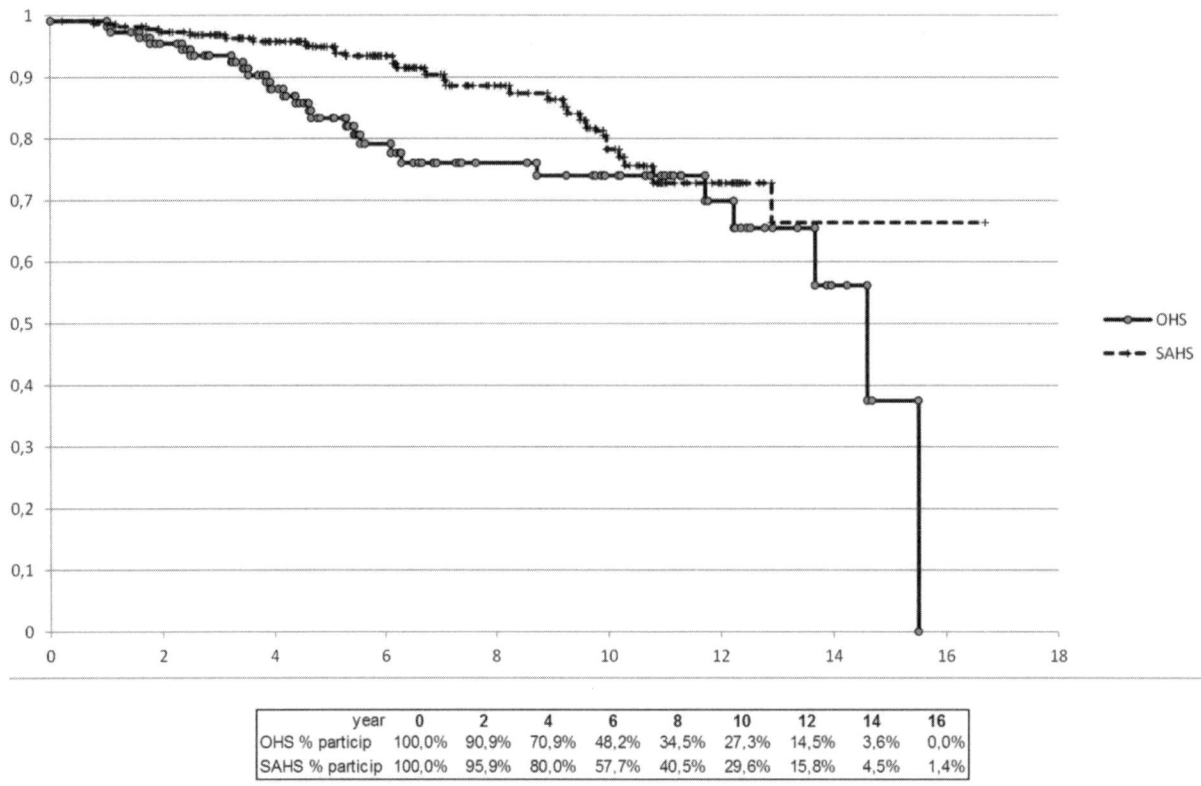

Figure 5.5 Kaplan-Meier survival curves
OHS=Obesity Hypoventilation Syndrome; SAHS=Sleep Apnoea-Hypopnoea Syndrome
Source: Castro-Añón et al.[65]

increased rates of mortality, chronic heart failure, pulmonary hypertension, and hospitalisation due to acute-on-chronic hypercapnic respiratory failure. Worryingly, patients with OHS have earlier cardiovascular events, and mortality for OHS is higher than for OSA[65] (see Figures 5.4, 5.5). Mainstays of therapy include PAP and weight loss, the latter of which can be influenced by PBDs, as discussed above.

Extra pulmonary restriction

Extra pulmonary or extra thoracic restriction, often noted on pulmonary function tests obtained to evaluate shortness of breath, can be due to factors such as muscle weakness or obesity. As discussed in previous sections, a PBD has been shown in multiple studies to be an effective weight loss strategy, and may even be superior to currently recommended diets, such as the Mediterranean diet.

A final note

Though this chapter largely deals with respiratory and sleep health, it must be noted that many respiratory physicians also practice critical care medicine (for example, in the US). As such, we must take into account the benefits of plant-based diets on commonly seen ailments in the intensive care unit (ICU). Most of these illnesses will be discussed in their relevant chapters. But for the ICU physician or other healthcare staff, the ICU represents an opportunity to begin introducing patients to the benefits of a plant-based diet. For the patient admitted with diabetic ketoacidosis, hyperosmolar non-ketosis, or cardiovascular diseases such as acute coronary syndrome, STEMI or NSTEMI, stroke, or congestive heart failure, it has been the author's experience that the earlier the initiation of nutrition interventions, the better. Continuing these interventions upon transfer to the regular ward and then arranging follow up with an appropriate healthcare provider (GP, dietician etc. who is well versed in lifestyle medicine) upon discharge is best to support patients as they embark on healthier, plant-based eating.

Conclusion

Whether in the inpatient or outpatient setting, clinicians have an opportunity to help patients better manage their respiratory health through nutrition counselling. From decreasing risk of COPD in smokers to helping achieve better control of asthma symptoms, to reducing risk of sleep disordered breathing, plant-based diets can play a significant role. Plant-based diets can be an inexpensive non-pharmacological intervention with minimal side effects. It behoves the clinician, then, to develop familiarity with the principles behind plant-based eating in order to offer all available therapeutic and preventative options to patients.

References

1. Wannamethee SG, Shaper AG, Whincup PH. Body fat distribution, body composition, and respiratory function in elderly men. *Am J Clin Nutr* 2005; 82(5): 996-1003. doi: 10.1093/ajcn/82.5.996
2. Mafort TT, Rufino R, Costa CH, Lopes AJ. Obesity: systemic and pulmonary complications, biochemical abnormalities, and impairment of lung function. *Multidisciplinary Respiratory Medicine* 2016; 11: 28. doi: 10.1186/s40248-016-0066-z
3. Tuso PJ, Ismail MH, Ha BP, Bartolotto C. Nutritional update for physicians: plant-based diets. *Perm J* 2013; 17(2): 61-66. doi: 10.7812/TPP/12-085
4. Berkow SE, Barnard N. Vegetarian Diets and Weight Status. *Nutrition Reviews* 2006; 64(4): 175-188. doi: 10.1111/j.1753-4887.2006.tb00200.x
5. Wang Y, Beydoun MA. Meat consumption is associated with obesity and central obesity among US adults. *Int J Obes* 2009; 33(6): 621-628. doi: 10.1038/ijo.2009.45
6. Estruch R, Ros E, Salas-Salvadó J, Covas M-I, Corella D, Arós F, et al. Primary Prevention of Cardiovascular Disease with a Mediterranean Diet. *New England Journal of Medicine* 2013; 368(14): 1279-1290. doi: 10.1056/NEJMoa1200303
7. Barnard ND, Alwarith J, Rembert E, Brandon L, Nguyen M, Goergen A, et al. A Mediterranean Diet and Low-Fat Vegan Diet to Improve Body Weight and Cardiometabolic Risk Factors: A Randomized, Cross-over Trial. *Journal of the American College of Nutrition* 2021; 1-13. doi: 10.1080/07315724.2020.1869625
8. Spencer EA, Appleby PN, Davey GK, Key TJ. Diet and body mass index in 38000 EPIC-Oxford meat-eaters, fish-eaters, vegetarians and vegans. *International Journal of Obesity and Related Metabolic Disorders* 2003; 27(6): 728-734. doi: 10.1038/sj.ijo.0802300
9. Rizzo NS, Jaceldo-Siegl K, Sabate J, Fraser GE. Nutrient Profiles of Vegetarian and Nonvegetarian Dietary Patterns. *Journal of the Academy of Nutrition and Dietetics* 2013; 113(12): 1610-1619. doi: 10.1016/j.jand.2013.06.349
10. WHO. WHO Newsroom Factsheets Top 10 Causes of Death. 9 December 2020. www.who.int/news-room/fact-sheets/detail/the-top-10-causes-of-death [Accessed 19 May 2022]
11. WHO. WHO Newsroom Factsheets Chronic

Obstructive Pulmonary Disease (COPD). 21 June 2021. www.who.int/news-room/fact-sheets/detail/chronic-obstructive-pulmonary-disease-(copd) [Accessed 19 May 2022]

12. Barnes P.J. SSD, Pauwels R.A. Chronic Obstructive Pulmonary Disease: Molecular and cellular mechanisms. *Eur Respir J* 2003; 22(4): 672-688. doi: 10.1183/09031936.03.00040703

13. Kessler R, Partridge MR, Miravitlles M, Cazzola M, Vogelmeier C, Leynaud D, et al. Symptom variability in patients with severe COPD: a pan-European cross-sectional study. *The European respiratory journal* 2011; 37(2): 264-272. doi: 10.1183/09031936.00051110

14. Jones J, Knipe, H. . COPD (summary): Radiopaedia. Available from: https://radiopaedia.org/articles/39654.

15. Mannino DM, Buist AS. Global burden of COPD: risk factors, prevalence, and future trends. *Lancet* 2007; 370(9589): 765–773. doi: 10.1016/S0140-6736(07)61380-4

16. Quint J. The Air We Breathe: Effect of Environmental Exposures on COPD. *Tanaffos* 2017; 16(Suppl 1): S14-S5.

17. American Thoracic Society/European Respiratory Society Statement Standards for the Diagnosis and Management of Individuals with Alpha-1 Antitrypsin Deficiency. *Am J Respir Crit Care Med* 2003; 168(7): 818-900. doi: 10.1164/rccm.168.7.818

18. Bruse S, Moreau, M., Bromberg, Y. et al. Whole exome sequencing identifies novel candidate genes that modify chronic obstructive pulmonary disease susceptibility. *Hum Genomics* 2016; 10(1). doi: 10.1186/s40246-015-0058-7

19. Kc R, Shukla SD, Gautam SS, Hansbro PM, O'Toole RF. The role of environmental exposure to non-cigarette smoke in lung disease. *Clinical and Translational Medicine* 2018; 7(1): 39. doi: 10.1186/s40169-018-0217-2

20. Zheng P-F, Shu L, Si C-J, Zhang X-Y, Yu X-L, Gao W. Dietary Patterns and Chronic Obstructive Pulmonary Disease: A Meta-analysis. *COPD* 2016; 13(4): 515-522. doi: 10.3109/15412555.2015.1098606

21. van Eeden SF, Sin DD. Oxidative stress in chronic obstructive pulmonary disease: a lung and systemic process. *Can Respir J* 2013; 20(1): 27-29. doi: 10.1155/2013/509130

22. Strachan DP, Cox BD, Erzinclioglu SW, Walters DE, Whichelow MJ. Ventilatory function and winter fresh fruit consumption in a random sample of British adults. *Thorax* 1991; 46(9): 624-629. doi: 10.1136/thx.46.9.624

23. Carey IM, Strachan DP, Cook DG. Effects of changes in fresh fruit consumption on ventilatory function in healthy British adults. *Am J Respir Crit Care Med* 1998; 158(3): 728-733. doi: 10.1164/ajrccm.158.3.9712065

24. Sargeant L, Jaeckel A, Wareham N. Interaction of vitamin C with the relation between smoking and obstructive airways disease in EPIC Norfolk. European Prospective Investigation into Cancer and Nutrition. *European Respiratory Journal* 2000; 16(3): 397-403. doi: 10.1034/j.1399-3003.2000.016003397.x

25. Jung YJ, Lee SH, Chang JH, Lee HS, Kang EH, Lee SW. The Impact of Changes in the Intake of Fiber and Antioxidants on the Development of Chronic Obstructive Pulmonary Disease. *Nutrients* 2021; 13(2): 580. doi: 10.3390/nu13020580

26. Ness AR, Khaw KT, Bingham S, Day NE. Vitamin C status and respiratory function. *European Journal of Clinical Nutrition* 1996; 50(9): 573-579.

27. Ahmad A, Shameem M, Husain Q. Altered oxidant-antioxidant levels in the disease prognosis of chronic obstructive pulmonary disease. The international journal of tuberculosis and lung disease. *The official journal of the International Union against Tuberculosis and Lung Disease* 2013; 17(8): 1104-1109. doi: 10.5588/ijtld.12.0512

28. Bajpai J, Prakash V, Kant S, Verma AK, Srivastava A, Bajaj DK, et al. Study of oxidative stress biomarkers in chronic obstructive pulmonary disease and their correlation with disease severity in north Indian population cohort. *Lung India* 2017; 34(4): 324-329. doi: 10.4103/lungindia.lungindia_205_16

29. Gouzi F, Maury J, Héraud N, Molinari N, Bertet H, Ayoub B, et al. Additional Effects of Nutritional Antioxidant Supplementation on Peripheral Muscle during Pulmonary Rehabilitation in COPD Patients: A Randomized Controlled Trial. *Oxid Med Cell Longev* 2019; 2019: 5496346. doi: 10.1155/2019/5496346

30. Kan H, Stevens J, Heiss G, Rose KM, London

SJ. Dietary fiber, lung function, and chronic obstructive pulmonary disease in the atherosclerosis risk in communities study. *Am J Epidemiol* 2008; 167(5): 570-578. doi: 10.1093/aje/kwm343
31. Varraso R, Fung TT, Barr RG, Hu FB, Willett W, Camargo CA, Jr. Prospective study of dietary patterns and chronic obstructive pulmonary disease among US women. *Am J Clin Nutr* 2007; 86(2): 488-495. doi: 10.1093/ajcn/86.2.488
32. Varraso R, Fung TT, Hu FB, Willett W, Camargo CA. Prospective study of dietary patterns and chronic obstructive pulmonary disease among US men. *Thorax* 2007; 62(9): 786-791. doi: 10.1136/thx.2006.074534
33. Varraso R, Willett WC, Camargo CA, Jr. Prospective study of dietary fiber and risk of chronic obstructive pulmonary disease among US women and men. *Am J Epidemiol* 2010; 171(7): 776-784. doi: 10.1093/aje/kwp455
34. Jiang R, Camargo CA, Jr., Varraso R, Paik DC, Willett WC, Barr RG. Consumption of cured meats and prospective risk of chronic obstructive pulmonary disease in women. *Am J Clin Nutr* 2008; 87(4): 1002-1008. doi: 10.1093/ajcn/87.4.1002
35. Varraso R, Jiang R, Barr RG, Willett WC, Camargo CA, Jr. Prospective study of cured meats consumption and risk of chronic obstructive pulmonary disease in men. *Am J Epidemiol* 2007; 166(12): 1438-1445. doi: 10.1093/aje/kwm235
36. Vermeeren MA, Wouters EF, Nelissen LH, van Lier A, Hofman Z, Schols AM. Acute effects of different nutritional supplements on symptoms and functional capacity in patients with chronic obstructive pulmonary disease. *Am J Clin Nutr* 2001; 73(2): 295-301. doi: 10.1093/ajcn/73.2.295
37. Collins PF, Elia M, Stratton RJ. Nutritional support and functional capacity in chronic obstructive pulmonary disease: A systematic review and meta-analysis. *Respirology* 2013; 18(4): 616-629. doi: 10.1111/resp.12070
38. Butland BK, Fehily AM, Elwood PC. Diet, lung function, and lung function decline in a cohort of 2512 middle aged men. *Thorax* 2000; 55(2): 102-108. doi: 10.1136/thorax.55.2.102
39. Vestbo J, Prescott E, Almdal T, Dahl M, Nordestgaard BG, Andersen T, et al. Body mass, fat-free body mass, and prognosis in patients with chronic obstructive pulmonary disease from a random population sample: findings from the Copenhagen City Heart Study. *Am J Respir Crit Care Med* 2006; 173(1): 79-83. doi: 10.1164/rccm.200506-969OC
40. Franssen FME, O'Donnell DE, Goossens GH, Blaak EE, Schols AMWJ. Obesity and the lung: 5. Obesity and COPD. *Thorax* 2008; 63(12) :1110-1117. doi: 10.1136/thx.2007.086827
41. LANDBO C, PRESCOTT E, LANGE P, VESTBO J, ALMDAL TP. Prognostic Value of Nutritional Status in Chronic Obstructive Pulmonary Disease. *American Journal of Respiratory and Critical Care Medicine* 1999; 160(6): 1856-1861. doi: 10.1164/ajrccm.160.6.9902115
42. Clarys P, Deliens T, Huybrechts I, Deriemaeker P, Vanaelst B, De Keyzer W, et al. Comparison of nutritional quality of the vegan, vegetarian, semi-vegetarian, pesco-vegetarian and omnivorous diet. *Nutrients* 2014; 6(3): 1318-1332. doi: 10.3390/nu6031318
43. Global Initiative for Asthma. Global Strategy for Asthma Management and Prevention, 2021.
44. Han Y-Y, Blatter J, Brehm JM, Forno E, Litonjua AA, Celedón JC. Diet and asthma: vitamins and methyl donors. *Lancet Respir Med* 2013; 1(10): 813-822. doi: 10.1016/S2213-2600(13)70126-7
45. Thorburn AN, Macia L, Mackay Charles R. Diet, Metabolites, and "Western-Lifestyle" Inflammatory Diseases. *Immunity* 2014; 40(6): 833-842. doi: 10.1016/j.immuni.2014.05.014
46. Misso NL, Brooks-Wildhaber J, Ray S, Vally H, Thompson PJ. Plasma concentrations of dietary and nondietary antioxidants are low in severe asthma. *The European Respiratory Journal* 2005; 26(2): 257-264. doi: 10.1183/09031936.05.00006705
47. Milan SJ, Hart A, Wilkinson M. Vitamin C for asthma and exercise-induced bronchoconstriction. *Cochrane Database Syst Rev* 2013; 2013(10): CD010391. doi: 10.1002/14651858.CD010391.pub2
48. Wood LG, Shivappa N, Berthon BS, Gibson PG, Hebert JR. Dietary inflammatory index is related to asthma risk, lung function and systemic inflammation in asthma. *Clin Exp Allergy* 2015; 45(1): 177-183. doi: 10.1111/cea.12323

49. Forastiere F, Pistelli R, Sestini P, Fortes C, Renzoni E, Rusconi F, et al. Consumption of fresh fruit rich in vitamin C and wheezing symptoms in children. SIDRIA Collaborative Group, Italy (Italian Studies on Respiratory Disorders in Children and the Environment). *Thorax* 2000; 55(4): 283-288. doi: 10.1136/thorax.55.4.283

50. Cook DG, Carey IM, Whincup PH, Papacosta O, Chirico S, Bruckdorfer KR, et al. Effect of fresh fruit consumption on lung function and wheeze in children. *Thorax* 1997; 52(7): 628-633. doi: 10.1136/thx.52.7.628

51. Buckley ST, Ehrhardt C. The Receptor for Advanced Glycation End Products (RAGE) and the Lung. *Journal of Biomedicine and Biotechnology* 2010; 2010: 917108. doi: 10.1155/2010/917108

52. Wang JG, Liu B, Kroll F, Hanson C, Vicencio A, Coca S, et al. Increased advanced glycation end product and meat consumption is associated with childhood wheeze: analysis of the National Health and Nutrition Examination Survey. *Thorax* 2021; 76(3): 292-294. doi: 10.1136/thoraxjnl-2020-216109

53. Uribarri J, Woodruff S, Goodman S, Cai W, Chen X, Pyzik R, et al. Advanced glycation end products in foods and a practical guide to their reduction in the diet. *J Am Diet Assoc* 2010; 110(6): 911-916.e12. doi: 10.1016/j.jada.2010.03.018

54. Bates JHT. Physiological Mechanisms of Airway Hyperresponsiveness in Obese Asthma. *Am J Respir Cell Mol Biol* 2016; 54(5): 618-623. doi: 10.1165/rcmb.2016-0019PS

55. McGoey-Smith KJ EC, McGoey-Smith AD. Reversal of Pulmonary Hypertension, Diabetes, and Retinopathy after Adoption of a Whole Food Plant-Based Diet. *IJDRP* 2021; 1(2). doi: 10.22230/ijdrp.2019v1n2a41

56. Patil SP, Schneider H, Schwartz AR, Smith PL. Adult obstructive sleep apnea: pathophysiology and diagnosis. *Chest* 2007; 132(1): 325-337. doi: 10.1378/chest.07-0040

57. Senaratna CV, Perret JL, Lodge CJ, Lowe AJ, Campbell BE, Matheson MC, et al. Prevalence of obstructive sleep apnea in the general population: A systematic review. *Sleep Medicine Reviews* 2017; 34: 70-81. doi: 10.1016/j.smrv.2016.07.002

58. Punjabi NM, Caffo BS, Goodwin JL, Gottlieb DJ, Newman AB, O'Connor GT, et al. Sleep-disordered breathing and mortality: a prospective cohort study. *PLoS Med* 2009; 6(8): e1000132-e. doi: 10.1371/journal.pmed.1000132

59. Epstein LJ, Kristo D, Strollo PJ, Jr., Friedman N, Malhotra A, Patil SP, et al. Clinical guideline for the evaluation, management and long-term care of obstructive sleep apnea in adults. *J Clin Sleep Med* 2009; 5(3): 263-276.

60. St-Onge M-P, Crawford A, Aggarwal B. Plant-based diets: Reducing cardiovascular risk by improving sleep quality? *Curr Sleep Med Rep* 2018; 4(1): 74-8.

61. Cui Y, Niu K, Huang C, Momma H, Guan L, Kobayashi Y, et al. Relationship between daily isoflavone intake and sleep in Japanese adults: a cross-sectional study. *Nutrition Journal* 2015; 14(1): 127. doi: 10.1186/s12937-015-0117-x

62. Cao Y, Taylor AW, Zhen S, Adams R, Appleton S, Shi Z. Soy Isoflavone Intake and Sleep Parameters over 5 Years among Chinese Adults: Longitudinal Analysis from the Jiangsu Nutrition Study. *Journal of the Academy of Nutrition and Dietetics* 2017; 117(4): 536-44.e2. doi: 10.1016/j.jand.2016.10.016

63. Mokhlesi B, Kryger MH, Grunstein RR. Assessment and management of patients with obesity hypoventilation syndrome. *Proc Am Thorac Soc* 2008; 5(2): 218-225. doi: 10.1513/pats.200708-122MG

64. Randerath W, Verbraecken J, Andreas S, Arzt M, Bloch KE, Brack T, et al. Definition, discrimination, diagnosis and treatment of central breathing disturbances during sleep. *The European respiratory journal* 2017; 49(1): 1600959. doi: 10.1183/13993003.00959-2016

65. Castro-Añón O, Pérez de Llano LA, De la Fuente Sánchez S, Golpe R, Méndez Marote L, Castro-Castro J, et al. Obesity-Hypoventilation Syndrome: Increased Risk of Death over Sleep Apnea Syndrome. *PLOS One* 2015; 10(2): e0117808. doi: 10.1371/journal.pone.0117808

Chapter 6
Plant-based nutrition and weight management

Sue Kenneally

Introduction

Obesity is a modern pandemic and its global prevalence has increased markedly in recent decades, from 3·2% (2·4–4·1) in 1975 to 10·8% (9·7–12·0) in 2014 in men, and from 6·4% (5·1–7·8) to 14·9% (13·6–16·1) in women. The rate of increase varies among countries: the prevalence of obesity continues to rise in high-income countries, but the rate of increase has slowed since 2010, whereas in middle-income countries the rate of increase is rising steadily and there is agreement that this global increase is expected to continue.[1,2]

This is of grave concern at both an individual and public health level, as obesity confers a considerable increased risk of excess morbidity and mortality. The Global BMI Mortality Collaboration reviewed 239 prospective studies from four continents, and their meta-analysis revealed an increased risk of mortality in the underweight, compared with those in the healthy range, and in those with overweight a steadily increasing risk of mortality with increasing BMI. Living with a BMI of 30 increases the relative risk of all-cause mortality to 1.45 compared with a BMI of 20; a BMI of between 40 and 60 raises this further to 2.76.[3]

Obesity is a risk factor for a significant burden of chronic disease, including oesophageal cancer, gallbladder and biliary tract cancer, pancreatic cancer, kidney and other urinary organ cancers, breast cancer, uterine cancer, colon and rectum cancers, diabetes mellitus, ischaemic heart disease, ischaemic stroke, cardiomyopathy, myocarditis, endocarditis (atrial fibrillation and flutter), peripheral vascular disease and other cardiovascular disease, chronic kidney disease, osteoarthritis and low back pain.[4] In extreme cases, the lifespan of people living with obesity can be reduced by up to 14 years.[5] An important contributor to this is the development of chronic low grade systemic inflammation associated with obesity and many of its comorbidities.[6]

BMI as a measure of obesity and risk of morbidity and mortality has limitations; it is possible to have a BMI in the overweight or obese range and not have excess body fat, or to have excess body fat but remain metabolically healthy. Equally it is possible to have a BMI in the healthy range, but to still have excess body fat relative to a low muscle mass (known as sarcopenic obesity).

Reversing obesity, and maintaining a healthy body weight, therefore, has many putative benefits at an individual and global level.

Causes of obesity

The causes, or determinants of obesity are many and complex, but can be summarised as an interaction of human biology and behaviour with an obesogenic environment, resulting in individuals consuming slightly more energy than they use over the long term, resulting in gradual weight gain. Obesity was once considered an issue of personal responsibility, but evidence increasingly demonstrates that wider societal issues are stronger drivers of the weight gain pandemic. This is unsurprising, as gaining and retaining body weight conferred a significant evolutionary advantage upon our hunter-gatherer ancestors, and our biology has not moved on from that era.

The physiological drive to eat is relatively a lot stronger than the drive to stop eating, with attempts at weight loss met with significant resistance at a physiological level. Appetite regulation can easily be overcome in the presence of drivers to overeat, including highly palatable energy-dense food, typically containing large quantities of fat, sugar and salt in various combinations. These foods are also heavily marketed by the food industry. Healthful foods associated with effective weight regulation are more difficult to obtain than those associated with weight gain because of availability and price, and physical activity is less necessary than previously with the increase in car ownership, less physically demanding jobs, labour-saving devices in work and at home, and more sedentary leisure time. Wider societal influences are also involved. A detailed review of the determinants of obesity is beyond the scope of this chapter but has been clearly documented elsewhere.[7]

Genetics

Obesity can also have a significant genetic component, with epidemiological and twin studies indicating that the heritability of body mass index is 40–70%.[8] Genes that regulate energy intake are primarily found in the leptin-melanocortin pathway, and a single gene mutation in this pathway can result in a significantly increased risk of obesity,[8] referred to as 'monogenic obesity'. There are medical syndromes associated with obesity, e.g., Prader-Willi syndrome, referred to as 'syndromic obesity', and lastly there is 'polygenic obesity', a result of a large number of genetic polymorphisms that promote weight gain by interacting with an obesogenic environment. This is the most common form of obesity in genetic terms.

The Genetic Investigation of Anthropometric Traits (GIANT) consortium has identified around 100 BMI-associated loci but concluded that these loci account for only 2.7% of BMI variation, leading to the concept of 'missing heritability'. The remaining heritability may be explained by epigenetic modification of the polymorphisms, or by other factors that remain poorly understood.[8]

Epigenetics describes the process by which the expression of genes is modified by external factors including lifestyle, so that some factors increase the expression of genes coding for obesity and therefore increase the risk of obesity in the individual. Conversely, other factors may decrease expression of these genes. Evidence regarding plant-based diets and epigenetic modification of genes coding for obesity is sparse, however, saturated fat, fried foods and sugar-sweetened beverages, all of which do not typically form a significant part of a whole food, plant-based diet, have been shown to epigenetically modify the expression of obesity related genes.[9]

Limitations of current lifestyle and pharmaceutical interventions

Weight loss medications can form an important part of a weight loss strategy, with evidence suggesting that losing 5% of starting body weight is sufficient to significantly reduce metabolic risk in individuals living with obesity,[10] and a number of pharmaceutical preparations are available that can effect this much change. These presently include orlistat, lorcaserin, liraglutide, phentermine/topiramate in combination and naltrexone/bupropion in combination, although other pharmaceutical agents continue to be researched and more options are likely to be approved in the future. The availability of these medications varies according to specific prescribing guidelines in different parts of the world.

All of these medications can result in clinically significant weight loss in terms of reducing metabolic risk, ranging from 1 to 6% of starting total body weight, but often greater weight loss than this is required to obtain optimal health, and weight regain is likely to occur upon cessation of the medication.[11]

Lifestyle interventions intended to result in weight loss are generally effective, particularly when reducing energy intake and increasing physical activity in combination, but recidivism is significant. The vast majority of people regain most of their lost weight after the end of the intervention, leading to obesity being deemed a chronic, relapsing condition.[11]

A dietary pattern that can be adhered to in the long term, such that there is permanent behaviour change rather than yo-yo dieting, is desirable. A whole food, plant-based diet is an example of this, being both acceptable in the long term and associated with a healthy body weight.

Bariatric surgery can be an effective management option for people living with obesity. It results in weight loss that far exceeds that achievable by medication, and is sustainable long term, with one study evaluating patients 20 years after surgery concluding that average long-term total weight loss was 22% of starting weight.[12] It is cost effective, and reduces all-cause mortality risk and comorbidity risk,[13] but is associated with significant risks and complications, and is not available to many who are suitable candidates because of limited resources. Furthermore, not all people living with obesity who qualify for surgery are willing to proceed. A sustainable lifestyle that results in long-term weight loss and weight loss maintenance therefore remains essential.

Concept of a plant-based diet

Plant-based diets can be healthful or unhealthful. A diet rich in fruits, vegetables, legumes, whole grains, nuts and seeds has many putative health benefits, whereas a diet based on plant foods that are highly processed and contain significant quantities of salt, fat and sugar confer little advantage over a standard Westernised diet in terms of weight and risk of other chronic diseases.[20] This chapter will review the benefits of a healthful entirely plant-based eating pattern.

Acceptability

One of the key factors determining the success of any weight loss diet is, unsurprisingly, the ability of the individual to adhere to the suggested dietary changes.[14] Evidence indicates that a low-fat plant-based diet is highly acceptable to participants,[15] and adherence to this dietary pattern is high, despite potentially involving a greater dietary change. Weight loss may also be superior in those following a low-fat plant-based diet compared with other diets when participants are relatively non-adherent.[15]

Observational evidence for plant-based diets and weight

Epidemiological evidence suggests that people who eat a plant-based diet have a lower BMI than those who follow other dietary patterns. In the USA, studies of the Seventh Day Adventist population suggest that vegetarians and vegans (grouped together for one study) had a significantly lower risk of obesity than non-vegetarians, with a mean BMI of 27 vs 30 respectively in Black participants, p<0.0001,[16] and BMI of 24 in vegans vs 28 in omnivores overall.[17] This is consistent with previous Adventist data that suggests that vegans were the only group with a BMI in the healthy range.[18]

In the UK, the baseline anthropometric data of the participants in the European Prospective Investigation into Cancer and Nutrition (EPIC) trial confirms that vegans as a group have a BMI of 22, the lowest of all dietary patterns, compared with non-vegetarians who had the highest with a BMI of 24.[19] Elsewhere a meta-analysis of observational data concluded that vegans have the lowest BMI overall.[20]

Prospective observational studies also suggest that plant-based diets are associated with a lower risk of obesity and weight gain. A review of the EPIC data confirmed that in five years of follow up, those following a vegan diet gained less weight than other groups, and in those who changed their diets during follow up, the ones who reduced their animal food intake the most gained the least weight.[21]

Elsewhere, in the Adventist studies, people eating a vegan diet gained less weight than non-vegetarians during the period of follow up.[22]

Intervention trials

A search of the literature identified 18 intervention trials comparing vegan diets with alternative dietary interventions or normal diet (see Table 6.1). Fourteen were randomised controlled trials, two had control groups but no randomisation, and two had no control groups. All reported significant weight loss in the intervention groups compared with controls where present. In trials comparing different dietary interventions, weight loss in vegan groups was at least equivalent, or greater than other groups. This is consistent with the findings of two systematic reviews, for example the one published by Medawar et al.[23] and meta-analyses, for example Huang et al., 2016.[24]

One of the earliest intervention trials assessing the effects of a vegan diet on weight was in 1984.[25] There were no controls, but 29 individuals with overweight and hypertension lost an average of 7.8 kg in 12 months. In a non-randomised but controlled intervention assessing a vegan diet vs normal diet over three months, those following the vegan diet reduced their BMI from 28 to 26, compared with no change in the control group, p<0.0001.[26]

Regarding randomised controlled trials, in 2005, overweight postmenopausal women followed either a low-fat vegan diet or the diet recommended by the USA National Cholesterol Education Programme. The vegan group lost 5.8 kg in 14 weeks vs 3.8 kg in the NCEP group, p=0.012.[27] The group were followed up at two years, where the vegan group were shown to have maintained a greater weight loss, particularly those who had attended regular support group meetings.[28]

A two-month intervention comparing the effects of the Atkins, Zone, Weight watchers and Ornish diets noted that the Ornish (vegan) arm of the trial lost 6.6 kg, p<0.01 compared with baseline, but all groups lost weight and there were no significant differences among groups.[29]

Elsewhere, in a 12-month intervention assessing a gluten-free vegan diet with a well-balanced omnivore diet in patients with rheumatoid arthritis, mean loss was 4.2 kg compared with no change in the controls, p<0,001. Notably, most of the participants had a healthy starting weight.[30]

Table 6.1: Trials comparing vegan diets with alternative dietary interventions or normal diet

Author, date, country	Design	Population, number of participants (% female)	Intervention	Primary and secondary outcomes	Weight outcomes Loss (range or 95% CI) vs controls where present
Barnard[27] 2005 USA	RCT	Overweight PM women, 64 (100%)	14-weeks, low-fat vegan vs NCEP	BW, EI, TEF, RMR, EE, IS	5.8 kg (2.6–9.0) vs 3.8 (1.0–6.4), p=0.012
Barnard[31] 2009 USA	RCT	Type 2 diabetes, any weight, 99 (60%)	74-weeks low-fat vegan vs ADA diet	HbA1c, BW, lipids, drugs	6.5 kg (2.2–10.8) vs 3.1 (-0.3–6.5), p=0.0001 (in those who did not change medication)
Dansinger[29] 2005 USA	RCT	Overweight or obesity with comorbidity, 160 (51%)	2-months following Atkins, Zone, Weight Watchers or Ornish	BW, BMI, WC, lipids, BP, glucose	6.6 kg in the Ornish group, p<0.01 for change from baseline, but no difference among groups
Elkan[30] 2008 Sweden	RCT	Rheumatoid arthritis, mostly healthy weight, 58 (89%)	12-months gluten-free vegan diet vs well-balanced omnivore diet	DAS28, HAQ, CRP, lipids, anti-PC, BMI, BW	4.2 kg, from 66.4 (61.7 to 71.1) to 62.2 (58.2 to 66.2) in the intervention group (p<0.001), no loss in controls
Ferdowsian[32] 2010 USA	RCT	GEICO, overweight or obesity and/or T2D, 113 (82%)	22-weeks low-fat vegan vs normal diet	BW, WC, HC, WHR, lipids, BP, HbA1c	5.3 kg (3.5–7.0) difference between groups (p<0.0001)
Jakse[38] 2017 Slovenia	Non-randomised controlled trial	Adults, 325 (87%)	10-weeks, low-fat vegan diet including meal replacement vs educational sessions	BW, FAT, muscle mass, water content	5.6 kg (5.2–6) vs 1.2 kg (0.8–1.6), p<0.001
Jenkins[34] 2014 Canada	RCT	Overweight men with raised cholesterol and PM women, 39 (61%)	6-months low-CHO vegan vs high-CHO LOV	BW, BMI, FAT, WC, GLC, INS, HbA1c, BP, HOMA-IR, lipids, APO, CRP, CHDR	5 kg (high-CHO) vs 6.8 kg (low-CHO vegan), p=0.047
Kaartinen[26] 2000 Finland	Non-randomised controlled trial	Fibromyalgia any weight, 33 (not given)	3-months raw vegan vs normal omnivorous diet	VAS, JS, QOS, HAQ, GHQ, BMI, lipids	BMI reduced from 28 to 26 in intervention, no change in controls, p<0.0001

Abbreviations for Table 6.1: ADA: American Diabetic Association; anti-PC: antiphosphatidylcholine antibodies: APO: apolipoproteins; BP: blood pressure: BMI: body mass index; BUN: blood urea nitrogen; BW: body weight; CHDR: coronary heart disease risk; CREAT: creatinine; CRP: C reactive protein; DAS28: disease activity score; EE: energy expenditure; EI: energy intake; FAT: fat mass; GEICO: Government Employees Insurance Company; GHQ: general health questionnaire; GLC: glucose; HAQ: health activity questionnaire; HC: hip circumference; INS: insulin; IS: insulin sensitivity; JS: joint stiffness; NCEP: National Cholesterol Education Programme; PI: protein intake; PM: post-menopausal; QOS: quality of sleep; RCT: randomised con-trolled trial; RMR: resting metabolic rate; TEF: thermic effect of food; VAS: visual ana-logue scores; WC: waist circumference; WHR: waist/hip ratio.

Author, date, country	Design	Population, number of participants (% female)	Intervention	Primary and secondary outcomes	Weight outcomes Loss (range or 95% CI) vs controls where present
Kahleova[39] 2018 USA	RCT	Overweight and obesity, 75 (89%)	16-weeks, low-fat vegan vs normal omnivorous diet	EI, PI, BMI, BW, FAT, HOMA-IR	6.5 kg (4.1–8.9), no loss in controls, p<0.001
Kahleova[40] 2018 USA	RCT (same cohort)	Overweight and obesity, 75 (89%)	16-weeks low-fat vegan vs normal omnivorous diet	BW, BMI, HOMA-IR, FAT	6.5 kg (4.1–8.9), no loss in controls, p<0.001
Lindahl[25] 1984 Sweden	Intervention, no control group	Raised BP, 29 (65%)	1-year, vegan diet	BW, BP	7.8 kg (SD 14), p<0.001
McDougall[35] 2014 USA	Intervention, no control group	McDougall pro-gramme complet-ers, 1,615 (65%)	7-days, vegan diet	BW, lipids, BP, GLC, CREAT, CHDR, BUN	1.4 kg (median, IQR 1.8)
Mishra[33] 2013 USA	RCT	GEICO employ-ees, overweight adults 291 (83%)	18-weeks, low-fat vegan diet vs normal diet	BW, BMI, lipids, BP, HbA1c	2.9 kg vs no loss in controls, p<0.001
Moore[15] 2015 USA	RCT	Overweight and obese adults 63 (73%)	6-months, vegan, vegetarian, pesco-vegetarian, semi-vegetarian or omnivore	BW and die-tary adherence	6 kg +/- 6.7% in vegans/vegetarians vs 0.4kg +/- 0.6 kg in omnivores, p=0.04
Sisay[41] 2020 Ethiopia	Intervention trial with no control group	Orthodox Christians observing Lent, 75 (45%)	7-week vegan diet analysed at week 7 and 7 weeks post intervention	BP, BW, WC, BMI, lipids	2.4 kg (M), 3.7 kg (F), p=0.02
Turner-McGrievy[28] 2007 USA	RCT	PM overweight women, 62	14 weeks, low-fat vegan vs NCEP diet, assessment at 2 years	BW	3.1 kg (0.0–6.0) intervention vs 0.8 kg (-3.1–4.2), p=0.022
Turner-McGrievy[36] 2015 USA	RCT (same cohort as Moore 2015)	Overweight and obese adults 63 (73%)	6-months, vegan, vegetarian, pesco-vegetarian, semi-vegetarian or omnivore	BW	7.5% +/- 4.5% greater loss than other groups, p=0.03
Wright[37] 2017 New Zealand	RCT	Overweight and obesity with comorbidity 65 (60%)	12-weeks vegan diet with twice weekly meetings, as-sessed at 6 months vs normal diet	BMI and cholesterol	4.4 kg in intervention, 0.4 kg in control, 95%CI for difference between groups is +/- 1 kg, p<0.0001

Abbreviations for Table 6.1: ADA: American Diabetic Association; anti-PC: antiphosphatidylcholine antibodies: APO: apolipoproteins; BP: blood pressure: BMI: body mass index; BUN: blood urea nitrogen; BW: body weight; CHDR: coronary heart disease risk; CREAT: creatinine; CRP: C reactive protein; DAS28: disease activity score; EE: energy expenditure; EI: energy intake; FAT: fat mass; GEICO: Government Employees Insurance Company; GHQ: general health questionnaire; GLC: glucose; HAQ: health activity questionnaire; HC: hip circumference; INS: insulin; IS: insu-lin sensitivity; JS: joint stiffness; NCEP: National Cholesterol Education Programme; PI: protein intake; PM: post-menopausal; QOS: quality of sleep; RCT: randomised controlled trial; RMR: resting metabolic rate; TEF: thermic effect of food; VAS: visual analogue scores; WC: waist circumference; WHR: waist/hip ratio.

A 74-week intervention comparing a low-fat vegan diet with the American Diabetic Association-recommended diet in participants with diabetes of any starting weight, found the mean loss in those who continued their medication throughout was 6.5 kg in the vegan group compared with 3.1 kg in the ADA group, p=0.0001.[31]

Another study assessed employees of the USA Government Employees Insurance Company. Participants followed either a low-fat vegan diet or their normal diet, and the intervention group lost 5.3 kg more in 22 weeks.[32] A similar study in a different cohort from the same company noted a 2.9 kg weight loss compared with no loss in controls over 18 weeks, p<0.001.[33]

In 2014 a 6-month intervention assessing the effects of a low-carbohydrate vegan diet and a high-carbohydrate lacto-ovo-vegetarian diet noted that both groups lost weight, although the vegan group lost more, p=0.047.[34] In the same year, patients undergoing an inpatient intervention that included a low-fat vegan diet, had a median weight loss at 7 days of 1.4 kg. There were no controls.[35]

Two articles discussed a randomised controlled trial, assessing the effects of vegan, vegetarian, pescatarian, semi-vegetarian and omnivore diets over six months. The vegan cohort lost significantly more weight than the other groups.[15, 36] even if they were not strongly adherent to the diet.

The BROAD study assessed a 12-week intervention, including a low-fat vegan diet and regular support meetings with normal diet in participants with overweight or obesity and ≥1 comorbidity. The intervention group lost 4.4 kg, p<0.0001.[37]

A non-randomised but controlled trial comparing a low-fat vegan diet, including regular meal replacements, with controls receiving regular educational material about the benefits of a plant-based diet, demonstrated a loss of 5.6 kg in 10 weeks compared with 1.2 kg in controls, p<0.001.[38]

In 2018, two articles discussing the same cohort, compared the effects of a low-fat vegan diet with the participants 'usual diet' over 16 weeks in patients with overweight, and noted a loss of 6.5 kg in 16 weeks compared with no weight change in controls, p<0.001.[39, 40]

Most recently, an assessment of Orthodox Christians voluntarily following a vegan diet for seven weeks during Lenten noted that males lost 2.4 kg and females 3.7 kg , (p=0.02) a significant change from baseline.[41]

Limitations of these trials are that they are heterogeneous in terms of size, duration, design, inclusion criteria, and in different populations, and the longest intervention was 74 weeks. Longer trials are needed in order to further substantiate the effects suggested by these and the epidemiological data.

In summary, all of the interventions noted significant weight loss, and the majority allowed *ad libitum* intakes of low-fat vegan food. In comparison with other dietary patterns, weight loss was at least equivalent, or significantly more in the low-fat vegan groups. Some of the trials also noted a reduction in fat mass as well as BMI, which is relevant in light of concerns about sarcopenic obesity. In light of the multiple other presumed health benefits of plant-based diets, and the environmental and ethical benefits, plant-based diets can be considered a viable intervention for sustainable weight loss.

Differences between plant-based diets and other eating patterns

Energy density

One of the great advantages of plant-based diets is that they are generally low in energy density. Energy density describes the amount of energy per weight or volume of food, so kcal per 100 g for example. People eat a consistent weight of food per day, typically about three pounds. It stands to reason that eating three pounds of food that contains a lot of calories will result in the absorption of a greater amount of energy than that obtained from three pounds of food containing fewer calories.

The foods with the lowest energy density are all plant foods. The lowest subgroups are the green, leafy vegetables and cruciferous vegetables, followed by non-starchy vegetables, fruits and then starchy vegetables. Whole grains and legumes have a slightly higher energy density, but as part of a mixed diet are consistent with weight loss. Meat and dairy, or meat and dairy substitutes, have a slightly higher energy density, followed by baked goods, sugars, nuts and seeds, oil-based spreads and lastly oils, which have the highest energy density of all foods. A diet that is based on vegetables, fruits, whole grains and legumes is naturally low-energy density. This is because of the high fibre and water content of these foods, with both fibre and water adding volume and weight to food without adding calories. Lowering the fat content of the diet also reduces energy density as fat is the most energy dense of the macronutrients, and plant-based diets tend to be lower in fat than other eating patterns.

There is agreement in the literature that reducing dietary energy density does result in reduced intake in practice, including cross sectional,[42, 43] observational[44] and intervention trial data. In one meta-analysis of randomised controlled trials, energy density was inversely correlated with body mass index,[45] and evidence suggests that reducing energy density both reduces energy intake and also results in weight loss that is superior to controls or other dietary patterns, for example the POUNDS LOST study.[46] Lower energy density diets are also effective for weight loss maintenance and compare favourably with other diets. Reducing dietary fat is effective but combining reduced fat with increased fibre is superior.[47] Reducing dietary energy density does not affect hunger or satiety.[48]

A high nutrient dense diet is associated with lower body weight, particularly a diet incorporating large quantities of vegetables,[49] with special focus being on the fruits and vegetables with the lowest energy densities,[47] and also pulses.[50] Plant-based diets have the highest levels of micronutrients,[51] and intervention trial evidence suggest that changing to a plant-based diet from a variety of other eating patterns improves dietary quality.[52]

Plant protein

Protein has been the focus of extensive research related to weight management as it is the most satiating of the three macronutrients.[53] Prospective observational evidence suggests that high intake of animal protein is associated with weight gain over time, whereas plant-based protein intake is not.[54] Plant-based diets typically include more pulses as a protein source than other dietary patterns, and intervention trials suggest that pulses are associated with weight loss.[50]

Trials comparing the effects of meals containing plant and animal proteins on hunger, satiety and weight have produced mixed results. No human trials have found that animal proteins are superior, but some have found no difference between animal and plant proteins in terms of weight, for example Nielsen et al., 2018,[55] while others have concluded that plant protein is superior for weight loss, for example Kristensen et al., 2016.[56]

Soya has been researched specifically because of its reputation as a 'complete' protein, and it does have apparent benefits for weight loss. This could be because foods containing soya also contain significant quantities of fibre, or because of the metabolic effects of the isoflavones in soya, but evidence suggests that the protein in soya does directly promote weight loss.[53]

A trial assessing the different effects of plant

and animal proteins in the diet for several weeks concluded that plant proteins were associated with greater weight loss, fat mass reduction and improvement in insulin sensitivity.[39]

There are potential mechanisms that may explain the superior effects of plant proteins compared with animal proteins in promoting weight loss. They have different effects on insulin and glucagon, with a diet rich in the essential amino acids found in animal proteins tending to increase insulin secretion, thereby promoting protein and muscle synthesis but also fat storage. In contrast, a diet relatively richer in plants and therefore nonessential amino acids favours glucagon secretion. Glucagon reduces hepatic *de novo* lipogenesis, and also promotes fatty acid oxidation and therefore a reduction in body fat stores. Fatty acid oxidation in particular is associated with improved satiety and reduced hunger, which may be a significant contributor to the effects of plant proteins on weight loss.[57, 58]

Lower fat

Another benefit of plant-based diets for weight loss is that they tend to contain less fat than other dietary patterns.[51] Fat has a higher energy density than other macronutrients, leading to speculation that reducing dietary energy density by reducing fat intake may lead to weight loss. It is also known that high fat intakes are associated with hyperphagia, and that in contrast with other macronutrients, dietary fat is not autoregulated so fat intake can continue without any compensatory mechanisms in the body to reduce further intake.[59]

Nuts are of particular interest as they are relatively high in fat, yet not associated with weight gain. This may be because they improve satiety overall,[60, 61] and they may increase resting energy expenditure.[60] Other potential mechanisms include reduction of less favourable nutrient intakes as a result of the nut intakes, increased dietary-induced thermogenesis, reduced availability of the calories, anti-obesity effects of the micronutrients in nuts, and beneficial effects on the microbiome.[61]

Saturated fat in the diet may also be implicated in weight gain, as saturated fat stimulates insulin secretion, which promotes fat storage.[62] A plant-based diet is naturally low in saturated fat, as saturated fat is found almost exclusively in animal food products.

Systematic reviews agree that a low-fat diet results in weight loss overall. Conclusions are mixed regarding whether a low-fat diet is superior to other dietary patterns, particularly a low carbohydrate diet, but low-fat diets are at least equivalent.[63] This suggests that the low-fat nature of a plant-based diet may be one of the reasons why it is associated with weight loss.

Fibre and whole grains

Plant-based diets contain the highest amount of fibre,[51] and this has reputed benefits in weight regulation. Fibre improves satiety[64] because it adds volume to food without increasing energy intake, and it also increases the production of short chain fatty acids in the colon which are known to reduce the risk of obesity.[65] In addition, If dietary fibre intake increases, it typically results in a decrease in dietary fat intake.[66]

Cross sectional data suggests that low fibre intake is one of the strongest predictors for weight gain over time,[19] and prospective evidence suggests that fibre and whole grain intake decreases weight gain.[67] The POUNDS LOST intervention trial concluded that fibre intake was the strongest predictor for weight loss.[68]

Pulses

Diets high in pulses are associated with a reduced risk of obesity according to observational data,[69] with a number of studies documenting an inverse relationship between pulse consumption and BMI or risk of obesity. Elsewhere, a meta-analysis of randomised controlled trials suggests that increasing consumption of pulses can have a small but significant effect on body weight, resulting in weight loss overall, and probably fat loss.[50]

There are several potential mechanisms to explain this. Pulses are high in fibre and protein, and are low glycaemic index foods, all factors that are known to increase satiety as discussed elsewhere in this chapter, and trials have suggested that dietary pulses are associated with increased satiety. Pulses also often have intact cell walls when they are eaten, which results in their energy content being relatively difficult to digest and absorb. As such, their caloric availability is relatively low, so the calories that are ingested when pulses are eaten are not only associated with increased satiety, but with an increased likelihood of the calories ingested not being absorbed, resulting in a lower net calorie absorption overall.[50]

Drinks

Green tea contains epigallocatechin gallate, a polyphenol compound that is associated with weight loss because it is a lipase inhibitor, reducing the digestion and absorption of dietary fat. A number of human RCTs suggest that regular green tea consumption can result in modest weight loss.[70] Coffee also has suggested weight loss benefits because of its chlorogenic acid content, and epidemiological studies suggest that it too has modest weight loss benefits.[71] Intervention trial data, however, is currently lacking.

Water

One reason why fruit and vegetable consumption may contribute to weight loss is their water content. Water contains no calories, but adds volume to food, thereby reducing its energy density. As individuals tend to consume the same weight of food daily,[72] and lower energy density of meals reduces overall energy intake,[72, 73] this is associated with weight loss.[73] Evidence from preloading studies suggests that the volume ingested has more of an effect than energy content on subsequent energy intake. A large volume drink prior to a meal reduces the energy intake in that meal compared with a smaller volume, whereas varying the energy content of that drink has no effect.[74] Water alone as a preload does not affect subsequent energy intake, whereas water incorporated into food does reduce energy intake.[75] Fruits and vegetables naturally contain water, and it is likely that this contributes to their effects on body weight.

Effects of a plant-based diet on different contributors to weight regulation

Microbiome

Plant-based diets may affect body weight via effects on the gut microbiome. People living with obesity typically have different microbiota compared with those with a healthy weight. The two types of gut bacteria related to body weight are the firmicutes and bacteroidetes. The ratio of firmicutes to bacteroidetes varies with body weight, and the proportion of bacteroidetes varies inversely with body weight.[76] Increased diversity of the microbiome is associated with a healthy body weight.[77] Alteration in diet rapidly alters the microbiome,[78] and vegan diets are associated with a greater prevalence of bacteroidetes and microbiome diversity, possibly because of the high fibre intake.[79] Intervention trial evidence suggests that changing to a plant-based dietary pattern results in these changes,[80] suggesting another mechanism by which plant-based diets may modify body weight.

Endocrinology

Insulin resistance is one of the most widely acknowledged comorbidities of obesity, and weight loss can reverse this. However, insulin resistance promotes further worsening of obesity because of the associated hyperinsulinaemia encouraging increased fat storage. Increasing insulin sensitivity has associated benefits in reducing fat storage.[81] Epidemiological data suggests that those eating a plant-based diet have superior insulin sensitivity, for example the Rotterdam study.[82] This could be because a plant-based diet lacks branched chain amino acids that are only found in animal foods and are associated with an increase in insulin resistance, or because plant-based diets promote a reduction in intramyocellular lipid that is strongly associated with insulin resistance.[83] Intervention trials suggest that changing from a standard Western diet to a plant-based diet improves insulin sensitivity.[39, 84]

Plant-based diets may also modify hormones related to appetite and satiety. Leptin promotes satiety and reduces energy intake but can be elevated in a state of obesity due to leptin resistance in the same way that insulin levels can be elevated in a state of insulin resistance. Glucacon-like peptide 1 (GLP-1) slows gastric emptying and promotes satiety, among others.[85] One study suggests that people eating a plant-based diet have lower serum leptin levels, indicating a lower risk of leptin resistance.[86] Elsewhere, a vegan meal promotes greater secretion of GLP-1 and satiety than a meat-based meal.[87] The evidence is somewhat limited currently, but suggests a small benefit overall.

Thermic effect of food

For weight loss to occur, a state of energy deficit must be achieved and maintained, so that the individual is using more energy than they are absorbing from their diet. This can be achieved by either reducing energy intake, or increasing energy expenditure, or a combination of both. Evidence suggests that a combination of both is the most effective intervention for weight loss.[88] On this basis, any behaviour that increases energy expenditure has theoretical weight loss benefits.

Daily energy expenditure includes resting energy expenditure, activity related energy expenditure, and the energy required to digest and absorb nutrients. After any energy intake, metabolic rate increases as the work of digestion and absorption is done. This has been termed 'dietary-induced thermogenesis', or the thermic effect of food. The thermic effect of food is small, around 10–12% of total energy expenditure.[89] but in an obesogenic environment and the presence of an internal milieu that will resist weight loss, even marginal increases in energy expenditure can be significant.

Intervention trials have demonstrated that a low-fat, plant-based diet results in an increase in the thermic effect of food in comparison with other dietary patterns, for example Kahleova et al., 2020,[97] probably by reducing the amount of intramyocellular lipid in muscle and thereby improving insulin sensitivity. This is likely to be another reason why plant-based foods are associated with weight loss.

TMAO

Trimethylamine N-oxide (TMAO) is a molecule created by the metabolism of foods of animal origin that contain L-carnitine, choline and phosphatidylcholine. The main dietary sources of these are egg yolks, milk, dairy products, organ and muscle meats, and seafood such as molluscs, crustaceans and fish. There are some plant sources, but the levels are lower in these foods. These provide the substrate for the gut microbiota to create trimethylamine, which is then metabolised in the liver to TMAO. It has been widely studied because of a putative role in the aetiology of cardiovascular disease and type 2 diabetes, but more recently it has become of interest as a potential cause of weight gain and obesity.

A meta-analysis of levels of TMAO in the blood and risk of obesity has found a significant positive association. Those with the lowest levels of circulating TMAO are at a low risk of obesity, and those with the highest levels of TMAO have a corresponding elevated risk. At time of writing there is no human data regarding a plausible mechanism for this, so TMAO has not yet been proven to have a causal role in the aetiology of obesity. It may be related to the effects of TMAO on insulin resistance.[90]

A plant-based diet is low in foods that provide substrates for the microbiota to synthesise trimethylamine, and vegans have lower circulating levels of TMAO than omnivores. They also synthesise less TMAO than omnivorous peers after consuming carnitine. This may be another reason why plant foods are associated with a lower risk of overweight and obesity.[91]

Anti-inflammatory effects

The chronic low grade inflammatory state associated with obesity is both a cause and a consequence of it. Oxidative stress increases adiposity and affects genetics, the microbiome, insulin and appetite regulation in ways that promote further increases in weight gain and adiposity.[92] Cross-sectional data and a review of intervention trials[93] suggest that a plant-based diet is associated with lower levels of pro-inflammatory molecules and a reduction in the obesity related pro-inflammatory state.

Effects on the reward system

Food can affect dopamine and opioid activity in the brain. Dopamine forms part of the mesolimbic system and is associated with reward, whereas opioids are associated with reduction in pain. Both are related to addiction type behaviours, and are dysfunctional in the presence of obesity.[94] The chronic low grade pro-inflammatory state associated with obesity may be implicated in this process, as reactive oxygen species contribute to the dysregulation of these systems, affecting appetite and satiety, and increasing addiction type behaviour.[92] Some foods contain exogenous opioids that can stimulate opioid receptors directly; these are mainly dairy products, but also include wheat and soya to a lesser extent.[95] One randomised controlled trial assessing this in vegan diets investigated the effects of a plant-based meal vs a conventional control meal on subsequent perfusion of the thalamus, which is a key part of the brain involved in appetite, satiety and reward. The plant-based diet resulted in significantly less thalamic perfusion based on MRI imaging in comparison with the conventional meal, suggesting less stimulation of the reward and appetite pathways.[96] This may be another reason why plant-based diets are associated with lower energy intake and lower body weight.

Conclusion

Evidence consistently demonstrates that plant-based diets are effective for weight loss and are usually more effective than other eating patterns. There are a number of physiological reasons for this, based on the differences between a whole food plant-based diet and other eating patterns. Plant-based diets also ameliorate the effects of a number of obesity-related comorbidities, as detailed elsewhere in this book, therefore there are many benefits that occur independently of weight loss.

References

1. Di Cesare M, Bentham J, Stevens GA, Zhou B, Danaei G, Lu Y, et al. Trends in adult body-mass index in 200 countries from 1975 to 2014: A pooled analysis of 1698 population-based measurement studies with 19.2 million participants. *Lancet* 2016; 387(10026): 1377–1396. doi: 10.1016/S0140-6736(16)30054-X
2. Ng M, Fleming T, Robinson M, Thomson B, Graetz N, Margono C, et al. Global, regional, and national prevalence of overweight and obesity in children and adults during 1980-2013: A systematic analysis for the Global Burden of Disease Study 2013. *Lancet* 2014; 384(9945): 766–781. doi: 10.1016/S0140-6736(14)60460-8
3. Di Angelantonio E, Bhupathiraju SN, Wormser D, Gao P, Kaptoge S, de Gonzalez AB, et al. Body-mass index and all-cause mortality: individual-participant-data meta-analysis of 239 prospective studies in four continents. *Lancet* 2016; 388(10046): 776–786. doi: 10.1016/S0140-6736(16)30175-1
4. Lim SS, Vos T, Flaxman AD, Danaei G, Shibuya K, Adair-Rohani H, et al. A comparative risk assessment of burden of disease and injury attributable to 67 risk factors and risk factor clusters in 21 regions, 1990-2010: A systematic analysis for the Global Burden of Disease Study 2010. *Lancet* 2012; 380(9859): 2224–2260. doi: 10.1016/S0140-6736(12)61766-8
5. Printz C. Extreme obesity may shorten life expectancy up to 14 years. *Cancer* 2014; 120(23): 3591–3591.
6. Tobore TO. Towards a comprehensive theory of obesity and a healthy diet: The causal role of oxidative stress in food addiction and obesity. *Behavioural Brain Research* 2020; 384: 112560. doi: 10.1016/j.bbr.2020.112560
7. Butland B, Jebb S, Kopelman P, Mcpherson K. Tackling Obesities: Future Choices-Project Report 2 nd Edition Government Office for Science Foresight Tackling Obesities: Future Choices-Project report.
8. Herrera BM, Keildson S, Lindgren CM. Genetics and epigenetics of obesity. *Maturitas* 2011; 69(1): 41–49. doi: 10.1016/j.maturitas.2011.02.018
9. Heianza Y, Qi L. Gene-diet interaction and precision nutrition in obesity. *International Journal of Molecular Sciences* 2017; 18(4): 787. doi: 10.3390/ijms18040787
10. Blackburn G. Effect of Degree of Weight Loss on Health Benefits. *Obes Res* 1995; 3(2 S): 211s-216s. doi: 10.1002/j.1550-8528.1995.tb00466.x
11. Bray GA, Kim KK, Wilding JPH. Obesity: a chronic relapsing progressive disease process. A position statement of the World Obesity Federation. *Obes Rev* 2017; 18(7): 715-723. doi: 10.1111/obr.12551
12. O'Brien PE, Hindle A, Brennan L, Skinner S, Burton P, Smith A, et al. Long-Term Outcomes After Bariatric Surgery: a Systematic Review and Meta-analysis of Weight Loss at 10 or More Years for All Bariatric Procedures and a Single-Centre Review of 20-Year Outcomes After Adjustable Gastric Banding. *Obes Surg* 2019; 29(1): 3–14. doi: 10.1007/s11695-018-3525-0
13. Wiggins T, Guidozzi N, Welbourn R, Ahmed AR, Markar SR. Association of bariatric surgery with all-cause mortality and incidence of obesity-related disease at a population level: A systematic review and meta-analysis. *PLoS Medicine* 2020; 17(7): e1003206. doi: 10.1371/journal.pmed.1003206
14. Acharya SD, Elci OU, Sereika SM, Music E, Styn MA, Turk MW, et al. Adherence to a behavioral weight loss treatment program enhances weight loss and improvements in biomarkers. *Patient Prefer Adherence* 2009; 3: 151–60. doi: 10.2147/ppa.s5802
15. Moore WJ, McGrievy ME, Turner-McGrievy GM. Dietary adherence and acceptability of five different diets, including vegan and vegetarian diets, for weight loss: The New DIETs study. *Eat Behav* 2015; 19: 33–38. doi: 10.1016/j.eatbeh.2015.06.011
16. Fraser G, Katuli S, Anousheh R, Knutsen S, Herring P, Fan J. Vegetarian diets and cardiovascular risk factors in black members of the Adventist Health Study-2. *Public Health Nutr* 2015; 18(3): 537–45. doi: 10.1017/S1368980014000263
17. Rizzo NS, Jaceldo-Siegl K, Sabate J, Fraser GE. Nutrient Profiles of Vegetarian and Nonvegetarian Dietary Patterns. *J Acad Nutr Diet*

2013; 113(12): 1610–9.
doi: 10.1016/j.jand.2013.06.349
18. Le LT, Sabaté J. Beyond meatless, the health effects of vegan diets: Findings from the Adventist cohorts. *Nutrients* 2014; 6(6):2131–47.
doi: 10.3390/nu6062131
19. Spencer EA, Appleby PN, Davey GK, Key TJ. Diet and body mass index in 38 000 EPIC-Oxford meat-eaters, fish-eaters, vegetarians and vegans. *Int J Obes* 2003 ; 27(6): 728–34.
doi: 10.1038/sj.ijo.0802300
20. Li J, Zhou R, Huang W, Wang J. Bone loss, low height, and low weight in different populations and district: a meta-analysis between vegans and non-vegans. *Food Nutr Res* 2020; 64: 1–14.
doi: 10.29219/fnr.v64.3315
21. Rosell M, Appleby P, Spencer E, Key T. Weight gain over 5 years in 21 966 meat-eating, fish-eating, vegetarian, and vegan men and women in EPIC-Oxford. *Int J Obes* 2006; 30(9): 1389–1396.
doi: 10.1038/sj.ijo.0803305
22. Japas C, Knutsen S, Dehom S, Dos Santos H, Tonstad S. Body mass index gain between ages 20 and 40 years and lifestyle characteristics of men at ages 40-60 years: The Adventist Health Study-2. *Obes Res Clin Pract* 2014; 8(6): e549–e557.
doi: 10.1016/j.orcp.2013.11.007
23. Medawar E, Huhn S, Villringer A, Veronica Witte A. The effects of plant-based diets on the body and the brain: a systematic review. *Translational Psychiatry* 2019; 9(266).
doi: 10.1038/s41398-019-0552-0
24. Huang RY, Huang CC, Hu FB, Chavarro JE. Vegetarian Diets and Weight Reduction: a Meta-Analysis of Randomized Controlled Trials. *J Gen Intern Med* 2016; 31(1): 109–116.
doi: 10.1007/s11606-015-3390-7
25. Lindahl O, Lindwall L, Spångberg A, Stenram Åk, Öckerman PA. A vegan regimen with reduced medication in the treatment of hypertension. *Br J Nutr* 1984; 52(1): 11–20.
doi: 10.1079/bjn19840066
26. Kaartinen K, Lammi K, Hypen M, Nenonen M, Hänninen O. Vegan diet alleviates fibromyalgia symptoms. *Scand J Rheumatol* 2000; 29(5): 308–313. doi: 10.1080/030097400447697
27. Barnard ND, Scialli AR, Turner-McGrievy G, Lanou AJ, Glass J. The effects of a low-fat, plant-based dietary intervention on body weight, metabolism, and insulin sensitivity. *Am J Med* 2005; 118(9): 991–997.
doi: 10.1016/j.amjmed.2005.03.039
28. Turner-McGrievy GM, Barnard ND, Scialli AR. A two-year randomized weight loss trial comparing a vegan diet to a more moderate low-fat diet. *Obesity* 2007;15(9): 2276–2281.
doi: 10.1038/oby.2007.270
29. Dansinger ML, Gleason JA, Griffith JL, Selker HP, Schaefer EJ. Comparison of the Atkins, Ornish, Weight Watchers, and Zone Diets for weight loss and heart disease risk reduction: A randomized trial. *J Am Med Assoc* 2005; 293(1): 43–53.
doi: 10.1001/jama.293.1.43
30. Elkan AC, Sjöberg B, Kolsrud B, Ringertz B, Hafström I, Frostegård J. Gluten-free vegan diet induces decreased LDL and oxidized LDL levels and raised atheroprotective natural antibodies against phosphorylcholine in patients with rheumatoid arthritis: A randomized study. *Arthritis Res Ther* 2008; 10(2): R34.
doi: 10.1186/ar2388
31. Barnard ND, Cohen J, Jenkins DJ, Turner-McGrievy G, Gloede L, Green A, Ferdowsian H. A low-fat vegan diet and a conventional diabetes diet in the treatment of type 2 diabetes: a randomized, controlled, 74-wk clinical trial. *Am J Clin Nutr* 2009; 89(5): 1588S-1596S.
doi: 10.3945/ajcn.2009.26736H..
32. Ferdowsian HR, Barnard ND, Hoover VJ, Katcher HI, Levin SM, Green AA, et al. A multicomponent intervention reduces body weight and cardiovascular risk at a GEICO corporate site. *Am J Heal Promot* 2010; 24(6): 384–387. doi: 10.4278/ajhp.081027-QUAN-255
33. Mishra S, Xu J, Agarwal U, Gonzales J, Levin S, Barnard ND. A multicenter randomized controlled trial of a plant-based nutrition program to reduce body weight and cardiovascular risk in the corporate setting: The GEICO study. *Eur J Clin Nutr* 2013; 67(7): 718–724. doi: 10.1038/ejcn.2013.92
34. Jenkins DJA, Wong JMW, Kendall CWC, Esfahani A, Ng VWY, Leong TCK, et al. Effect of a 6-month vegan low-carbohydrate ('Eco-Atkins') diet on cardiovascular risk factors and body weight in hyperlipidaemic adults: A randomised

controlled trial. *BMJ Open* 2014; 4(2). doi: 10.1136/bmjopen-2013-003505
35. McDougall J, Thomas LE, McDougall C, Moloney G, Saul B, Finnell JS, et al. Effects of 7 days on an ad libitum low-fat vegan diet: The McDougall Program cohort. *Nutr J* 2014; 13(1): 99. doi: 10.1186/1475-2891-13-99
36. Turner-McGrievy GM, Davidson CR, Wingard EE, Wilcox S, Frongillo EA. Comparative effectiveness of plant-based diets for weight loss: A randomized controlled trial of five different diets. *Nutrition* 2015; 31(2): 350–358. doi: 10.1016/j.nut.2014.09.002
37. Wright N, Wilson L, Smith M, Duncan B, McHugh P. The BROAD study: A randomised controlled trial using a whole food plant-based diet in the community for obesity, ischaemic heart disease or diabetes. *Nutr Diabetes* 2017; 7(3): e256. doi: 10.1038/nutd.2017.3
38. Jakše B, Pinter S, Jakše B, Bučar Pajek M, Pajek J. Effects of an Ad Libitum Consumed Low-Fat Plant-Based Diet Supplemented with Plant-Based Meal Replacements on Body Composition Indices. *Biomed Res Int* 2017. doi: 10.1155/2017/9626390
39. Kahleova H, Fleeman R, Hlozkova A, Holubkov R, Barnard ND. A plant-based diet in overweight individuals in a 16-week randomized clinical trial: metabolic benefits of plant protein. *Nutr Diabetes* 2018; 8(1): 58. doi: 10.1038/s41387-018-0067-4
40. Kahleova H, Dort S, Holubkov R, Barnard ND. A plant-based high-carbohydrate, low-fat diet in overweight individuals in a 16-week randomized clinical trial: The role of carbohydrates. *Nutrients* 2018; 10(9): 1302. doi: 10.3390/nu10091302
41. Sisay T, Tolessa T, Mekonen W. Changes in biochemical parameters by gender and time: Effect of short-term vegan diet adherence. *PLoS One* 2020; 15(8): e0237065. doi: 10.1371/journal.pone.0237065
42. Ledikwe JH, Blanck HM, Khan LK, Serdula MK, Seymour JD, Tohill BC, et al. Dietary energy density is associated with energy intake and weight status in US adults. *American Journal of Clinical Nutrition* 2006; 83(6): 1362-1268. doi: 10.1093/ajcn/83.6.1362
43. Vernarelli JA, Mitchell DC, Rolls BJ, Hartman TJ. Dietary energy density and obesity: how consumption patterns differ by body weight status. *Eur J Nutr* 2018; 57(1): 351–361. doi: 10.1007/s00394-016-1324-8
44. Stelmach-Mardas M, Rodacki T, Dobrowolska-Iwanek J, Brzozowska A, Walkowiak J, Wojtanowska-Krosniak A, et al. Link between food energy density and body weight changes in obese adults. *Nutrients* 2016; 8(4): 229. doi: 10.3390/nu8040229
45. Rouhani MH, Haghighatdoost F, Surkan PJ, Azadbakht L. Associations between dietary energy density and obesity: A systematic review and meta-analysis of observational studies. *Nutrition* 2016; 32(10): 1037-1047. doi: 10.1016/j.nut.2016.03.017
46. Champagne C, Burton J, DeCesare L, Johnson C, Talbot G, Sacks F, et al. Energy Density and Adherence as Predictors of Weight Loss in the POUNDS LOST Study. *FASEB J* 29: 117.5.
47. Bertoia ML, Mukamal KJ, Cahill LE, Hou T, Ludwig DS, Mozaffarian D, et al. Changes in Intake of Fruits and Vegetables and Weight Change in United States Men and Women Followed for Up to 24 Years: Analysis from Three Prospective Cohort Studies. Razak F, editor. *PLOS Med* 2015; 12(9): e1001878. doi: 10.1371/journal.pmed.1001878
48. Bell EA, Castellanos VH, Pelkman CL, Thorwart ML, Rolls BJ. Energy density of foods affects energy intake in normal-weight women. *Am J Clin Nutr* 1998; 67(3): 412–420. doi: 10.1093/ajcn/67.3.412
49. Tapsell LC, Batterham MJ, Thorne RL, O'Shea JE, Grafenauer SJ, Probst YC. Weight loss effects from vegetable intake: A 12-month randomised controlled trial. *Eur J Clin Nutr* 2014; 68(7): 778–785. doi: 10.1038/ejcn.2014.39
50. Kim SJ, de Souza RJ, Choo VL, Ha V, Cozma AI, Chiavaroli L, et al. Effects of dietary pulse consumption on body weight: a systematic review and meta-analysis of randomized controlled trials. *Am J Clin Nutr* 2016; 103(5): 1213–1223. doi: 10.3945/ajcn.115.124677
51. Davey GK, Spencer EA, Appleby PN, Allen NE, Knox KH, Key TJ. EPIC–Oxford:lifestyle characteristics and nutrient intakes in a cohort of 33 883 meat-eaters and 31 546 non meat-eaters in the UK. *Public Health Nutr* 2003; 6(3): 259–69.

doi: 10.1079/PHN2002430

52. Dewell A, Weidner G, Sumner MD, Chi CS, Ornish D. A Very-Low-Fat Vegan Diet Increases Intake of Protective Dietary Factors and Decreases Intake of Pathogenic Dietary Factors. *J Am Diet Assoc* 2008; 108(2): 347–356. doi: 10.1016/j.jada.2007.10.044

53. Velasquez MT, Bhathena SJ. Role of dietary soy protein in obesity. *International Journal of Medical Sciences* 2007; 4(2): 72-82. doi: 10.7150/ijms.4.72

54. Halkjær J, Olsen A, Overvad K, Jakobsen MU, Boeing H, Buijsse B, et al. Intake of total, animal and plant protein and subsequent changes in weight or waist circumference in European men and women: The Diogenes project. *Int J Obes* 2011; 35(8): 1104–1113. doi: 10.1038/ijo.2010.254

55. Nielsen L V., Kristensen MD, Klingenberg L, Ritz C, Belza A, Astrup A, et al. Protein from meat or vegetable sources in meals matched for fiber content has similar effects on subjective appetite sensations and energy intake—A randomized acute cross-over meal test study. *Nutrients* 2018; 10(1): 96. doi: 10.3390/nu10010096

56. Kristensen MD, Bendsen NT, Christensen SM, Astrup A, Raben A. Meals based on vegetable protein sources (beans and peas) are more satiating than meals based on animal protein sources (veal and pork) - A randomized crossover meal test study. *Food Nutr Res* 2016; 60: 32634. doi: 10.3402/fnr.v60.32634

57. McCarty MF. Vegan proteins may reduce risk of cancer, obesity, and cardiovascular disease by promoting increased glucagon activity. *Med Hypotheses* 1999; 53(6): 459–485. doi: 10.1054/mehy.1999.0784

58. McCarty MF. The origins of Western obesity: A role for animal protein? *Med Hypotheses* 2000; 54(3): 488–494. doi: 10.1054/mehy.1999.0882

59. Prentice AM. Manipulation of dietary fat and energy density and subsequent effects on substrate flux and food intake. In: American Journal of Clinical Nutrition. *American Society for Nutrition* 1998; 67(3): 535S-541S. doi: 10.1093/ajcn/67.3.535S

60. Tan SY, Dhillon J, Mattes RD. A review of the effects of nuts on appetite, food intake, metabolism, and body weight. In: American Journal of Clinical Nutrition. *American Society for Nutrition* 2014; 100(1): 412S-22S. doi: 10.3945/ajcn.113.071456

61. Tindall AM, Petersen KS, Lamendella R, Shearer GC, Murray-Kolb LE, Proctor DN, et al. Tree nut consumption and adipose tissue mass: Mechanisms of action. *Current Developments in Nutrition* 2018; 2(11): nzy069 doi: 10.1093/cdn/nzy069.

62. McCarty MF. Dietary saturate/unsaturate ratio as a determinant of adiposity. *Med Hypotheses* 2010; 75(1): 14–16. doi: 10.1016/j.mehy.2009.12.021

63. Johnston BC, Kanters S, Bandayrel K, Wu P, Naji F, Siemieniuk RA, et al. Comparison of weight loss among named diet programs in overweight and obese adults: A meta-analysis. *J Am Med Assoc* 2014; 312(9): 923–933. doi: 10.1001/jama.2014.10397

64. Samra RA, Anderson GH. Insoluble cereal fiber reduces appetite and short-term food intake and glycemic response to food consumed 75 min later by healthy men. *Am J Clin Nutr* 2007; 86(4): 972–979. doi: 10.1093/ajcn/86.4.972

65. McNabney SM, Henagan TM. Short chain fatty acids in the colon and peripheral tissues: A focus on butyrate, colon cancer, obesity and insulin resistance. *Nutrients* 2017; 9(12): 1348. doi: 10.3390/nu9121348

66. Lattimer JM, Haub MD. Effects of Dietary Fiber and Its Components on Metabolic Health. *Nutrients* 2010; 2(12): 1266–1289. doi: 10.3390/nu2121266

67. Ye EQ, Chacko SA, Chou EL, Kugizaki M, Liu S. Greater Whole-Grain Intake Is Associated with Lower Risk of Type 2 Diabetes, Cardiovascular Disease, and Weight Gain. *J Nutr* 2012; 142(7): 1304–1313. doi: 10.3945/jn.111.155325

68. Miketinas D, Bray G, Sacks F, Champagne C. Fiber Intake, Dietary Energy Density, and Adherence to Diet Assignment are Positively Associated with Weight-Loss in Free-Living Adults Consuming Calorie-Restricted Diets at 6-Month Follow-Up: The POUNDS LOST Study. FASEB J 2018; 31: 796.2-796.2. doi: 10.1096/fasebj.31.1_supplement.796.2

69. McCrory MA, Hamaker BR, Lovejoy JC, Eichelsdoerfer PE. Pulse consumption, satiety, and weight management. *Advances in Nutrition* 2010; 1(1): 17–30. doi: 10.3945/an.110.1006

70. Suzuki T, Pervin M, Goto S, Isemura M, Nakamura Y. Beneficial effects of tea and the green tea catechin epigallocatechin-3-gallate on obesity. *Molecules* 2016; 21(10): 1305. doi: 10.3390/molecules21101305
71. Lee A, Lim W, Kim S, Khil H, Cheon E, An S, et al. Coffee intake and obesity: A meta-analysis. *Nutrients* 2019; 11(6): 1274. doi: 10.3390/nu11061274
72. Rolls BJ. The relationship between dietary energy density and energy intake. *Physiol Behav* 2009; 97(5): 609–615. doi: 10.1016/j.physbeh.2009.03.011
73. de Oliveira MC, Sichieri R, Venturim Mozzer R. A low-energy-dense diet adding fruit reduces weight and energy intake in women. *Appetite* 2008; 51(2): 291–295. doi: 10.1016/j.appet.2008.03.001
74. Rolls BJ, Castellanos VH, Halford JC, Kilara A, Panyam D, Pelkman CL, et al. Volume of food consumed affects satiety in men. *Am J Clin Nutr* 1998; 67(6): 1170–1177. doi: 10.1093/ajcn/67.6.1170
75. Rolls BJ, Bell EA, Thorwart ML. Water incorporated into a food but not served with a food decreases energy intake in lean women. *Am J Clin Nutr* 1999; 70(4): 448–455. doi: 10.1093/ajcn/70.4.448
76. Tseng CH, Wu CY. The gut microbiome in obesity. *Journal of the Formosan Medical Association* 2019; 118(1): S3-S9. doi: 10.1016/j.jfma.2018.07.009
77. Menni C, Jackson MA, Pallister T, Steves CJ, Spector TD, Valdes AM. Gut microbiome diversity and high-fibre intake are related to lower long-term weight gain. *Int J Obes* 2017; 41(7): 1099–1105. doi: 10.1038/ijo.2017.66
78. David LA, Maurice CF, Carmody RN, Gootenberg DB, Button JE, Wolfe BE, et al. Diet rapidly and reproducibly alters the human gut microbiome. *Nature* 2014; 505(7484): 559–563. doi: 10.1038/nature12820
79. Glick-Bauer M, Yeh MC. The health advantage of a vegan diet: Exploring the gut microbiota connection. *Nutrients* 2014; 6(11): 4822-4838. doi: 10.3390/nu6114822
80. Kahleova H, Rembert E, Alwarith J, Yonas WN, Tura A, Holubkov R, et al. Effects of a low-fat vegan diet on gut microbiota in overweight individuals and relationships with body weight, body composition, and insulin sensitivity. A randomized clinical trial. *Nutrients* 2020; 12(10): 1–16. doi: 10.3390/nu12102917
81. Barazzoni R, Gortan Cappellari G, Ragni M, Nisoli E. Insulin resistance in obesity: an overview of fundamental alterations. *Eating and Weight Disorders* 2018; 23(2): 149-157. doi: 10.1007/s40519-018-0481-6
82. Chen Z, Zuurmond MG, van der Schaft N, Nano J, Wijnhoven HAH, Ikram MA, et al. Plant versus animal based diets and insulin resistance, prediabetes and type 2 diabetes: the Rotterdam Study. *Eur J Epidemiol* 2018; 33(9): 883–893. doi: 10.1007/s10654-018-0414-8
83. Adeva-Andany MM, Gonz Alez-Luc M, Fern Andez-Fern Andez C, Carneiro-Freire N, Onica Seco-Filgueira M, María Pedre-Pi A. Effect of diet composition on insulin sensitivity in humans. *Clin Nutr ESPEN* 2019; 33: 29-38. doi: 10.1016/j.clnesp.2019.05.014
84. Goff LM, Bell JD, So PW, Dornhorst A, Frost GS. Veganism and its relationship with insulin resistance and intramyocellular lipid. *Eur J Clin Nutr* 2005; 59(2): 291–298. doi: 10.1038/sj.ejcn.1602076
85. Perry B, Wang Y. Appetite regulation and weight control: The role of gut hormones. *Nutrition and Diabetes* 2012; 2(1): e26. doi: 10.1038/nutd.2011.21
86. Gogga P, Śliwińska A, Aleksandrowicz-Wrona E, Małgorzewicz S. Association between different types of plant-based diets and leptin levels in healthy volunteers. *Acta Biochim Pol* 2019; 66(1): 77–82. doi: 10.18388/abp.2018_2725
87. Klementova M, Thieme L, Haluzik M, Pavlovicova R, Hill M, Pelikanova T, et al. A plant-based meal increases gastrointestinal hormones and satiety more than an energy-and macronutrient-matched processed-meat meal in t2d, obese, and healthy men: A three-group randomized crossover study. *Nutrients* 2019; 11(1): 157. doi: 10.3390/nu11010157
88. Franz MJ, VanWormer JJ, Crain AL, Boucher JL, Histon T, Caplan W, et al. Weight-Loss Outcomes: A Systematic Review and Meta-Analysis of Weight-Loss Clinical Trials with a Minimum

1-Year Follow-Up. *J Am Diet Assoc* 2007; 107(10): 1755–1767. doi: 10.1016/j.jada.2007.07.017
89. Vermorel M, Lazzer S, Bitar A, Ribeyre J, Montaurier C, Fellmann N, et al. Contributing factors and variability of energy expenditure in non-obese, obese, and post-obese adolescents. *Reproduction Nutrition Development* 2005; 45(2): 129-142. doi: 10.1051/rnd:2005014
90. Dehghan P, Farhangi MA, Nikniaz L, Nikniaz Z, Asghari-Jafarabadi M. Gut microbiota-derived metabolite trimethylamine N-oxide (TMAO) potentially increases the risk of obesity in adults: An exploratory systematic review and dose-response meta- analysis. *Obes Rev* 2020; 21(5): e12993. doi: 10.1111/obr.12993
91. Koeth RA, Wang Z, Levison BS, Buffa JA, Org E, Sheehy BT, et al. Intestinal microbiota metabolism of l-carnitine, a nutrient in red meat, promotes atherosclerosis. *Nat Med* 2013; 19(5): 576–585. doi: 10.1038/nm.3145
92. Tobore TO. Towards a comprehensive theory of obesity and a healthy diet: The causal role of oxidative stress in food addiction and obesity. *Behavioural Brain Research* 2020; 384: 112560. doi: 10.1016/j.bbr.2020.112560
93. Eichelmann F, Schwingshackl L, Fedirko V, Aleksandrova K. Effect of plant-based diets on obesity-related inflammatory profiles: a systematic review and meta-analysis of intervention trials. *Obes Rev* 2016; 17(11): 1067–1079. doi: 10.1111/obr.12439
94. Leigh SJ, Morris MJ. The role of reward circuitry and food addiction in the obesity epidemic: An update. *Biol Psychol* 2018; 131: 31–42. doi: 10.1016/j.biopsycho.2016.12.013
95. Tyagi A, Daliri EBM, Ofosu FK, Yeon SJ, Oh DH. Food-derived opioid peptides in human health: A review. *International Journal of Molecular Sciences* 2020; 21(22): 8825. doi: 10.3390/ijms21228825
96. Kahleova H, Tintera J, Thieme L, Veleba J, Klementova M, Kudlackova M, et al. A plant-based meal affects thalamus perfusion differently than an energy- and macronutrient-matched conventional meal in men with type 2 diabetes, overweight/obese, and healthy men: A three-group randomized crossover study. *Clin Nutr* 2020; 40(4): 1822-1833. doi: 10.1016/j.clnu.2020.10.005
97. Kahleova H, Petersen KF, Shulman GI, Alwarith J, Rembert E, Tura A, Hill M, Holubkov R, Barnard ND. Effect of a Low-Fat Vegan Diet on Body Weight, Insulin Sensitivity, Postprandial Metabolism, and Intramyocellular and Hepatocellular Lipid Levels in Overweight Adults: A Randomized Clinical Trial. *JAMA Netw Open* 2020; 3(11): e2025454. doi:10.1001/jamanetworkopen.2020.25454

Chapter 7

Plant-based nutrition for the prevention and treatment of diabetes

Gemma Newman and Shireen Kassam

Introduction

Diabetes is a leading and growing cause of chronic disease globally. In 2019, the global prevalence of diabetes was 9.3% (463 million people), 90% of which is accounted for by type 2 diabetes.[1] It is predicted that by 2045, the prevalence will have increased to 10.9% (700 million people) with a more rapid rate of rise in middle- and low-income countries.[1,2] Similar numbers of people are living with impaired glucose tolerance.[1] Diabetes not only reduces life expectancy, particularly due to cardiovascular disease, but also adversely impacts quality of life.[3] Diet and lifestyle factors are responsible for the majority of cases of type 2 diabetes, especially the typical Western-style diet pattern, which is high in animal-derived and processed foods, and a sedentary lifestyle and thus it is a condition that is almost entirely preventable.[4] This chapter will review the evidence for the role of plant-based diets for the prevention and treatment of diabetes.

Plant-based diets for prevention of type 2 diabetes

Large prospective cohort studies demonstrate that the incidence of type 2 diabetes is significantly lower amongst those following a predominantly or exclusively plant-based diet pattern, including vegetarian and vegan diets. The EPIC-Oxford study included 45,314 participants who were free of diabetes at recruitment. Dietary data were correlated with linked hospital admissions and death data during the 17.6 years of follow-up in which 1,224 cases of diabetes were documented.[5] Participants were categorised as regular meat eaters, low meat eaters, fish eaters and vegetarian/vegan. Compared with regular meat eaters, the low meat eaters, fish eaters, and vegetarians and vegans were significantly less likely to develop diabetes (37–53% reduced risk) although these associations were substantially attenuated after adjusting for body mass index (BMI).

The Adventist Health Study 2 examined the prevalence of diabetes in 60,903 health-conscious participants living in the USA and Canada. The prevalence decreased in line with the degree of reduction in consumption of animal-derived foods from 7.6% in non-vegetarians, 6.1% in semi-vegetarians, 4.8% in pesco-vegetarians, 3.2% in lacto-ovo vegetarians and 2.9% in vegans.[6] Even after adjustment for BMI, the vegan group had half the rate of type 2 diabetes compared with non-vegetarians. In a prospective analysis from this same study cohort including 41,387 participants, those following a vegan or lacto-ovo vegetarian diet had a 77% and 54% reduction in the risk of developing diabetes, respectively. In the study's Black population (17%), the degree of the protection associated with vegetarian and vegan diets was as great as the excess risk associated with Black ethnicity.[7] It is worth noting that the non-vegans in this cohort ate meat and poultry relatively infrequently (once a week or more for non-vegetarians; less than once a week for semi-vegetarians), suggesting that even small increases in red meat and poultry consumption can disproportionately increase the risk of type 2 diabetes.

In a cohort of 4384 Taiwanese Buddhists, vegetarian men had approximately half the rate of diabetes, and vegetarian women one-quarter of the rate of diabetes compared with their omnivorous counterparts.[8] There were no cases of diabetes recorded amongst the 69 vegan participants. These findings were significant despite statistical adjustment for BMI and other factors. Interestingly, the omnivores in this study consumed a predominantly plant-based diet with little meat or fish, again implying that a small amount of meat consumption can contribute significantly to the development of type 2 diabetes.

In an analysis from the Nurses' Health Study and the Health Professionals Follow-up Study including 200,727 men and women, the plant-based diet index was used to assess the impact of a plant-based dietary pattern on the risk of developing diabetes during the more than 20 year follow-up.[9] Adherence to a healthy plant-based diet comprising predominantly healthy whole plant foods, whilst minimising all animal and processed foods was associated with a 34% reduction in the risk of diabetes. In contrast, an unhealthy plant-based diet, including more refined plant-based foods, was associated with a 16% increased risk of diabetes. A further updated analysis from the same study cohorts showed that improvement in diet quality over time can reduce the risk of developing type 2 diabetes, with every 10% increase in adherence to a healthy plant-based diet reducing subsequent risk of diabetes by 7–9% during the following 4 years.[10] The converse was also true, with a 10% decrease in plant-based diet quality resulting in a subsequent 12–23% higher risk of diabetes. This provides evidence that diet change is beneficial regardless of age and stage of life.

Results from the Rotterdam Study, a prospective cohort from the Netherlands including 6798 participants followed for 7.3 years, also demonstrated benefits of a more plant-based dietary pattern for prevention of insulin resistance, pre-diabetes and type 2 diabetes.[11] Higher adherence to a plant-based diet was associated with a 11% and 18% reduction in the risk of pre-diabetes and diabetes, respectively.

Other predominantly plant-based dietary patterns, including the Mediterranean and DASH (Dietary Approaches to Stop Hypertension) diets have also been associated with a reduced risk of type 2 diabetes.[12]

Individual foods and the risk of type 2 diabetes

Studies have clearly demonstrated the positive impact of individual components of a healthy plant-based diet on the risk of developing type 2 diabetes. Conversely, meat, particularly processed and unprocessed red meat, eggs and animal protein consumption in general is associated with an increased risk of type 2 diabetes.

Data from the Nurses' Health Study and the Health Professionals follow-up study have shown a significant association between the consumption of red and processed meat and an increased risk of developing type 2 diabetes.[13] In the study, a standard serving size was 85 g for unprocessed red meat, 45 g for one hot dog, 28 g for two slices of bacon, or 45 g for one piece of other processed red meat. For a one serving per day increase in unprocessed, processed, and total red meat consumption, the risk of diabetes was increased by 12%, 32% and 14% respectively. When food substitutions were examined, one serving of nuts, low-fat dairy, and whole grains per day instead of one serving of red meat per day was associated with a 16–35% lower risk of type 2 diabetes. Essentially, substituting any food for red and processed meat in the diet resulted in a significant reduction in risk of developing type 2 diabetes. These results have been confirmed with an updated analysis from the same study cohorts in which replacing processed and unprocessed red meat with any other source of protein (be it poultry, seafood, legumes, nuts) resulted in significant reductions in the risk of type 2 diabetes in the order of 11–18%.[14]

In the Dutch component of the EPIC (European Prospective Investigation into Cancer and Nutrition) study, during 10-year follow-up of 38,094 participants, 918 cases of type 2 diabetes were documented. The consumption of animal protein, but not vegetable protein, was associated with an increased risk of type 2 diabetes. For every 5% of calories derived from animal protein there was a 30% increased risk of developing type 2 diabetes.[15] In the EPIC-InterAct study, including 340,234 adults from eight European countries followed for almost 12 years, increasing quantities of red meat consumption was associated with an increased risk of type 2 diabetes.[16] For every 50 g increase in total, red and processed red meat consumption, there was an 8%, 8% and 12% increase in the risk of type 2 diabetes, respectively. For women, there was also a positive association with poultry consumption.

There is accumulating evidence to show that egg consumption increases the risk of developing type 2 diabetes in Caucasian and non-Caucasian populations. In people with type 2 diabetes, eggs cause further harm by significantly increasing the risk of cardiovascular disease. There have been three meta-analyses assessing the impact of egg consumption on the risk of type 2 diabetes which together confirm an 18–42% increased risk in those eating one or more eggs per day.[17, 18, 19] In people living with type 2 diabetes, those consuming the most eggs were shown to have a 40% increased risk of cardiovascular disease.[18]

In contrast to animal-derived foods, plant foods and plant-derived protein are protective, with numerous meta-analyses confirming these benefits. For example, the consumption of 45 g per day of whole grains has the potential to reduce the risk of type 2 diabetes by 20%.[20] Fruit and vegetable consumption has consistently been associated with a lower risk of type 2 diabetes. A paper from the EPIC-InterAct study analysed fruit and vegetable consumption in 9,754 participants with and 13,662 participants without type 2 diabetes.[21] The novel aspect of this study was that plasma biomarkers of fruit and vegetable consumption were measured, such as vitamin C and carotenoids, to a give a more accurate indication of consumption. The results showed that higher fruit and vegetable consumption (six portions a day) was associated with a significantly reduced risk of type 2 diabetes, in the order of 20–30%, and that even small to moderate increases in consumption were beneficial. Interestingly, consumption of legumes appear to be of more benefit to those with established type 2 diabetes rather than for prevention per se, with legume consumption associated with better glycaemic control.[22] The exception to this appears to be soya consumption, which is consistently associated with a reduced risk of type 2 diabetes.[23]

Plant-based diets for treatment and remission of type 2 diabetes

For decades, type 2 diabetes has been considered a chronic and progressive condition. However, recent progress in management has demonstrated that remission is possible for most people, especially early on in the disease course. Thus, the optimal management should be aimed at achieving remission. The definition of remission has long been discussed. In 2021, a consensus statement was published by the American Diabetes Association (ADA), the Endocrine Society, the European Association for the Study of Diabetes and Diabetes UK. It defined remission as a return of HbA1c to less than 6.5%, that occurs spontaneously, or following an intervention and that persists for at least three months in the absence of usual glucose-lowering pharmacotherapy.[24]

Diet and lifestyle interventions have been demonstrated to be essential for remission of diabetes. These are mostly aimed at weight loss, yet the positive impact of a plant-based diet has been observed even in the absence of weight loss. One metabolic ward trial involving 20 lean men with long standing insulin-dependent diabetes (up to 20 years) investigated the impact of a high carbohydrate, high fibre, plant-based diet designed to maintain body weight for an average of 16 days.[25] Some participants did lose weight, but caloric intake was increased to compensate. All participants were able to lower their dose of insulin, with nine participants being able to come off insulin completely. The same study team has shown that a high-fibre (35–40 g per 1,000 calories), high carbohydrate (70% of calories), plant-based diet results in significant reductions in body weight, blood glucose and need for insulin or diabetes medications.[26, 27, 28]

In the 1970s, Nathan Pritikin pioneered a diet and lifestyle approach for reversal of common chronic conditions, including diabetes. The Pritikin Program continues to this day and uses a low-fat, high fibre, predominantly plant-based diet, although fish, low-fat dairy and small amounts of lean meat are included. The results of this intervention have shown benefits for weight loss and glycaemic control with the ability to discontinue insulin or oral medications in people with type 2 diabetes.[29] The clues for these results were already present in the literature in the 1950s when physician Walter Kempner demonstrated reversal of diabetic retinopathy in his patients on a high-carbohydrate diet without caloric restriction, using white rice, fruit and fruits juices.[30]

Recent studies, mainly from the USA, with a more robust study design have demonstrated that a vegetarian or 100% plant-based or vegan diet can improve body weight, fat mass, insulin sensitivity and induce remission of type 2 diabetes. A study of 75 people with diabetes were randomised to follow a vegetarian (n = 38) or a conventional diabetes diet (n = 37), with both groups reducing energy intake by 500 calories per day.[31] Researchers assessed body composition and insulin resistance and found that only the vegetarian group showed significant reductions in body weight and a reduction in sub-fascial and intramuscular fat. Both groups lost subcutaneous fat equally. Changes in sub-fascial fat correlated with changes in HbA1c, fasting plasma glucose, and β-cell insulin sensitivity. In a subsequent study using a vegan diet, the same researchers showed that these metabolic improvements were associated with an increased intake of plant protein and decreased intake of animal protein (in particular the amino acid leucine). Reduced histidine intake on the plant-based diet was associated with a decrease in insulin resistance, independent of changes in BMI and energy intake.[32]

A study of 99 individuals with type 2 diabetes randomised participants to a low-fat vegan diet (n=49) or a diet based on the ADA guidelines (n=50). Participants were evaluated at baseline and 22 weeks. The results showed that 43% of the vegan group and 26% of the ADA group reduced their diabetes medications. There were also greater reductions in HBA1c, body weight (6.5 kg versus 3.1 kg) and LDL-cholesterol (21.2% versus 10.7%) in the vegan group.[33] A further study by the same research team lasting for 74 weeks follow up, showed similar results.[34]

Studies conducted outside of the USA have also shown similar results. A randomised study from the Czech Republic involving 74 participants over 24 weeks compared a vegetarian whole foods diet with a conventional diabetes diet. The vegetarian group achieved greater weight loss (6.2 kg versus 3.2 kg), insulin sensitivity (30% greater versus 20% greater) and reductions in diabetes medications (43% versus 5% reduction) compared to the conventional diet.[35] Another study from South Korea included 93 participants with type 2 diabetes and compared the Korean Diabetes Association diet with a vegan diet over 12 weeks.[36] Glycaemic control was better with the vegan diet (0.9% HBA1c reduction versus 0.3%).

Weight loss is required for most people with type 2 diabetes to induce remission and as discussed in Chapter 6, a plant-based diet is the optimal way to achieve a healthy weight. This was clearly demonstrated in the Broad Study, from New Zealand, which included 65 patients in a primary care setting with elevated BMI plus at least one of type 2 diabetes, ischaemic heart disease, hypertension or hypercholesterolaemia. They were randomised to normal care group or a whole food plant-based (WFPB) diet group which included a community-based education group that met twice weekly for 12 weeks.[37] After one year follow up, the mean weight loss for the WFPB diet group was 4.2 kg/m^2 BMI points with improvements in glycaemic control. These are in fact the best weight-loss results in a randomised setting with an intervention that did not mandate energy restriction or regular exercise.

The benefits of using a plant-based diet for inducing remission of type 2 diabetes is that it is composed of foods that are naturally low in calorie density yet high in essential, health promoting nutrients. There is usually no requirement to count calories or restrict carbohydrates or portion size, which makes it more acceptable and sustainable for patients.[38] In addition, this way of eating is associated with substantial reductions in the risk of other common chronic conditions such as cardiovascular diseases, renal failure and cancer.

The strength of evidence for this dietary approach is such that it been incorporated into national and international guidelines. For example, the American Association of Clinical Endocrinologists recommend a primarily plant-based meal plan[39] and the American College of Lifestyle Medicine recommend a whole food plant-based diet as the optimal approach for inducing diabetes remission.[40]

Clinicians need to be aware that a plant-based diet has the ability to improve glycaemic control and hence the requirement for glucose lowering medications within days to weeks, so patients will need to be supported to appropriately reduce their medications doses and ultimately stop them. There is a requirement for further guidelines development for de-prescribing in this setting.

Benefits of a plant-based diet for complications of type 2 diabetes

The benefits of a plant-based diet for prevention of cardiovascular disease and its risk factors and renal failure are discussed in Chapters 3 and 8 respectively and are applicable to people living with type 2 diabetes.

Specific to type 2 diabetes, a plant-based diet has been shown to improve many of the microvascular complications. Peripheral neuropathy is a well-known consequence of diabetes, and can impact multiple parts of the body causing gastroparesis, erectile dysfunction, neuralgic pain, insensitivity to injury leading to complications such as amputation (as well as increased risk of peripheral vascular disease), sleep disturbances, anxiety and depression.[41] More than 50% of individuals with diabetes can suffer from neuropathy and current management strategies include medications for improving glycaemic control in an attempt to slow disease progression and to ease the neuropathic pain that ensues.

Dietary approaches for the management of neuropathy are underutilised and under-researched. A 20-week randomised controlled trial, including 35 participants with diabetes, used a low-fat, vegan dietary intervention and demonstrated improved nerve function and reduced pain, compared with an untreated control group.[42] A small study which used a vegan diet demonstrated the elimination of neuropathic symptoms in 17 out of 21 participants.[43]

There is some evidence that dietary interventions are effective for prevention and treatment of retinopathy associated with diabetes. The first indication of the reversibility of retinopathy came from Dr Walter Kempner and the results of his rice diet intervention.[30] There have not been many interventional studies for diabetic retinopathy but from the available data, mostly observational, it seems a high fibre and a Mediterranean diet are protective.[44]

An important consideration is the psychological impact of a diagnosis of diabetes and people living with diabetes commonly report poor psychological wellbeing. A systematic review of 11 interventional studies specifically investigated the impact of plant-based diets on psychological and physical wellbeing.[45] The results demonstrated that plant-based diets were associated with significant improvement in emotional wellbeing, physical wellbeing, depression, quality of life and general health when compared to several official dietary guidelines and other comparator diets. This was in addition to improvements in markers of diabetes control and other cardiovascular risk factors.

Mechanisms by which plant-based diet prevent insulin resistance

The underlying cause of type 2 diabetes is insulin resistance, whereby the liver and muscle cells are no longer responsive to the effects of insulin secreted from the pancreas. In addition, there is impairment of pancreatic β-cell function.[46] Insulin resistance is caused by the accumulation of fat in the liver, muscle and pancreatic cells that precedes the onset of type 2 diabetes. Obesity is an independent causal factor for type 2 diabetes, increasing the risk of insulin resistance. The majority of people living with type 2 diabetes do carry excess body weight, but 10–15% have a normal body weight. It is predominantly visceral rather than subcutaneous fat that leads to insulin resistance and different people have different fat thresholds or tolerance.[47] This is a particular problem in people of South Asian and Asian origin who for every equivalent BMI point have a 2–4 fold increased risk of developing type 2 diabetes compared to Caucasians.[48] Thus a normal BMI for South Asians and Asians is considered to be 18.5–23 kg/m2.

Dietary components that promote the accumulation of intracellular fat are saturated fat and fructose. Saturated fat is mainly found in animal-derived foods and high fat diets such as the Western-style diet pattern can impair insulin sensitivity both acutely and in the longer-term even in the absence of excess body fat. An interesting study evaluated intramyocellular fat and insulin sensitivity in 24 vegans and 25 omnivores of normal body weight and showed that vegans had lower intramuscular fat and better β-cell function.[49] A larger study amongst 273 vegetarians, including 73 vegans, demonstrated better insulin sensitivity compared to 273 matched omnivores and this was independent of body weight.[50] Excessive intracellular fat has a toxic effect on mitochondria through the generation of reactive oxygen species thus increasing metabolic stress, resulting in impaired insulin signalling and insulin resistance.[51]

A plant-based or vegan intervention is particularly effective due to the low saturated fat content. Palmitic acid, a saturated fat found in meat and dairy, has been shown to be directly toxic to pancreatic cells, whereas unsaturated fatty acids are not.[52] Acute increases in fatty acids in the blood that would occur after the consumption of a high fat diet have also been shown to impair insulin.[53, 54] One mechanism by which this may occur is by downregulating genes necessary for mitochondrial function.[55] Another mechanism by which saturated fats in particular induce acute insulin resistance is by disrupting the intestinal barrier and allowing entry of endotoxins into the blood stream, which in turn induce insulin resistance.[56]

In the clinical setting, a vegan diet has been shown to reduce intracellular fat and insulin resistance. A randomised 16-week study of a low-fat vegan diet in 244 overweight, but non-diabetic, participants demonstrated significant reductions in intramyocellular and intrahepatic fat, which correlated with improvements in insulin sensitivity.[57] A similar randomised 16-week study using a low-fat vegan diet in 75 overweight participants demonstrated improved β-cell function and improved insulin sensitivity.[58]

Another form of cellular stress that occurs in type 2 diabetes is thought to be the formation of dicarbonyl compounds (molecules containing two carbonyl (C=O) groups), toxic reactive metabolites formed from glucose and lipids, that may be involved in the development of vascular complications of diabetes. Dicarbonyls interact with proteins to form advanced glycation end products (AGEs), which can damage the endothelium and impair vascular function. A vegan meal with tofu when compared to a meat-based meal was shown to result in less oxidative and dicarbonyl stress in people with type 2 diabetes, and thus may further explain the benefits seen with a plant-based diet.[59]

Fructose consumption is another factor to consider for diet-induced insulin resistance and the development of diabetes. The main sources of fructose in the diet that are contributing to harm are from table sugar (or sucrose, which is 50% glucose and 50% fructose) and high fructose corn syrup (sweetener made from corn starch and ubiquitous in processed foods and soft drinks). This free fructose can for the most part only be metabolised in the liver. Some is converted to glucose and also stored as glycogen but when in excess of calorie requirements, it is also converted to triglycerides and uric acid. The conversion to triglycerides increases blood triglyceride levels and is stored in the liver, contributing to fatty liver and insulin resistance. In addition, excess fructose promotes the liver to produce more glucose and fatty acids.[60] The insulin resistance induced by fructose is also associated with resistance to the hunger hormone leptin, decreasing satiety and increasing the feeling of hunger and thus promotes the consumption of excess calories.

A plant-based diet promotes the health of the gut microbiome, which in turn promotes glucose regulation and insulin sensitivity.[61] When intestinal microbes ferment and digest fibre, they produce short chain fatty acids (SCFAs) such as proprionate and butyrate, which act to reduce post-prandial glucose levels not only after the meal but also in response to the subsequent meal.[62] SCFA's also reduce the post-prandial levels of free fatty acids thus reducing insulin resistance[63] and proprionate has been shown to directly improve β-cell function and protect against the damage caused by free fatty acids.[64] Dietary fibre has the additional benefit of reducing the energy density of foods, promoting satiety, and has been associated with weight loss, which in turn reduces insulin resistance. Fibre has also been associated with decreased markers of inflammation, which may also ameliorate insulin resistance.[65] Plant-based diets also have a beneficial impact on the secretion of gut hormones that promote satiety, regulate glucose metabolism, insulin secretion and energy homeostasis. A vegan meal with tofu was shown to increase gut hormones such as glucagon-like peptide-1 (GLP-1), amylin, and peptide YY (PYY) and promote better satiety when compared to a matched meat-based meal.[66]

Further benefits of plant foods include the abundance of antioxidant compounds such as polyphenols, which may inhibit glucose absorption, stimulate insulin secretion, reduce hepatic glucose output, and enhance glucose uptake.[67]

It is likely that some of the benefits of a plant-based diet for prevention and treatment of type 2 diabetes are attributable to the reduction or avoidance of certain exposures from meat and meat products.[68] For example, processed meat is cured or salted with nitrates or nitrites, which are converted in the intestine to nitrosamines and have been shown to be toxic to the β-cells of the pancreas and impair insulin response through generation of reactive oxygen species and pro-inflammatory cytokines.[69] Cooking meat produces AGEs, which are pro-oxidant compounds that are high in meat (especially when cooked at high, dry temperatures) and lower in plant-based foods such as fruit, vegetables, legumes and whole grains. AGEs have been associated with insulin resistance.[69, 70] High levels of haem iron, a pro-oxidant molecule, found particularly in red meat promotes insulin resistance through various likely mechanisms.[71] Observational and Mendelian randomisation studies have also suggested an association with serum ferritin levels and the development of diabetes.[72] Several meta-analyses have demonstrated a strong association between serum ferritin, dietary haem iron and the risk of type 2 diabetes.[73]

The amino acid content of animal protein differs from that of plant protein. One difference is the higher amounts of branched chain amino acids (valine, leucine and isoleucine) in animal protein. These amino acids have been implicated in the promotion of insulin resistance and hence an increased risk of type 2 diabetes.[74] Choline and carnitine present in meat and eggs is converted by gut microbiota into trimethylamine (TMA), which the liver subsequently converts to trimethylamine N-oxide (TMAO). TMAO has been implicated in the development of insulin resistance and type 2 diabetes.[75]

Alternative dietary approaches for treatment of type 2 diabetes

Very low-calorie diets

The President of the Academy of Medicine in France in 1866, Apollinaire Bouchardat, was one of the first physicians to understand a link between the disease of excess urination, glycosuria and diet. He described the phenomenon of improvement during the food shortage in the 4-month siege of Paris in the Franco-Prussian war in 1870, noting that his patients who suffered from starvation presented diminished glucose in their urine.[76] He went on to experiment with periodic fasting. He had also observed that exercise seemed to increase the tolerance of carbohydrate in people with diabetes. More recently, a number of trials have demonstrated the efficacy of very low-calorie diet for achieving remission of diabetes. These include the eight-year long 'Look Ahead' study,[77] the Counterpoint Trial[78] and the Direct trial.[79] This approach relies on rapid weight loss as a means of reversing type 2 diabetes and the outcomes are directly proportional to the degree of weight loss achieved. In addition, the studies demonstrate the ability to restore β-cell pancreatic function.

It is worth considering the DIRECT trial in more detail as this approach has been incorporated into treatment guidelines in the UK's National Health Service. The trial was a randomised study conducted within 49 primary care practices in the UK and recruited 306 patients diagnosed with diabetes within six years, who were overweight or obese but were not receiving insulin. The intervention group received a very low calorie (850 kcal/day) total meal replacement formula diet for 3–5 months. The 1-year results showed that diabetes remission was achieved in 46% of patients. Remission was dependent on the degree of weight loss achieved, with 86% of patients losing 15 kg or more achieving remission.[80] The limitations of this approach are seen with the 2-year follow-up where only 36% of participants remain in remission highlighting the need for a sustainable dietary approach.[79]

Low-carbohydrate diets

The threshold for low-carbohydrate intake is usually accepted as less than 130 g/day, equivalent to less than 26% of total energy from carbohydrates. Some use a very low-carbohydrate diet definition of less than 20 g a day, equivalent to about 10% of total energy intake. Carbohydrate intakes of more than 50 g per day are not usually sufficient for ketogenesis to occur. Hence, 'low-carbohydrate' and 'ketogenic' are not synonymous dietary terms but do overlap. Studies have shown glycaemic control can be improved and remission of diabetes achieved using a low-carbohydrate approach, but there is very little evidence to support efficacy of this approach beyond 12 months or that such a diet is sustainable for patients.[81]

The SACN (Scientific Advisory Commission on Nutrition in the UK) reviewed all the available evidence on low-carbohydrate diets for type 2 diabetes in recognition of the fact that such diets are increasingly being promoted.[82] Several limitations were identified, including no agreed definition of a low-carbohydrate diet and overlap in the reported mean carbohydrate intakes between lower (13 to 47%) and higher (41 to 55%) carbohydrate groups, as well as variation in the type and amount of macronutrient that replaced carbohydrate (fat and/or protein). The report also noted a lack of detail on the types of carbohydrate consumed (for example, whole grain, refined grain, free sugars, fibre) or consideration of how this could affect outcomes. Most of the studies included did not report outcomes beyond 12 months. The authors concluded that for adults living with type 2 diabetes and obesity, a lower carbohydrate diet could be recommended by clinicians as an effective short-term option (up to six months) for improving glycaemic control and serum triacylglycerol concentrations, with the caveat that they should include whole grain or higher fibre foods, a variety of fruits and vegetables and limits intakes of saturated fats, reflecting current dietary advice for the general population.

Although studies suggest low-carbohydrate approaches can induce weight loss and resultant improvement in glycaemic control and medication reduction, we do not have evidence that they can improve insulin resistance or β-cell function. Dr Kevin Hall's team at the National Institute of Health has conducted a number of metabolic ward trials to better understand the metabolic impact of different macronutrient combinations. One such study of 20 overweight adults comparing a low-fat plant-based diet (75% carbohydrate, 10% fat) with an animal-based ketogenic diet (10% carbohydrate, 75% fat) in a two-week crossover design with unrestricted food intake.[83] On the plant-based diet, participants consumed significantly fewer calories. Both diets led to improvements in fasting glucose and insulin levels, but the plant-based diet resulted in greater weight and body fat loss and improvements in cholesterol levels. The ketogenic group lost mainly water weight and muscle mass, developed a degree of insulin resistance and a rise in LDL-cholesterol levels. The low-carbohydrate diet did improve triglyceride levels, which worsened on the plant-based diet. A previous metabolic ward study conducted in 17 participants found that a ketogenic diet was associated with an increase in markers of inflammation and in LDL-cholesterol and did not improve insulin sensitivity or glucose regulation.[84] These results are not able to support the carbohydrate–insulin model of obesity hypothesis which suggests that high carbohydrate diets result in excess insulin secretion, thus promoting fat accumulation and increased calorie intake.

What is sometimes forgotten is that protein-rich foods can also affect insulin secretion. One useful study investigated the insulin response to a variety of common foods and correlated this with the nutrient content.[85] Protein-rich foods stimulated a large amount of insulin secretion relative to their glycaemic response. A standard portion size of 1000 kJ was chosen for the study because this resulted in realistic serving sizes for most of the foods. Although some protein-rich foods may normally be eaten in smaller quantities, fish, beef, cheese, and eggs still had larger insulin responses per gram than many of the foods consisting predominantly of carbohydrate. In fact, they induced as much insulin secretion as some carbohydrate-rich foods (e.g., beef was equal to brown rice and fish was equal to grain bread). So, not only are the protein-rich foods on a high-fat low-carbohydrate diet specifically insulinogenic, the saturated fat, as previously discussed, promotes insulin resistance.

The main concern with the low-carbohydrate approach is that in the longer-term it may increase the risk of cardiovascular disease and some cancers and have been associated with an increased risk of developing type 2 diabetes. The Health Professionals Follow up study included 40,475 men of whom 2689 developed diabetes during the 20 years of follow-up. Those participants consuming the most animal protein and fat and thus lower amounts of carbohydrates had a 37% increased risk of diabetes, with processed and red meat associated with the greatest. In contrast, higher intakes of plant protein and fat were associated with a 22% decreased risk of diabetes.[86] Similar associations have been reported in women.[87]

A large study examined the relationship between low-carbohydrate diets, all-cause death, and deaths from coronary heart disease, cerebrovascular disease (including stroke), and cancer in a nationally representative sample of 24,825 participants of the US National Health and Nutrition Examination Survey (NHANES) during 1999 to 2010.[88] Compared to participants with the highest carbohydrate consumption, those with the lowest intake had a 32% higher risk of all-cause death over an average 6.4-year follow-up. In addition, risks of death from coronary heart disease, cerebrovascular disease, and cancer were increased by 51%, 50%, and 35%, respectively. The results were confirmed in a meta-analysis of seven prospective cohort studies with 462,934 participants followed for an average of 16.1 years, which found 22%, 13%, and 8% increased risk in total, cardiovascular, and cancer mortality with low (compared to high) carbohydrate diets. The mechanism for some of these adverse long-term impacts may be explained by studies that have shown that an animal protein rich low-carbohydrate approach can reduce flexibility of peripheral arteries,[89] reduce blood flow to the heart,[90] increase insulin resistance[91] and increase oxidative stress from gut-derived endotoxins, the entry of which is promoted by saturated fat.[92]

It is of course possible to design a low-carbohydrate plant-based diet, such as the Eco-Atkins diet pioneered by Dr David Jenkins, but these have not been studied for the treatment of type 2 diabetes.[93]

Type 1 and type 1.5 diabetes

Type 1 diabetes is an autoimmune disease in which insulin is functionally absent because of the destruction of the β-cells in the pancreas by the immune system. The triggers for the autoimmune attack are not fully understood, but it is now widely accepted that both environmental and genetic factors contribute to it. One potential environmental factor is the consumption of cow's milk.[94] There is less evidence for the role of plant-based nutrition in the management of type 1 diabetes, but published case reports show that the same mechanisms that can result in improvements in insulin sensitivity, insulin dose and cardiovascular risk factors in type 2 diabetes work well for type 1 diabetes.[95] This is because people with type 1 diabetes can also develop insulin resistance, with the risk increased by carrying excess body weight and a diet high in animal-derived and processed foods.[96] A plant-based diet may help to mitigate against this.

Type 1.5 diabetes, which is also known as type 3 diabetes or latent autoimmune diabetes in adults (LADA), is a form of type 1 diabetes that is diagnosed during adulthood. Type 1.5 diabetes also has a slow onset and is an autoimmune disease that will almost certainly require insulin therapy. Interestingly, around 15–20% of people diagnosed with type 2 diabetes may actually have type 1.5 diabetes.[97] Medications designed to reduce insulin resistance do not work, as people with type 1.5 diabetes have little or no resistance to insulin. Some other oral medications may be effective at first, which, alongside adult-onset symptoms, makes misdiagnosis as type 2 diabetes more common. Amongst those with type 1.5 diabetes, insulin is required on average within four years. Clinical features to note at diagnosis include a normal BMI, an absence of issues such as metabolic syndrome, onset of diabetes at ≥25 years of age, a fast evolution to insulin necessity within months, and some features of type 1 diabetes such as low fasting C-peptide and positive glutamic acid decarboxylase autoantibodies.[98] More research is needed on the role of diet in type 1.5 diabetes, but the principles discussed are broadly relevant to maintaining pancreatic function and improving insulin sensitivity in these patients.

Conclusion

A whole food plant-based diet, rich in fibre and phytonutrients whilst being low in saturated fat and absent in animal protein, is an optimal choice for prevention and treatment of diabetes, particularly type 2 diabetes. As clinicians, our primary treatment goal should be to achieve a sustained remission when treating people with type 2 diabetes. If that is not possible, we should strive for minimising medications and optimising health outcomes and longevity. A tertiary outcome would be improving insulin sensitivity and aiming to maintain a healthier body weight. Any dietary pattern, including very low-calorie, low-carbohydrate and ketogenic diets, can produce weight loss, which is required in most patients with type 2 diabetes. The most sustainable, accessible and culturally appropriate approach for our patients is the ultimate goal, and a plant-based dietary pattern is a way to offer satiety, ad libitum eating and optimal results for these specified treatment goals.

References

1. Saeedi P, Petersohn I, Salpea P, Malanda B, Karuranga S, Unwin N, et al. Global and regional diabetes prevalence estimates for 2019 and projections for 2030 and 2045: Results from the International Diabetes Federation Diabetes Atlas, 9th edition. *Diabetes Res Clin Pract* 2019; 157: 107843. doi: 10.1016/j.diabres.2019.107843
2. Lin X, Xu Y, Pan X, Xu J, Ding Y, Sun X, et al. Global, regional, and national burden and trend

of diabetes in 195 countries and territories: an analysis from 1990 to 2025. *Sci Rep* 2020; 10(1): 14790. doi: 10.1038/s41598-020-71908-9
3. Raghavan S, Vassy JL, Ho YL, Song RJ, Gagnon DR, Cho K, et al. Diabetes mellitus–related all-cause and cardiovascular mortality in a national cohort of adults. *J Am Heart Assoc* 2019; 8(4): e011295. doi: 10.1161/JAHA.118.011295
4. Uusitupa M, Khan TA, Viguiliouk E, Kahleova H, Rivellese AA, Hermansen K, et al. Prevention of type 2 diabetes by lifestyle changes: A systematic review and meta-analysis. *Nutrients* 2019; 11(11): 2611. doi: 10.3390/nu11112611
5. Papier K, Appleby PN, Fensom GK, Knuppel A, Perez-Cornago A, Schmidt JA, et al. Vegetarian diets and risk of hospitalisation or death with diabetes in British adults: results from the EPIC-Oxford study. *Nutr Diabetes* 2019; 9(1): 7. doi: 10.1038/s41387-019-0074-0
6. Tonstad S, Butler T, Yan R, Fraser GE. Type of vegetarian diet, body weight, and prevalence of type 2 diabetes. *Diabetes Care* 2009; 32(5): 791-6. doi: 10.2337/dc08-1886
7. Tonstad S, Stewart K, Oda K, Batech M, Herring RP, Fraser GE. Vegetarian diets and incidence of diabetes in the Adventist Health Study-2. *Nutr Metab Cardiovasc Dis* 2013; 23(4): 292-9. doi: 10.1016/j.numecd.2011.07.004
8. Chiu THT, Huang HY, Chiu YF, Pan WH, Kao HY, Chiu JPC, et al. Taiwanese vegetarians and omnivores: Dietary composition, prevalence of diabetes and IFG. *PLoS One* 2014; 9(2): e88547. doi: 10.1371/journal.pone.0088547
9. Satija A, Bhupathiraju SN, Rimm EB, Spiegelman D, Chiuve SE, Borgi L, et al. Plant-Based Dietary Patterns and Incidence of Type 2 Diabetes in US Men and Women: Results from Three Prospective Cohort Studies. *PLoS Med* 2016; 13(6): e1002039. doi: 10.1371/journal.pmed.1002039
10. Chen Z, Drouin-Chartier JP, Li Y, Baden MY, Manson JAE, Willett WC, et al. Changes in Plant-Based Diet Indices and Subsequent Risk of Type 2 Diabetes in Women and Men: Three U.S. Prospective Cohorts. *Diabetes Care* 2021; 44(3): 663-671. doi: 10.2337/dc20-1636
11. Chen Z, Zuurmond MG, van der Schaft N, Nano J, Wijnhoven HAH, Ikram MA, et al. Plant versus animal based diets and insulin resistance, prediabetes and type 2 diabetes: the Rotterdam Study. *Eur J Epidemiol* 2018; 33(9): 883-893. doi: 10.1007/s10654-018-0414-8
12. Toi PL, Anothaisintawee T, Chaikledkaew U, Briones JR, Reutrakul S, Thakkinstian A. Preventive role of diet interventions and dietary factors in type 2 diabetes mellitus: An umbrella review. *Nutrients* 2020; 12(9): 2722. doi: 10.3390/nu12092722
13. Pan A, Sun Q, Bernstein AM, Schulze MB, Manson JAE, Willett WC, et al. Red meat consumption and risk of type 2 diabetes: 3 Cohorts of US adults and an updated meta-analysis. *Am J Clin Nutr* 2011; 94(4): 1088-96. doi: 10.3945/ajcn.111.018978
14. Würtz AML, Jakobsen MU, Bertoia ML, Hou T, Schmidt EB, Willett WC, et al. Replacing the consumption of red meat with other major dietary protein sources and risk of type 2 diabetes mellitus: a prospective cohort study. *Am J Clin Nutr* 2021; 113(3): 113(3): 612-621. doi: 10.1093/ajcn/nqaa284
15. Sluijs I, Beulens JWJ, Van Der A DL, Spijkerman AMW, Grobbee DE, Van Der Schouw YT. Dietary intake of total, animal, and vegetable protein and risk of type 2 diabetes in the European Prospective Investigation into Cancer and Nutrition (EPIC)-NL study. *Diabetes Care* 2010; 33(1): 43-8. doi: 10.2337/dc09-1321
16. Bendinelli B, Palli D, Masala G, Sharp SJ, Schulze MB, Guevara M, et al. Association between dietary meat consumption and incident type 2 diabetes: The EPIC-InterAct study. *Diabetologia* 2013; 56(1): 47-59. doi: 10.1007/s00125-012-2718-7
17. Wallin A, Forouhi NG, Wolk A, Larsson SC. Egg consumption and risk of type 2 diabetes: a prospective study and dose–response meta-analysis. *Diabetologia* 2016; 59(6): 1204-1213. doi: 10.1007/s00125-016-3923-6
18. Drouin-Chartier JP, Chen S, Li Y, Schwab AL, Stampfer MJ, Sacks FM, et al. Egg consumption and risk of cardiovascular disease: Three large prospective US cohort studies, systematic review, and updated meta-analysis. *BMJ* 2020; 368: m513. doi: 10.1136/bmj.m513
19. Shin JY, Xun P, Nakamura Y, He K. Egg consumption in relation to risk of cardiovascular disease

and diabetes: A systematic review and meta-analysis. *Am J Clin Nutr* 2013; 98(1): 146-159. doi: 10.3945/ajcn.112.051318
20. Chanson-Rolle A, Meynier A, Aubin F, Lappi J, Poutanen K, Vinoy S, et al. Systematic review and meta-analysis of human studies to support a quantitative recommendation for whole grain intake in relation to type 2 diabetes. *PLoS One* 2015; 10(6): e0131377.
doi: 10.1371/journal.pone.0131377
21. Zheng JS, Sharp SJ, Imamura F, Chowdhury R, Gundersen TE, Steur M, et al. Association of plasma biomarkers of fruit and vegetable intake with incident type 2 diabetes: EPIC-InterAct case-cohort study in eight European countries. *BMJ* 2020; 370: m2194. doi: 10.1136/bmj.m2194
22. Bielefeld D, Grafenauer S, Rangan A. The effects of legume consumption on markers of glycaemic control in individuals with and without diabetes mellitus: A systematic literature review of randomised controlled trials. *Nutrients* 2020; 12(7): 2123. doi: 10.3390/nu12072123
23. Li W, Ruan W, Peng Y, Wang D. Soy and the risk of type 2 diabetes mellitus: A systematic review and meta-analysis of observational studies. *Diabetes Research and Clinical Practice* 2018; 137: 190-199. doi: 10.1016/j.diabres.2018.01.010
24. Riddle MC, Cefalu WT, Evans PH, Gerstein HC, Nauck MA, Oh WK, et al. Consensus report: definition and interpretation of remission in type 2 diabetes. *Diabetologia* 2021; 44(10): 2438-2444. doi: 10.2337/dci21-0034
25. Anderson JW, Ward K. High-carbohydrate, high-fiber diets for insulin-treated men with diabetes mellitus. *Am J Clin Nutr* 1979; 32(11): 2312-21. doi: 10.1093/ajcn/32.11.2312
26. Anderson JW, Ward K. Long-term effects of high-carbohydrate, high-fiber diets on glucose and lipid metabolism: a preliminary report on patients with diabetes. *Diabetes Care* 1978; 1(2): 77-82. doi: 10.2337/diacare.1.2.77
27. Anderson JW. High carbohydrate, high fiber diets for patients with diabetes. *Adv Exp Med Biol* 1979; 119: 263-273. doi: 10.1007/978-1-4615-9110-8_38
28. Anderson JW, Zeigler JA, Deakins DA, Floore TL, Dillon DW, Wood CL, et al. Metabolic effects of high-carbohydrate, high-fiber diets for insulin-dependent diabetic individuals. Am J Clin Nutr 1991; 54(5): 936-943. doi: 10.1093/ajcn/54.5.936
29. Rosenthal MB, Barnard RJ, Rose DP, Inkeles S, Hall J, Pritikin N. Effects of a high-complex-carbohydrate, low-fat, low-cholesterol diet on levels of serum lipids and estradiol. *Am J Med* 1985; 78(1): 23-27.
doi: 10.1016/0002-9343(85)90456-5
30. Kempner W, Peschel RL, Schlayer C. Effect of rice diet on diabetes mellitus associated with vascular disease. *Postgrad Med* 1958; 24(4): 359-371.
doi: 10.1080/00325481.1958.11692236
31. Kahleova H, Klementova M, Herynek V, Skoch A, Herynek S, Hill M, et al. The Effect of a Vegetarian vs Conventional Hypocaloric Diabetic Diet on Thigh Adipose Tissue Distribution in Subjects with Type 2 Diabetes: A Randomized Study. *J Am Coll Nutr* 2017; 36(5): 364-369.
doi: 10.1080/07315724.2017.1302367
32. Kahleova H, Fleeman R, Hlozkova A, Holubkov R, Barnard ND. A plant-based diet in overweight individuals in a 16-week randomized clinical trial: metabolic benefits of plant protein. *Nutr Diabetes* 2018; 8(1): 58. doi: 10.1038/s41387-018-0067-4
33. Barnard ND, Cohen J, Jenkins DJA, Turner-McGrievy G, Gloede L, Jaster B, et al. A low-fat vegan diet improves glycemic control and cardiovascular risk factors in a randomized clinical trial in individuals with type 2 diabetes. *Diabetes Care* 2006; 29(8): 1777-83.
doi: 10.2337/dc06-0606
34. Barnard ND, Cohen J, Jenkins DJA, Turner-McGrievy G, Gloede L, Green A, et al. A low-fat vegan diet and a conventional diabetes diet in the treatment of type 2 diabetes: A randomized, controlled, 74-wk clinical trial. *American Journal of Clinical Nutrition* 2009; 89(5): 1588S-1596S.
doi: 10.3945/ajcn.2009.26736H
35. Kahleova H, Matoulek M, Malinska H, Oliyarnik O, Kazdova L, Neskudla T, et al. Vegetarian diet improves insulin resistance and oxidative stress markers more than conventional diet in subjects with Type 2 diabetes. *Diabet Med* 2011; 28(5): 549-559. doi: 10.1111/j.1464-5491.2010.03209.x
36. Lee YM, Kim SA, Lee IK, Kim JG, Park KG, Jeong JY, et al. Effect of a brown rice based vegan diet and conventional diabetic diet on glycemic control of patients with type 2 diabetes: A 12-week randomized clinical trial. *PLoS One*

37. Wright N, Wilson L, Smith M, Duncan B, McHugh P. The BROAD study: A randomised controlled trial using a whole food plant-based diet in the community for obesity, ischaemic heart disease or diabetes. *Nutr Diabetes* 2017; 7(3): e256. doi: 10.1038/nutd.2017.3
38. Jardine MA, Kahleova H, Levin SM, Ali Z, Trapp CB, Barnard ND. Perspective: Plant-Based Eating Pattern for Type 2 Diabetes Prevention and Treatment: Efficacy, Mechanisms, and Practical Considerations. *Adv Nutr* 2021; 12(6): 2045-2055. doi: 10.1093/advances/nmab063
39. Garber AJ, Handelsman Y, Grunberger G, Einhorn D, Abrahamson MJ, Barzilay JI, et al. Consensus statement by the American Association of clinical Endocrinologists and American College of Endocrinology on the comprehensive type 2 diabetes management algorithm - 2020 executive summary. *Endocrine Practice* 2020; 26(1): 107-139. doi: 10.4158/CS-2019-0472
40. Kelly J, Karlsen M, Steinke G. Type 2 Diabetes Remission and Lifestyle Medicine: A Position Statement From the American College of Lifestyle Medicine. *American Journal of Lifestyle Medicine* 2020; 14(4): 406-419. doi: 10.1177/1559827620930962
41. Alleman CJM, Westerhout KY, Hensen M, Chambers C, Stoker M, Long S, et al. Humanistic and economic burden of painful diabetic peripheral neuropathy in Europe: A review of the literature. *Diabetes Research and Clinical Practice* 2015; 109(2): 215-225. doi: 10.1016/j.diabres.2015.04.031
42. Bunner AE, Wells CL, Gonzales J, Agarwal U, Bayat E, Barnard ND. A dietary intervention for chronic diabetic neuropathy pain: A randomized controlled pilot study. *Nutr Diabetes* 2015; 5(5): e158. doi: 10.1038/nutd.2015.8
43. Crane MG, Sample C. Regression of diabetic neuropathy with total vegetarian (vegan) diet. *J Nutr Med* 1994; 4(4): 431-439. doi: 10.3109/13590849409003592
44. Wong MYZ, Man REK, Fenwick EK, Gupta P, Li LJ, van Dam RM, et al. Dietary intake and diabetic retinopathy: A systematic review. *PLoS One* 2018; 13(1): e0186582. doi: 10.1371/journal.pone.0186582
45. Toumpanakis A, Turnbull T, Alba-Barba I. Effectiveness of plant-based diets in promoting well-being in the management of type 2 diabetes: A systematic review. *BMJ Open Diabetes Research and Care* 2018; 6(1): e000534. doi: 10.1136/bmjdrc-2018-000534
46. American Diabetes Association. 2. Classification and diagnosis of diabetes: Standards of medical care in diabetes-2021. *Diabetes Care* 2021; 44(Suppl 1): S15-S33. doi: 10.2337/dc21-S002
47. Taylor R, Ramachandran A, Yancy WS, Forouhi NG. Nutritional basis of type 2 diabetes remission. *BMJ* 2021; 374(9): n1449. doi: 10.1136/bmj.n1449
48. Ntuk UE, Gill JMR, Mackay DF, Sattar N, Pell JP. Ethnic-specific obesity cutoffs for diabetes risk: Cross-sectional study of 490,288 uk biobank participants. *Diabetes Care* 2014; 37(9): 2500-2507. doi: 10.2337/dc13-2966
49. Goff LM, Bell JD, So PW, Dornhorst A, Frost GS. Veganism and its relationship with insulin resistance and intramyocellular lipid. *Eur J Clin Nutr* 2005; 59(2): 291-8. doi: 10.1038/sj.ejcn.1602076
50. Cui X, Wang B, Wu Y, Xie L, Xun P, Tang Q, et al. Vegetarians have a lower fasting insulin level and higher insulin sensitivity than matched omnivores: A cross-sectional study. *Nutr Metab Cardiovasc Dis* 2019; 29(5): 467-473. doi: 10.1016/j.numecd.2019.01.012
51. Meex RCR, Blaak EE, van Loon LJC. Lipotoxicity plays a key role in the development of both insulin resistance and muscle atrophy in patients with type 2 diabetes. *Obesity Reviews* 2019; 20(9): 1205-1217. doi: 10.1111/obr.12862
52. Nemecz M, Constantin A, Dumitrescu M, Alexandru N, Filippi A, Tanko G, et al. The distinct effects of palmitic and oleic acid on pancreatic beta cell function: The elucidation of associated mechanisms and effector molecules. *Front Pharmacol* 2019; 9: 1554. doi: 10.3389/fphar.2018.01554
53. Lee S, Boesch C, Kuk JL, Arslanian S. Effects of an overnight intravenous lipid infusion on intramyocellular lipid content and insulin sensitivity in African-American versus Caucasian

adolescents. *Metabolism* 2013; 62(3): 417-423. doi: 10.1016/j.metabol.2012.09.007
54. Wolpert HA, Atakov-Castillo A, Smith SA, Steil GM. Dietary fat acutely increases glucose concentrations and insulin requirements in patients with type 1 diabetes: Implications for carbohydrate-based bolus dose calculation and intensive diabetes management. *Diabetes Care* 2013; 36(4): 810-816. doi: 10.2337/dc12-0092
55. Sparks LM, Xie H, Koza RA, Mynatt R, Hulver MW, Bray GA, et al. A high-fat diet coordinately downregulates genes required for mitochondrial oxidative phosphorylation in skeletal muscle. *Diabetes* 2005; 54(7): 1926-1933. doi: 10.2337/diabetes.54.7.1926
56. Anderson AS, Haynie KR, McMillan RP, Osterberg KL, Boutagy NE, Frisard MI, et al. Early skeletal muscle adaptations to short-term high-fat diet in humans before changes in insulin sensitivity. *Obesity* 2015; 23(4): 720-724. doi: 10.1002/oby.21031
57. Kahleova H, Petersen KF, Shulman GI, Alwarith J, Rembert E, Tura A, et al. Effect of a Low-Fat Vegan Diet on Body Weight, Insulin Sensitivity, Postprandial Metabolism, and Intramyocellular and Hepatocellular Lipid Levels in Overweight Adults: A Randomized Clinical Trial. *JAMA Netw Open* 2020; 3(11): e2025454. doi: 10.1001/jamanetworkopen.2020.25454
58. Kahleova H, Tura A, Hill M, Holubkov R, Barnard ND. A plant-based dietary intervention improves beta-cell function and insulin resistance in overweight adults: A 16-week randomized clinical trial. *Nutrients* 2018; 10(2): 189. doi: 10.3390/nu10020189
59. Malinska H, Klementová M, Kudlackova M, Veleba J, Hoskova E, Oliyarnyk O, et al. A plant-based meal reduces postprandial oxidative and dicarbonyl stress in men with diabetes or obesity compared with an energy- and macronutrient-matched conventional meal in a randomized crossover study. *Nutr Metab* 2021; 18(1): 84. doi: 10.1186/s12986-021-00609-5
60. Mai BH, Yan LJ. The negative and detrimental effects of high fructose on the liver, with special reference to metabolic disorders. *Diabetes, Metabolic Syndrome and Obesity: Targets and Therapy* 2019; 12: 821-826. doi: 10.2147/DMSO. S198968
61. Tomova A, Bukovsky I, Rembert E, Yonas W, Alwarith J, Barnard ND, et al. The Effects of Vegetarian and Vegan Diets on Gut Microbiota. *Frontiers in Nutrition* 2019; 6: 47. doi: 10.3389/fnut.2019.00047
62. Higgins JA. Whole grains, legumes, and the subsequent meal effect: Implications for blood glucose control and the role of fermentation. *Journal of Nutrition and Metabolism* 2012; 2012: 829238. doi: 10.1155/2012/829238
63. Tarini J, Wolever TMS. The fermentable fibre inulin increases postprandial serum short-chain fatty acids and reduces free-fatty acids and ghrelin in healthy subjects. *Appl Physiol Nutr Metab* 2010; 35(1): 9-16. doi: 10.1139/H09-119
64. Pingitore A, Chambers ES, Hill T, Maldonado IR, Liu B, Bewick G, et al. The diet-derived short chain fatty acid propionate improves beta-cell function in humans and stimulates insulin secretion from human islets in vitro. *Diabetes, Obes Metab* 2017; 19(2): 257-265. doi: 10.1111/dom.12811
65. Wannamethee SG, Whincup PH, Thomas MC, Sattar N. Associations between dietary fiber and inflammation, hepatic function, and risk of type 2 diabetes in older men: Potential mechanisms for the benefits of fiber on diabetes risk. *Diabetes Care* 2009; 32(10): 1823-1825. doi: 10.2337/dc09-0477
66. Klementova M, Thieme L, Haluzik M, Pavlovicova R, Hill M, Pelikanova T, et al. A plant-based meal increases gastrointestinal hormones and satiety more than an energy-and macronutrient-matched processed-meat meal in t2d, obese, and healthy men: A three-group randomized crossover study. *Nutrients* 2019; 11(1): 157. doi: 10.3390/nu11010157
67. Kim YA, Keogh JB, Clifton PM. Polyphenols Polyphenols and Glycemic Control. *Nutrients* 2016; 8(1): 17. doi: 10.3390/nu8010017
68. Wolk A. Potential health hazards of eating red meat. *Journal of Internal Medicine* 2017; 281(2): 106-122. doi: 10.1111/joim.12543
69. Fretts AM, Follis JL, Nettleton JA, Lemaitre RN, Ngwa JS, Wojczynski MK, et al. Consumption of meat is associated with higher fasting glucose and insulin concentrations regardless of glucose

and insulin genetic risk scores: A meta-analysis of 50,345 Caucasians. *Am J Clin Nutr* 2015; 102(5): 1266-1278. doi: 10.3945/ajcn.114.101238
70. Uribarri J, Woodruff S, Goodman S, Cai W, Chen X, Pyzik R, et al. Advanced Glycation End Products in Foods and a Practical Guide to Their Reduction in the Diet. *J Am Diet Assoc* 2010; 110(6): 911-916.e12. doi: 10.1016/j.jada.2010.03.018
71. White DL, Collinson A. Red meat, dietary heme iron, and risk of type 2 diabetes: The involvement of advanced lipoxidation endproducts. *Advances in Nutrition* 2013; 4(4): 403-411. doi: 10.3945/an.113.003681
72. Abbasi A, Sahlqvist AS, Lotta L, Brosnan JM, Vollenweider P, Giabbanelli P, et al. A systematic review of biomarkers and risk of incident type 2 diabetes: An overview of epidemiological, prediction and aetiological research literature. *PLoS One* 2016; 11(10): e0163721. doi: 10.1371/journal.pone.0163721
73. Zhao Z, Li S, Liu G, Yan F, Ma X, Huang Z, et al. Body iron stores and heme-iron intake in relation to risk of type 2 diabetes: A systematic review and meta-analysis. *PLoS One* 2012; 7(7): e41641. doi: 10.1371/journal.pone.0041641
74. Flores-Guerrero J, Osté M, Kieneker L, Gruppen E, Wolak-Dinsmore J, Otvos J, et al. Plasma Branched-Chain Amino Acids and Risk of Incident Type 2 Diabetes: Results from the PREVEND Prospective Cohort Study. *J Clin Med* 2018; 7(12): 513. doi: 10.3390/jcm7120513
75. Zhuang R, Ge X, Han L, Yu P, Gong X, Meng Q, et al. Gut microbe–generated metabolite trimethylamine N-oxide and the risk of diabetes: A systematic review and dose-response meta-analysis. *Obesity Reviews* 2019; 20(6): 883-894. doi: 10.1111/obr.12843
76. Chast F, Slama G. Apollinaire Bouchardat and diabetes. *Hist Sci Med* 2007; 41(3): 287-301.
77. Wadden TA. Eight-year weight losses with an intensive lifestyle intervention: The look AHEAD study. *Obesity* 2014; 22(1): 5-13. doi: 10.1002/oby.20662
78. Lim EL, Hollingsworth KG, Aribisala BS, Chen MJ, Mathers JC, Taylor R. Reversal of type 2 diabetes: Normalisation of beta cell function in association with decreased pancreas and liver triacylglycerol. *Diabetologia* 2011; 54(10): 2506-2514. doi: 10.1007/s00125-011-2204-7
79. Lean MEJ, Leslie WS, Barnes AC, Brosnahan N, Thom G, McCombie L, et al. Durability of a primary care-led weight-management intervention for remission of type 2 diabetes: 2-year results of the DiRECT open-label, cluster-randomised trial. *Lancet Diabetes Endocrinol* 2019; 7(5): 344-355. doi: 10.1016/S2213-8587(19)30068-3
80. Lean ME, Leslie WS, Barnes AC, Brosnahan N, Thom G, McCombie L, et al. Primary care-led weight management for remission of type 2 diabetes (DiRECT): an open-label, cluster-randomised trial. *Lancet* 2018; 391(10120): 541-551. doi: 10.1016/S0140-6736(17)33102-1
81. Goldenberg JZ, Day A, Brinkworth GD, Sato J, Yamada S, Jönsson T, et al. Efficacy and safety of low and very low carbohydrate diets for type 2 diabetes remission: systematic review and meta-analysis of published and unpublished randomized trial data. *BMJ* 2021; 372: m4743. doi: 10.1136/bmj.m4743
82. The Scientific Advisory Committee on Nutrition. SACN report: lower carbohydrate diets for type 2 diabetes. 2021. Available from: www.gov.uk/government/publications/sacn-report-lower-carbohydrate-diets-for-type-2-diabetes
83. Hall KD, Guo J, Courville AB, Boring J, Brychta R, Chen KY, et al. Effect of a plant-based, low-fat diet versus an animal-based, ketogenic diet on ad libitum energy intake. *Nat Med* 2021; 27(2): 344-353. doi: 10.1038/s41591-020-01209-1
84. Hall KD, Chen KY, Guo J, Lam YY, Leibel RL, Mayer LES, et al. Energy expenditure and body composition changes after an isocaloric ketogenic diet in overweight and obese men. *Am J Clin Nutr* 2016; 104(2): 324-333. doi: 10.3945/ajcn.116.133561
85. Holt SHA, Brand Miller JC, Petocz P. An insulin index of foods: The insulin demand generated by 1000-kJ portions of common foods. *Am J Clin Nutr* 1997; 66(5): 1264-1276. doi: 10.1093/ajcn/66.5.1264
86. De Koning L, Fung TT, Liao X, Chiuve SE, Rimm EB, Willett WC, et al. Low-carbohydrate diet scores and risk of type 2 diabetes in men. *Am J Clin Nutr* 2011; 93(4): 844-850. doi: 10.3945/ajcn.110.004333

87. Bao W, Li S, Chavarro JE, Tobias DK, Zhu Y, Hu FB, et al. Low Carbohydrate-Diet Scores and Long-term Risk of Type 2 Diabetes Among Women with a History of Gestational Diabetes Mellitus: A Prospective Cohort Study. *Diabetes Care* 2016; 39(1): 43-49. doi: 10.2337/dc15-1642
88. Mazidi M, Katsiki N, Mikhailidis DP, Sattar N, Banach M. Lower carbohydrate diets and all-cause and cause-specific mortality: A population-based cohort study and pooling of prospective studies. *Eur Heart J* 2019; 40(34): 2870-2879. doi: 10.1093/eurheartj/ehz174
89. Merino J, Kones R, Ferré R, Plana N, Girona J, Aragonés G, et al. Negative effect of a low-carbohydrate, high-protein, high-fat diet on small peripheral artery reactivity in patients with increased cardiovascular risk. *Br J Nutr* 2013; 109(7): 1241-1247.
doi: 10.1017/S0007114512003091
90. Fleming RM. The effect of high-protein diets on coronary blood flow. *Angiology* 2000; 51(10): 817-826. doi: 10.1177/000331970005101003
91. Roden M, Krssak M, Stingl H, Gruber S, Hofer A, Fürnsinn C, et al. Rapid impairment of skeletal muscle glucose transport/phosphorylation by free fatty acids in humans. *Diabetes* 1999; 48(2): 358-364. doi: 10.2337/diabetes.48.2.358
92. González F, Considine R V., Abdelhadi OA, Acton AJ. Saturated Fat Ingestion Promotes Lipopolysaccharide-Mediated Inflammation and Insulin Resistance in Polycystic Ovary Syndrome. *J Clin Endocrinol Metab* 2018; 104(3): 934-946.
doi: 10.1210/jc.2018-01143
93. Jenkins DJA, Wong JMW, Kendall CWC, Esfahani A, Ng VWY, Leong TCK, et al. Effect of a 6-month vegan low-carbohydrate ('Eco-Atkins') diet on cardiovascular risk factors and body weight in hyperlipidaemic adults: A randomised controlled trial. *BMJ Open* 2014; 4(2).
doi: 10.1136/bmjopen-2013-003505
94. Chia JSJ, McRae JL, Kukuljan S, Woodford K, Elliott RB, Swinburn B, et al. A1 beta-casein milk protein and other environmental pre-disposing factors for type 1 diabetes. *Nutr Diabetes* 2017; 7(5): e274. doi: 10.1038/nutd.2017.16
95. Kahleova H, Carlsen B, Berrien Lopez R, Barnard ND. Plant-Based Diets for Type 1 Diabetes. *Diabetes Metab Case* 2020; 11(7).
doi: 0.35248/2155-6156.20.11.847
96. Wolosowicz M, Lukaszuk B, Chabowski A. The causes of insulin resistance in type 1 diabetes mellitus: Is there a place for quaternary prevention? *International Journal of Environmental Research and Public Health* 2020; 17(22): 8651. doi: 10.3390/ijerph17228651
97. Brahmkshatriya PP, Mehta AA, Saboo BD, Goyal RK. Characteristics and Prevalence of Latent Autoimmune Diabetes in Adults (LADA). *ISRN Pharmacol* 2012; 2012: 580202.
doi: 10.5402/2012/580202
98. Falorni A, Calcinaro F. Autoantibody profile and epitope mapping in latent autoimmune diabetes in adults. *Annals of the New York Academy of Sciences* 2002; 958: 99-106.
doi: 10.1111/j.1749-6632.2002.tb02951.x

Chapter 8
Plant-based nutrition and clinical nephrology

Leonie Dupuis and Shivam Joshi

Introduction

Whole-food plant-based diets have become widely recognised as the foundation for the prevention and treatment of many diseases. As of recently, the utility of these diets in chronic kidney disease (CKD) has becoming increasingly clear.[1] In this chapter, we consider a plant-based diet to be any dietary pattern focused on whole, unprocessed plant-based foods such as flexitarian, vegetarian, Mediterranean, and vegan diets. We will review the data discussing the use of plant-based diets in the incidence and progression of CKD, complications of CKD, and potential concerns for clinicians.

Plant-based diets and CKD incidence and progression

The data supporting plant-based diets' role in the prevention of CKD development (and albuminuria) ranges from observational studies to randomised control trials (RCTs). The Tehran Lipid and Glucose Study (TLGS) (n = 5316) is a cross-sectional study that investigated the association between macronutrients and CKD in non-diabetic adults.[2] They observed that the odds for CKD were 30% lower in those in the highest quartile of *plant* protein intake when compared to those in the lowest quartile (OR, 0.70; 95% CI, 0.51–0.97). Conversely, those in the highest quartile of *animal* protein intake had a 37% higher odds of CKD (OR, 1.37; 95% CI, 1.05–1.79). In the Multiethnic Study of Atherosclerosis (MESA) (n = 5042), Nettleton et al. assessed the relationship between microalbuminuria and the intake of plant and animal foods.[3] They found that eating high amounts of whole grains, fruits, vegetables, and low-fat dairy foods was associated with a 20% lower albumin-to-creatinine ratio (ACR) across quintiles (P for trend = 0.004). They also found that non-dairy animal food consumption was associated with 11% higher ACR across quintiles (P for trend = 0.03). A smaller cross-sectional study (n = 420) found that higher intake of plant protein (when adjusting for lifestyle and dietary factors) was associated with a lower prevalence of renal function impairment.[4] They also used theoretical replacement models to show that replacing 3% of energy from animal protein to plant protein lowered the prevalence ratio of renal function impairment to 0.20 (reference of 1) (95% CI: 0.06–0.63, P = 0.01).

Prospective studies show similar results. The Singapore Chinese Health Study (n = 63, 527) followed participants for a median of 15.5 years.[5] This study stands out due to its large cohort. They found that red meat intake was associated with ESRD (end stage renal disease) in a dose-dependent manner. Those in the highest quartile of red meat intake had a 40% higher risk for developing ESRD compared to those in the lowest quartile (HR, 1.40; 95% CI, 1.15–1.71). No association was found with intakes of poultry, fish, eggs, or dairy products, whereas soya and legumes appeared to be slightly protective. In their substitution analyses, they found that replacing one serving of red meat per day with other sources of protein, like soya and legumes was associated with a relative risk reduction of 50.4% (95% CI, 33.1–78.9%; P<0.01).

The Atherosclerosis Risk in Communities study followed a total of 11,952 adults over 1987 to 2013 to study the risk for incident chronic disease and dietary protein sources.[6] They found that the odds for CKD were 19% lower in those within the highest quintile of dietary consumption of nuts, legumes, and low-fat dairy when compared to the lowest quintile (OR, 0.81; 95% CI, 0.72–0.92). Mirmiran et al. conducted a prospective study to investigate the association of different meat intake with risk of CKD incidence in 4881 participants of the TLGS who were free of CKD.[7] After adjusting for confounders, they found that the OR of CKD incidence in members of the highest quartile of total red meat intake was 1.73 (95% CI: 1.33–2.24) and 1.99 (95% CI: 2.54–2.56) when comparing the highest quartile to the lowest quartile. They also conducted substitution analyses and found that replacing one serving of total red meat and processed meat with one serving of whole grains was associated with a 21% lower odds of CKD incidence (OR: 0.79; 95% CI, 0.73–0.86), 16% for one serving of nuts (OR: 0.84; 95% CI: 0.74–0.95), and 19% for one serving of legumes (OR: 0.81; 95% CI: 0.68–0.97).

In terms of end stage renal disease, a multinational cohort study of 8078 patients on haemodialysis found that increased intake of fruits and vegetables was associated with reduced all-cause and non-cardiovascular death.[8] In this study, participants were asked to complete a food frequency questionnaire for a median follow-up of 2.7 years totalling 18,586 person-years. Despite such a large sample size, only 4% of the participants consumed the minimum recommended four servings of fruit and vegetables per day. Furthermore, a meta-analysis found that polyphenol-rich interventions (such as plant-based diets) in patients on haemodialysis can improve diastolic blood pressure, triglycerides, and myeloperoxidase, reducing cardiovascular disease risk in patients on haemodialysis.[9] Studies also suggest that plant-based diets, rich in linoleic acid, are inversely associated with IL-6 and all-cause mortality in haemodialysis patients.[10]

Several RCTs exist regarding diet and kidney disease, but so far only three corrected for the total amount of protein consumed, an important confounder when comparing plant-based diets to other diets.[11] All three RCTs were conducted in patients with albuminuria and type 2 diabetes mellitus.[12, 13, 14] In this patient population, Azadbakht et al. (n = 14) found that soya-protein consumption reduces proteinuria, Teixeira et al. (n = 14) found that soya protein consumption improves albumin excretion and other markers, and Azadbakht et al. (n = 41) also found that soya protein consumption improved kidney-related biomarkers (proteinuria, urinary creatinine). These three studies show statistically significant reductions in albuminuria when partially substituting animal protein with plant protein.

Animal-based foods are composed of substances that may impair kidney health and function (saturated fats, sodium, phosphorus, dietary acid load (DAL), higher protein content, advanced glycation end products, haem iron, carnitine, and choline). Carnitine and choline, specifically, lead to the generation of trimethylamine N-oxide (TMAO), a toxic, pro-inflammatory compound that promotes the development of atherosclerosis and possibly kidney disease.[15, 16] The lack of these substances and the presence of dietary fibre, phytochemicals, vitamins, minerals, and antioxidants substantiate most theories on the mechanism of diet on kidney health.[17, 18, 19, 20]

Complications of CKD

Metabolic acidosis

Metabolic acidosis in kidney disease stimulates production of paracrine hormones such as angiotensin II, aldosterone, and endothelin 1. These hormones upregulate kidney acid excretion acutely but cause chronic inflammation and fibrosis. Increased acid retention (which can lead to metabolic acidosis) has been associated with an increased dietary acid load (DAL). The African American Study of Kidney Disease and Hypertension (AASK) (n = 1,044) found that lower urinary ammonium excretion (which is important in the pathogenesis of acidosis) was associated with an increased risk for death or dialysis (HR, 1.36; C=95% CI, 1.09–1.71) even in the absence of metabolic acidosis.

Traditional Western diets tend to emphasise animal products, acid-inducing foods due to the presence of organic sulphur which is oxidised to inorganic sulphate.[21] Most of human non-volatile acid production is a direct result of dietary consumption of acid-inducing foods. Contrarily, plant-based diets have an innate alkaline quality in the form of citrate, malate, and other bases, which can then be used to produce bicarbonate. In an average person consuming a traditional Western diet, about 50 to 75 mEq/d of DAL is produced daily. In comparison, an average person following a vegan diet has a close to neutral DAL.[21]

With this background on diet's effect on acid production, it makes sense that administering alkali can reduce the DAL, acid retention, and kidney function decline.[22] A randomised control trial (n = 134) showed that patients with CKD receiving alkali therapy experienced a slowing of GFR decline from 5.93 to 1.88 mL/min/1.73 m^2 per year.[23] In this trial, supplements were used to supply the alkali, but in a series of trials, Goraya et al. utilised fruits and vegetables to manage metabolic acidosis in those with CKD and found significant benefit in their use.[24, 25, 26] In an RCT (n = 108), they randomised stage 3 CKD patients to receive either standard care or sodium bicarbonate (0.3 mEq/kg per day) or base-producing fruits and vegetables (typically 2–4 cups per day) for three years.[24] GFR decline was slowed in both the sodium bicarbonate and fruits and vegetables groups suggesting that the two may share the same efficacy in preserving renal function. Furthermore, the fruits and vegetables group lost an average of 3.7 kg and had an average 7.4 mm Hg decrease in systolic blood pressure after three years when compared to the sodium bicarbonate supplementation group. Goraya et al. also conducted a similar RCT (n = 71) in individuals with stage 4 CKD and found that fruits and vegetables improve metabolic acidosis and reduce kidney injury in stage 4 CKD.[25]

As a result of the growing evidence in favour of patients with CKD consuming fruits and vegetables, the recently published National Kidney Foundation's Kidney Disease Outcomes Quality Initiative (KDOQI) guidelines include the recommendation that increased consumption of fruits and vegetables 'may decrease body weight, blood pressure, and net acid production'.[27]

Hypertension

Hypertension is a unique component of kidney disease because it can be both a cause and a consequence of the disease. It is the second most common cause of kidney failure and comorbid in 60 to 90% of patients with CKD with higher prevalence rates among those with advanced CKD.

Neurohormonal activation and sodium retention in kidney disease contribute to the development of hypertension.[28] Whether diagnosed with kidney disease or not, the benefits of plant-based diets for hypertension have been observed for at least a century.[29]

In a meta-analysis of 32 observational studies (n = 21,604) in patients without CKD, it was found that plant-based diets were associated with a lower mean systolic and diastolic blood pressure when compared with omnivorous diets (−6.9 [95% CI, −9.1 to −4.7] mm Hg and −4.7 [95% CI, −6.3 to −3.1] mm Hg, respectively).[30] A prospective study (n = 188,518) found that consuming one or more servings of animal-based flesh per day was associated with a 30% increased risk (HR, 1.30; 95% CI, 1.16–1.47) for hypertension when compared with eating less than one serving per month.[31]

For those with CKD, Goraya et al. found that consuming 2–4 cups of fruits and vegetables per day reduced blood pressure in those with CKD stage 3 when compared to those using a sodium bicarbonate supplement.[24] Similar findings were shown in patients with stage 4 CKD where their systolic blood pressure decreased by a mean of 4.3 mm Hg after one year of including 2–4 cups of fruits and vegetables compared to a group consuming a sodium bicarbonate supplement.[25]

The explanation for plant-based diets' effect on blood pressure is multifactorial. The most common explanation is that plant-based diets cause a reduction in weight that thereby causes a decrease in blood pressure, but several observational studies have shown reduction in blood pressure on plant-based diets even when adjusting for weight.[31, 32, 33] The European Prospective Investigation into Cancer and Nutrition (EPIC)-Oxford cohort study found that only half of blood pressure variation can be attributed to weight.[34] Other explanations for the observed changes in blood pressure include reduced dietary sodium content, increased dietary potassium content, microbiome changes, and reduced oxidative stress.[29]

Hyperphosphataemia

Hyperphosphataemia is an independent risk factor for mortality in patients with CKD and kidney failure.[35, 36] Because of this risk, traditional dietary recommendations for patients with severe kidney disease have promoted avoiding plant-based foods. Plant-based foods can be high in phosphate content, especially nuts, seeds, and legumes, but this quantitative approach to phosphate content fails to consider the reduced bioavailability of phosphate found in plant-based foods. Plant food phosphates are bound to phytate, a substance that requires phytase to be separated from the phosphates. Humans lack phytase, reducing the bioavailability of phosphate found in plant-based foods to between 10 and 30%.[37] The bioavailability of phosphates in animal foods, however, has been estimated to be between 40 and 60% but can reach up to 80 %.[38] Furthermore, many animal-based foods are processed with phosphate-containing additives that increase the bioavailable phosphate by 7 to 100%.[39] However, it should be noted that processing of plant foods, like legumes and grains, can increase the amount of bioavailable phosphorus.

Nonetheless, studies have shown that consuming a plant-based diet results in reduced serum phosphate levels when compared to an animal-based diet despite controlling for dietary phosphate intake. Moe et al. performed a crossover study (n = 9) in patients with CKD stages 3–4 and found that patients who were fed a vegetarian diet had a lower serum phosphate level and urinary phosphate excretion when compared to patients following an animal-based diet with equivalent nutrients.[40] In another cross-over study (n = 14), a decrease in serum phosphate levels was seen in patients with CKD with only partial replacement of animal-based protein with plant-based protein.[12] Prospective and retrospective cohort studies have also shown the same result – eating plant-based foods can lower serum phosphate levels in kidney failure.[41] A small observational study also found that, in patients on haemodialysis, phosphate levels were significantly lower in vegetarian patients than in nonvegetarian patients.[42]

Uraemic toxins, dietary fibres, microbiome

Dietary fibre can reduce uraemic toxin production.[43] Uraemic toxins are toxic substances that accumulate in bodily fluids during the progression of chronic kidney disease. Along with worsening kidney disease, uraemic toxins have been shown to increase inflammation, insulin resistance, and cardiovascular disease.[41] In kidney disease, uraemic toxins may promote glomerular filtration rate losses by increasing levels of transforming growth factor beta which then increases fibrogenesis of the kidney.[10]

A meta-analysis of controlled feeding trials in patients with CKD showed that as fibre intake increases, urea and creatinine decrease in a dose-dependent function.[44] In a cross-sectional study, vegetarians undergoing haemodiafiltration had 47% and 67% lower levels of indoxyl sulphate and p-cresyl sulphate when compared to nonvegetarians underdoing haemodiafiltration, respectively.[45] Despite the many benefits of dietary fibre, the average fibre intake of patients on haemodialysis is 20 to 30% less than controls at about 11 g per day, which is less than the standard recommended guidelines for daily intake, for example 22–28 g for women and 28–34 g for men each day in the *Dietary Guidelines for Americans, 2020–2025*.[46] In patients on haemodialysis, fibre supplementation has also been associated with decreased uraemic toxins, reduced inflammatory markers such tumour necrosis factor-alpha, interleukin-6, and C-reactive protein, improved lipid profiles and oxidative status, and reduced all-cause mortality.[10]

Mortality

In the general population, diets high in plant foods and low in animal foods are associated with significantly reduced mortality risk. This observation was shown using data from the Atherosclerosis Risk in Communities study of 12,168 individuals who were followed from 1987 to 2016, including information about their diet.[47] Kelly et al. conducted a meta-analysis of six prospective cohort studies of patients with CKD (n = 14,000) and found that eating diets with more fruits, vegetables, cereals, whole grains, fibre, and fish and less red meat, salt, and refined sugars was associated with a reduced mortality risk (RR, 0.73; 95% CI, 0.63–0.83).[48] A prospective study (n = 8078) across 11 countries in Europe and South America found that patients in the highest tertile of fruit and vegetable intake had a significantly lower risk for all-cause (HR, 0.80; 95% CI, 0.71–0.91) and non-cardiovascular (HR, 0.77; 95% CI, 0.66–0.91) mortality when compared to those in the lowest tertile.[8]

Potential concerns

Hyperkalaemia

Hyperkalaemia has been an oft-cited reason for the avoidance of plant foods. Indeed, plant-based items have been identified as causes of hyperkalaemia in a case series of patients with and without CKD.[49] However, the bulk of these causes were attributed to juices, sauces, or dried fruit with only a minority of causes attributable to unprocessed plant foods. Juices, sauces and dried fruit are all processed foods in a way that concentrates the rate and quantity of potassium consumed when compared to its whole food form. Juices, sauces, and dried fruit also have less fibre or water than their whole-food counterparts which can result in the consumption of greater amounts of potassium per unit of time. Fibre also increases faecal bulk which facilitates potassium excretion, thus potentially mitigating the risk for hyperkalaemia.

Although case reports have previously presented a relationship between plant-based foods and hyperkalaemia, several prospective observational and experimental studies have only shown the same connection in one instance.[41] Joshi et al. reviewed previous studies on plant-based diets and their relationship to serum potassium in patients with CKD. They reported that in that one instance, the patient with hyperkalaemia had a pre-existing type IV renal tubular acidosis and was consuming raw edamame, one of the most potassium-rich foods. In this case, the patient swapped edamame for tofu and the hyperkalaemia resolved.

In the case of patients on haemodialysis, the overall paucity in clinical trials examining dietary potassium intake limits the ability to draw a definitive conclusion on the need for potassium restriction in patients on dialysis. In a study by Saglimbene et al, it was found that predialysis potassium levels across a wide quantity of fruit and vegetable serving intake (0–5.5, 5.6–10, and >10 per week) were 5.1, 5.0, and 5.0, respectively.[8] In other words, the predialysis potassium levels did not show fluctuation despite the differences in dietary plant consumption. Plant-based foods have built in factors to help mitigate the risk of hyperkalaemia, such as fibre discussed earlier. The natural alkali of plant foods can also help facilitate intracellular movement of potassium, especially in states of metabolic acidosis. Other mitigatory factors include improved insulin sensitivity and better blood pressure control, reducing the need for hypertensive medications known to cause hyperkalaemia (beta blockers, angiotensin II receptor blockers, and angiotensin-converting enzyme inhibitors). Thus, it is reasonable to advise that patients with kidney disease avoid plant-based juices, sauces, dried fruits, potassium-containing supplements, and foods unusually high in potassium like molasses and raw legumes when eating plant-based diets. Although the incidence of hyperkalaemia is rare in the literature, it is wise to be cautious with any dietary changes and regularly monitor serum electrolytes in this patient population.

Protein adequacy and beyond

Protein adequacy is a common concern when approaching plant-based diets, both in terms of quantity and quality. Studies consistently show more than adequate levels of protein consumption both in patients with and without kidney disease consuming plant-based diets.[41] Recent KDOQI guidelines recommend that those with CKD consume between 0.55 to 0.80 g/kg/d of dietary protein. In several studies of patients with kidney disease, patients were readily able to attain 0.7 to 0.9 g/kg/d without signs of nutritional inadequacy.[50] The lower – but not inadequate – intake of protein among those eating plant-based diets may also help reduce the effects of hyperfiltration and, thus, help reduce the progression of kidney disease.

Dialysis considerations: constipation and vitamin K

More specific to patients on haemodialysis is the possible sequelae of vitamin deficiencies and constipation. Although vitamin deficiencies can be the result of a wide range of factors from decreased appetite or smell to difficulty cooking or obtaining certain ingredients, there is good reason to closely look at dietary pattern and micronutrient content to prevent worsening of the deficiency. Like anyone following a plant-based diet, a vitamin B12 supplement is strongly recommended, but patients on dialysis also are at risk of vitamin K deficiency which has been associated with cardiovascular calcification, bleeding risk, and cardiovascular risk in both the general population and patients on dialysis.[51] Vitamin K can be found in green vegetables such as spinach, kale, brussels sprouts, and broccoli. Thus, dietary regimens poor in plant foods (such as the ones currently recommended to many patients on dialysis) may inadvertently result in vitamin K deficiency. On the other end, guidelines recommending a 'stable intake' of vitamin-K-rich foods are sometimes interpreted as 'no intake' of vitamin-K-rich foods which might further increase the prevalence of vitamin K deficiency in this patient population.[10]

Another complication to look out for in haemodialysis patients is that of constipation. A 2013 cross-sectional study of 478 patients on dialysis noted 71.7% of patients to have constipation (using the Roma III criteria).[52] It is possible that the historical guidance to minimise fibre-rich foods when on dialysis may have contributed to the prevalence of constipation in patients on dialysis, but further studies are needed on this subject in the population of patients on haemodialysis.

Special topic: kidney stones

The oxalate content of plant-based food is another possible concern when eating plant-based foods with kidney disease. However, excess oxalate can lead to nephrolithiasis, especially when other risk factors are involved.[53] When risk factors are absent, studies are inconsistent in regard to the effect of dietary oxalate on urinary oxalate excretion. In one study, the consumption of high-oxalate foods like spinach, rhubarb, nuts, and beets resulted in increased urinary oxalate excretion.[54] In other studies, dietary oxalate restriction only minimally reduced urinary oxalate excretion.[55] Despite the concern for oxalate stones, observational studies have shown that vegetarians are linked with a lower risk for kidney stones.[56] One mediating mechanism for a lower risk of kidney stones may be the presence of gut bacterium *Oxalobacter formigenes*, a gram-negative, obligate anaerobe that requires oxalate for its survival. Studies have shown that *O. formigenes* can increase by 10-fold with a 10-fold increase in dietary oxalate, and those with *O. formigenes* colonisation have been associated with a lower risk of kidney stones.[57]

Conclusion

Evidence is mounting to show the possible benefits of plant-based foods in renal disease. From reducing the incidence and progression of CKD to mitigating complications of CKD, evidence in the form of observational studies, prospective studies, and randomised controlled trials exists to suggest that plant-based diets may provide a benefit in these scenarios. Furthermore, plant-based foods may contribute to reduced uraemic toxin production and reduce the risk of mortality in CKD. Potential concerns of hyperkalaemia, protein quality, and protein quantity are addressed in this chapter as well as plant-based foods to reduce the risk for nephrolithiasis.

Acknowledgements

The authors would like to thank Dr Michelle McMacken for connecting them and for her invaluable guidance and mentorship.

References

1. Joshi S, Hashmi S, Shah S, Kalantar-Zadeh K. Plant-based diets for prevention and management of chronic kidney disease. *Curr Opin Nephrol Hypertens* 2020; 29(1): 16-21. doi: 10.1097/MNH.0000000000000574
2. Institute of Medicine. Dietary Reference Intakes for Energy, Carbohydrate, Fiber, Fat, Fatty Acids, Cholesterol, Protein, and Amino Acids (Macronutrients). National Academy of Sciences 2005. doi: 10.17226/10490

3. Nettleton JA, Steffen LM, Palmas W, Burke GL, Jacobs DR, Jr. Associations between microalbuminuria and animal foods, plant foods, and dietary patterns in the Multiethnic Study of Atherosclerosis. *The American Journal of Clinical Nutrition* 2008; 87(6): 1825-1836. doi: 10.1093/ajcn/87.6.1825

4. Oosterwijk MM, Soedamah-Muthu SS, Geleijnse JM, Bakker SJL, Navis G, Binnenmars SH, et al. High Dietary Intake of Vegetable Protein Is Associated With Lower Prevalence of Renal Function Impairment: Results of the Dutch DIALECT-1 Cohort. *Kidney International Reports* 2019; 4(5): 710-719. doi: 10.1016/j.ekir.2019.02.009

5. Lew QJ, Jafar TH, Koh HW, Jin A, Chow KY, Yuan JM, et al. Red Meat Intake and Risk of ESRD. *J Am Soc Nephrol* 2017; 28(1): 304-312. doi: 10.1681/ASN.2016030248

6. Haring B, Selvin E, Liang M, Coresh J, Grams ME, Petruski-Ivleva N, et al. Dietary Protein Sources and Risk for Incident Chronic Kidney Disease: Results From the Atherosclerosis Risk in Communities (ARIC) Study. *J Ren Nutr* 2017; 27(4): 233-242. doi: 10.1053/j.jrn.2016.11.004

7. Mirmiran P, Yuzbashian E, Aghayan M, Mahdavi M, Asghari G, Azizi F. A Prospective Study of Dietary Meat Intake and Risk of Incident Chronic Kidney Disease. *J Ren Nutr* 2020; 30(2): 111-118. doi: 10.1053/j.jrn.2019.06.008

8. Saglimbene VM, Wong G, Ruospo M, Palmer SC, Garcia-Larsen V, Natale P, et al. Fruit and Vegetable Intake and Mortality in Adults undergoing Maintenance Hemodialysis. *Clinical Journal of the American Society of Nephrology* 2019; 14(2): 250-260. doi: 10.2215/CJN.08580718

9. Marx W, Kelly J, Marshall S, Nakos S, Campbell K, Itsiopoulos C. The Effect of Polyphenol-Rich Interventions on Cardiovascular Risk Factors in Haemodialysis: A Systematic Review and Meta-Analysis. *Nutrients* 2017; 9(12): 1345. doi: 10.3390/nu9121345

10. Dupuis L, Brown-Tortorici A, Kalantar-Zadeh K, Joshi S. A Mini Review of Plant-Based Diets in Hemodialysis. *Blood Purif* 2021; 50(4-5): 672-677. doi: 10.1159/000516249

11. Clarys P, Deliens T, Huybrechts I, Deriemaeker P, Vanaelst B, De Keyzer W, et al. Comparison of Nutritional Quality of the Vegan, Vegetarian, Semi-Vegetarian, Pesco-Vegetarian and Omnivorous Diet. *Nutrients* 2014; 6(3): 1318-1332. doi: 10.3390/nu6031318

12. Azadbakht L, Esmaillzadeh A. Soy-protein consumption and kidney-related biomarkers among type 2 diabetics: a crossover, randomized clinical trial. *J Ren Nutr* 2009; 19(6): 479-486. doi: 10.1053/j.jrn.2009.06.002

13. Teixeira SR, Tappenden KA, Carson L, Jones R, Prabhudesai M, Marshall WP, et al. Isolated Soy Protein Consumption Reduces Urinary Albumin Excretion and Improves the Serum Lipid Profile in Men with Type 2 Diabetes Mellitus and Nephropathy. *The Journal of Nutrition* 2004; 134(8): 1874-1880. doi: 10.1093/jn/134.8.1874

14. Azadbakht L, Atabak S, Esmaillzadeh A. Soy Protein Intake, Cardiorenal Indices, and C-Reactive Protein in Type 2 Diabetes With Nephropathy. *A longitudinal randomized clinical trial* 2008; 31(4): 648-654. doi: 10.2337/dc07-2065

15. Ufnal M, Zadlo A, Ostaszewski R. TMAO: A small molecule of great expectations. *Nutrition* 2015; 31(11-12): 1317-1323. doi: 10.1016/j.nut.2015.05.006

16. Fogelman AM. TMAO is both a biomarker and a renal toxin. Circ Res. 2015;116(3):396-7.

17. Gluba-Brzózka A, Franczyk B, Rysz J. Vegetarian Diet in Chronic Kidney Disease-A Friend or Foe. *Nutrients* 2017; 9(4): 374. doi: 10.3390/nu9040374

18. Chauveau P, Koppe L, Combe C, Lasseur C, Trolonge S, Aparicio M. Vegetarian diets and chronic kidney disease. *Nephrology Dialysis Transplantation* 2018; 34(2): 199-207. doi: 10.1093/ndt/gfy164

19. Cases A, Cigarrán-Guldrís S, Mas S, Gonzalez-Parra E. Vegetable-Based Diets for Chronic Kidney Disease? It Is Time to Reconsider. *Nutrients* 2019; 11(6): 1263. doi: 10.3390/nu1106126

20. Kalantar-Zadeh K, Joshi S, Schlueter R, Cooke J, Brown-Tortorici A, Donnelly M, et al. Plant-Dominant Low-Protein Diet for Conservative Management of Chronic Kidney Disease. *Nutrients* 2020; 12(7): 1931. doi: 10.3390/nu12071931

21. Scialla JJ, Anderson CA. Dietary acid load: a novel nutritional target in chronic kidney disease?

Adv Chronic Kidney Dis 2013; 20(2): 141-149. doi: 10.1053/j.ackd.2012.11.001

22. Wesson DE, Buysse JM, Bushinsky DA. Mechanisms of Metabolic Acidosis–Induced Kidney Injury in Chronic Kidney Disease. *J Am Soc Nephrol* 2020; 31(3): 469-482. doi: 10.1681/ASN.2019070677

23. de Brito-Ashurst I, Varagunam M, Raftery MJ, Yaqoob MM. Bicarbonate supplementation slows progression of CKD and improves nutritional status. *J Am Soc Nephrol* 2009; 20(9): 2075-2084. doi: 10.1681/ASN.2008111205

24. Goraya N, Simoni J, Jo C-H, Wesson DE. Treatment of metabolic acidosis in patients with stage 3 chronic kidney disease with fruits and vegetables or oral bicarbonate reduces urine angiotensinogen and preserves glomerular filtration rate. *Kidney Int* 2014; 86(5): 1031-1038. doi: 10.1038/ki.2014.83

25. Goraya N, Simoni J, Jo CH, Wesson DE. A comparison of treating metabolic acidosis in CKD stage 4 hypertensive kidney disease with fruits and vegetables or sodium bicarbonate. *Clin J Am Soc Nephrol* 2013; 8(3): 371-381. doi: 10.2215/CJN.02430312

26. Goraya N, Simoni J, Jo C, Wesson DE. Dietary acid reduction with fruits and vegetables or bicarbonate attenuates kidney injury in patients with a moderately reduced glomerular filtration rate due to hypertensive nephropathy. *Kidney Int* 2012; 81(1): 86-93. doi: 10.1038/ki.2011.313

27. Ikizler TA, Burrowes JD, Byham-Gray LD, Campbell KL, Carrero JJ, Chan W, et al. KDOQI Clinical Practice Guideline for Nutrition in CKD: 2020 Update. *Am J Kidney Dis* 2020; 76(3 Suppl 1): S1-S107. doi: 10.1053/j.ajkd.2020.05.006

28. Saran R, Robinson B, Abbott KC, Agodoa LYC, Bragg-Gresham J, Balkrishnan R, et al. US Renal Data System 2018 Annual Data Report: Epidemiology of Kidney Disease in the United States. *Am J Kidney Dis* 2019; 73(3 Suppl 1): A7-A8. doi: 10.1053/j.ajkd.2019.01.001

29. Joshi S, Ettinger L, Liebman SE. Plant-Based Diets and Hypertension. *Am J Lifestyle Med* 2019; 14(4): 397-405.

30. Yokoyama Y, Nishimura K, Barnard ND, Takegami M, Watanabe M, Sekikawa A, et al. Vegetarian Diets and Blood Pressure: A Meta-analysis. *JAMA Internal Medicine* 2014; 174(4): 577-587. doi: 10.1001/jamainternmed.2013.14547

31. Borgi L, Curhan GC, Willett WC, Hu FB, Satija A, Forman JP. Long-term intake of animal flesh and risk of developing hypertension in three prospective cohort studies. *J Hypertens* 2015; 33(11): 2231-2238. doi: 10.1097/HJH.0000000000000722

32. Pettersen BJ, Anousheh R, Fan J, Jaceldo-Siegl K, Fraser GE. Vegetarian diets and blood pressure among white subjects: results from the Adventist Health Study-2 (AHS-2). *Public Health Nutr* 2012; 15(10): 1909-1916. doi: 10.1017/S1368980011003454

33. Spencer EA, Appleby PN, Davey GK, Key TJ. Diet and body mass index in 38000 EPIC-Oxford meat-eaters, fish-eaters, vegetarians and vegans. *Int J Obes Relat Metab Disord* 2003; 27(6): 728-734. doi: 10.1038/sj.ijo.0802300

34. Davey GK, Spencer EA, Appleby PN, Allen NE, Knox KH, Key TJ. EPIC-Oxford: lifestyle characteristics and nutrient intakes in a cohort of 33 883 meat-eaters and 31 546 non meat-eaters in the UK. *Public Health Nutr* 2003; 6(3): 259-269. doi: 10.1079/PHN2002430

35. Hou Y, Li X, Sun L, Qu Z, Jiang L, Du Y. Phosphorus and mortality risk in end-stage renal disease: A meta-analysis. *Clin Chim Acta* 2017; 474: 108-113. doi: 10.1016/j.cca.2017.09.005

36. Palmer SC, Hayen A, Macaskill P, Pellegrini F, Craig JC, Elder GJ, et al. Serum Levels of Phosphorus, Parathyroid Hormone, and Calcium and Risks of Death and Cardiovascular Disease in Individuals With Chronic Kidney Disease: A Systematic Review and Meta-analysis. *JAMA* 2011; 305(11): 1119-1127. doi: 10.1001/jama.2011.308

37. Noori N, Sims JJ, Kopple JD, Shah A, Colman S, Shinaberger CS, et al. Organic and inorganic dietary phosphorus and its management in chronic kidney disease. *Iran J Kidney Dis* 2010; 4(2): 89-100.

38. González-Parra E, Gracia-Iguacel C, Egido J, Ortiz A. Phosphorus and nutrition in chronic kidney disease. *Int J Nephrol* 2012; 2012: 597605. doi: 10.1155/2012/597605

39. Sherman RA, Mehta O. Phosphorus and

potassium content of enhanced meat and poultry products: implications for patients who receive dialysis. *Clin J Am Soc Nephrol* 2009; 4(8): 1370-1373. doi: 10.2215/CJN.02830409

40. Moe SM, Zidehsarai MP, Chambers MA, Jackman LA, Radcliffe JS, Trevino LL, et al. Vegetarian compared with meat dietary protein source and phosphorus homeostasis in chronic kidney disease. *Clin J Am Soc Nephrol* 2011; 6(2): 257-264. doi: 10.2215/CJN.05040610

41. Joshi S, McMacken M, Kalantar-Zadeh K. Plant-Based Diets for Kidney Disease: A Guide for Clinicians. *Am J Kidney Dis* 2021; 77(2): 287-296. doi: 10.1053/j.ajkd.2020.10.003

42. Wu TT, Chang CY, Hsu WM, Wang IK, Hsu CH, Cheng SH, et al. Nutritional status of vegetarians on maintenance haemodialysis. *Nephrology (Carlton)* 2011; 16(6): 582-587. doi: 10.1111/j.1440-1797.2011.01464.x

43. Rampton DS, Cohen SL, Crammond VD, Gibbons J, Lilburn MF, Rabet JY, et al. Treatment of chronic renal failure with dietary fiber. *Clin Nephrol* 1984; 21(3): 159-163.

44. Chiavaroli L, Mirrahimi A, Sievenpiper JL, Jenkins DJA, Darling PB. Dietary fiber effects in chronic kidney disease: a systematic review and meta-analysis of controlled feeding trials. *Eur J Clin Nutr* 2015; 69(7): 761-768. doi: 10.1038/ejcn.2014.237

45. Kandouz S, Mohamed AS, Zheng Y, Sandeman S, Davenport A. Reduced protein bound uraemic toxins in vegetarian kidney failure patients treated by haemodiafiltration. *Hemodial Int* 2016; 20(4): 610-617. doi: 10.1111/hdi.12414

46. Khoueiry G, Waked A, Goldman M, El-Charabaty E, Dunne E, Smith M, et al. Dietary intake in hemodialysis patients does not reflect a heart healthy diet. *J Ren Nutr* 2011; 21(6): 438-447. doi: 10.1053/j.jrn.2010.09.001

47. Kim H, Caulfield LE, Garcia-Larsen V, Steffen LM, Coresh J, Rebholz CM. Plant-Based Diets Are Associated With a Lower Risk of Incident Cardiovascular Disease, Cardiovascular Disease Mortality, and All-Cause Mortality in a General Population of Middle-Aged Adults. *J Am Heart Assoc* 2019; 8(16): e012865. doi: 10.1161/JAHA.119.012865

48. Kelly JT, Palmer SC, Wai SN, Ruospo M, Carrero JJ, Campbell KL, et al. Healthy Dietary Patterns and Risk of Mortality and ESRD in CKD: A Meta-Analysis of Cohort Studies. *Clin J Am Soc Nephrol* 2017; 12(2): 272-279. doi: 10.2215/CJN.06190616

49. Te Dorsthorst RPM, Hendrikse J, Vervoorn MT, van Weperen VYH, van der Heyden MAG. Review of case reports on hyperkalemia induced by dietary intake: not restricted to chronic kidney disease patients. *Eur J Clin Nutr* 2019; 73(1): 38-45. doi: 10.1038/s41430-018-0154-6

50. Joshi S, Shah S, Kalantar-Zadeh K. Adequacy of Plant-Based Proteins in Chronic Kidney Disease. *J Ren Nutr* 2019; 29(2): 112-117. doi: 10.1053/j.jrn.2018.06.006

51. Carrero JJ, González-Ortiz A, Avesani CM, Bakker SJL, Bellizzi V, Chauveau P, et al. Plant-based diets to manage the risks and complications of chronic kidney disease. *Nat Rev Nephrol* 2020; 16(9): 525-542. doi: 10.1038/s41581-020-0297-2

52. Zhang Y, Zhou Z, Gao J, Wang D, Zhang Q, Zhou Z, et al. Health-related quality of life and its influencing factors for patients with hypertension: evidence from the urban and rural areas of Shaanxi Province, China. *BMC Health Serv Res* 2016; 16: 277. doi: 10.1186/s12913-016-1536-x

53. Makkapati S, D'Agati VD, Balsam L. "Green Smoothie Cleanse" Causing Acute Oxalate Nephropathy. *Am J Kidney Dis* 2018; 71(2): 281-286. doi: 10.1053/j.ajkd.2017.08.002

54. Massey LK, Roman-Smith H, Sutton RAL. Effect of dietary oxalate and calcium on urinary oxalate and risk of formation of calcium oxalate kidney stones. *J Am Diet Assoc* 1993; 93(8): 901-906. doi: 10.1016/0002-8223(93)91530-4

55. Taylor EN, Curhan GC. Determinants of 24-hour urinary oxalate excretion. *Clin J Am Soc Nephrol* 2008; 3(5): 1453-1460. doi: 10.2215/CJN.01410308

56. Turney BW, Appleby PN, Reynard JM, Noble JG, Key TJ, Allen NE. Diet and risk of kidney stones in the Oxford cohort of the European Prospective Investigation into Cancer and Nutrition (EPIC). *Eur J Epidemiol* 2014; 29(5): 363-369. doi: 10.1007/s10654-014-9904-5

57. Joshi S, Goldfarb DS. The use of antibiotics and risk of kidney stones. *Curr Opin Nephrol Hypertens* 2019; 28(4): 311-315.

Chapter 9
Plant-based nutrition and non-alcoholic fatty liver disease

Divya Devabhaktuni and Meagan Gray

Disease overview

What is NAFLD?

Over the last 30 years, non-alcoholic fatty liver disease (NAFLD) has become the most common cause of chronic liver disease globally.[1] NAFLD is defined by the presence of >5% hepatic steatosis with a lack of secondary cause for hepatic fat accumulation. NAFLD can be further divided into two entities based on liver histology: non-alcoholic fatty liver (NAFL) and non-alcoholic steatohepatitis (NASH). NAFL represents 75% of NAFLD cases and is defined by simple steatosis with or without lobular inflammation, while NASH is defined as steatosis in addition to lobular inflammation and cellular ballooning.[2] The distinction is important as NASH confers approximately a 20% risk of progression to cirrhosis while <4% of NAFL cases will progress.[3] Compared to matched controls, those with NAFLD have increased overall mortality,[4] with cardiovascular disease being the most common cause of death, followed by malignancy.[5] In patients with NASH, the stage of fibrosis, which, using the Metavir scoring system ranges from stage 0 (no fibrosis) to stage 4 (cirrhosis), is closely associated with both liver- and all-cause mortality,[5] which highlights the desperate need for treatment strategies to resolve NASH and reverse fibrosis.

Pathophysiology

The hallmark of NAFLD is the development of hepatic steatosis, or the abnormal accumulation of excess lipids, including free fatty acids (FFAs) and triglycerides, in the liver (see Figure 9.1). This occurs as a result of alterations in pathways of lipid metabolism that result in excess FFAs in the liver through increased lipolysis, *de novo* lipogenesis (DNL), excess hepatic import of dietary FFAs, and decreased export of FFA by very low-density lipoprotein (VLDL).[6] Although the pathogenesis of NAFLD is multifaceted, insulin resistance is thought to play a key role in the development of hepatic steatosis through its effects on lipid metabolism, primarily through ineffective suppression of peripheral lipolysis and increased uptake of FFA into the liver.[7] The effect of insulin resistance in NAFLD can be seen even in the absence of obesity or diabetes.[8] The accumulation of FFAs in the liver overwhelm hepatic oxidation processes, which then leads to increased oxidative stress, resulting in the hepatocellular injury and inflammation characteristic of NASH. Excess visceral fat increases the production of free fatty acids influxing into the liver, further increasing *de novo* lipogenesis, and contributing to the formation of a pro-inflammatory environment through the release of pro-fibrotic adipokines and inflammatory cytokines.[9] Lipotoxicity, with the resulting chronic inflammatory state, leads to fibrosis in the liver, which can be irreversible in the advanced stages.

(Growing) Prevalence of NAFLD and disease burden in the US and worldwide

Worldwide prevalence of NAFLD ranges from 13.5–31.8%, with resource-poor areas having much lower rates compared to industrialised countries.[10] Across the United States, Europe and Asia, prevalence rates are similar between 23.7–31.8%.[10] The rapid rise in NAFLD cases globally parallels the rise in obesity and chronic metabolic conditions, including type 2 diabetes mellitus (T2DM), hypertension, dyslipidaemia, and polycystic ovarian syndrome, all of which represent NAFLD risk factors (see Table 9.1, page 157).[1] Other risk factors, including polymorphisms in the Patatin-like Phospholipase Domain Containing 3 (PNPLA3) and Transmembrane 6 Superfamily Member 2 (TM6SF2) genes, which are more prevalent in Hispanic populations, help explain the high rates (30.5%) of disease in South America.[1] In fact, Hispanics have the highest prevalence of NAFLD compared to Caucasians and African Americans, likely in part due to these genetic factors, which also confer risk for progressive NASH.[1]

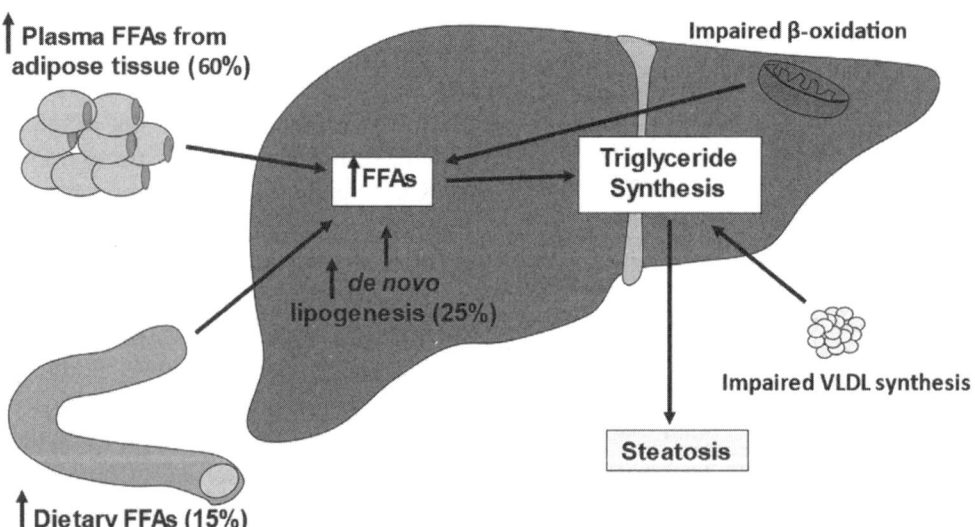

Figure 9.1 Mechanisms by which excess free fatty acids (FFAs) lead to NAFLD. The main source of FFAs come from adipose tissue (60%), following by *de novo* lipogenesis (25%) and dietary intake (15%). In the liver, FFAs are then either oxidised, exported as very low-density lipoprotein (VLDL), or stored as triglycerides in the hepatocyte. Excess FFAs also impair beta-oxidation and impair VLDL synthesis, further increasing triglyceride synthesis and steatosis in the liver.

Where are we now?

To date, there are no approved pharmacologic therapies for NASH. Current recommendations are for weight loss of 7–10% of total body weight, achieved via a daily caloric deficit of 500–1,000 kilocalories (kcal) and moderate-intensity exercise.[11] This degree of weight loss has been shown not only to lead to NASH resolution in a large proportion of patients (~45%), but may also lead to fibrosis regression.[12] While the American Association for the Study of Liver Disease (AASLD) does not offer any specific guidance regarding optimal diet for patients with NAFLD,[11] the European Association for the Study of the Liver (EASL) advises patients with NAFLD to follow a Mediterranean diet with avoidance of processed foods and added fructose.[13] Excellent control of other metabolic comorbidities is also recommended, with strong data for the use of statins in those with dyslipidemia.[11] Pioglitazone and Vitamin E can improve liver histology in patients with type 2 diabetes and biopsy-proven NASH, and can be considered in this population.[11]

The standard American diet in disease development and progression

The United States Department of Agriculture (USDA) Dietary Guidelines have consistently shown poor diet quality across Americans of all ages.[14] Based on the 'Analysis of What We Eat in America' from the *National Health and Nutrition Examination Survey*, Americans consistently exceed recommended limits on daily amounts of added sugars, saturated fat, and sodium, while consistently falling well below recommendations for fruits, vegetables, and whole grains.[14] Industrialised countries globally have adopted similar dietary habits. This eating pattern, high in processed and fast foods, and low in plant-based foods, drives the development of NAFLD in several distinct ways.

Red and processed meats

The consumption of red and processed meats contributes to the development of NAFLD by promoting insulin resistance and increasing oxidative stress in the liver. Red and processed meats are naturally high in saturated fat and cholesterol, known to worsen NAFLD, in addition to haem-iron, sodium, preservatives, and advanced glycation end products, which may also be harmful.[15] In addition, unhealthy cooking methods such as grilling or frying of these meats, produce heterocyclic amines which may promote insulin resistance, further contributing to NAFLD development.[15] Branched-chain amino acids (BCAAs), found in higher concentrations in animal proteins, lead to impaired insulin sensitivity by inducing the formation of mammalian target of rapamycin (mTOR) complex 1, formed by mTOR and insulin, leading to *de novo* lipogenesis in the liver through its activation of sterol regulatory element-binding protein-1c (SREBP-1).[16, 17] Additionally, the metabolism of phosphatidylcholine and L-carnitine, both present in high amounts in red and processed meats, to trimethylamine (TMA) by gut microbiota, can promote the development of NAFLD.[18] TMA is oxidised in the liver to trimethylamine N-oxide (TMAO), which has been hypothesised to alter bile acid synthesis and transport, leading to reversal of the direction of cholesterol transport and glucose energy and homeostasis. Indeed, circulating TMAO levels are associated with the presence and severity of NAFLD on liver biopsy.[18]

High animal protein intake is associated with NAFLD in overweight Caucasians independent of sociodemographic, lifestyle and metabolic traits.[19] In a cross-sectional study, patients with NAFLD ate 27% more animal protein compared to controls (p <0.001), with 46% of those in the highest quartile of consumption having NAFLD, compared with only 17% in the lowest quartile (p = 0.001).[20] Total and red and/or processed meat consumption has also been strongly associated (p = 0.028 and p = 0.031, respectively) with NAFLD and insulin resistance even after adjustment for body mass index (BMI), physical activity, alcohol, energy, saturated fat and cholesterol intake.[15]

Only one study has prospectively evaluated animal versus plant protein on liver fat and lipogenic indices in patients with T2DM and NAFLD.[21] In a 6-week, isocaloric, high-protein diet using either plant or animal protein (unspecified whether red, processed or lean) the high animal protein diet led to large postprandial increases in BCAA and methionine compared to the plant protein group, however both groups experienced significant reductions in liver fat and down-regulation of lipolysis.[21] The study was limited due to small sample size and significant weight loss in both groups. Larger, prospective studies which clearly define the source of animal protein and have histologic endpoints are needed.

Saturated fats

Saturated fatty acids (SFA) are mainly found in fatty animal products such as fatty meats, eggs, dairy, butter and cheese. Similar to red and processed meats, saturated fats also exert their effects on the liver through the promotion of insulin resistance and oxidative stress. They induce hepatic steatosis by increasing lipolysis as well as *de novo* lipogenesis, which occurs through the promotion of the transcription of peroxisome proliferator-activated receptor (PPAR) γ coactivator-1β and SREBP-1c (Figure 9.2).[22] In addition, they promote lipotoxicity through activating the formation of ceramides and diacylglycerols, which leads to hepatocyte apoptosis and increased oxidative stress, which may promote the development of NASH.[23]

Overfeeding studies highlight the impact of SFA in the diet. In a study comparing 38 subjects eating 1,000 extra kcal daily of saturated fat, unsaturated fat, or simple sugars for three weeks, those in the saturated fat group had significantly greater increases in intrahepatic triglyceride content (+55%) compared to those in the unsaturated fat group (+15%) and simple sugar group (+33%) (p <0.05) despite similar weight gain across all groups.[24] Similarly, when comparing 39 healthy subjects randomised to eat 750 extra kcal daily of muffins either high in SFA (palm oil) or polyunsaturated fatty acids (PUFA) (sunflower oil) for seven weeks, the saturated fat group had significant increases in liver fat (p = 0.033) and visceral adipose tissue (p = 0.035) compared to the PUFA group, while the PUFA group had significant increases in lean tissue (p = 0.015) compared to the saturated fat group.[25] Prospective studies evaluating isolated reduction in SFA content in the diet aside from more comprehensive dietary interventions are not available.

Added sugars

Added sugars make up a significant proportion of the standard adult diet, and comprise sweetened beverages, refined carbohydrates, sweet bakery products, candy and other desserts. These sugars, mainly encompassing glucose and fructose, induce *de novo* lipogenesis through activation of the carbohydrate responsive transcription factor, carbohydrate response element binding protein (ChREBP) (see Figure 9.2).[26] Fructose is metabolised predominantly in the liver where it is converted into glyceraldehyde-3-phosphate, which can be used for gluconeogenesis or acetyl-CoA production. Breakdown of glucose can additionally be used for acetyl-CoA production or glycogen synthesis. In times of calorie abundance, excess acetyl-CoA is shunted toward *de novo* lipogenesis, simultaneously reducing fatty acid oxidation and promoting triglyceride synthesis (see Figure 9.3).[27] Fructose can also activate fatty acid synthase and stearoyl-CoA-desaturase-1, which promotes inflammation and may lead to the development of NASH.[28]

Epidemiologic studies evaluating the association between carbohydrates and NAFLD have had heterogenous results, likely as a result of generalising all carbohydrates rather than separating simple and complex carbohydrates, therefore overfeeding studies may highlight the impact better. After overfeeding 16 overweight adults with 1,000 kcal/day of candy or sugar sweetened beverages for three weeks, liver fat increased by 27% (p = 0.005) despite body weight only increasing by 2% (p < 0.0001) when compared to baseline.[29] The increase in liver fat was proportional to increase in *de novo* lipogenesis, measured using the ratio of palmitate to linoleate in serum and VLDL triglycerides. In a separate study, 47 overweight adults were randomised to one litre daily of sugar sweetened soda, skim milk, diet soda, or water for six months.[30] There were no significant weight changes across any of the cohorts during the intervention. Compared to the milk, diet cola, and water group, accumulation of liver fat was significantly greater in the regular cola group (143% [95% CI: 50, 236] p <0.05, 139% [95% CI: 50, 227] p <0.05, and 132% [95% CI: 43, 222] p <0.025, respectively). Those consuming the regular cola also had significant increases in visceral fat (p <0.05), and skeletal muscle fat (p <0.05), compared to no changes in the other groups.[30]

Prospective data is limited to one 8-week

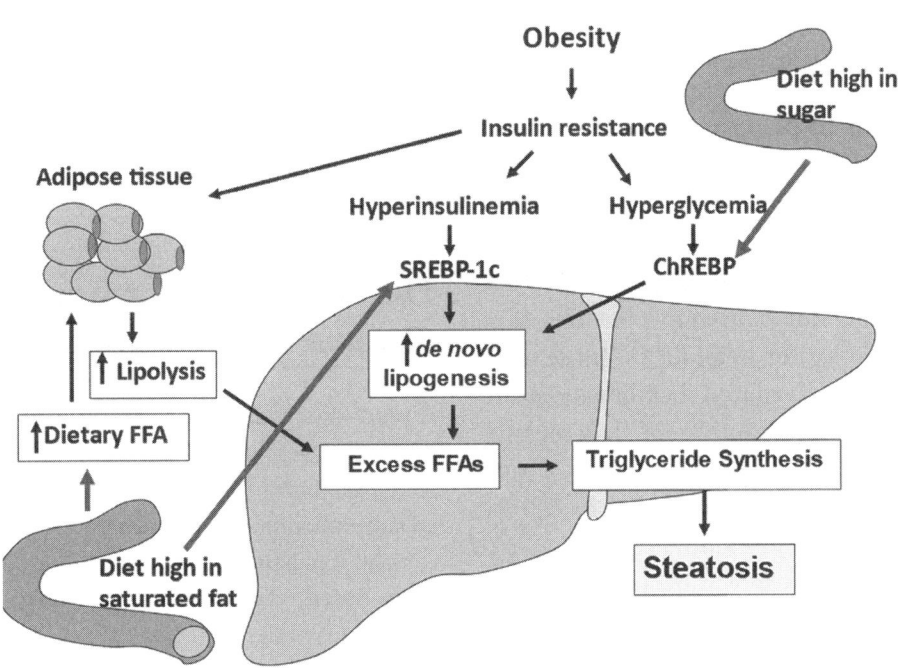

Figure 9.2 Diets high in saturated fat increases triglyceride accumulation and steatosis in the liver through two main mechanisms: (1) Increased lipolysis of adipose tissue, (2) Activation of sterol regulatory element binding protein-1c (SREBP-1c), which promotes *de novo* lipogenesis. Diets high in sugar (fructose and glucose) activate the carbohydrate response element binding protein (ChREBP), which further increase *de novo* lipogenesis.

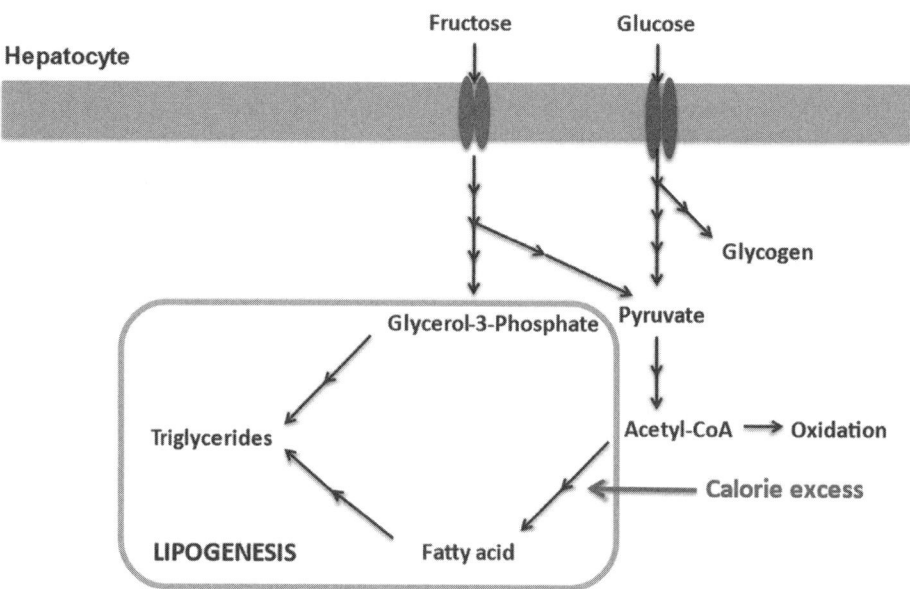

Figure 9.3 Metabolism of fructose leads to *de novo* lipogenesis and triglyceride synthesis either through the glycerol-3-phosphate pathway or the acetyl-CoA pathway. Additionally, glucose leads to *de novo* lipogenesis through pyruvate and acetyl-CoA synthesis. In times of calorie abundance, acetyl-CoA is shunted towards triglyceride synthesis instead of oxidation, increasing fatty acid synthesis and causing or worsening NAFLD.

clinical trial of adolescent boys aged 11 to 16 years old with NAFLD randomised to a low free-sugar (<3% daily calories) or usual diet.[31] Those in the sugar restricted arm reduced their hepatic steatosis (25% to 17%) significantly more than the usual diet (21% to 20%) group, with an adjusted mean difference of -6.23% [95% CI -9.45% to -3.02%], p <0.001). Serum alanine aminotransferase levels also decreased significantly more in the intervention group (103 U/L to 61 U/L) vs the usual diet group (82 U/L to 75 U/L) with an adjusted ratio of the geometric means of 0.65 U/L [95% CI: 0.53, 0.81 U/L], p <0.001. Larger, prospective studies are still needed in both adult and pediatric populations in order to be able to generalise results.

The role of a plant-based diet in disease reversal and prevention

A plant-based diet is one based heavily on fruits, vegetables, legumes, nuts, and whole grains with minimal, if any, red and processed meats, saturated fat, and refined carbohydrates. Multiple diets can be considered plant-based: a whole-food, plant-based, vegan diet, the Dietary Approaches to Stop Hypertension (DASH) diet, and a Mediterranean diet, in addition to others. The inherent reduction in disease promoting foods in all of these diets makes them ideal for patients with NAFLD, in addition to weight loss and increase in disease-fighting foods.

Weight loss

Improvement in hepatic steatosis on histologic evaluation has been shown with weight loss of at least 5%, with resolution of NASH and improvement in fibrosis seen with weight loss of 7% and 10%, respectively.[12] Many diets, including a plant-based diet, can be an effective means to achieve weight loss. Indeed, when compared to an *ad libitum* omnivore, semi-vegetarian, or pesco-vegetarian diet, those randomised to a vegan diet lost significantly more weight at six months (p = 0.03) and had significantly lower saturated fat intake (p <0.05).[32] More important than weight loss alone, however, for disease reversal and prevention, is the sustainability of the weight reduction. Weight loss experienced on a plant-based diet has been demonstrated to be sustainable at one- and two-year intervals after initial intervention.[33] Other dietary weight loss strategies, likely due to their inherently restrictive nature, tend to be challenging to maintain for prolonged periods of time and often lead to weight regain.

Reduction in disease promoting foods

Plant-based diets are inherently low in red and processed meats, saturated fats, and added sugars. By reducing or eliminating these foods in the diet, many of the mechanisms for steatosis accumulation are eliminated. In addition, plant-based diets tend to be lower in certain essential amino acids, specifically methionine and lysine. It is postulated that a methionine-restricted diet may up-regulate fibroblast growth factor 21 (FGF21), which can inhibit SREBP-1 and *de novo* lipogenesis while promoting hepatic free fatty acid oxidation.[34]

Increase in disease fighting foods

Plant-based diets are naturally high in monounsaturated fats (MUFAs) and PUFAs which can be found in foods such as nuts, seeds, avocados, and plant-based oils such as olive, soybean, and sunflower oil. These fats activate peroxisome proliferator-activated receptor α (PPARα), which promotes fatty acid oxidisation and downregulation of *de novo* lipogenesis through suppression of SREBP-1 (see Figure 9.4).[35] In addition, MUFAs activate transcription factor PPARγ, which promotes safe fatty acid storage in adipose tissue. In a cross-sectional analysis of 1,624 patients who were classified as either meat-eaters, fish-eaters, vegetarians, or vegans, those in the vegan groups showed the highest intake of PUFAs and lowest intake of SFAs with similar intake of MUFAs across all groups.[36] The positive impact of unsaturated fats on hepatic steatosis have been evaluated in several small prospective randomised trials, which have been summarised previously.[37] The results consistently show a reduction in liver fat in subjects fed isocaloric diets high in MUFA or PUFAs, in addition to improvements in total and LDL cholesterol, serum triglycerides, and insulin resistance. In addition, during calorie excess, PUFAs may promote lean tissue formation instead of liver and visceral fat promoted by SFAs.[25]

Plant-based diets are also very high in fibre. Not surprisingly, vegans and vegetarians have been shown to have higher levels of fibre consumption when compared to meat- and fish-eaters.[36] Higher soluble fibre intake may play a protective role against NAFLD through its effect on reduction of serum low-density lipoprotein (LDL) levels, possibly by binding to bile acids or cholesterol during the formation of micelles, lowering the cholesterol concentration in hepatocytes, leading to up-regulation of LDL receptors and clearance of LDL-cholesterol.[38] Soluble fibre can also slow the rate at which carbohydrates are absorbed into the circulation reducing

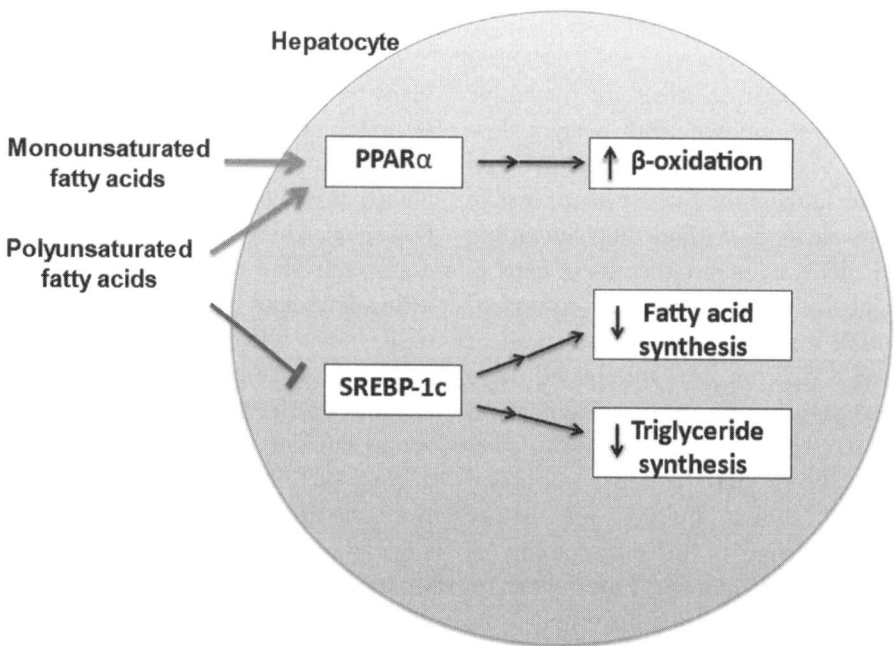

Figure 9.4 Mono- and polyunsaturated fatty acids increase fatty acid oxidation through activation of PPARα, which upregulates transcription of fatty acid oxidation genes, thereby increasing both peroxisome and mitochondrial β-oxidation. In addition, polyunsaturated fatty acids suppress sterol regulatory element binding protein-1c (SREBP-1c), which suppresses transcription of lipogenic genes and leads to downregulation of fatty acid and triglyceride synthesis within the hepatocyte.

post-prandial hyperglycaemia and improving glucose tolerance.[39] When 70 obese individuals with features of the metabolic syndrome were randomised to two energy-restricted diets for six months, participants who consumed higher levels of fibre from fruit experienced improvements in their non-invasive liver fat scores (Fatty Liver Index, Hepatic Steatosis Index, and NAFLD Liver Fat Score) and liver enzymes compared to those with lower fibre intake.[40] Additionally, in a small, randomised double-blind crossover trial of patients with NASH, 16 g/day of oligofructose (a prebiotic fibre) for eight weeks led to a significant reduction in insulin levels and liver enzymes compared to control, independent of a significant effect on plasma lipids.[41] Larger studies are needed in patients with NASH and fibrosis to determine effect.

Plant-based diets also offer beneficial effects due to their phytochemicals and subset, polyphenols. These are secondary metabolites of plants found in high amounts in fruits and vegetables, and have been studied for their potent anti-inflammatory effects, which may mitigate the oxidative stress generated during the pathologic pathways activated in NAFLD.[42] Polyphenols have been implicated in preventing hepatocellular damage through reduction of *de novo* lipogenesis and increased fatty acid oxidation.

What does the data show?

Studying dietary determinants of disease is notoriously challenging due the confounding effects of other dietary components and lifestyle factors in addition to the short-term nature of such interventions. The American Association for the Study of Liver Disease (AASLD) specifically cites the lack of longer-term, prospective trials as their reason to not make specific dietary recommendations.[11] More recently, however, a few high-quality large, randomised controlled trials evaluating various plant-based dietary interventions over 18–24 months have been published. The results repeatedly show an advantage in participants following plant-based styles of eating, which are high in fruits and vegetables, whole grains, unsaturated fats, and may incorporate limited lean meats and low-fat dairy products. Besides the Mediterranean diet, other diets evaluated include the Dietary Approach to Stop Hypertension (DASH) diet,[43] Fatty Liver in Obesity (FLiO) diet,[44] and the green-Mediterranean (green-MED) diet.[45] The DASH diet is a vegetable- and fruit-rich diet that allows fish and poultry while limiting sodium, total fat, saturated fat, and added sugars.[43] The FLiO diet focuses on plant-based sources of protein, low glycaemic index carbohydrates, and increased PUFA consumption while the green-MED diet adds polyphenols (via green tea and Mankai green shake) to a traditional Mediterranean diet. Limitations to these studies include the lack of histologic data, and therefore inability to comment on the resolution of NASH or fibrosis with dietary intervention.

Table 9.1 Risk factors for non-alcoholic fatty liver disease

Obesity
Type 2 diabetes mellitus
Hypertension
Dyslipidaemia
Polycystic ovarian syndrome
Smoking
Ethnicity
Older age
Male gender
PNPLA3 gene polymorphism
TM6SF2 genetic polymorphism

Conclusion

Overall, there is evidence that a plant-based diet results not only in improvement of the biochemical features of NAFLD but also improves the underlying aberrant state of insulin resistance. Furthermore, the benefit of these diets has been demonstrated even in the absence of weight loss, indicating that the composition of plant-based diets have their own role in improving the pathologic features of NAFLD. The specific mechanism for benefits of a plant-based diet in the management of NAFLD has not yet been fully elucidated, however several ideas regarding their effectiveness in the management of NAFLD have been stated. The inherent energy deficits due to higher intake of vegetables and fruits, which can provide satiety with lower energy dense foods, results in effective long-term weight management. In addition, the natural reduction in disease promoting foods such as saturated fat, simple sugars, and red and processed meats, and increase in disease fighting foods such as unsaturated fat, fibre and polyphenols leads to a reduction in fatty acid and triglyceride synthesis while stimulating fatty acid oxidation. The Mediterranean, DASH, FLiO, green-MED and whole-food, plant-based diets all represent healthy dietary patterns to improve steatosis in patients with NAFLD. We await further studies with histologic endpoints to further define the benefits of these diets on NASH resolution and fibrosis regression.

References

1. Younossi Z, Anstee QM, Marietti M, Hardy T, Henry L, Eslam M, et al. Global burden of NAFLD and NASH: trends, predictions, risk factors and prevention. *Nature Reviews Gastroenterology & Hepatology* 2018; 15(1): 11-20.
2. Chalasani N, Younossi Z, Lavine JE, Diehl AM, Brunt EM, Cusi K, et al. The diagnosis and management of non-alcoholic fatty liver disease: practice guideline by the American Gastroenterological Association, American Association for the Study of Liver Diseases, and American College of Gastroenterology. *Gastroenterology* 2012; 142(7): 1592-1609. doi: 10.1053/j.gastro.2012.04.001
3. Singh S, Allen AM, Wang Z, Prokop LJ, Murad MH, Loomba R. Fibrosis progression in nonalcoholic fatty liver vs nonalcoholic steatohepatitis: a systematic review and meta-analysis of paired-biopsy studies. Clinical gastroenterology and hepatology : the official clinical practice journal of the American Gastroenterological Association. *Clin Gastroenterol Hepatol* 2015; 13(4): 643-654.e1-9. doi: 10.1016/j.cgh.2014.04.014
4. Adams LA, Lymp JF, St. Sauver J, Sanderson SO, Lindor KD, Feldstein A, et al. The Natural History of Nonalcoholic Fatty Liver Disease: A Population-Based Cohort Study. *Gastroenterology* 2005; 129(1): 113-121. doi: 10.1053/j.gastro.2005.04.014
5. Dulai PS, Singh S, Patel J, Soni M, Prokop LJ, Younossi Z, et al. Increased risk of mortality by fibrosis stage in nonalcoholic fatty liver disease: Systematic review and meta-analysis. *Hepatology* 2017; 65(5): 1557-1565. doi: 10.1002/hep.29085
6. Donnelly KL, Smith CI, Schwarzenberg SJ, Jessurun J, Boldt MD, Parks EJ. Sources of fatty acids stored in liver and secreted via lipoproteins in patients with nonalcoholic fatty liver disease. *Journal of Clinical Investigation* 2005; 115(5): 1343-1351. doi: 10.1172/JCI23621
7. Sanyal AJ, Campbell–Sargent C, Mirshahi F, Rizzo WB, Contos MJ, Sterling RK, et al. Nonalcoholic steatohepatitis: Association of insulin resistance and mitochondrial abnormalities. *Gastroenterology* 2001; 120(5): 1183-1192. doi: 10.1053/gast.2001.23256
8. Huang MA, Greenson JK, Chao C, Anderson L, Peterman D, Jacobson J, et al. One-year intense nutritional counseling results in histological improvement in patients with non-alcoholic steatohepatitis: a pilot study. *The American Journal of Gastroenterology* 2005; 100(5): 1072-1081. doi: 10.1111/j.1572-0241.2005.41334.x
9. Abenavoli L, Peta V. Role of adipokines and cytokines in non-alcoholic fatty liver disease. *Reviews on recent clinical trials* 2014; 9(3): 134-140. doi: 10.2174/1574887109666141216102458
10. Rinella M, Charlton M. The globalization of nonalcoholic fatty liver disease: Prevalence and impact on world health. *Hepatology* 2016; 64(1): 19-22. doi: 10.1002/hep.28524
11. Chalasani N, Younossi Z, Lavine JE, Charlton M, Cusi K, Rinella M, et al. The diagnosis and management of nonalcoholic fatty liver disease: Practice guidance from the American Association for the Study of Liver Diseases. *Hepatology* 2018; 67(1): 328-357. doi: 10.1002/hep.29367
12. Vilar-Gomez E, Martinez-Perez Y, Calzadilla-Bertot L, Torres-Gonzalez A, Gra-Oramas B, Gonzalez-Fabian L, et al. Weight Loss Through Lifestyle Modification Significantly Reduces Features of Nonalcoholic Steatohepatitis. *Gastroenterology* 2015; 149(2): 367-378.e5. doi: 10.1053/j.gastro.2015.04.005
13. Ando Y, Jou JH. Nonalcoholic Fatty Liver Disease and Recent Guideline Updates. *Clinical Liver Disease* 2021; 17(1): 23-28. doi: 10.1002/cld.1045
14. Dietary Guidelines for Americans, 2020-2025, 9th Edition [press release]. December, 2020.
15. Zelber-Sagi S, Ivancovsky-Wajcman D, Fliss Isakov N, Webb M, Orenstein D, Shibolet O, et

al. High red and processed meat consumption is associated with non-alcoholic fatty liver disease and insulin resistance. *Journal of Hepatology* 2018; 68(6): 1239-1246. doi: 10.1016/j.jhep.2018.01.015

16. Menon S, Dibble CC, Talbott G, Hoxhaj G, Valvezan AJ, Takahashi H, et al. Spatial control of the TSC complex integrates insulin and nutrient regulation of mTORC1 at the lysosome. *Cell* 2014; 156(4): 771-785. doi: 10.1016/j.cell.2013.11.049

17. Kim JB, Sarraf P, Wright M, Yao KM, Mueller E, Solanes G, et al. Nutritional and insulin regulation of fatty acid synthetase and leptin gene expression through ADD1/SREBP1. *The Journal of Clinical Investigation* 1998; 101(1): 1-9. doi: 10.1172/JCI1411

18. Chen YM, Liu Y, Zhou RF, Chen XL, Wang C, Tan XY, et al. Associations of gut-flora-dependent metabolite trimethylamine-N-oxide, betaine and choline with non-alcoholic fatty liver disease in adults. *Sci Rep* 2016; 6: 19076. doi: 10.1038/srep19076

19. Alferink LJ, Kiefte-de Jong JC, Erler NS, Veldt BJ, Schoufour JD, de Knegt RJ, et al. Association of dietary macronutrient composition and non-alcoholic fatty liver disease in an ageing population: the Rotterdam Study. *Gut* 2019; 68(6): 1088-1098. doi: 10.1136/gutjnl-2017-315940

20. Zelber-Sagi S, Nitzan-Kaluski D, Goldsmith R, Webb M, Blendis L, Halpern Z, et al. Long term nutritional intake and the risk for non-alcoholic fatty liver disease (NAFLD): a population based study. *Journal of hepatology* 2007; 47(5): 711-717. doi: 10.1016/j.jhep.2007.06.020

21. Markova M, Pivovarova O, Hornemann S, Sucher S, Frahnow T, Wegner K, et al. Isocaloric Diets High in Animal or Plant Protein Reduce Liver Fat and Inflammation in Individuals With Type 2 Diabetes. *Gastroenterology* 2017; 152(3): 571-585. e8. doi: 10.1053/j.gastro.2016.10.007

22. Lin J, Yang R, Tarr PT, Wu PH, Handschin C, Li S, et al. Hyperlipidemic effects of dietary saturated fats mediated through PGC-1beta coactivation of SREBP. *Cell* 2005; 120(2): 261-273. doi: 10.1016/j.cell.2004.11.043

23. Leamy AK, Egnatchik RA, Young JD. Molecular mechanisms and the role of saturated fatty acids in the progression of non-alcoholic fatty liver disease. *Prog Lipid Res* 2013; 52(1): 165-174.

doi: 10.1016/j.plipres.2012.10.004

24. Luukkonen PK, Sadevirta S, Zhou Y, Kayser B, Ali A, Ahonen L, et al. Saturated Fat Is More Metabolically Harmful for the Human Liver Than Unsaturated Fat or Simple Sugars. *Diabetes Care* 2018; 41(8): 1732-1739. doi: 10.2337/dc18-0071

25. Rosqvist F, Iggman D, Kullberg J, Cedernaes J, Johansson HE, Larsson A, et al. Overfeeding polyunsaturated and saturated fat causes distinct effects on liver and visceral fat accumulation in humans. *Diabetes* 2014; 63(7): 2356-2368. doi: 10.2337/db13-1622

26. Ma L, Tsatsos NG, Towle HC. Direct role of ChREBP.Mlx in regulating hepatic glucose-responsive genes. *The Journal of Biological Chemistry* 2005; 280(12): 12019-12027. doi: 10.1074/jbc.M413063200

27. Dirlewanger M, Schneiter P, Jequier E, Tappy L. Effects of fructose on hepatic glucose metabolism in humans. *American Journal of Physiology Endocrinology and Metabolism* 2000; 279(4): E907-911. doi: 10.1152/ajpendo.2000.279.4.E907

28. Renaud HJ, Cui JY, Lu H, Klaassen CD. Effect of diet on expression of genes involved in lipid metabolism, oxidative stress, and inflammation in mouse liver-insights into mechanisms of hepatic steatosis. *PloS One* 2014; 9(2): e88584. doi: 10.1371/journal.pone.0088584

29. Sevastianova K, Santos A, Kotronen A, Hakkarainen A, Makkonen J, Silander K, et al. Effect of short-term carbohydrate overfeeding and long-term weight loss on liver fat in overweight humans. *The American Journal of Clinical Nutrition* 2012; 96(4): 727-734. doi: 10.3945/ajcn.112.038695

30. Maersk M, Belza A, Stodkilde-Jorgensen H, Ringgaard S, Chabanova E, Thomsen H, et al. Sucrose-sweetened beverages increase fat storage in the liver, muscle, and visceral fat depot: a 6-mo randomized intervention study. *The American Journal of Clinical Nutrition* 2012; 95(2): 283-289. doi: 10.3945/ajcn.111.022533

31. Schwimmer JB, Ugalde-Nicalo P, Welsh JA, Angeles JE, Cordero M, Harlow KE, et al. Effect of a Low Free Sugar Diet vs Usual Diet on Nonalcoholic Fatty Liver Disease in Adolescent Boys. *JAMA* 2019; 321(3): 256-265. doi: 10.1001/jama.2018.20579

32. Moore WJ, McGrievy ME, Turner-McGrievy GM. Dietary adherence and acceptability of five different diets, including vegan and vegetarian diets, for weight loss: The New DIETs study. *Eat Behav* 2015; 19: 33-38. doi: 10.1016/j.eatbeh.2015.06.011
33. Turner-Mcgrievy GM, Barnard ND, Scialli AR. A Two-Year Randomized Weight Loss Trial Comparing a Vegan Diet to a More Moderate Low-Fat Diet. *Obesity* 2007; 15(9): 2276-2281. doi: 10.1038/oby.2007.270
34. McCarty MF. The moderate essential amino acid restriction entailed by low-protein vegan diets may promote vascular health by stimulating FGF21 secretion. *Horm Mol Biol Clin Investig* 2016; 30(1). doi: 10.1515/hmbci-2015-0056
35. Yokoi H, Mizukami H, Nagatsu A, Tanabe H, Inoue M. Hydroxy monounsaturated fatty acids as agonists for peroxisome proliferator-activated receptors. *Biol Pharm Bull* 2010; 33(5): 854-861. doi: 10.1248/bpb.33.854
36. Bradbury KE, Crowe FL, Appleby PN, Schmidt JA, Travis RC, Key TJ. Serum concentrations of cholesterol, apolipoprotein A-I and apolipoprotein B in a total of 1694 meat-eaters, fish-eaters, vegetarians and vegans. *European Journal of Clinical Nutrition* 2014; 68(2): 178-183. doi: 10.1038/ejcn.2013.248
37. Hydes TJ, Ravi S, Loomba R, M EG. Evidence-based clinical advice for nutrition and dietary weight loss strategies for the management of NAFLD and NASH. *Clin Mol Hepatol* 2020; 26(4): 383-400. doi: 10.3350/cmh.2020.0067
38. Anderson JW, Tietyen-Clark J. Dietary fiber: hyperlipidemia, hypertension, and coronary heart disease. *Am J Gastroenterol* 1986; 81(10): 907-919.
39. Bjorck I, Elmstahl HL. The glycaemic index: importance of dietary fibre and other food properties. *The Proceedings of the Nutrition Society* 2003; 62(1): 201-206. doi: 10.1079/pns2002239
40. Cantero I, Abete I, Monreal JI, Martinez JA, Zulet MA. Fruit Fiber Consumption Specifically Improves Liver Health Status in Obese Subjects under Energy Restriction. *Nutrients* 2017; 9(7): 667. doi: 10.3390/nu9070667
41. Daubioul CA, Horsmans Y, Lambert P, Danse E, Delzenne NM. Effects of oligofructose on glucose and lipid metabolism in patients with nonalcoholic steatohepatitis: results of a pilot study. *Eur J Clin Nutr* 2005; 59(5): 723-726. doi: 10.1038/sj.ejcn.1602127
42. Rodriguez-Ramiro I, Vauzour D, Minihane AM. Polyphenols and non-alcoholic fatty liver disease: impact and mechanisms. *Proceedings of the Nutrition Society* 2016; 75(1): 47-60. doi: 10.1017/S0029665115004218
43. Razavi Zade M, Telkabadi MH, Bahmani F, Salehi B, Farshbaf S, Asemi Z. The effects of DASH diet on weight loss and metabolic status in adults with non-alcoholic fatty liver disease: a randomized clinical trial. *Liver International* 2016; 36(4): 563-71. doi: 10.1111/liv.12990
44. Marin-Alejandre BA, Cantero I, Perez-Diaz-Del-Campo N, Monreal JI, Elorz M, Herrero JI, Cantero I, Perez-Diaz-Del-Campo N, Monreal JI, Elorz M, Herrero JI, Benito-Boillos A, et al. Effects of two personalized dietary strategies during a 2-year intervention in subjects with nonalcoholic fatty liver disease: A randomized trial. *Liver Int* 2021; 41(7): 1532-1544. doi: 10.1111/liv.14818
45. Yaskolka Meir A, Rinott E, Tsaban G, Zelicha H, Kaplan A, Rosen P, et al. Effect of green-Mediterranean diet on intrahepatic fat: the DIRECT PLUS randomised controlled trial. *Gut* 2021; 70(11): 2085-2095. doi: 10.1136/gutjnl-2020-323106
46. Ryan MC, Itsiopoulos C, Thodis T, Ward G, Trost N, Hofferberth S, et al. The Mediterranean diet improves hepatic steatosis and insulin sensitivity in individuals with non-alcoholic fatty liver disease. *Journal of Hepatology* 2013; 59(1): 138-143. doi: 10.1016/j.jhep.2013.02.012
47. Kani AH, Alavian SM, Esmaillzadeh A, Adibi P, Azadbakht L. Effects of a novel therapeutic diet on liver enzymes and coagulating factors in patients with non-alcoholic fatty liver disease: A parallel randomized trial. *Nutrition* 2014; 30(7-8): 814-821. doi: 10.1016/j.nut.2013.11.008
48. Properzi C, O'Sullivan TA, Sherriff JL, Ching HL, Jeffrey GP, Buckley RF, et al. Ad Libitum Mediterranean and Low-Fat Diets Both Significantly Reduce Hepatic Steatosis: A Randomized Controlled Trial. *Hepatology* 2018; 68(5): 1741-1754. doi: 10.1002/hep.30076

49. Garousi N, Tamizifar B, Pourmasoumi M, Feizi A, Askari G, Clark CCT, et al. Effects of lacto-ovo-vegetarian diet vs. standard-weight-loss diet on obese and overweight adults with non-alcoholic fatty liver disease: a randomised clinical trial. Archives of Physiology and Biochemistry 2021; 1-9. doi: 10.1080/13813455.2021.1890128

50. Gepner Y, Shelef I, Komy O, Cohen N, Schwarzfuchs D, Bril N, et al. The beneficial effects of Mediterranean diet over low-fat diet may be mediated by decreasing hepatic fat content. *Journal of Hepatology* 2019; 71(2): 379-388. doi: 10.1016/j.jhep.2019.04.013

Chapter 10
Plant-based nutrition and gastrointestinal disorders

Alan Desmond and Rosie Martin

Introduction

A large number of people globally suffer with one or more gastrointestinal (GI) conditions and the impact on both patients and health care systems is significant. In addition to high mortality rates and disease burden, there are also major economic effects on health care systems and it is therefore imperative that solutions are found to reduce these impacts.

This chapter will discuss the role of the microbiome in maintaining gut health and will focus on the following: gastro-oesophageal reflux disease (GORD), diverticular disease, colorectal cancer, coeliac disease, irritable bowel syndrome (IBS), food intolerances, and inflammatory bowel disease (IBD). The majority of these GI diseases/conditions are associated with poor diet and lifestyle choices, specifically diets low in plant foods and therefore fibre, and high in animal foods and associated saturated fat, cholesterol and other health-harming components.

The gut microbiome and digestive health

The term 'gut microbiome' was first coined in 2001 to describe the approximately 100 trillion microbial cells which exist within each human being, residing largely within the large intestine.[1] New genetic sequencing and bioinformatic technologies have allowed a rapid expansion in our knowledge of the structure and function of the gut microbiome in last two decades.[2] The gut microbiome plays a crucial role in the development of the rapidly developing digestive tract and is established in its mature form by the age of three years.[3] Throughout the hosts' lifetime, the micro-organisms which inhabit the human digestive tract play a crucial role in maintaining our gut health and overall health and have been described as a 'control centre for human biology'. Whether our gut microbiome helps us maintain a healthy digestive system, or contributes to increased risk of chronic disease states, is very much dependant on the environmental factors we are exposed to each day. The most important of these factors may well be the food we eat.[4]

Among the key benefits of a healthy gut

microbiome is the efficient production of the short-chain fatty acids (SCFAs) by the bacteria that thrive in a high fibre environment. The main SCFAs are acetate, butyrate and propionate.[4]

The efficient production of SCFAs has numerous gut-health benefits:
- Butyrate is the primary energy source for human colonocytes.[5]
- Intestinal homeostasis and the integrity of the gut barrier depend on a steady supply of SCFAs.[5]
- SCFAs stimulate the production of colonic mucin, an important defence against pathogenic bacteria.[6]
- SCFAs are important regulators of intestinal inflammation and combat mechanisms implicated in the development of Crohn's disease and ulcerative colitis.[6,7]
- Butyrate remarkably inhibits the glucose metabolism and DNA synthesis of colorectal cancer cells, leading to cell apoptosis and prevention of colorectal cancer.[6]

Overall, it almost appears that our gut microbes produce SCFAs to help ensure that their human digestive system home remains as healthy as possible, for as long as possible. Making the transition to a high-fibre, plant-based diet can favourably influence the production of these incredibly beneficial SCFAs within days, increasing production by 250% within two weeks.[8,9] Given the importance of a fibre-rich diet in promoting gut microbial health, it is not surprising that the gut microbiomes of long-term vegans and vegetarians produce substantially more SCFAs than omnivores.[10]

Fibre-deficiency is just one of the mechanisms whereby a standard Western diet adversely effects our gut microbial health. A diet that depends on saturated fats, refined sugars, animal products, and ultra-processed foods, promotes a state of gut microbiome dysfunction or 'dysbiosis', which contributes to both poor digestive health and to numerous disease states beyond the gut.[4, 11, 12]

Gastro-oesophageal reflux disease (GORD)

Most people experience episodic and physiological reflux of gastric contents into their oesophagus. GORD develops when this reflux causes troublesome symptoms and/or complications.[13] Manifestations may be oesophageal (such as heartburn, oesophagitis and structuring etc), or extra-oesophageal (wheeze, laryngitis, chronic cough, dental erosions, and laryngo-pharyngeal reflux). The prevalence in adults ranges from 30% in some Western populations to below 10% in East Asian populations, but GORD is prevalent worldwide, and the disease burden is increasing.[14]

The treatment of GORD is primarily by medication with antacids, H2-receptor antagonists and proton pump inhibitors, while surgery (typically with fundoplication) is used in selected patients. While proton pump inhibitors remain one of the world's most prescribed medications,[15] effective diet and lifestyle advice should always be discussed.[16]

Avoidance of trigger foods

Patients often identify common trigger foods which can be avoided. Coffee, alcohol, chocolate, peppermint, citrus, carbonated drinks and spicy foods are common culprits.

Meal size and timing

Patients with GORD should aim for smaller meals taken more frequently and avoiding eating within two hours of bedtime.

Smoking cessation

Tobacco use aggravates GORD symptoms and increases the risk of associated malignancies. Patients should be encouraged to stop smoking and signposted to available smoking cessation services where they can be given ongoing support.

Elevating the head of the bed

The use of 'bed blocks' or 'mattress wedges' to elevate the head whilst sleeping can be effective for nocturnal reflux. The ideal height of bed head elevation is at least 6–8 inches (15–20 cm).[17]

Weight loss

In overweight individuals, a four-point reduction in BMI over six months may lead to resolution of GORD symptoms in up to 60% of cases.[18] Even patients who are at the upper limit of a healthy BMI can achieve a reduction in GORD symptoms with healthy weight loss.[19] The Nurses' Health Study, an observational cohort study of 10,545 women, showed a dose-dependently reduced risk of reflux symptoms among women who had decrease in BMI compared to women with no BMI change.[20]

Increased dietary fibre

Low fibre intake is associated with decreased stomach and gut motility, delayed gastric emptying, and increased risk of symptomatic GORD.[21, 22] A fibre-enriched diet (baseline fibre <20 g/day increased by 15 g/day) has been shown to resolve GORD symptoms in 57% of cases.[22]

Reduced dietary fat

High fat meals are known to provoke the production of potentially irritant bile salts and to activate neurohormonal mediators that reduce lower oesophageal tone (e.g., cholecystokinin).[23] Daily intakes of total fat, saturated fat, cholesterol, percentage of energy from dietary fat, and average fat servings are significantly higher in individuals with GORD symptoms.[18] Although more studies examining dietary fat reduction as a treatment for GORD are needed, a whole-food, plant-focused, Mediterranean diet has been reported to be as effective as proton pump inhibitor therapy in one case series of 85 patients with laryngo-pharyngeal reflux.[23]

Diverticular disease

Diverticula of the large bowel are outpouchings of the mucosa and submucosal layers of the mucosa which protrude via deficits in the muscularis layers. The accumulation of multiple diverticula gives rise to diverticular disease, or 'diverticulosis'. When these pouches become inflamed or infected, it gives rise to 'diverticulitis'.[24] Diverticular disease is commonly found in high-income countries, including the USA and Europe, but is a rare condition in rural Africa.[25] In European countries, diverticular disease is present in 40% of adults aged 70–79, and almost 60% of adults aged above 80.[26]

While many patients may be asymptomatic or encounter occasional mild abdominal pain, potentially life-threatening complicated disease such as abscess, perforation or haemorrhage do occur.[27] Diverticular disease has been traditionally viewed as a disease affecting elderly patients, but acute admissions of middle-aged and younger patients have become more common.[28]

The role of dietary fibre in the prevention of diverticular disease and diverticulitis was proposed by Dr Denis Burkitt half a century ago. During his time as a surgeon in rural Uganda he documented the associations between high fibre consumption (50–120 g/day) and a relative absence of colonic diseases common in high income countries, including diverticular disease, diverticulitis, and colon cancer. He also observed that this high-fibre diet was low in red meat and animal fat but high in starch and fibre-rich foods, such as colourful fruits and vegetables, leafy greens, tubers, potatoes, beans, nuts, and whole grains. Dr Burkitt reported daily fibre intake for adults in rural Uganda averaged 100 g, compared with just 15 g in the UK, and recommended that residents of high-income countries should strive to achieve a daily intake of at least 50 g.[29] The 'fibre hypothesis' – that a fibre-deficient diet contributes to unfavourable changes in stool bulk and content, bacterial flora, total transit time, and intraluminal pressures, leading to diverticulosis and other disease has subsequently been validated by dozens of groups and remains incredibly relevant in the 21st century.[30] Consumption of insoluble fibre (legumes, fruit skins, whole wheat etc) may be particularly protective, reducing the risk of symptomatic diverticular disease by 40%.[31]

These findings are consistent with the Health Professional Follow-up Study, which showed that as little as one serving of meat per week is associated with increased risk.[32] In that study, men in the highest quintile for meat consumption were 58% more likely to develop acute diverticulitis.[45]

The prevalence of diverticular disease in British vegetarians in the late 1970s was reported to be approximately one-third that of meat eaters.[33] The more recent EPIC prospective study showed that the relative risk of diverticular disease was found to be 27% less for British vegetarians and 72% less for vegans compared to meat eaters. High dietary fibre intake was again shown to be an independent factor, reducing the relative risk of diverticular disease by 41%. Other important variables were obesity, hypertension, cigarette smoking, hormone replacement therapy and oral contraceptives.[34]

Colorectal cancer

More than 42,000 new cases of colorectal cancer (CRC) are diagnosed in the UK each year. It is the third most common cancer diagnosis in both males and females, responsible for approximately 16,500 deaths each year.[35] CRC incidence and mortality rates vary up to 10-fold worldwide. The highest incidences are found in Australasia, high-income Asia Pacific, North America, and Europe. As more countries move towards a more Western diet and lifestyle, it is projected that the global burden of CRC will increase by 60% to more than 2.2 million new cases and 1.1 million deaths by 2030.[36] While effective screening programmes have led to plateaus or reductions in incidence among older adults, CRC rates in young people have continued to rise.[37]

There is a strong scientific consensus that plant-derived fibre intake is protective against the development of CRC. The 2010 Continuous Update Report from the World Cancer Research Fund systematic review and meta-analysis graded the evidence linking high dietary fibre with a decreased risk of colorectal cancer as 'convincing'.[38] Consumption of whole grains offers substantial protection, with every 10 g of whole grain fibre consumed per day associated with a risk reduction of 10–17%. Epidemiological data from high income countries suggests that high intake of fruits and vegetables alone is associated with a risk reduction of up to 52%, while high consumption of legumes, cabbage, and cruciferous vegetables is associated with a risk reduction of between 9–24%. Meta-analyses indicate a clear dose-response relationship, with CRC incidence diminishing by 11% for every 100 g of fruits and vegetables consumed daily.[39]

The only food group that has been consistently linked to increased CRC risk is meat. Meta-analyses of observational studies indicate a significant association with between meat consumption and CRC, with increased risk ranging from 12–21%. Dose-effect studies report a 10–30% increased risk for each increment of 100 g per day or total or red meat consumption, with no limit threshold identifiable.[39]

Prospective studies on CRC risk in omnivores, vegans, and vegetarians have generally reported significant or non-significant trends to reduced risk. The low meat consuming Seventh Day Adventist populations have CRC rates of 30% lower than the US national average. Its notable that even among this lower CRC risk population, vegans and vegetarians are 16–18% less likely to develop CRC than non-vegetarians.[40] While early results from the EPIC-Oxford study reported an approximately 50% increased risk of CRC in vegetarians, this surprisingly adverse association did not persist with longer duration of follow-up.[41, 42, 43, 44, 45, 46]

The Nurses' Health Study reported a 250% greater CRC incidence among participants who consumed beef, pork, or lamb daily, compared to those who consumed those meats less frequently than once per month.[45] Red and processed meats are especially linked to increased CRC risk, at the current levels of consumption (76 g per day), it is estimated that these two food groups account for 20% of CRC cases diagnosed in the UK each year.[46]

Numerous components of meat have been identified which help explain these epidemiological findings. Haem iron, heterocyclic amines, polycyclic aromatic hydrocarbons, the nitrates that naturally occur in red meats, and the nitrites that are added to processed meats, are all known to directly contribute to inflammation, DNA damage, and carcinogenesis.[47, 48, 49, 50, 51] The consumption of meats and animal fats also contribute negatively to gut microbial health, driving the production of secondary bile acids, ammonia, and hydrogen sulphide gases, all of which combine to provide a gut microbial environment that is conducive to chronic inflammation and carcinogenesis. In contrast, the consumption of whole plants contributes to a gut microbial environment that supports healthy cell metabolism and defences.[52]

Based on the available scientific data, in 2015 the International Agency for Research on Cancer took the landmark decision to classify processed meats such as bacon, sausages and lunch meats as 'group 1 agents – carcinogenic to humans'. At the same time, unprocessed meats were classified as 'group 2a agents – probably carcinogenic to humans'.[53] This is crucial information to share with any patient who wishes to act to reduce their personal risk of developing CRC. The high-risk changes found in the colorectal mucosa and gut microbiome of individuals who consume a standard Western diet can be reversed within 14 days of adapting a high-fibre, plant-predominant diet.[9] A healthier diet and lifestyle, with higher intakes of fruits, vegetables, and wholegrains, may also offer substantial benefits in terms of CRC survivorship.[54]

Do dairy and fish consumption reduce CRC risk?

Several large meta-analyses have demonstrated that milk consumption is associated with reduced CRC risk.[39] This is most likely accounted for by the role of dietary calcium, which combats the carcinogenic effects of secondary bile acids and ionised fatty acids. Daily calcium intake >700 mg has been linked to a 35% reduction in distal CRC.[55] While acknowledging the evidence on dairy and CRC, the World Cancer Research Fund has stated that 'because we are unsure about the effect on other cancers, we don't make any recommendations about dairy products'.[56] A pragmatic approach may be to advise patients to increase their intake of calcium, fibre, and legumes simultaneously by eating beans, greens (such as broccoli, kale, and rocket), dates, calcium-set tofu, and other healthy sources of dietary calcium.

Despite significant enthusiasm, meta-analyses

of observational studies and site-specific subgroup analyses fail to support any effect for fish and omega-3 consumption in pre-cancerous adenoma or CRC prevention.[39]

Coeliac disease

Coeliac disease (CD) is an immune-mediated multisystem disorder, characterised by enteropathy in the lining of the small intestine following the ingestion of gluten in those with a genetic predisposition. Gluten is a protein that is present in wheat, rye and barley. Correct diagnosis is crucial, as the only effective treatment is strict, life-long elimination of dietary gluten.[57] CD is estimated to affect 1% of the population.

Clinical suspicion of CD is predominantly based on symptoms or associated conditions. Symptoms can be intestinal or extra-intestinal, but around 20% of patients are asymptomatic.[57] Initial investigation uses tTG IgA serology testing, with total IgA to rule out IgA deficiency. With a positive serology, a biopsy is performed to test duodenal histology for associated damage. A gluten-free diet (GFD) prior to coeliac screening will provide a false negative result in both serology and biopsy. The requirement for gluten ingestion prior to testing is likely to have contributed to underdiagnosis due to a resistance to gluten reintroduction in those whom experience symptom relief on a GFD.

Well-defined areas of CD include its genetic elements (human leukocyte antigen (HLA)-DQ2 and HLA DQ8), the antigen involved (tissue transglutaminase (tTG)), and the environmental trigger (gluten). Additional factors involved in CD appear to be loss of intestinal barrier function, inappropriate innate and adaptive immune response, and an imbalanced gut microbiome.[57]

Undiagnosed CD or continued gluten ingestion leads to complications predominantly resulting from gut inflammation, leading to villous atrophy and malabsorption of key nutrients. Nutrients at risk include calcium, vitamin D, folate, B12 and iron. Associated conditions therefore include iron deficiency anaemia, osteopenia or osteoporosis, delayed development and rarely T-cell lymphoma and small bowel adenocarcinoma. Other manifestations of CD include dermatitis herpetiformis and reduced fertility.[58]

The role of microbial factors in the development of CD has been suggested, with early life exposure to a variety of commensal, non-pathogenic microorganisms found to associated with protection.[59] Observational data has also identified alterations towards a pathogenic profile in the gut microbiota of participants with CD, which appears to be persistent in those in remission on a GFD. Alterations may be due to a reduction in polysaccharides associated with following a GFD, leading to weakened host defences against inflammation and infection.[60] Increased dietary fibre may promote increased microbial colonisation through greater SCFA production. Due to varying findings, however, evidence-based conclusions on CD and the gut microbiome cannot yet be made, particularly regarding cause and effect.

Specialised gluten-free (GF) products are often found to be higher in fat, sugar and salt, and lower in fibre than many gluten-containing (GC) products, and an intentional reduction of dietary gluten may result in the reduced consumption of whole grains.[61] This nutrient comparison between GFD and GC diets highlights the importance of choosing whole foods over popular and often ultra-processed GF alternatives. Increased intake of ultra-processed 'free-from' foods may put CD patients at greater risk of increased BMI, cardiovascular disease and metabolic syndrome; further research into this area is required.[61]

On diagnosis of CD, patients require comprehensive education and support from a specialist dietitian to cover all aspects of a strict, permanent and balanced GFD. Patients should also be encouraged to ensure a diversity of plant foods, and therefore plant fibre, to promote a gut microbiota beneficial for health. Whole food alternatives to wheat, rye and barley-based products should be encouraged to ensure sufficient micronutrients and fibre, for example brown rice, millet, corn, quinoa and buckwheat. Some patients may need to avoid oats based on individualised dietetic advice. For those following a plant-based diet, education on supplementary sources of calcium, iron, vitamin D and vitamin B12 should be provided alongside wider advice relevant for plant-based diets.

Irritable bowel syndrome

Irritable bowel syndrome (IBS) is a common multifactorial disorder of gut-brain interaction resulting in gastrointestinal symptoms.[62] IBS symptoms specifically include abdominal pain or discomfort associated with a change in bowel habit. Symptom severity varies widely and can considerably impact quality of life.[63] IBS is estimated to affect more than 11% of the global population. Prevalence ranges between countries however and the condition is thought to impact up to 20% of people UK and USA with female predominance. Data suggests that IBS diagnosis occurs 25% less in people over 50 and it does not appear to be correlated with socioeconomic status.[63]

IBS is diagnosed using symptom criteria (Rome IV), and after the exclusion of underlying conditions including inflammatory bowel disease (IBD), coeliac disease (CD) and malignancy.[64] IBS can be categorised into subtypes based on predominant symptoms: constipation (IBS-C), diarrhoea (IBS-D), and mixed (IBS-M). There is currently no cure for IBS, and treatments therefore target symptom management.[62] As a multifactorial disease with the potential to involve factors including psychology, genetics and epigenetics, neuroendocrine function, post infectious plasticity, bile acids and gut health, the pathophysiology is considered complex and not yet fully understood.[64]

Food ingestion is a powerful stimulus of gut motility, enzyme secretion and microbial status and could therefore impact IBS through a number of primary osmotic, chemical and mechanical mechanisms, or secondary mechanisms involving products of fermentation, luminal pH and gut microbial alterations.[62] Postprandial exacerbation of symptoms has been reported in 80% of patients and one study found epithelial breaks and increased intervillous spaces in patients with IBS following ingestion of foods to which they reported to be intolerant.[62, 65] Interestingly, a 2019 study demonstrated that individuals with severe IBS symptoms have a higher consumption of low-quality food products during their main meals,[66] highlighting a potential association between food choices and symptom severity.

Alteration in the gut microbiota has been associated with compromised epithelial permeability, immune system activation, low grade inflammation and pain in IBS.[64] There has been much interest in substances produced by gut bacteria that interact with both host brain and gut function; these postbiotics include fatty acids, tryptophan and neurotransmitters. A 2021 study by Bolte et al. found that the association between diet and the gut microbiome appears to be consistent with intestinal diseases including IBS.[67] The gut microbiota is subject to influences from factors including diet quality, antibiotic usage, infection and stress; factors that have been implicated in the pathophysiology of IBS. These findings provide the foundations for an exciting area of future study.[68]

Manipulation of food intake can support symptom management. Table 10.1 presents first line advice from the British Dietetic Association (BDA) current patient guidelines,[69] which is also available as a patient factsheet.[70] Second-line advice includes elimination diets including the low FODMAP (fermentable oligo-di-mono-saccharides and polyols) diet. The low FODMAP diet is designed to support the identification of highly fermentable dietary carbohydrates that may be

Table 10.1 Current IBS first-line advice (BDA, 2016)[69, 70]

Dietary advice	<ul><li>Aim for three meals at regular times each day</li><li>Avoid missing meals or eating close to bedtime</li><li>Stick to no more than two units of alcohol each day with at least two alcohol-free days a week</li><li>Limit caffeine-containing drinks e.g. no more than three cups a day</li><li>Minimise or avoid carbonated drinks</li><li>Drink plenty of fluid aiming for at least eight cups of non-caffeinated drinks daily e.g. water, herbal tea</li><li>Reduce rich and fatty foods for example chips, pies, batter, cheese, creamy sauces, crisps, chocolate, cakes, biscuits, cooking oils, burgers, sausages and other fatty meats</li><li>Cook from fresh ingredients where possible</li><li>Limit fresh fruit to three portions (80 g) each day</li><li>Seek advice from a healthcare professional about the amount of dietary fibre that is right for you</li></ul>
Lifestyle advice	<ul><li>Include regular relaxing activities such as yoga, meditation, massage or aromatherapy</li><li>Keep active with activities such as walking, swimming or cycling</li><li>Slow down at meals by sitting at a table, chewing food thoroughly and avoiding distractions</li><li>Log your food and symptoms whilst making changes so you can see what has helped</li></ul>
Symptom-targeted advice	<ul><li>Bloating and wind:</li><li>Reduce intake of gas-producing foods e.g. beans and pulses, Brussels sprouts, cauliflower and sugar-free mints/chewing gum</li><li>Increase intake of oats and add linseeds (up to 1 tbsp per day with an extra 150 ml of fluid)</li></ul>
Constipation:	<ul><li>Drink six to eight glasses of uncaffeinated fluid daily</li><li>Increase fibre intake gradually with foods such as wholegrains, vegetables, fruit and linseeds</li><li>Add 1 tbsp of linseed daily with an extra 150 ml of fluid</li><li>Avoid any extra wheat bran</li></ul>
Diarrhoea:	<ul><li>Keep fluid up to replace lost fluid</li><li>Limit caffeine to three caffeinated drinks daily</li><li>Trial a temporary reduction of high-fibre food</li><li>Avoid sugar-free foods containing sorbitol, mannitol or xylitol</li></ul>

resulting in osmotic changes and fermentation in the gut leading to IBS symptom exacerbation. Following a low FODMAP diet shows symptom improvement in 50–80% of patients working with a specialist dietitian.[71]

Fibre is specifically lacking in increasingly Westernised diets where IBS is on the rise. In contrast, a whole food, plant-based diet provides an abundance and variety of fibre that is beneficial for the gut microbiome. When moving to a plant-predominant, fibre-rich diet however, the initial increase in fermentable carbohydrates, or FODMAPs, may result in short-term abdominal symptoms, particularly in those with IBS. Increasing fermentable carbohydrates gradually is a sensible option here to improve tolerance and ensure sufficient dietary prebiotics for optimal gut microbial health. A healthy and balanced low FODMAP, plant-based diet plan is possible, but seeking support from an experienced dietitian specialising in this area is encouraged. The low FODMAP diet is a short-term programme to support symptom relief and identification of trigger foods and is not suitable for long-term adherence due to the potential negative impact on gut microbial number and diversity with unknown longer-term effects.[72] If a low FODMAP diet is not possible, specialised gut-directed hypnotherapy has been found to have a similar success rate on IBS symptoms as the low FODMAP diet, highlighting the role of psychological factors in IBS and providing an alternative for some patients.[73]

It remains crucial to encourage those with gut symptoms to seek specialist advice and pursue a positive IBS diagnosis. Establishing an effective doctor-patient relationship and shared understanding of IBS is key in condition management.[62] Patients with an IBS diagnosis are recommended to follow healthy eating guidelines alongside the first line advice outlined in Table 10.1. Lifestyle factors such as sleep, exercise, stress, and anxiety or depression should also be addressed prior to considering dietitian-led exclusion diets.

Long-term diets with a higher intake of plant foods over animal foods have the potential to prevent intestinal inflammatory processes via the gut microbiome.[74] Gradual progression towards a plant-predominant diet alongside standard treatment may therefore have a role to play in IBS symptom relief and improved quality of life.

Food intolerances

Food hypersensitivity, or an adverse reaction following food ingestion, can be categorised into food intolerance and food allergy. In contrast to food allergy, food intolerances are non-allergic reactions, and therefore do not involve a detectable immune response.[75]

Food intolerances are thought to affect up to 20% of the population, in contrast to only 1–2% with a true food allergy.[75] Although reactions vary in severity and are rarely life-threatening, food intolerance can significantly impact on quality of life. Common symptoms include abdominal pain, bloating, wind, constipation, diarrhoea, skin rashes and itching among others and symptoms crossover with those of food allergy. On diagnosis of a food intolerance, it is important to rule out allergy as well as potential underlying disease processes for example inflammatory bowel disease, coeliac disease, lymphoma, mastocytosis or tumours.[76]

Despite the prevalence of food intolerance, diagnosis can be complex and requires specialist investigation of clinical symptoms, symptom severity and timing of food in relation to symptoms. Although skin prick tests can be part of the diagnostic pathway for allergy, there are currently no validated diagnostic tests for food intolerance, despite the array of tests available on the market.[77]

Mechanisms involved in food intolerances are varied and may relate to enzyme deficiencies, pharmacological food components, or individual gastrointestinal function. Common triggers include gluten/wheat, caffeine, amines, fermentable carbohydrates, sulphites, as well as food additives such as sweeteners, sodium glutamate, colourings and preservatives.[76]

An example of a common food intolerance is carbohydrate malabsorption. The absorption of carbohydrates requires enzymatic breakdown (e.g., galactosidase in the breakdown of galacto-oligosaccharides) and efficient transport across the wall of the small intestine (e.g., GLUT 5 in fructose transport). Defects in these processes results in carbohydrates reaching the large intestine intact leading to changes in osmotic pressure and bacterial fermentation inducing gas production, wind, visceral sensitivity and changes in stool frequency and consistency. The short-term low FODMAP (fermentable oligo-, di-, mono- saccharides and polyols) diet can be utilised to address intolerances in otherwise healthy diets, particularly within IBS) and is found to be effective in 50–80% of patients.[71]

In suspected wheat or gluten intolerance in the absence of coeliac disease, both the protein and carbohydrates components of wheat grains are proposed causes. The carbohydrates (fructans) are subject to malabsorption as described above, and the proteins that triggers a reaction in coeliac disease and wheat allergy has also been suspected to cause symptoms in non-coeliac gluten sensitivity (NCGS). One theory suggests that dysbiosis can lead to alterations in intestinal permeability and impair protection against inflammatory stimuli. Balance and quality of the diet is strongly related to the gut microbial community, as well as epigenetic components.[78]

With any suspected food hypersensitivity, expertise from a specialist dietitian is required to ensure appropriate and personalised implementation of exclusion diets followed by reintroduction and diversification of the diet to protect long term health. Unsupported exclusion of foods may result in nutritional deficiencies as well as reduction in gut microbial number and diversity.[71, 78]

Diet is an important regulator of gastro-intestinal tract homeostasis and intestinal permeability through the interaction of dietary factors, the immune system and gut microbiota on the mucosal barrier. Diet quality should form an important part of initial investigation. Fibre from plant-based foods is integral to gastrointestinal health and it is therefore it is important to ensure food intolerances and food exclusion does not compromise intake of these healthful foods. A diet based around high fibre and high FODMAP foods may however cause some initial symptoms that may be mistaken for intolerance. Working on a gradual increase of these foods can improve tolerance on a plant-based diet and working with a specialist dietitian will support identification of food-based triggers.

Inflammatory bowel disease

Inflammatory bowel disease (IBD), including Crohn's disease and ulcerative colitis (UC) is characterised by chronic relapsing intestinal inflammation. It has been a worldwide healthcare problem with a continually increasing incidence.[79] In common with many chronic digestive disorders, IBD can be considered a disease of high-income nations. At the national level, the USA is known to have the highest age-standardised prevalence rate in the world (0.46% of the population), followed closely by the UK (0.45% of the population).[80] However, recent studies suggest that the true prevalence of IBD in the UK is likely to exceed 1% of the adult population.[81, 82]

In the early 21st century, IBD has emerged as a global disease with accelerating incidence in newly-industrialised countries[83] Multiple epidemiological studies have found associations between dietary intakes and IBD, with diets higher in refined carbohydrates, animal protein, total fat and dairy fat being positively associated with IBD prevalence.[12, 83, 84, 85, 86, 87, 88, 89] IBD is also more common in populations with higher intakes of ultra-processed foods.[89] Conversely, higher intakes of fruits, vegetables, whole grains, and legumes may have a protective effect.[10, 11]

The gut microbiota may be a crucial mediator between diet and IBD pathogenesis.[90] For example, common food emulsifiers and artificial flavour enhancers have been shown to promote the growth and pathogenic action of adherent invasive *E. coli*; harmful bacteria found in the microbiota of patients with Crohn's disease.[91, 92] In contrast, dietary concentrations of soluble plant polysaccharides have been shown to down-regulate adherence.[15] A diet high in animal products and low in fibre can induce rapid changes in the human gut microbiota and provoke an outgrowth of bacterial subtypes that have been associated with IBD pathogenesis.[8]

Prospective case series have shown that a diet which eliminates or restricts dairy foods, animal protein, animal fat, emulsifiers and other artificial food additives can induce Crohn's disease remission. This dietary intervention is effective in patients with newly diagnosed, active Crohn's disease and in patients with established Crohn's disease who have failed to respond to standard medical therapy, with reported clinical remission rates of 78.7% and 90.4%, respectively.[91, 92] Whole food dietary intervention is also well tolerated by patients with Crohn's disease, with excellent adherence.[93, 94] A case series of 22 patients demonstrated a remission rate of 92% in Crohn's disease patients who adhered to a whole food, semi-vegetarian diet for two years, compared to 25% in patients who continued with a standard omnivorous diet.[95]

Dietary intervention with exclusive enteral nutrition or elemental feeding is a well-established treatment for both adults and children with Crohn's disease.[96] Recent advances in our understanding of Crohn's disease pathogenesis suggest that this mode of treatment is successful because it excludes the common dietary components which may aggravate the disease process. A dietary approach which minimises highly processed foods, animal products, and dairy fat while emphasising plant-based sources of nutrition may be able to deliver the same therapeutic benefit.[97] One small prospective dietary intervention has shown that among patients with UC, a low-fat, high-fibre diet (26 g of fibre per day, 11% of calories from fat) out-performed an 'improved standard Western diet' (18 g of fibre per day, 36% of calories from fat) in reducing intestinal inflammation, improving markers of dysbiosis, and improving reported quality of life.[98]

In 2020, the International Organisation for the Study of Inflammatory Bowel Diseases published the first comprehensive and evidence-based dietary guidance for patients with Crohn's disease and ulcerative colitis, designed to help them better control their disease and prevent relapses. The foods that should be increased, where possible, are fruits, vegetables, and sources of omega-3 fatty acids. The foods and food components that should be limited or avoided are sources of saturated and trans fats, emulsifiers, carageenans, artificial sweeteners, titanium dioxide, red and processed meats, and dairy fats.[99] Although a whole-food, plant-based diet was not specifically recommended, it does naturally meet these specifications (if coconut oil and palm oil are avoided as sources of saturated fats). In clinical practice, most patients with IBD can benefit from dietetic review to ensure their dietary needs are met.[100] This support is especially important while making the transition to a healthier approach to food.

Meat consumption and digestive health

In 2021, the UK Biobank study published health outcomes among almost 475,000 middle-aged adults followed for up to eight years.[101] The goal of this analysis had been to assess the associations between meat consumption and the incidence of the 25 most common non-cancerous causes of hospital admission in this large population. Having corrected for variables including body mass index, dietary fibre intake, education, employment, alcohol use, smoking, physical activity and other health-related behaviours, the findings on meat and digestive health were striking.

For every 70 g increase in red and processed

meat consumption (separately or combined) they reported:
- 19% increased risk of diverticular disease
- 10% increased risk in colonic polyps.

For every 60 g increase in poultry consumption they found:
- 34% increased risk of GORD
- 24% increased risk of gastritis and duodenitis
- 20% increased risk of diverticular disease
- 22% increased risk of gallbladder disease.

The authors highlighted the many constituents of meat – including the presence of *H. pylori* in the poultry supply chain and adverse effects of animal products on gut microbial health – as potential explanations for these findings. However, the lesson from this finding of this large, prospective study is clear: meat consumption is significantly associated with poorer digestive health.

Conclusion

A whole food plant-based diet offers significant benefits for digestive health, both for day-to-day symptoms and longer-term prognosis. Health care professionals advising gastroenterology patients should ensure they base their guidance on the ever-growing evidence base demonstrating the beneficial effects of following a plant-based diet, not only in helping to protect against the development of gastrointestinal conditions but also as an integral part of treatment for existing conditions.

References

1. Marchesi JR, Ravel J. The vocabulary of microbiome research: a proposal. *Microbiome* 2015; 3(1): 31. doi: 10.1186/s40168-015-0094-5
2. Mullish BH, Quraishi MN, Segal JP, Ianiro G, Iqbal TH. The gut microbiome: what every gastroenterologist needs to know. *Frontline Gastroenterol* 2021; 12(2): 118–127. doi: 10.1136/flgastro-2019-101376
3. Gritz EC, Bhandari V. The human neonatal gut microbiome: a brief review. *Front Pediatr* 2015; 3: 17. doi: 10.3389/fped.2015.00017
4. Sonnenburg ED, Sonnenburg JL. Starving our microbial self: the deleterious consequences of a diet deficient in microbiota-accessible carbohydrates. *Cell Metab* 2014; 20(5): 779–786. doi: 10.1016/j.cmet.2014.07.003
5. De Angelis M, Ferrocino I, Calabrese FM, De Filippis F, Cavallo N, Siragusa S, et al. Diet influences the functions of the human intestinal microbiome. *Sci Rep* 2020; 10(1): 4247. doi: 10.1038/s41598-020-61192-y
6. Donohoe DR, Garge N, Zhang X, Sun W, O'Connell TM, Bunger MK, et al. The microbiome and butyrate regulate energy metabolism and autophagy in the mammalian colon. *Cell Metab* 2011; 13(5): 517–526. doi: 10.1016/j.cmet.2011.02.018
7. Parada Venegas D, De la Fuente MK, Landskron G, González MJ, Quera R, Dijkstra G, et al. Short Chain Fatty Acids (SCFAs)-Mediated Gut Epithelial and Immune Regulation and Its Relevance for Inflammatory Bowel Diseases. *Front Immunol* 2019; 10: 277. doi: 10.3389/fimmu.2019.00277
8. David LA, Maurice CF, Carmody RN, Gootenberg DB, Button JE, Wolfe BE, et al. Diet rapidly and reproducibly alters the human gut microbiome. *Nature* 2014; 505(7484): 559–563. doi: 10.1038/nature12820
9. O'Keefe SJD, Li JV, Lahti L, Ou J, Carbonero F, Mohammed K, et al. Fat, fibre and cancer risk in African Americans and rural Africans. *Nat Commun* 2015; 6(1): 6342. doi: 10.1038/ncomms7342
10. De Angelis M, Ferrocino I, Calabrese FM, De Filippis F, Cavallo N, Siragusa S, et al. Diet influences the functions of the human intestinal microbiome. *Sci Rep* 2020; 10(1): 4247. doi: 10.1038/s41598-020-61192-y
11. Cani PD. Human gut microbiome: hopes, threats and promises. *Gut* 2018; 67(9): 1716–1725. doi: 10.1136/gutjnl-2018-316723
12. Dong TS, Gupta A. Influence of Early Life, Diet,

and the Environment on the Microbiome. *Clin Gastroenterol Hepatol* 2019; 17(2): 231–242. doi: 10.1016/j.cgh.2018.08.067

13. Vakil N, van Zanten SV, Kahrilas P, Dent J, Jones R, Global Consensus Group. The Montreal definition and classification of gastroesophageal reflux disease: a global evidence-based consensus. Am J Gastroenterol. 2006; 101(8): 1900–1920; quiz 1943. doi: 10.1111/j.1572-0241.2006.00630.x

14. El-Serag HB, Sweet S, Winchester CC, Dent J. Update on the epidemiology of gastro-oesophageal reflux disease: a systematic review. *Gut* 2014; 63(6): 871–880. doi: 10.1136/gutjnl-2012-304269

15. Liu Y, Zhu X, Li R, Zhang J, Zhang F. Proton pump inhibitor utilisation and potentially inappropriate prescribing analysis: insights from a single-centred retrospective study. *BMJ Open* 2020; 10(11): e040473. doi: 10.1136/bmjopen-2020-040473

16. Kahrilas PJ, Shaheen NJ, Vaezi MF, Hiltz SW, Black E, Modlin IM, et al. American Gastroenterological Association Medical Position Statement on the management of gastroesophageal reflux disease. *Gastroenterology* 2008; 135(4): 1383–1391, 1391.e1-5. doi: 10.1053/j.gastro.2008.08.045

17. Albarqouni L, Moynihan R, Clark J, Scott AM, Duggan A, Del Mar C. Head of bed elevation to relieve gastroesophageal reflux symptoms: a systematic review. *BMC Family Practice* 2021; 22(1): 24. doi: 10.1186/s12875-021-01369-0

18. El-Serag HB, Satia JA, Rabeneck L. Dietary intake and the risk of gastro-oesophageal reflux disease: a cross sectional study in volunteers. *Gut* 2005; 54(1): 11–17. doi: 10.1136/gut.2004.040337

19. Fraser-Moodie CA, Norton B, Gornall C, Magnago S, Weale AR, Holmes GK. Weight loss has an independent beneficial effect on symptoms of gastro-oesophageal reflux in patients who are overweight. *Scand J Gastroenterol* 1999; 34(4): 337–340. doi: 10.1080/003655299750026326

20. Jacobson BC, Somers SC, Fuchs CS, Kelly CP, Camargo CA. Body-Mass Index and Symptoms of Gastroesophageal Reflux in Women. *New England Journal of Medicine* 2006; 354(22): 2340–2348. doi: 10.1056/NEJMoa054391

21. Nilsson M, Johnsen R, Ye W, Hveem K, Lagergren J. Lifestyle related risk factors in the aetiology of gastro-oesophageal reflux. *Gut* 2004; 53(12): 1730–1735. doi: 10.1136/gut.2004.043265

22. Morozov S, Isakov V, Konovalova M. Fiber-enriched diet helps to control symptoms and improves esophageal motility in patients with non-erosive gastroesophageal reflux disease. *World J Gastroenterol* 2018; 24(21): 2291–2299. doi: 10.3748/wjg.v24.i21.2291

23. Newberry C, Lynch K. The role of diet in the development and management of gastroesophageal reflux disease: why we feel the burn. *J Thorac Dis* 2019; 11(Suppl 12): S1594–S1601. doi: 10.21037/jtd.2019.06.42

24. Matrana MR, Margolin DA. Epidemiology and pathophysiology of diverticular disease. *Clin Colon Rectal Surg* 2009; 22(3): 141–146. doi: 10.1055/s-0029-1236157

25. Imaeda H, Hibi T. The Burden of Diverticular Disease and Its Complications: West versus East. *Inflamm Intest Dis* 2018; 3(2): 61–68. doi: 10.1159/000492178

26. Tursi A. Diverticulosis today: unfashionable and still under-researched. *Therap Adv Gastroenterol* 2016; 9(2): 213–228. doi: 10.1177/1756283X15621228

27. Weizman AV, Nguyen GC. Diverticular disease: Epidemiology and management. *Can J Gastroenterol* 2011; 25(7): 385–389. doi: 10.1155/2011/795241

28. Etzioni DA, Mack TM, Beart RW, Kaiser AM. Diverticulitis in the United States: 1998-2005: changing patterns of disease and treatment. *Ann Surg* 2009; 249(2): 210–217. doi: 10.1097/SLA.0b013e3181952888

29. Burkitt DP, Trowell HC. Refined Carbohydrate Foods and Disease—Some Implications of Dietary Fibre. *Postgrad Med J* 1976; 52(609): 476.

30. O'Keefe SJ. The association between dietary fibre deficiency and high-income lifestyle-associated diseases: Burkitt's hypothesis revisited. *Lancet Gastroenterol Hepatol* 2019; 4(12): 984–996. doi: 10.1016/S2468-1253(19)30257-2

31. Aldoori WH, Giovannucci EL, Rockett HR, Sampson L, Rimm EB, Willett WC. A prospective study of dietary fiber types and symptomatic diverticular disease in men. *J Nutr* 1998; 128(4): 714–719. doi: 10.1093/jn/128.4.714

32. Cao Y, Strate LL, Keeley BR, Tam I, Wu K, Giovannucci EL, et al. Meat intake and risk of diverticulitis among men. *Gut*. 2018 Mar;67(3):466–72.
33. Gear JS, Ware A, Fursdon P, Mann JI, Nolan DJ, Brodribb AJ, et al. Symptomless diverticular disease and intake of dietary fibre. *Lancet* 1979; 1(8115): 511–514. doi: 10.1016/s0140-6736(79)90942-5
34. Crowe FL, Appleby PN, Allen NE, Key TJ. Diet and risk of diverticular disease in Oxford cohort of European Prospective Investigation into Cancer and Nutrition (EPIC): prospective study of British vegetarians and non-vegetarians. *BMJ* 2011; 343: d4131. doi: 10.1136/bmj.d4131
35. Cancer Research, UK. Bowel cancer statistics. Cancer Research UK. 2015 [cited 2021 Nov 10]. https://www.cancerresearchuk.org/health-professional/cancer-statistics/statistics-by-cancer-type/bowel-cancer
36. Arnold M, Sierra MS, Laversanne M, Soerjomataram I, Jemal A, Bray F. Global patterns and trends in colorectal cancer incidence and mortality. *Gut* 2017; 66(4): 683–691. doi: 10.1136/gutjnl-2015-310912
37. Vuik FE, Nieuwenburg SA, Bardou M, Lansdorp-Vogelaar I, Dinis-Ribeiro M, Bento MJ, et al. Increasing incidence of colorectal cancer in young adults in Europe over the last 25 years. *Gut* 2019; 68(10): 1820–1826. doi: 10.1136/gutjnl-2018-317592
38. World Cancer Research Fund/American Institute for Cancer Research. Continuous Update Project Expert Report 2018. Diet, nutrition, physical activity and colorectal cancer. https://www.wcrf.org/diet-activity-and-cancer/
39. Chapelle N, Martel M, Toes-Zoutendijk E, Barkun AN, Bardou M. Recent advances in clinical practice: colorectal cancer chemoprevention in the average-risk population. *Gut* 2020; 69(12): 2244–2255. doi: 10.1136/gutjnl-2020-320990
40. Orlich MJ, Singh PN, Sabaté J, Fan J, Sveen L, Bennett H, et al. Vegetarian dietary patterns and the risk of colorectal cancers. *JAMA Intern Med* 2015; 175(5): 767–776. doi: 10.1001/jamainternmed.2015.59
41. Key TJ, Appleby PN, Spencer EA, Travis RC, Roddam AW, Allen NE. Cancer incidence in vegetarians: results from the European Prospective Investigation into Cancer and Nutrition (EPIC-Oxford). *Am J Clin Nutr* 2009; 89(5): 1620S-1626S. doi: 10.3945/ajcn.2009.26736M
42. Appleby PN, Thorogood M, Mann JI, Key TJ. The Oxford Vegetarian Study: an overview. *Am J Clin Nutr* 1999; 70(3 Suppl): 525S-531S. doi: 10.1093/ajcn/70.3.525s
43. Sanjoaquin MA, Appleby PN, Thorogood M, Mann JI, Key TJ. Nutrition, lifestyle and colorectal cancer incidence: a prospective investigation of 10998 vegetarians and non-vegetarians in the United Kingdom. *Br J Cancer* 2004; 90(1): 118–121. doi: 10.1038/sj.bjc.6601441
44. Key TJ, Appleby PN, Crowe FL, Bradbury KE, Schmidt JA, Travis RC. Cancer in British vegetarians: updated analyses of 4998 incident cancers in a cohort of 32,491 meat eaters, 8612 fish eaters, 18,298 vegetarians, and 2246 vegans. *Am J Clin Nutr* 2014; 100 Suppl 1: 378S-85S. doi: 10.3945/ajcn.113.071266
45. Willett WC, Stampfer MJ, Colditz GA, Rosner BA, Speizer FE. Relation of meat, fat, and fiber intake to the risk of colon cancer in a prospective study among women. *N Engl J Med* 1990; 323(24): 1664–1672. doi: 10.1056/NEJM199012133232404
46. Bradbury KE, Murphy N, Key TJ. Diet and colorectal cancer in UK Biobank: a prospective study. *Int J Epidemiol* 2020; 49(1): 246–258. doi: 10.1093/ije/dyz064
47. Cross AJ, Pollock JRA, Bingham SA. Haem, not protein or inorganic iron, is responsible for endogenous intestinal N-nitrosation arising from red meat. *Cancer Res* 2003; 63(10): 2358–2360.
48. Sinha R, Rothman N, Brown ED, Mark SD, Hoover RN, Caporaso NE, et al. Pan-fried meat containing high levels of heterocyclic aromatic amines but low levels of polycyclic aromatic hydrocarbons induces cytochrome P4501A2 activity in humans. *Cancer Res* 1994; 54(23): 6154–6159.
49. Bingham SA, Hughes R, Cross AJ. Effect of white versus red meat on endogenous N-nitrosation in the human colon and further evidence of a dose response. *J Nutr* 2002; 132(11 Suppl): 3522S-3525S. doi: 10.1093/jn/132.11.3522S
50. Gurjao C, Zhong R, Haruki K, Li YY, Spurr LF,

Lee-Six H, et al. Discovery and Features of an Alkylating Signature in Colorectal Cancer. *Cancer Discov* 2021; 11(10): 2446–2455. doi: 10.1158/2159-8290.CD-20-1656

51. Joosen AMCP, Kuhnle GGC, Aspinall SM, Barrow TM, Lecommandeur E, Azqueta A, et al. Effect of processed and red meat on endogenous nitrosation and DNA damage. *Carcinogenesis* 2009; 30(8): 1402–1407. doi: 10.1093/carcin/bgp130

52. Yang J, Yu J. The association of diet, gut microbiota and colorectal cancer: what we eat may imply what we get. *Protein Cell* 2018; 9(5): 474–487. doi: 10.1007/s13238-018-0543-6

53. IARC Working Group on the Evaluation of Carcinogenic Risks to Humans, Centre international de recherche sur le cancer, Organisation mondiale de la sante Red meat and processed meat. 2018.

54. Van Blarigan EL, Fuchs CS, Niedzwiecki D, Zhang S, Saltz LB, Mayer RJ, et al. Association of Survival With Adherence to the American Cancer Society Nutrition and Physical Activity Guidelines for Cancer Survivors After Colon Cancer Diagnosis: The CALGB 89803/Alliance Trial. *JAMA Oncol* 2018; 4(6): 783–790. doi: 10.1001/jamaoncol.2018.0126

55. Wu K, Willett WC, Fuchs CS, Colditz GA, Giovannucci EL. Calcium intake and risk of colon cancer in women and men. *J Natl Cancer Inst* 2002; 94(6): 437–446. doi: 10.1093/jnci/94.6.437

56. Protect yourself against bowel cancer | World Cancer Research Fund UK. World Cancer Research Fund. 2019 [cited 2021 Nov 10]. https://www.wcrf-uk.org/health-advice-and-support/health-advice-booklets/protect-yourself-against-bowel-cancer/

57. Caio G, Volta U, Sapone A, Leffler DA, De Giorgio R, Catassi C, et al. Celiac disease: a comprehensive current review. *BMC Med* 2019; 17(1): 142. doi: 10.1186/s12916-019-1380-z

58. Goddard CJR, Gillett HR. Complications of coeliac disease: are all patients at risk? *Postgrad Med J* 2006; 82(973): 705–712. doi: 10.1136/pgmj.2006.048876

59. Verdu EF, Galipeau HJ, Jabri B. Novel players in coeliac disease pathogenesis: role of the gut microbiota. *Nat Rev Gastroenterol Hepatol* 2015; 12(9): 497–506. doi: 10.1038/nrgastro.2015.90

60. Melini V, Melini F. Gluten-Free Diet: Gaps and Needs for a Healthier Diet. *Nutrients* 2019; 11(1): 170. doi: 10.3390/nu11010170

61. Lebwohl B, Cao Y, Zong G, Hu FB, Green PHR, Neugut AI, et al. Long term gluten consumption in adults without celiac disease and risk of coronary heart disease: prospective cohort study. *BMJ* 2017; 357: j1892. doi: 10.1136/bmj.j1892

62. Vasant DH, Paine PA, Black CJ, Houghton LA, Everitt HA, Corsetti M, et al. British Society of Gastroenterology guidelines on the management of irritable bowel syndrome. *Gut* 2021; 70(7): 1214–1240. doi: 10.1136/gutjnl-2021-324598

63. Enck P, Aziz Q, Barbara G, Farmer AD, Fukudo S, Mayer EA, et al. Irritable bowel syndrome. *Nat Rev Dis Primers* 2016; 2(1): 16014. doi: 10.1038/nrdp.2016.14

64. Lacy BE, Patel NK. Rome Criteria and a Diagnostic Approach to Irritable Bowel Syndrome. *J Clin Med* 2017; 6(11): 99. doi: 10.3390/jcm6110099

65. Fritscher-Ravens A, Schuppan D, Ellrichmann M, Schoch S, Röcken C, Brasch J, et al. Confocal endomicroscopy shows food-associated changes in the intestinal mucosa of patients with irritable bowel syndrome. *Gastroenterology* 2014; 147(5): 1012-1020.e4. doi: 10.1053/j.gastro.2014.07.046

66. Wang L, Alammar N, Singh R, Nanavati J, Song Y, Chaudhary R, et al. Gut Microbial Dysbiosis in the Irritable Bowel Syndrome: A Systematic Review and Meta-Analysis of Case-Control Studies. *J Acad Nutr Diet* 2020; 120(4): 565–586. doi: 10.1016/j.jand.2019.05.015

67. Bolte LA, Vila AV, Imhann F, Collij V, Gacesa R, Peters V, et al. Long-term dietary patterns are associated with pro-inflammatory and anti-inflammatory features of the gut microbiome. *Gut* 2021; 70(7): 1287–1298. doi: 10.1136/gutjnl-2020-322670

68. Collins SM. A role for the gut microbiota in IBS. *Nat Rev Gastroenterol Hepatol* 2014; 11(8): 497–505. doi: 10.1038/nrgastro.2014.40

69. McKenzie YA, Bowyer RK, Leach H, Gulia P, Horobin J, O'Sullivan NA, et al. British Dietetic Association systematic review and evidence-based practice guidelines for the dietary management of irritable bowel syndrome in

adults (2016 update). *J Hum Nutr Diet* 2016; 29(5): 549–575. doi: 10.1111/jhn.12385
70. British Dietetic Association (BDA). Irritable Bowel Syndrome Food Fact Sheet. 2019 [cited 2021 Nov 10]. https://www.bda.uk.com/resource/irritable-bowel-syndrome-diet.html
71. Staudacher HM, Whelan K. The low FODMAP diet: recent advances in understanding its mechanisms and efficacy in IBS. *Gut* 2017; 66(8): 1517–1527. doi: 10.1136/gutjnl-2017-313750
72. Vandeputte D, Joossens M. Effects of Low and High FODMAP Diets on Human Gastrointestinal Microbiota Composition in Adults with Intestinal Diseases: A Systematic Review. *Microorganisms* 2020; 8(11): 1638.
doi: 10.3390/microorganisms8111638
73. Peters SL, Yao CK, Philpott H, Yelland G, Muir J, Gibson P. Randomised clinical trial: the efficacy of gut-directed hypnotherapy is similar to that of the low FODMAP diet for the treatment of irritable bowel syndrome. *Alimentary pharmacology & therapeutics* 2016; 44(5): 447-459.
doi: 10.1111/apt.13706
74. Tap J, Störsrud S, Le Nevé B, Cotillard A, Pons N, Doré J, et al. Diet and gut microbiome interactions of relevance for symptoms in irritable bowel syndrome. *Microbiome* 2021; 9(1): 74.
doi: 10.1186/s40168-021-01018-9
75. Tuck CJ, Biesiekierski JR, Schmid-Grendelmeier P, Pohl D. Food Intolerances. *Nutrients* 2019; 11(7): 1684. doi: 10.3390/nu11071684
76. Zopf Y, Hahn EG, Raithel M, Baenkler H-W, Silbermann A. The Differential Diagnosis of Food Intolerance. *Dtsch Arztebl Int* 2009; 106(21): 369–370. doi: 10.3238/arztebl.2009.0359
77. British Dietetic Association (BDA). Allergy Food Fact Sheet 2021 [cited 2021 Nov 10]. https://www.bda.uk.com/resource/food-allergy-food-intolerance.html
78. Leccioli V, Oliveri M, Romeo M, Berretta M, Rossi P. A New Proposal for the Pathogenic Mechanism of Non-Coeliac/Non-Allergic Gluten/Wheat Sensitivity: Piecing Together the Puzzle of Recent Scientific Evidence. *Nutrients* 2017; 9(11): 1203. doi: 10.3390/nu9111203
79. Zhang Y-Z, Li Y-Y. Inflammatory bowel disease: Pathogenesis. *World J Gastroenterol* 2014; 20(1): 91–99. doi: 10.3748/wjg.v20.i1.91
80. GBD 2017 Inflammatory Bowel Disease Collaborators. The global, regional, and national burden of inflammatory bowel disease in 195 countries and territories, 1990-2017: a systematic analysis for the Global Burden of Disease Study 2017. *Lancet Gastroenterol Hepatol* 2020; 5(1): 17–30. doi: 10.1016/S2468-1253(19)30333-4
81. Freeman K, Ryan R, Parsons N, Taylor-Phillips S, Willis BH, Clarke A. The incidence and prevalence of inflammatory bowel disease in UK primary care: a retrospective cohort study of the IQVIA Medical Research Database. *BMC Gastroenterol* 2021; 21(1): 139.
doi: 10.1186/s12876-021-01716-6
82. Jones G-R, Lyons M, Plevris N, Jenkinson PW, Bisset C, Burgess C, et al. IBD prevalence in Lothian, Scotland, derived by capture–recapture methodology. *Gut* 2019; 68(11): 1953–1960.
doi: 10.1136/gutjnl-2019-318936
83. Ng SC, Shi HY, Hamidi N, Underwood FE, Tang W, Benchimol EI, et al. Worldwide incidence and prevalence of inflammatory bowel disease in the 21st century: a systematic review of population-based studies. *Lancet* 2017; 390(10114): 2769–2778. doi: 10.1016/S0140-6736(17)32448-0
84. DeClercq V, Langille MGI, Limbergen JV. Differences in adiposity and diet quality among individuals with inflammatory bowel disease in Eastern Canada. *PLOS One* 2018; 13(7): e0200580. doi: 10.1371/journal.pone.0200580
85. Jantchou P, Morois S, Clavel-Chapelon F, Boutron-Ruault M-C, Carbonnel F. Animal protein intake and risk of inflammatory bowel disease: The E3N prospective study. *Am J Gastroenterol* 2010; 105(10): 2195–2201.
doi: 10.1038/ajg.2010.192
86. Sakamoto N, Kono S, Wakai K, Fukuda Y, Satomi M, Shimoyama T, et al. Dietary risk factors for inflammatory bowel disease: a multicenter case-control study in Japan. *Inflamm Bowel Dis* 2005; 11(2): 154–163.
doi: 10.1097/00054725-200502000-00009
87. Reif S, Klein I, Lubin F, Farbstein M, Hallak A, Gilat T. Pre-illness dietary factors in inflammatory bowel disease. *Gut* 1997; 40(6): 754–760. doi: 10.1136/gut.40.6.754
88. Burisch J, Pedersen N, Cukovic-Cavka S, Turk N, Kaimakliotis I, Duricova D, et al. Environmental

factors in a population-based inception cohort of inflammatory bowel disease patients in Europe-an ECCO-EpiCom study. *J Crohns Colitis* 2014; 8(7): 607–616. doi: 10.1016/j.crohns.2013.11.021

89. Niewiadomski O, Studd C, Wilson J, Williams J, Hair C, Knight R, et al. Influence of food and lifestyle on the risk of developing inflammatory bowel disease. *Intern Med J* 2016; 46(6): 669–676. doi: 10.1111/imj.13094

90. Eom T, Kim YS, Choi CH, Sadowsky MJ, Unno T. Current understanding of microbiota- and dietary-therapies for treating inflammatory bowel disease. *J Microbiol* 2018; 56(3): 189–198. doi: 10.1007/s12275-018-8049-8

91. Roberts CL, Keita AV, Duncan SH, O'Kennedy N, Söderholm JD, Rhodes JM, et al. Translocation of Crohn's disease Escherichia coli across M-cells: contrasting effects of soluble plant fibres and emulsifiers. *Gut* 2010; 59(10): 1331–1339. doi: 10.1136/gut.2009.195370

92. Nickerson KP, McDonald C. Crohn's disease-associated adherent-invasive Escherichia coli adhesion is enhanced by exposure to the ubiquitous dietary polysaccharide maltodextrin. *PLoS One* 2012; 7(12): e52132. doi: 10.1371/journal.pone.0052132

91. Sigall-Boneh R, Pfeffer-Gik T, Segal I, Zangen T, Boaz M, Levine A. Partial enteral nutrition with a Crohn's disease exclusion diet is effective for induction of remission in children and young adults with Crohn's disease. *Inflamm Bowel Dis* 2014; 20(8): 1353–1360. doi: 10.1097/MIB.0000000000000110

92. Sigall Boneh R, Sarbagili Shabat C, Yanai H, Chermesh I, Ben Avraham S, Boaz M, et al. Dietary Therapy with the Crohn's Disease Exclusion Diet is a Successful Strategy for Induction of Remission in Children and Adults Failing Biological Therapy. *J Crohns Colitis* 2017; 11(10): 1205–1212. doi: 10.1093/ecco-jcc/jjx071

93. Van Limbergen J, Wine E, Assa A, Sigall Boneh R, Shaoul R, Kori M, et al. OP05 Crohn's disease exclusion diet is equally effective but better tolerated than exclusive enteral nutrition for induction of remission in mild-to-moderate active paediatric Crohn's disease: a prospective randomised controlled trial. *Journal of Crohn's and Colitis* 2019; 13(1): S003. doi: 10.1093/ecco-jcc/jjy222.004

94. Sandefur K, Kahleova H, Desmond AN, Elfrink E, Barnard ND. Crohn's Disease Remission with a Plant-Based Diet: A Case Report. *Nutrients* 2019; 11(6): 1385. doi: 10.3390/nu11061385

95. Chiba M, Abe T, Tsuda H, Sugawara T, Tsuda S, Tozawa H, et al. Lifestyle-related disease in Crohn's disease: Relapse prevention by a semi-vegetarian diet. *World J Gastroenterol* 2010; 16(20): 2484–2495. doi: 10.3748/WJG.V16.I20.2484

96. Narula N, Dhillon A, Zhang D, Sherlock ME, Tondeur M, Zachos M. Enteral nutritional therapy for induction of remission in Crohn's disease. *Cochrane Database Syst Rev* 2018; 4: CD000542. doi: 10.1002/14651858.CD000542.pub3

97. Levine A, Sigall Boneh R, Wine E. Evolving role of diet in the pathogenesis and treatment of inflammatory bowel diseases. *Gut* 2018; 67(9): 1726–1738. doi: 10.1186/s12916-020-01815-3

98. Fritsch J, Garces L, Quintero MA, Pignac-Kobinger J, Santander AM, Fernández I, et al. Low-Fat, High-Fiber Diet Reduces Markers of Inflammation and Dysbiosis and Improves Quality of Life in Patients with Ulcerative Colitis. Clin Gastroenterol Hepatol 2021; 19(6): 1189-1199.e30. doi: 10.1016/j.cgh.2020.05.026

99. Levine A, Rhodes JM, Lindsay JO, Abreu MT, Kamm MA, Gibson PR, et al. Dietary Guidance from the International Organization for the Study of Inflammatory Bowel Diseases. *Clin Gastroenterol Hepatol* 2020; 18(6): 1381–1392. doi: 10.1016/j.cgh.2020.01.046

100. Casanova MJ, Chaparro M, Molina B, Merino O, Batanero R, Dueñas-Sadornil C, et al. Prevalence of Malnutrition and Nutritional Characteristics of Patients With Inflammatory Bowel Disease. *J Crohns Colitis* 2017; 11(12): 1430–1439. doi: 10.1093/ecco-jcc/jjx102

101. Papier K, Fensom GK, Knuppel A, Appleby PN, Tong TYN, Schmidt JA, et al. Meat consumption and risk of 25 common conditions: outcome-wide analyses in 475,000 men and women in the UK Biobank study. *BMC Medicine* 2021; 19(1): 53. doi: 10.1186/s12916-021-01922-9

Chapter 11
Plant-based nutrition for mental health and wellbeing

Arvind Kaur Maheru

Introduction

The human brain is easily the most intricate organ in the body and utilises a substantial proportion of the body's caloric and nutrient intake. In a diseased state it can alter how a person perceives the world. Psychiatric disorders contribute significantly to the global burden of disease, and depression is the leading cause of disability worldwide in those aged 15–44 years. Depression and anxiety symptoms co-exist with many chronic physical diseases. By all estimates, psychiatric disorders will continue to rise globally over the coming decades.[1] Effective preventative strategies are vital for public health. Furthermore, existing psychiatric medications typically have many side-effects. Therefore, adjunctive strategies that are simple to implement and sustainable, such as dietary interventions, have compelling clinical utility.

Although associations between diet and mental disorders were being observed long before the availability of drug treatments, such research was largely curtailed with the advent of targeted psychotropic medications for specific mental disorders. Fortunately, nutritional psychiatry is experiencing a renaissance, with some intriguing findings, although much of the current literature involves non-clinical populations.[2] Plant-based diets (PBDs) in particular, show promise for improving mental health, through both the protective effects of fruits and vegetables, as well as the reduced harm from excluding animal foods.

This chapter will cover the evidence for optimising nutrition to enhance wellbeing and mental health and explore how this may be applied to clinical practice. It will examine how healthful diets can assist prevention and treatment of the common mental disorders of depression and anxiety and explore how the practice of nutritional psychiatry might impact the disease burden of severe and enduring mental disorders such as psychosis. The chapter starts by examining more closely how diet may exert effects on mental health by exploring some possible underlying biological mechanisms of action.

Diet and mental health: biological mechanisms

The proposed mechanisms of action linking diet with mental health are complex, multifaceted, interacting, and not restricted to any one biological pathway. Modulation by the diet of numerous mechanistic pathways has been suggested, including those involving the gut microbiota, inflammation, oxidative stress, obesity, epigenetics, mitochondrial dysfunction, tryptophan–kynurenine metabolism, the hypothalamo-pituitary-adrenal (HPA) axis neuro-genesis and brain derived neurotrophic factor (BDNF).[3] We will look briefly at the first four of these in turn. Importantly, each pathway may exert effects on several other pathways.

Microbiota-gut-brain axis

The gut microbiota are integral to human health. The gut-brain axis (GBA) (see Figure 11.1) is now established as a bi-directional communication channel between the central nervous system (CNS) and the enteric nervous system, with the majority of signals passing from gut to brain.[4] The gut can influence mental health by communicating with the brain via the vagus nerve (the main route), by regulating hormones, and by

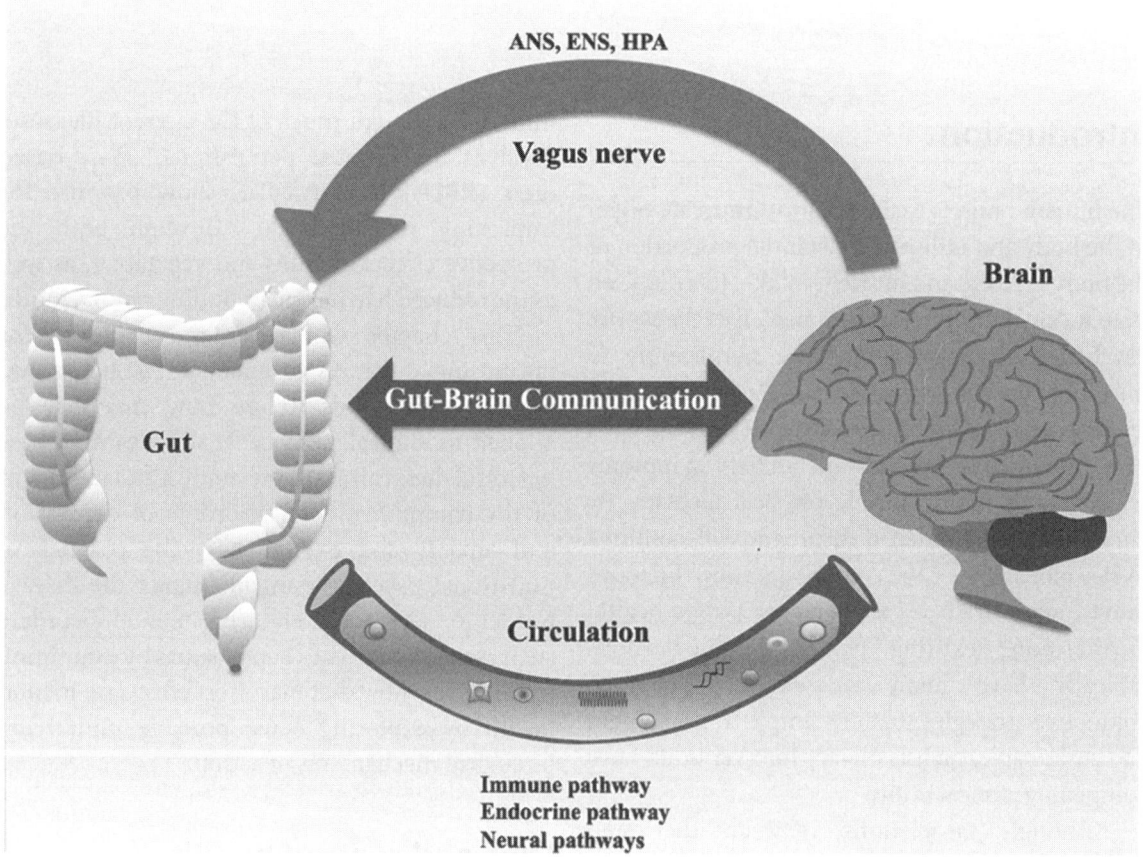

Figure 11.1 The gut-brain axis: schematic diagram showing the communication between the gut and brain. This is a bidirectional relationship that is strongly influenced by multiple pathways, including the autonomic nervous system (ANS), enteric nervous system (ENS), hypothalamic-pituitary-adrenal (HPA), immune pathways, endocrine pathways, and neural pathway.[61]

influencing inflammation. The gut microbiota are also vital to these interactions.[5]

Diet, in turn, is key for gut microbial health and although the fibre within whole plant foods is highly sought after by the gut's beneficial microbes, modern diets are frequently low in fibre, resulting in a disturbed balance of gut microbiota. In addition, dietary saturated fats reduce beneficial *Bifidobacteria* species and increase the pro-inflammatory *Bilophila* bacteria, with the same change also seen in studies of people with depression. Both a reduction in the quantity and the balance of microbial species (dysbiosis) has been reported in many mental disorders, including depression and anxiety.[6, 7, 8]

As the gut microbiota are modifiable, this has led to a hypothesis that neuropsychiatric disorders may be prevented and treated by altering the gut microbiota with so-called psychobiotics.[9] The term 'psychobiotics' refers to both the beneficial bacteria and their food sources (prebiotics) that when ingested, confer mental health benefits. Beneficial microbes ferment prebiotic fibre to produce short chain fatty acids (SCFAs), which are themselves neuroprotective and anti-inflammatory. Some SCFAs such as butyrate have been shown to reduce depression and sadness.[10] So SCFAs may be the mediators of the effects of microbiota on mental health.

As well as SCFAs acting as signalling molecules, the gut microbes also make other chemicals which talk to each other, including molecules that we know already as neurotransmitters such as serotonin, dopamine and GABA (gamma-aminobutyric acid), all of which can have antidepressant effects. It is thought that these neurotransmitters signal to the CNS via the GBA. This is likely the main way that gut bacteria influence mood. The vagus nerve is essential for the GBA. If the vagus is severed, the microbially produced neurotransmitters cannot reach the brain.[11]

People consuming PBDs have a more diverse gut microbiome. A whole food plant-based diet with a wide range of plant foods is recommended for the flourishing of diverse beneficial gut microbes and for supplying these microbes with crucial prebiotic fibre sources, such as resistant starches (e.g., oats, cooked and cooled rice and potatoes), and alliums (e.g., leeks, onions, garlic) and mushrooms.[12]

Manipulating the gut microbiota via additional dietary strategies, such as consuming fermented foods, (e.g., plant-based yoghurt, pickles, sauerkraut, kimchi and miso) as a means of modulating the GBA also has potential, but as yet the impact of such probiotic foods on mental health is unclear, and whether any effect is sustained beyond a short-term intervention is unknown.

Inflammation

Around 25% of patients with psychiatric conditions, including mood disorders, anxiety disorders and schizophrenia, show higher levels of chronic inflammation.[13] Additionally, the blood-brain barrier (BBB) was previously thought to prevent proteins like pro-inflammatory cytokines from crossing into the brain, but we now know that cytokines can cross, damage or send signals across the BBB. Although psychosocial stressors (both current and early-life) can cause inflammation, and regular physical activity can down-regulate systemic inflammation, arguably the most under-utilised modifier of inflammation is habitual diet quality.

Plant foods such as the beta-glucan fibre in whole grains appear to have immune-modulating functions.[14] In the Nurses' Health Study of over 43,000 participants a healthy ('prudent') dietary pattern, with higher intake of vegetables, fruit, whole grains, fish and legumes, was associated with lower levels of inflammatory markers, including C-reactive protein (CRP) and interleukin-6 (IL-6), and a lower risk of depression. In contrast, an unhealthy ('Western') dietary pattern, high in processed foods, red and processed meats, was associated with raised inflammatory markers and a higher risk of depression.[15] Western diets may impair the intestinal barrier and promote translocation of endotoxin-producing gram-negative bacteria into the blood (via so-called leaky gut) which may then trigger brain inflammation.[16]

In general, patients with severe mental illness have higher levels of 'dietary inflammation' than the general population, associated with greater intakes of pro-inflammatory foods, such as refined carbohydrates, refined vegetable oils and saturated fats; and lower intakes of anti-inflammatory nutrients, mostly derived from whole plant foods.[17] It has been proposed that resultant circulating inflammatory chemicals can damage the BBB and lead to mental illness, but the causal role of diet has not yet been established.[10]

Another proposed pro-inflammatory dietary pathway to depression is via the arachidonic acid cascade. People who virtually eliminated arachidonic acid from the diet (by following a vegetarian diet) reported happier, more positive mood compared to omnivores,[18] and in a further study, vegan diets were associated with less self-reported stress and anxiety than omnivorous diets.[19] A 3-arm randomised controlled trial (RCT) showed that over a 2-week period, scores on a depression, anxiety and stress scale in those on a vegetarian diet significantly improved, whilst those in the fish group and omnivore diet group showed no improvement.[20]

By manipulating diets towards a plant-based dietary pattern we have a potential tool for managing the inflammation associated with many mental health disorders. A useful dietary inflammation scoring-tool used in research is the Dietary Inflammatory Index (DII).[21] Key anti-inflammatory dietary constituents include phytochemicals such as polyphenols in fruit (especially berries), spices and legumes and omega-3 fatty acids. A systematic review and meta-analysis of 16 studies examined the relationship between the DII and mental health.[22] The results showed that compared to the lowest DII category, participants in the highest DII category had a significantly increased risk of several mental health disorders including depression, anxiety and schizophrenia.

Oxidative stress

Ongoing oxidative stress has also been suggested as a mechanism of cellular injury in mental health disorders. Inflammation and oxidative stress go together in that inflammatory processes unavoidably trigger and generate reactive oxygen species. Diet can both exacerbate and counteract oxidative stress with its balance of pro-oxidant and antioxidant food compounds. It has been postulated that high fat and high sugar Western-style diets could increase markers of oxidative stress, while a plant-based diet can supply powerful antioxidants.[23]

Obesity and weight gain

Adipose tissue is inflammatory. The complex relationship between diet, mood disorders and obesity is bi-directional. Meta-analyses show that both men and women with obesity have a 55% increased risk of developing depression, while those with depression have a 58% increased risk of developing obesity.[24] Higher levels of inflammation have been reported in both mood disorders and obesity, suggesting a common mediating effect. Interestingly, the SMILES clinical trial showed that a 12-week Mediterranean dietary intervention was effective for reducing depressive symptoms in the absence of weight change.[25] Nevertheless, it would seem prudent to manipulate diet to stabilise weight in people with depression, and indeed in those with severe mental illnesses. A whole food plant-based diet can facilitate weight loss, with its emphasis on nutrient density rather than calorie density.[26]

Now that we have outlined possible mechanisms by which diet affects mental health, next we will address which dietary interventions may be useful and in which health or disease states.

Whole diet interventions versus individual foods and nutrients

Dietary interventions can include nutrient interventions (e.g., zinc, omega-3 fatty acids), food interventions (e.g., increased fruit and vegetable intake, fermented foods), and whole diet interventions (e.g., whole food plant-based diet, Mediterranean diet). Studies of single nutrient interventions in mental illness have yielded inconsistent results. This reductionist approach fails to consider the complex interactions between nutrients. Accordingly, the evidence linking mental illness and diet has pivoted in the last decade to a focus on whole dietary patterns. Protective effects of whole food diets may come from the cumulative and synergistic effects of phytonutrients from diverse plant sources.

Nevertheless, there is still a role for investigating individual nutrients within the healthful whole diet context. People with depression have poor dietary habits[27] and it is already known that dietary vitamin deficiencies can cause depressive symptoms e.g., B12, B9 (folate) and zinc, presenting as low mood, fatigue, poor concentration and irritability. Importantly, folate is involved in the metabolism of monoamines such as serotonin in the brain. Maintaining adequate levels of vitamin B12, folate and zinc would appear prudent to protect against emergent depression. Although studies have investigated the link between other nutrients and mental illness, and despite biological plausibility, the results remain equivocal. For depression, adjunctive supplemental zinc, selenium, magnesium, calcium, vitamin C and vitamin D have been studied but evidence is inconclusive, although vitamin D supplementation may be beneficial.[28, 29] Overall, most studies conclude that individual nutrients are important but are best incorporated through the adoption of a healthy and varied diet.

Omega-3 fatty acids

Given the anti-inflammatory properties of omega-3 fatty acids, a plausible hypothesis arose that polyunsaturated fats could protect against and treat depression and anxiety. Some observational studies have suggested a link between low dietary intake of omega-3 fatty acids and depression. Yet a systematic review of 33 randomised trials with over 40,000 participants failed to show that supplementation with long chain omega-3 fatty acids has any benefit in preventing depression or anxiety.[30] There may be some evidence that omega-3 fatty acids are useful for treatment of depression, but the strength of evidence remains low.[31]

It remains unclear whether specific dietary sources of omega-3 fats are beneficial for mental health and whether fish sources are better. Reverse causation could explain the findings to date. In addition, people who eat fish generally have a healthier diet overall, often consuming less processed and red meat, yet more fruit and vegetables. So the results of observational studies may merely reflect the fact that people with depression are more likely to eat a lower quality diet.

A note on plant-based omega-3 sources. Data from nearly 5000 subjects (EPIC-Norfolk) found that although dietary omega-3 intake was lower in non-fish-eating vegetarians, their circulating omega-3 status was higher than expected, suggesting that those following plant-based diets may have a higher conversion of plant-derived alpha-linolenic acid (ALA) to longer chain omega-3 fatty acids.[32] A whole food plant-based source of dietary omega-3 fatty acids, such as ground flax or chia seeds is essential, and whether an algae-based source of long-chain omega-3 fatty acids is required for optimal mental health and wellbeing remains an area of active research.

Plant-based diets, wellbeing and general mental health

High psychological wellbeing is more than the absence of mental illness. It is a sense that we are functioning well in our life. People with high psychological wellbeing also report feeling capable, well-supported, and satisfied with life and are more likely to live healthier and longer lives. Accumulating data now show that PBDs, or simply increasing fruit and vegetable (FV) consumption, are associated with gains in wellbeing.

A study that used data on over 45,000 individuals followed over time, found that wellbeing increased in a dose-response fashion with the number of portions of FV consumed or with the frequency of FV consumption. Even modest increases in FV intake had substantive positive effects on wellbeing.[33]

Similarly, a novel 2-week study in New Zealand showed that providing high-quality FV to young adults resulted in short-term improvements in mental wellbeing, specifically vitality, flourishing, and motivation.[34] Consumption of raw FV may also be important in optimising better mental health wellbeing, with a high level of correlation with consumption of carrots, bananas, apples, leafy greens, citrus fruits, fresh berries, cucumber, and kiwi fruit in one study.[35]

In another longitudinal study of over 12,000 Australian adults, increased FV consumption was predictive of increased happiness, life satisfaction, and wellbeing. The gain was up to 0.24 life-satisfaction points (for an increase of eight portions a day), which is equal in size to the psychological gain of moving from unemployment to employment.[36] In a systematic review of 30 studies examining the association between FV consumption and general (broad) mental health in women, a positive influence of FV was seen using measures of wellbeing, quality of life, positive and negative affect, self-esteem, anxiety, distress, depressive symptoms, depression, and suicide.[37]

Wellbeing and diet have also been studied in the context of type 2 diabetes. Diabetes has significant co-morbidity with depressive illness, which itself places high demands on the individual's inner resources. A large longitudinal study of patients with diabetes has shown improved outcomes for 5-year mental health and wellbeing associated with higher intakes of FV and specifically FV-derived dietary fibre and resistant starch, such as that found in cereals and whole grains.[38] A systematic review of 11 controlled trials concluded that a plant-based diet can significantly improve psychological wellbeing and quality of life in people with type 2 diabetes.[39] The studies included were conducted in several different countries suggesting broad clinical applicability. Specifically, PBDs were associated with significant improvement in emotional wellbeing, physical wellbeing, depression, quality of life, general health, pain perception, weight, diabetes control and lipids, compared with several diabetes associations' official guidelines and other comparator diets.

In children and adolescents, a systematic review of 12 epidemiological studies reported a significant relationship between unhealthy dietary patterns (including higher intake of foods with saturated fat, refined carbohydrates and processed food products) and worse mental health.[40] They also observed an association between good-quality diet and better mental health. Since mental disorders often begin in youth, the implications are far-reaching.

A worksite-based pilot study using a whole food plant-based diet intervention resulted in significant improvements in the psychological subscale of quality of life, alongside other wellbeing improvements and is an early indicator that such interventions are both feasible and effective.[41]

Healthy dietary patterns for prevention of depression

Data from observational studies support the role of healthy diet patterns in the prevention of depression. There have been several systematic reviews and meta-analyses exploring the relationship between nutrition and incident depression. A large systematic review combining a total of 20 longitudinal and 21 cross-sectional studies provided strong evidence that a plant-rich Mediterranean diet can confer a protective effect against depression.[42] Another systematic review and meta-analysis demonstrated that a healthy/prudent diet, regardless of type (Mediterranean, vegetarian or Tuscan) reduced incidence of depression in a linear dose-dependent manner.[43] Analysis of data from a large (Whitehall II) cohort study showed that emergent depression was more likely with a processed food dietary pattern than a whole food dietary pattern.[44] An umbrella study bringing together data from 28 meta-analyses demonstrated that healthy diet patterns, characterised by high quality, nutrient-dense foods, were associated with a lower risk of depression.[31] Regarding individual foods, ultra-processed, sugar-sweetened beverages and red and processed meat were associated with a higher risk of depression. Higher intakes of fish, fruit, vegetables, tea and coffee were associated with a lower risk.

In a unique, large prospective cohort study from Japan, (n=89,000) a lower rate of suicide was associated with a high-quality 'prudent dietary pattern', characterised by high intake of vegetables, fruits, soya products, potatoes, seaweed, mushrooms and fish.[45] The comparison diets were a Westernised dietary pattern and a traditional Japanese dietary pattern, characterised by high intake of salmon, salty fish, oily fish, seafoods other than fish and pickles, neither of which affected suicide risk.

> **Box 11.1 Evidence-based dietary recommendations for prevention of depression[46]**
> - Follow 'traditional' dietary patterns, such as the Mediterranean, Norwegian, or Japanese diet.
> - Increase consumption of fruits, vegetables, legumes, whole grain cereals, nuts, and seeds.
> - Include a high consumption of foods rich in omega-3 polyunsaturated fatty acids.
> - Replace unhealthy foods with wholesome nutritious foods.
> - Limit intake of processed foods, 'fast' foods, commercial bakery goods, and sweets.

In summary, we have consistent epidemiological evidence suggesting an association between measures of diet quality and depression, across multiple populations and age groups. Box 11.1 provides summary recommendations for prevention of depression compiled by an international nutritional psychiatry expert group.[46] All the recommendations are compatible with a plant-based diet. More studies that control for confounding factors, such as obesity, are needed and we must remain vigilant to the potential for reverse causality in the findings thus far. Population-based studies provide information on diets that are associated with mental health and disease, but they do not confirm their role in treatment.

Dietary interventions in the treatment of depression

Existing treatments for depression fail to achieve remission for a significant proportion of people and the search continues for effective alternative approaches. There is growing evidence from RCTs to support dietary interventions as adjuvant therapy for depression. Recently a meta-analysis of 16 RCTs (total sample size, n = 45,826) primarily in participants with non-clinical depression concluded that dietary interventions can effect a small-to-moderate reduction in depressive symptoms.[47]

In patients with clinical depression, several RCTs have now shown moderate-to-large symptom improvements with a Mediterranean diet-based intervention compared to control conditions. The SMILES trial (see Box 11.2) was the landmark RCT in 2017 to report significant reductions in depressive symptoms following an adjunctive Mediterranean diet intervention in adults with depression compared to controls.[25] This was followed by similar results in The Healthy Eating for Life with a Mediterranean Diet (HELFIMED) trial,[48] which used adjunctive supplemental omega-3 fish oil in addition to diet and delivered fortnightly group cooking workshops for the dietary group participants, as well as food hampers. In both RCTs existing psychiatric treatments were continued and a dose-response effect was seen. The more that patients improved their diet, the fewer depressive and anxiety symptoms they had and the better they rated their quality of life.

A novel RCT that used a healthy diet in young adults with elevated depression symptoms also showed a moderate effect size, despite a small sample size (n=72).[49] Participants in the Diet Change group received the diet intervention instructions from a registered dietitian via a 13-minute video, available for re-watching online as needed, as well as paper resources and minimal telephone support. The diet was based on the *Australian Guide to Healthy Eating* (2003) and included fruit, vegetables, whole grains and cereals, dairy products, lean protein, fish and other seafood, olive oil, nuts and seeds, olives or avocado and spices. Within the Diet Change group, increased intake of recommended foods was associated with correlated spectrophotometer readings. These provided objective evidence to support the participants' self-reported dietary adherence by measuring skin carotenoid response (i.e. skin yellowness and the light reflected by the participant's skin). It allowed estimation of the quantity of flavonoids (from fruit and vegetables) in their diet and showed good compliance with the dietary intervention. The fact that this relatively low-cost intervention resulted in a population of young adults adhering to diet recommendations is encouraging, although longer-term studies are needed.

> **Box 11.2 The SMILES randomised controlled trial of dietary improvement in depression**
>
> The SMILES trial (sample size, n=56) was a 12-week study conducted in patients with established depressive disorder who were already on treatment (either antidepressant therapy, psychotherapy or both) and had a poor baseline diet. Researchers used an *ad libitum* modified Mediterranean diet (comprising a mostly plant-based diet with fish, low-fat dairy, eggs and meat permitted less frequently, and processed foods discouraged) versus a social support (befriending) intervention in the control group. Considerable dietary support was given, including seven dietitian-administered support sessions, written diet support, a food hamper and meal plans/ recipes. Dietitians used Motivational Interviewing techniques. Disease remission was achieved in 32% of diet intervention patients versus 8% of controls as measured on validated scales. The size of the effect was moderate with a number needed to treat (NNT) of 4.1, comparable to NNTs seen with antidepressant medication. The SMILES trial thus demonstrated that well-designed dietary interventions are feasible, acceptable to patients and effective in clinical practice.

Dietary interventions in the treatment of anxiety

Anxiety disorders are some of the most common mental illnesses worldwide. Yet medications and psychotherapy are only successful in treating about half of patients, and only one-quarter experience complete symptomatic resolution. Anxiety and depression often go hand-in-hand, with about half of those with depression also experiencing anxiety.

Most people have experience of nervousness manifesting in the gut and can appreciate a link between gut and anxiety. For those with anxiety disorders, aside from counselling on the dietary triggers (high intakes of refined sugar, alcohol, and caffeine), advice can extend to maintaining regular meal intake for a more consistent blood glucose, to lower the risk of panic symptoms. A whole food plant-based diet rich in low glycaemic index (GI) foods, such as intact whole grains, legumes, vegetables, and intact fruits will enable stable glucose metabolism.[50]

Poor quality, low fibre diets may act via modulating the microbiome to induce anxiety.[7] The relationship is bi-directional, as anxiety can in turn shift the balance of the microbial ecosystem by release of stress hormones that reach the gut lining and disturb equilibrium. Whilst plant-based diets have plausibility in principle, data on dietary interventions for treatment of clinical anxiety are few and as yet inconclusive. In a plant-based RCT of nearly 300 GEICO employees over 18 weeks, significant reductions in anxiety and depressive measures were seen on a validated health status profile (SF-36). Although the study did not sample a clinical population of patients with anxiety, its findings warrant further investigation.[51]

Dietary interventions in the treatment of severe mental illness

Patients with severe mental illness (SMI) such as psychosis and bipolar disorder, die 10 to 20 years earlier than the general population. In addition to unnatural causes of death such as suicide and accidents, preventable co-morbid cardiometabolic diseases are common and add to the higher mortality rates. To address these health inequalities an international working group and declaration, Healthy Active Lives (HeAL) was set up in 2011.[52] In the UK a positive cardiometabolic health resource was created with a motto 'don't just screen, intervene' and whilst it does mention dietary counselling, few mental health teams have access to specialist dietitians.[53] Hence, there remains considerable scope for PBDs to address physical co-morbidities and it is hoped an ambitious clinical research team would be motivated to advance the field of nutritional psychiatry within this patient group.

All types of SMI show heightened levels of peripheral inflammatory markers, which are linked to worse prognosis in these conditions. However, whilst we have preliminary observational data, there is currently no experimental evidence showing beneficial effects of dietary interventions on inflammation and mental health symptoms in schizophrenia or bipolar disorder.[47] Due to the considerable weight gain that antipsychotic medications can cause, so far studies to assess diet in patients with psychosis have focused on improving metabolic and physical health outcomes.

Treatment for psychosis is based on antipsychotic medication which targets the so-called *positive symptoms*, namely hallucinations and delusions. It is notable that the *negative symptoms* (such as amotivation, social withdrawal, lethargy, low mood, poor concentration) and cognitive and functional impairment often improve little with medication. There is clearly an unmet need to improve quality of life for patients with psychosis and their families.

When studying the effects of healthy diets in people with psychosis, it is encouraging that *negative and cognitive symptoms* have shown some attenuation with dietary interventions, including improvements in concentration, motivation and volition, energy and mood.[54] Individual phytonutrients that have shown some evidence of benefit to cognition include sulforaphane found in cruciferous vegetables such as broccoli, cabbage, kale; resveratrol found in red and black grapes, blueberries and raspberries; quercetin found in onions, berries, kale, grapes, plums; and polyphenols found in many fruits and vegetables.

There can be a clinical perception that patients with psychosis will find healthy diets unacceptable, but a recent systematic review showed that nutrition interventions are acceptable and effective in this patient population.[55] Dietary interventions delivered by dietitians, and those aiming to prevent weight gain at antipsychotic initiation had the largest effect sizes. A systematic review has also shown that there is scope for multimodal lifestyle interventions, including nutrition, for managing co-morbid conditions in those with bipolar disorder.[56]

Antipsychotic medications, weight gain and microbiota

A clinically significant side-effect of drug treatments for severe mental illness is weight gain. Antipsychotic medications induce greatly increased hunger, decreased satiety, and increased cravings for sweet foods and drinks. Antipsychotics appear to disturb the gut microbiome although the observed findings could be mediated by other effects related to the antipsychotic drugs.[57] An increase in the *Firmicutes* to *Bacteroidetes* ratio (similar to that seen in obesity) following use of olanzapine or risperidone has been consistently reported in several studies.[58] There are ongoing clinical trials testing the efficacy of probiotics in alleviating antipsychotic-induced weight gain, although we need better understanding of the precise roles of microbes to develop such specific microbial treatments. Fibre-rich whole food plant-based diets have clear potential to mitigate medication-associated weight gain, but this has not yet been tested in clinical settings.

Clinical applications of nutritional psychiatry

So how might we use the data on dietary manipulation in the clinical setting? Sometimes people consult clinicians seeking advice to avoid familial mental illness or to tackle weight gain from psychotropic medications, while others may be looking for ways to improve their mental health or to reduce medication use. It is important to be clear that dietary interventions for existing mental health conditions cannot yet be recommended as stand-alone treatments, and nor should they be a substitute for existing therapeutic approaches that have proven effective for an individual patient. Psychiatric disorders require careful assessment, including awareness of suicide risk and other psychiatric emergencies.

For enhancing psychological wellbeing, preventing depressive illness, or delivering adjuvant (complementary) treatment of depressive illness, dietary intervention warrants consideration. It is worth noting that we do not know yet which patient characteristics inform response to dietary intervention. Response is likely to depend on quality and constituents of baseline diet, as well as personal and familial history of co-existing

---

* Research data suggest that patients with a CRP >1 mg/L are less likely to respond to selective serotonin reuptake inhibitor (SSRI) antidepressants. Consider using CRP as a measure to track inflammatory load.[59]

obesity or inflammatory/ autoimmune disorders, making clinical skill and an exploratory mindset essential to the assessment. Box 11.3 outlines pointers for clinical practice.

> **Box 11.3 Suggestions for clinical practice**
> - Take a dietary history, alongside a past medical and family history.
> - Example questions (tailor to individual need): How often do you eat out? Number of meals and snacks a day. How many servings of vegetables a day? Frequency of desserts, sugar-sweetened drinks. How many hours of TV do you watch? (snacking linked to weight gain).
> - Assess patient's food literacy, including food and nutrition knowledge and skills and common terms (e.g., fibre, saturated fats, omega-3 fatty acids).
> - Assess patient's confidence and readiness to change diet and any cultural factors.
> - Devise a Change Plan, if ready. Ask 'What could you change?' (See Chapter 19).
> - Use a Nutrition History proforma that stays on file and is added to, as nutritional status improves, for use by all multi-disciplinary team staff.
> - Provide psycho-education with nutrition information, highlighting gut health, the pro-inflammatory nature of saturated fats and refined sugars. Emphasise that the main sources of saturated fats in Western diets are dairy, meat, fried foods, snack and baked foods.
> - Inform patient of the key role of plant-based foods in reducing inflammatory load and supplying antioxidant foods.
> - Ensure adequate intake of omega 3-rich plant foods.
> - Supplement B12 and Vitamin D on a PBD.

Suggested baseline work-up:
- Weight, body mass index (BMI), blood pressure, mood scales, CRP*, full blood count, folate, vitamins B12 and D, fasting glucose and lipids.

Interventions:
- Pictorial representations of a PBD in a handout to patients e.g., the Plant-based Eatwell Guide, Whole food Plant-based Food Pyramid.
- Referral to a dietitian, health coach, group intervention or multi-component dietary intervention if available, especially if BMI ≥25 kg/m2 (≥23 kg/m2 if South Asian or Chinese) and/or weight gain >5 kg over 3-month period, co-morbid type 2 diabetes, uncontrolled hypertension, raised cholesterol.[53]
- Suggest a trial to remove processed foods/add plant-based foods.
- Encourage patient to keep a mood and wellbeing diary. Review in 3–4 weeks. Wellbeing can increase within days.

Multi-component dietary interventions

Given the propensity for psychotropic medications to cause weight gain, as well as the mounting evidence for plant-rich diets to improve mood and wellbeing, mental health and primary care settings would benefit from a multi-component patient education intervention to support individual patient recommendations. Video, telephone and other modes of delivery at a group or individual level could be piloted, as in the work by Francis and colleagues.[49] In their study, resources were made available to patients to troubleshoot cravings, deal with social pressures and explain how to save money while eating healthier. They showed that in addition to increasing healthful food intake, reduction of processed food intake seemed to have an independent beneficial effect on mood symptoms. The Complete Health Improvement Programme (CHIP) is an existing group intervention that could be adapted to this setting.[60]

Conclusion

Nutritional psychiatry is an evolving field. In addition to well-documented positive effects of plant-based diets on psychological wellbeing, growing evidence now supports the use of plant-based dietary interventions for depressive symptoms. Diet is a modifiable risk factor for depression and could be targeted as an early intervention for prevention. Several positive RCTs now support the use of healthful (largely plant-based) diets as adjunctive treatment alongside existing interventions for established depressive disorders. The challenge will be to develop effective programmes to deliver these interventions within clinical and public health domains.

Research into dietary effects on other mental disorders is still in its infancy. Although more evidence is needed, whole-of-diet and targeted nutritional interventions are low-risk, easy to use, additive and acceptable to patients. As with many chronic diseases, the disease pathogenesis of psychiatric disorders is multifactorial, with multiple biopsychosocial contributors. Providing nutritional advice and dietary coaching should form part of our approach to tackling the biological contributors to mental illness. Since inflammation has been implicated in many mental disorders, the anti-inflammatory effects of a PBD could plausibly be exploited to achieve better outcomes. Medication-associated weight gain is a particular health threat to the mental health patient population and a whole food plant-based diet would go a long way to mitigating the co-morbid cardiometabolic disorders that cause disability and cut lives short.

Thus far we are lacking intervention studies using wholly plant-based diets in patients with clinical depression, anxiety disorders or other psychiatric disorders. Importantly, each of the healthy dietary interventions so far studied have common core features and involve decreasing intake of refined calorie-dense foods, while increasing intake of nutrient-dense fibre-filled foods and vegetables. Whole food PBDs are inherently nutrient-dense without being calorie-dense.

Clinicians can begin to add this underused tool to their therapeutic and preventative armamentarium. As research evolves, we will more clearly establish whether specific nutrients or specific dietary patterns of whole foods exert beneficial effects on mental health. Further RCTs may also identify individual demographic (e.g., sex, BMI, comorbid medical disorders) and biological (e.g., inflammation) factors to inform when to use a dietary intervention approach and which patients are most likely to respond.

Within an existing biopsychosocial framework, there is a valid case for enhancing a patient's nutrition, alongside standard-of-care treatments such as medication, psychotherapy and social care. At the very least, we can make it routine clinical practice to take a dietary history and highlight to patients the link between a plant-predominant diet, inflammation, gut health and wellbeing, to empower them to support their own recovery.

References

1. Rehm J, Shield KD. Global Burden of Disease and the Impact of Mental and Addictive Disorders. *Current Psychiatry Reports* 2019; 21(2): 10. doi: 10.1007/s11920-019-0997-0
2. Adan RAH, van der Beek EM, Buitelaar JK, Cryan JF, Hebebrand J, Higgs S, et al. Nutritional psychiatry: Towards improving mental health by what you eat. *European Neuropsychopharmacology* 2019; 29(12): 1321-1332. doi: 10.1016/j.euroneuro.2019.10.011

3. Marx W, Lane M, Hockey M, Aslam H, Berk M, Walder K, et al. Diet and depression: exploring the biological mechanisms of action. *Molecular Psychiatry* 2021; 26: 134-150. doi: 10.1038/s41380-020-00925-x
4. Cryan JF, Dinan TG. Mind-altering microorganisms: The impact of the gut microbiota on brain and behaviour. *Nature Reviews Neuroscience* 2012; 13(10): 701-712. doi: 10.1038/nrn3346
5. Mörkl S, Wagner-Skacel J, Lahousen T, Lackner S, Holasek SJ, Bengesser SA, et al. The role of nutrition and the gut-brain axis in psychiatry: A review of the literature. *Neuropsychobiology* 2018; 17: 1-9. doi: 10.1159/000492834
6. Jiang H, Ling Z, Zhang Y, Mao H, Ma Z, Yin Y, et al. Altered fecal microbiota composition in patients with major depressive disorder. *Brain Behav Immun* 2015; 48: 186-194. doi: 10.1016/j.bbi.2015.03.016
7. Jiang H yin, Zhang X, Yu Z he, Zhang Z, Deng M, Zhao J hua, et al. Altered gut microbiota profile in patients with generalized anxiety disorder. *J Psychiatr Res* 2018; 104: 130-136. doi: 10.1016/j.jpsychires.2018.07.007
8. Barandouzi ZA, Starkweather AR, Henderson WA, Gyamfi A, Cong XS. Altered composition of gut microbiota in depression: A systematic review. *Frontiers in Psychiatry* 2020; 11: 541. doi: 10.3389/fpsyt.2020.00541
9. Dinan TG, Stanton C, Cryan JF. Psychobiotics: A novel class of psychotropic. *Biological Psychiatry* 2013; 74(10): 720-6. doi: 10.1016/j.biopsych.2013.05.001
10. Noble EE, Hsu TM, Kanoski SE. Gut to brain dysbiosis: Mechanisms linking western diet consumption, the microbiome, and cognitive impairment. *Front Behav Neurosci* 2017; 11: 9. doi: 10.3389/fnbeh.2017.00009
11. Breit S, Kupferberg A, Rogler G, Hasler G. Vagus nerve as modulator of the brain-gut axis in psychiatric and inflammatory disorders. *Frontiers in Psychiatry* 2018; 9: 44. doi: 10.3389/fpsyt.2018.00044
12. Carlson JL, Erickson JM, Lloyd BB, Slavin JL. Health effects and sources of prebiotic dietary fiber. *Current Developments in Nutrition* 2018; 2(3): nzy005. doi: 10.1093/cdn/nzy005
13. Bauer ME, Teixeira AL. Inflammation in psychiatric disorders: What comes first? *Annals of the New York Academy of Sciences* 2019; 1437(1): 57-67. doi: 10.1111/nyas.13712
14. Berk M, Williams LJ, Jacka FN, O'Neil A, Pasco JA, Moylan S, et al. So depression is an inflammatory disease, but where does the inflammation come from? *BMC Med* 2013; 11(1): 200. doi: 10.1186/1741-7015-11-200
15. Lucas M, Chocano-Bedoya P, Shulze MB, Mirzaei F, O'Reilly ÉJ, Okereke OI, et al. Inflammatory dietary pattern and risk of depression among women. *Brain Behav Immun* 2014; 36: 46-53. doi: 10.1016/j.bbi.2013.09.014
16. Maes M, Kubera M, Leunis JC, Berk M. Increased IgA and IgM responses against gut commensals in chronic depression: Further evidence for increased bacterial translocation or leaky gut. *J Affect Disord* 2012; 141(1): 55-62. doi: 10.1016/j.jad.2012.02.023
17. Firth J, Veronese N, Cotter J, Shivappa N, Hebert JR, Ee C, et al. What is the role of dietary inflammation in severe mental illness? A review of observational and experimental findings. *Front Psychiatry* 2019; 10: 350. doi: 10.3389/fpsyt.2019.00350
18. Beezhold BL, Johnston CS, Daigle DR. Vegetarian diets are associated with healthy mood states: a cross-sectional study in seventh day adventist adults. *Nutr J* 2010; 9(26). doi: 10.1186/1475-2891-9-26
19. Beezhold B, Radnitz C, DiMatteo J. Large vegan sample reports less anxiety and stress than omnivores (823.3). *FASEB J* 2014; 28(1). doi:10.1096/fasebj.28.1_supplement.823.3
20. Beezhold BL, Johnston CS. Restriction of meat, fish, and poultry in omnivores improves mood: A pilot randomized controlled trial. *Nutr J* 2012; 11: 9. doi: 10.1186/1475-2891-11-9
21. Shivappa N, Steck SE, Hurley TG, Hussey JR, Hébert JR. Designing and developing a literature-derived, population-based dietary inflammatory index. *Public Health Nutr* 2014; 17(8): 1689-1696. doi: 10.1017/S1368980013002115
22. Chen GQ, Peng CL, Lian Y, Wang BW, Chen PY, Wang GP. Association Between Dietary Inflammatory Index and Mental Health: A Systematic Review and Dose–Response

Meta-Analysis. *Frontiers in Nutrition* 2021; 8: 662357. doi: 10.3389/fnut.2021.662357
23. Huang Q, Liu H, Suzuki K, Ma S, Liu C. Linking what we eat to our mood: A review of diet, dietary antioxidants, and depression. *Antioxidants* 2019; 8(9): 376. doi: 10.3390/antiox8090376
24. Luppino FS, De Wit LM, Bouvy PF, Stijnen T, Cuijpers P, Penninx BWJH, et al. Overweight, obesity, and depression: A systematic review and meta-analysis of longitudinal studies. *Archives of General Psychiatry* 2010; 67(3): 220-229. doi: 10.1001/archgenpsychiatry.2010.2
25. Jacka FN, O'Neil A, Opie R, Itsiopoulos C, Cotton S, Mohebbi M, et al. A randomised controlled trial of dietary improvement for adults with major depression (the 'SMILES' trial). *BMC Med* 2017; 15(1): 23. doi: 10.1186/s12916-017-0791-y
26. Wright N, Wilson L, Smith M, Duncan B, McHugh P. The BROAD study: A randomised controlled trial using a whole food plant-based diet in the community for obesity, ischaemic heart disease or diabetes. *Nutr Diabetes* 2017; 7(3): e256. doi: 10.1038/nutd.2017.3
27. Lai JS, Hiles S, Hure AJ, McEvoy M, Attia J. Systematic review and meta-analysis of dietary patterns and depression in commutiy-dwelling adults. *Am J Clin Nutr* 2014; 99(1): 181-197. doi: 10.3945/ajcn.113.069880
28. Sarris J, Murphy J, Mischoulon D, Papakostas GI, Fava M, Berk M, et al. Adjunctive nutraceuticals for depression: A systematic review and meta-analyses. *American Journal of Psychiatry* 2016; 173(6): 575-587. doi: 10.1176/appi.ajp.2016.15091228
29. Muscaritoli M. The Impact of Nutrients on Mental Health and Well-Being: Insights From the Literature. *Frontiers in Nutrition* 2021; 8: 656290. doi: 10.3389/fnut.2021.656290
30. Deane KHO, Jimoh OF, Biswas P, O'Brien A, Hanson S, Abdelhamid AS, et al. Omega-3 and polyunsaturated fat for prevention of depression and anxiety symptoms: Systematic review and meta-analysis of randomised trials. British Journal of Psychiatry 2021; 218(3): 135-142. doi: 10.1192/bjp.2019.234
31. Xu Y, Zeng L, Zou K, Shan S, Wang X, Xiong J, et al. Role of dietary factors in the prevention and treatment for depression: an umbrella review of meta-analyses of prospective studies. *Translational Psychiatry* 2021; 11(1): 478. doi: 10.1038/s41398-021-01590-6
32. Welch AA, Shakya-Shrestha S, Lentjes MAH, Wareham NJ, Khaw KT. Dietary intake and status of n-3 polyunsaturated fatty acids in a population of fish-eating and non-fish-eating meat-eaters, vegetarians, and vegans and the precursor-product ratio of α-linolenic acid to long-chain n-3 polyunsaturated fatty acids: results from the EPIC-Norfolk cohort. *Am J Clin Nutr* 2010; 92(5): 1040-1051. doi: 10.3945/ajcn.2010.29457
33. Ocean N, Howley P, Ensor J. Lettuce be happy: A longitudinal UK study on the relationship between fruit and vegetable consumption and well-being. *Soc Sci Med* 2019; 222: 335-345. doi: 10.1016/j.socscimed.2018.12.017
34. Conner TS, Brookie KL, Carr AC, Mainvil LA, Vissers MCM. Let them eat fruit! the effect of fruit and vegetable consumption on psychological well-being in young adults: A randomized controlled trial. *PLoS One* 2017;12(2): e0171206. doi: 10.1371/journal.pone.0171206
35. Brookie KL, Best GI, Conner TS. Intake of raw fruits and vegetables is associated with better mental health than intake of processed fruits and vegetables. *Front Psychol* 2018; 9: 487. doi: 10.3389/fpsyg.2018.00487
36. Mujcic R, Oswald AJ. Evolution of well-being and happiness after increases in consumption of fruit and vegetables. *Am J Public Health* 2016; 106(8): 1504-1510. doi: 10.2105/AJPH.2016.303260
37. Guzek D, Głąbska D, Groele B, Gutkowska K. Fruit and Vegetable Dietary Patterns and Mental Health in Women: A Systematic Review. *Nutr Rev* 2021; 1-14. doi: 10.1093/nutrit/nuab007
38. Rees J, Bagatini SR, Lo J, Hodgson JM, Christophersen CT, Daly RM, et al. Association between Fruit and Vegetable Intakes and Mental Health in the Australian Diabetes Obesity and Lifestyle Cohort. *Nutrients* 2021; 13(5): 1447. doi: 10.3390/nu13051447
39. Toumpanakis A, Turnbull T, Alba-Barba I. Effectiveness of plant-based diets in promoting well-being in the management of type 2 diabetes: A systematic review. *BMJ Open Diabetes Research and Care* 2018; 6(1). doi: 10.1136/bmjdrc-2018-000534

40. O'Neil A, Quirk SE, Housden S, Brennan SL, Williams LJ, Pasco JA, et al. Relationship between diet and mental health in children and adolescents: A systematic review. *American Journal of Public Health* 2014; 104(10): e31-42. doi: 10.2105/AJPH.2014.302110
41. Sutliffe JT, Carnot MJ, Fuhrman JH, Sutliffe CA, Scheid JC. A Worksite Nutrition Intervention is Effective at Improving Employee Well-Being: A Pilot Study. *Journal of Nutrition and Metabolism* 2018: 8187203. doi: 10.1155/2018/8187203
42. Lassale C, Batty GD, Baghdadli A, Jacka F, Sánchez-Villegas A, Kivimäki M, et al. Healthy dietary indices and risk of depressive outcomes: a systematic review and meta-analysis of observational studies. *Molecular Psychiatry* 2019; 24(7): 965-986. doi: 10.1038/s41380-018-0237-8
43. Molendijk M, Molero P, Ortuño Sánchez-Pedreño F, Van der Does W, Angel Martínez-González M. Diet quality and depression risk: A systematic review and dose-response meta-analysis of prospective studies. *Journal of Affective Disorders* 2018; 226: 346-354. doi: 10.1016/j.jad.2017.09.022
44. Akbaraly TN, Brunner EJ, Ferrie JE, Marmot MG, Kivimaki M, Singh-Manoux A. Dietary pattern and depressive symptoms in middle age. *Br J Psychiatry* 2009; 195(5): 408-413. doi: 10.1192/bjp.bp.108.058925
45. Nanri A, Mizoue T, Poudel-Tandukar K, Noda M, Kato M, Kurotani K, et al. Dietary patterns and suicide in Japanese adults: The Japan Public Health Center-based Prospective Study. *Br J Psychiatry* 2013; 203(6): 422-427. doi: 10.1192/bjp.bp.112.114793
46. Opie RS, Itsiopoulos C, Parletta N, Sanchez-Villegas A, Akbaraly TN, Ruusunen A, et al. Dietary recommendations for the prevention of depression. *Nutr Neurosci* 2017; 20(3): 161-171. doi: 10.1179/1476830515Y.0000000043
47. Firth J, Marx W, Dash S, Carney R, Teasdale SB, Solmi M, et al. The Effects of Dietary Improvement on Symptoms of Depression and Anxiety: A Meta-Analysis of Randomized Controlled Trials. *Psychosom Med* 2019; 81(3): 265-280. doi: 10.1097/PSY.0000000000000673
48. Parletta N, Zarnowiecki D, Cho J, Wilson A, Bogomolova S, Villani A, et al. A Mediterranean-style dietary intervention supplemented with fish oil improves diet quality and mental health in people with depression: A randomized controlled trial (HELFIMED). *Nutr Neurosci* 2019; 22(7): 474-487. doi: 10.1080/1028415X.2017.1411320
49. Francis HM, Stevenson RJ, Chambers JR, Gupta D, Newey B, Lim CK. A brief diet intervention can reduce symptoms of depression in young adults – A randomised controlled trial. *PLoS One* 2019; 14(10): e0222768. doi: 10.1371/journal.pone.0222768
50. Gangwisch JE, Hale L, Garcia L, Malaspina D, Opler MG, Payne ME, et al. High glycemic index diet as a risk factor for depression: Analyses from the Women's Health Initiative. *Am J Clin Nutr* 2015; 102(2): 454-463. doi: 10.3945/ajcn.114.103846
51. Agarwal U, Mishra S, Xu J, Levin S, Gonzales J, Barnard ND. A multicenter randomized controlled trial of a nutrition intervention program in a multiethnic adult population in the corporate setting reduces depression and anxiety and improves quality of life: The GEICO study. *Am J Heal Promot* 2015; 29(4): 245-254. doi: 10.4278/ajhp.130218-QUAN-72
52. Healthy Active Lives (HeAL). Available from: www.iphys.org.au
53. Shiers D, Rafi I, Cooper S, Holt R. Positive Cardiometabolic Health Resource: an intervention framework for patients with psychosis and schizophrenia. *R Coll Psychiatr* 2014; www.rcpsych.ac.uk/docs/default-source/improving-care/ccqi/national-clinical-audits/ncap-library/ncap-e-version-nice-endorsed-lester-uk-adaptation.pdf? (Accessed 15 June 2022)
54. Aucoin M, Lachance L, Cooley K, Kidd S. Diet and psychosis: A scoping review. *Neuropsychobiology* 2020; 79(1): 20-42. doi: 10.1159/000493399
55. Teasdale SB, Ward PB, Rosenbaum S, Samaras K, Stubbs B. Solving a weighty problem: Systematic review and meta-analysis of nutrition interventions in severe mental illness. *British Journal of Psychiatry* 2017; 210(2): 110-118. doi: 10.1192/bjp.bp.115.177139
56. Bauer IE, Gálvez JF, Hamilton JE, Balanzá-Martínez V, Zunta-Soares GB, Soares JC, et al. Lifestyle interventions targeting dietary habits and exercise in bipolar disorder: A systematic

review. *J Psychiatr Res* 2016; 74: 1-7. doi: 10.1016/j.jpsychires.2015.12.006

57. Le Bastard Q, Al-Ghalith GA, Grégoire M, Chapelet G, Javaudin F, Dailly E, et al. Systematic review: human gut dysbiosis induced by non-antibiotic prescription medications. *Alimentary Pharmacology and Therapeutics* 2018; 47(3): 332-345. doi: 10.1111/apt.14451

58. Bahr SM, Tyler BC, Wooldridge N, Butcher BD, Burns TL, Teesch LM, et al. Use of the second-generation antipsychotic, risperidone, and secondary weight gain are associated with an altered gut microbiota in children. *Transl Psychiatry* 2015; 5(10): e652. doi: 10.1038/tp.2015.135

59. Jha MK, Minhajuddin A, Gadad BS, Greer T, Grannemann B, Soyombo A, et al. Can C-reactive protein inform antidepressant medication selection in depressed outpatients? Findings from the CO-MED trial. *Psychoneuroendocrinology* 2017; 78: 105-113. doi: 10.1016/j.psyneuen.2017.01.023

60. Kent L, Morton D, Hurlow T, Rankin P, Hanna A, Diehl H. Long-term effectiveness of the community-based Complete Health Improvement Program (CHIP) lifestyle intervention: a cohort study. *BMJ Open* 2013; 3: e003751. doi:10.1136/bmjopen-2013-003751

61. Suganya, K.; Koo, B.-S. Gut–Brain Axis: Role of Gut Microbiota on Neurological Disorders and How Probiotics/Prebiotics Beneficially Modulate Microbial and Immune Pathways to Improve Brain Functions. *Int J Mol Sci* 2020; 21: 7551. doi: 10.3390/ijms21207551

Chapter 12
Plant-based nutrition for male and female health

Nitu Bajekal and Lisa Simon

Introduction

When discussing male and female health, there is no aspect that does not benefit from dietary and lifestyle changes. This applies to men and women of all ages and stages in their lives.

The average life expectancy for women in the UK is 83.1 years, with dementia and Alzheimer's disease being the biggest killer, followed by ischaemic heart disease. The average life expectancy for men is 79.3 years, with ischaemic heart disease being the biggest killer, followed by dementia and Alzheimer's disease.[36]

With this in mind, it is vital for both men and women to look after their physical and mental health, and each will benefit from adopting a fibre-rich, plant predominant way of eating, even when conventional Western medicine or surgical approaches are needed for particular conditions.

By the term 'men' and 'women', we wish to be inclusive, as people assigned male or female at birth may now identify as non-binary, intersex, and transgender people.

Women's health

Endometriosis

What is endometriosis?
Endometriosis is a chronic inflammatory oestrogen-dependent condition. Not much is known about the aetiology or risk factors, although there appears to be a familial link. Treatment approaches have often been unsatisfactory, yet a lifelong management plan is needed for many women who struggle with endometriosis.

Tissue similar to the endometrial lining that grows and bleeds with each menstrual cycle is found outside the uterus. These endometriotic deposits cause scarring, pelvic adhesions and ovarian chocolate cysts with symptoms that include painful and/or heavy periods, pelvic pain, painful sex, bowel involvement, urinary symptoms and infertility. Rarely, endometriosis can be found in distant places such as the lung, nose, or on caesarean section scars.

How common is endometriosis?
The actual prevalence of endometriosis is as yet unknown, since a laparoscopic diagnosis is

usually required.

The condition affects up to 15% of women of reproductive age and up to 70% of those with chronic pelvic pain.[1] It is more common in certain subgroups, with 20% of women being investigated for infertility or having a hysterectomy found to have endometriosis, compared to 1 in 20 women having a sterilisation. Increasing prevalence of endometriosis may be attributed to a combination of delayed childbirth, better diagnosis, environmental factors, pesticides and changes in diets.[2]

How is endometriosis diagnosed?
It takes an average of 6.7 years to diagnose endometriosis.[1] Diagnosis may be delayed because of overlap with irritable bowel syndrome or pelvic inflammatory disease.

A pelvic ultrasound or an MRI scan may be helpful to diagnose endometriomas, adenomyosis (deep internal endometriosis) and bigger endometriotic deposits. A laparoscopy remains the gold standard diagnostic test for endometriosis for now.

What are the available treatments for endometriosis?
Treatment depends on a number of factors including age, symptoms, fertility wishes, location and severity of disease. Medical treatment using hormonal medications are the most popular, as are pain killers (NSAIDS). Laparoscopic treatment of endometriosis can improve fertility, relieve pain and delay further invasive treatment. Extensive pelvic surgery and hysterectomy may need to be offered to some but are not without complications.

Can diet help with endometriosis?
There are no consistent dietary recommendations for prevention or treatment of endometriosis.[3] There is, however, growing evidence to suggest avoiding meat and eating a high fibre plant-based diet can help with the symptoms of endometriosis. Consumption of animal products has the potential to influence endometriosis risk through their effects on steroid hormones levels.

How do plant-based diets help with endometriosis?
Standard Western diets are associated with higher levels of oestradiol and lower levels of sex hormone binding globulin (SHBG). In contrast, plant-based diets tend to reduce blood oestrogen concentrations and increase SHBG concentration, effects that may be attributable to an increase in fibre intake, or the weight loss that typically results from these diet changes. Endometrial tissue can convert cholesterol to oestradiol, raising concerns about dietary cholesterol and saturated fat, which are almost exclusively found in animal derived products.

Adopting an anti-inflammatory, whole food plant-based diet, rich in vegetables, fruits, beans, whole grains, nuts, seeds, herbs and spices tends to improve symptoms. The higher fibre content of plant-based diets can lower oestrogen levels by increasing excretion and can also lower blood insulin levels. This is important due to insulin's agonistic effects for oestrogen production and endometrial cell proliferation.

Studies have shown a significant reduction in the risk of developing endometriosis with high intakes of green vegetables and fruit. Women consuming ≥1 servings of citrus fruits/day had a 22% lower endometriosis risk. Women having 13 or more servings per week of green leafy vegetables had a 70% lower risk of endometriosis compared with those who ate fewer than six servings per week. Those eating 14 or more servings of fruit, especially citrus fruit (rich in beta cryptoxanthin) per week had a 20% lower risk compared with women having fewer than six servings per week.[4,5]

Soya, green tea, turmeric, seaweed, omega-3 fatty acids can all help as part of a healthy varied phytonutrient-rich diet and promotes a healthy gut microbiome.[3,6]

However, care should be taken to not consume seaweed regularly due to the variable amounts of iodine contained therein, which can have deleterious effects on the thyroid, particularly in those with underlying disease. Curcumin in turmeric may have an effect by inhibiting angiogenesis in endometriosis.[6, 7] Phytoestrogens are able to interact with oestrogen receptors, either with oestrogenic or anti-oestrogenic effect. Soya food consumption and perhaps milled flaxseed powder through the same phytoestrogen mechanism can minimise the risk of endometriosis. In a case control study, Japanese women with a higher urinary concentration of daidzein and genistein, two isoflavones in soya, were found to have the lowest risk of severe endometriosis.[8]

A large study with 12 years of prospective data (n=70,709) found a relatively strong association between endometriosis and trans-fatty acid consumption, and a lower risk of endometriosis with increased consumption of long-chain omega-3 fatty acids.[9] Dietary sources include chia, flax and hemp seed and their oils, and walnuts. Green, leafy vegetables, soya, and avocadoes contain much smaller quantities, but if eaten regularly can make useful contributions.

The link between meat and endometriosis

There is an increased risk of endometriosis with intakes of beef or other red meat, or ham. The increased incidence of endometriosis in women consuming animal products may be attributed to the oxidative stress caused by the organic pollutants, haem iron found in red and processed meats, and other inflammatory compounds.

Yamamoto et al. published a prospective cohort study of meat and fish consumption and endometriosis risk. A total of 81,908 participants of the prospective Nurses' Health Study II were followed up from 1991 through 2013. Diet was assessed via food frequency questionnaire every four years. Women consuming >2 servings/d of red meat/d had a 56% higher risk of endometriosis compared to women having <1 serving/week. Even 2–4 servings per week elicited a modest increase in endometriosis risk. Processed red meat was also associated with higher risk. The effect of red meat was independent of animal fat or its most common saturated fatty acid, palmitic acid. Haem iron, a major component, may be responsible for the negative effects of red meat consumption. Poultry was associated with a rise in risk of endometriosis but the link was not as robust as for red meat.[10] The authors concluded from their analysis of premenopausal US nurses that red meat consumption may be an important modifiable risk factor for endometriosis, particularly among women with endometriosis who had not reported infertility and thus were more likely to present with pain symptoms.

Alcohol and other foods and supplements

A meta-analysis has suggested an association with greater alcohol intake with endometriosis, although it is unclear whether it exacerbates existing disease or is related to the severity of the condition.[11] A higher intake of dairy has been associated with a lower risk of endometriosis diagnosis,[12, 13] but it is unclear whether this is due to the vitamin D immunomodulator effect.[3] However, given the other negative effects of dairy on general health, this should ideally be replaced by plant milks, especially soya. In other studies, consumption of milk, liver, carrots, cheese, fish, olive oil, vegetable oils and whole-grain foods, as well as coffee consumption, were not significantly or consistently related to endometriosis.

What about complementary therapies for treating endometriosis?

Acupuncture, breathing techniques, yoga, acupressure, heat packs and regular exercise can all help with pain management. Herbal painkillers for the pelvis and abdomen can be used individually or in combination, such as Echinacea and medicinal fungi like cordyceps.[14] Certain herbal products such as *Agnus castus* (Chaste Berry) may help with premenstrual symptoms. Green tea, grape seed extract, pine bark and cocoa polyphenols (procyanidin being the active ingredient) may help with pain as part of a proper management plan, including surgery, chronic pain management and an anti-inflammatory diet. However, none of these have met rigorous testing standards.

No consistent recommendation can be made with regards to vitamins A, C, E supplements in reducing the risk of endometriosis.[3]

Recommendation
To see benefits for individual patients, a plant predominant diet along with lifestyle modifications should be advised, at least as a trial.[15] Simple dietary changes incorporating more whole plant foods may allow for the management of the complex condition of endometriosis alongside conventional treatments and provides a compelling case for women of reproductive age to re-evaluate their dietary habits for the prevention of this distressing condition.[16]

Fibroids

What are the symptoms and risk factors for fibroids?
Fibroids or uterine leiomyomas are oestrogen-dependent smooth muscle tumours, affecting at least 50% of women of reproductive age. Fibroids are associated with severe reproductive morbidity and are the primary indication for hysterectomy worldwide. They are almost always benign and cause symptoms depending on their location. Some women may have no symptoms from their fibroids, but a significant number will suffer from a range of complaints including heavy and/or painful periods, irregular bleeding, pelvic mass, pressure symptoms, pelvic pain, infertility, recurrent miscarriages and pregnancy complications. Fibroids tend to shrink with menopause due to falling levels of oestrogen.

Higher levels of oestrogen found in women with excess body weight increase the risk of fibroids. Nulliparity, a sedentary lifestyle and hypertension are associated with an increased risk of myomas. There appears to be a familial link and there are racial differences, with Black and Asian women found to have fibroids more often. There appears to be a link between a history of physical or sexual abuse and fibroids, especially in Black patients.[17]

How can diet influence fibroids?
Women eating a diet high in red and processed meat and low in fibre rich foods such as fruits and vegetables have an increased incidence of fibroids. This is thought to be partly because of the lack of fibre that binds oestrogen in the gut. Red meat has been shown in studies to promote the growth of fibroids, due to mammalian hormones and saturated fats. Significant consumption of beef and other red meats (1.7-fold) or ham (1.3-fold) is associated with an increased relative risk of fibroids and consumption of green vegetables (0.5-fold) and fruit (especially citrus fruit) with a decreased risk.[18, 19]

Intake of fish was found to be associated with an increased risk of fibroids. It was unclear as to whether persistent environmental pollutants or the marine fatty acids were driving the association. This was the conclusion from a five-year prospective cohort study of premenopausal Black women undergoing serial pelvic ultrasound, although similar effects have been in seen in White women in smaller studies.[20]

Soya intake does not appear to increase risk and may be protective for fibroids, by virtue of its phytoestrogens, although flaxseeds, whole grains and green tea may be better at shrinking overall size.[21, 22]

There is some evidence to suggest adequate vitamin D levels is associated with a reduced risk of uterine fibroids.[23] In a review article of current data, vitamins A and D deserve mention. No firm recommendations can be made regarding vitamins B3, C, and E.[24]

Alcohol appears to increase the risk for fibroids.

In US Black women, risk of uterine leiomyomata was positively associated with current consumption of alcohol, particularly beer.[25] This risk is positively correlated with the number of years of alcohol intake and specifically with beer consumption. Compared with women who abstained from alcohol, those who drank one or more beers per day had a greater than 50% increased risk for fibroids. Cigarette smoking and caffeine consumption were unrelated to risk overall.

Recommendation
Given the available evidence, eating a diet packed with fibre-rich fruit, green leafy vegetables and whole grains, while consuming green tea and avoiding alcohol, fish, red and processed meat appear to be sensible strategies for managing fibroids alongside medical management where indicated.

Heavy and painful periods

Menstrual symptoms including pain, heavy bleeding and low mood may be linked to nearly nine days of lost productivity per woman every year.[26]

Heavy menstrual bleeding (HMB)
Periods are considered heavy if they interfere with daily life, last longer than seven days, are associated with clots or flooding, or come more frequently (normal range of the menstrual cycle is 24–35 days). The medical criterion of blood loss of >80 ml is rarely used.

Fibroids, endometriosis, adenomyosis, endometrial polyps, pelvic inflammatory disease (PID) and PCOS are common causes of heavy periods and more uncommonly, endometrial or cervical cancer, bleeding disorders or thyroid dysfunction. Investigation with blood tests, appropriate imaging techniques (pelvic ultrasound, MRI) and diagnostic procedures such as laparoscopy or hysteroscopy may be needed to arrive at a diagnosis. Dysfunctional uterine bleeding (DUB) is the terminology used when no underlying cause is found after appropriate investigations. Treatment of heavy periods with pharmacotherapy (e.g., hormonal, NSAIDS) or surgery depends on the underlying cause and has a high success rate.

Dysmenorrhoea
Primary dysmenorrhoea refers to painful periods with no underlying cause. The release of prostaglandins from the endometrial lining as it sheds is responsible for pain and the other symptoms such as nausea, bowel upsets and headache often noticed during periods. Secondary dysmenorrhoea refers to period pain that has an underlying cause such as endometriosis, adenomyosis, PID or fibroids. Many of these women have both heavy and painful periods. Treatment depends upon the underlying cause in secondary dysmenorrhoea along with pain management, while primary dysmenorrhoea is usually treated with NSAID pain killers or hormonal medication.

Management of heavy and painful periods through diet and lifestyle
A fibre-rich, plant-based diet can help with period pains and also with heavy periods. The anti-inflammatory nature of the diet has positive effects on arachidonic acid and prostaglandin synthesis, which in turn is intimately related to both the flow and pain of menstruation.

A low-fat vegetarian diet was associated with increased serum sex-hormone binding globulin concentration and reductions in body weight, dysmenorrhea duration and intensity, as well as premenstrual symptom duration in a crossover study by Barnard et al. The symptom effects might be mediated by dietary influences on oestrogen activity.[27]

Vitamin D helps with the absorption of calcium, the lack of which can increase menstrual cramps.[28] Ensuring satisfactory levels of vitamin

D is important. There is no indication or benefit to taking calcium or magnesium supplements. Instead, it is better to suggest increasing the intake of foods naturally rich in calcium such as sesame seeds, soya, figs, beans, almonds and green leafy vegetables.

Ginger is a spice with anti-inflammatory properties that has a beneficial effect on the menstrual cycle, most likely from its action on prostaglandin synthesis and on inflammatory leukotrienes. Ginger can help with reducing period pain.[29] Treatment of primary dysmenorrhea in 120 students in a randomised controlled trial with ginger for five days had a statistically significant effect on relieving intensity and duration of pain.[30] Ginger may also be helpful for heavy periods.[31]

Chamomile tea possesses anti-spasmodic properties, which can relieve the painful cramps associated with the menstrual periods.[32] Vitamins E, D, B1, B6 can be helpful in reducing primary dysmenorrhea,[33] but studies with herbal supplements in general were found to be of low quality and cannot be routinely recommended.[34]

It is important to address iron deficiency anaemia caused by heavy periods with both iron supplementation and a plant-based diet. Green leafy vegetables, beans, lentils, tofu, nuts, blackstrap molasses and apricots will help to keep iron levels up. Vitamin C-rich foods such as oranges, sweet peppers and broccoli help to increase iron absorption while germination of grains and legumes improves the bioavailability of non-haem iron.

Lifestyle advice
Regular exercise, use of heat or cold treatment, yoga, acupuncture and acupressure have been shown to be helpful in reducing painful periods. It is important to also address the other lifestyle pillars, including stress management, the avoidance of toxic substances, and forming and maintaining healthy relationships.

Recommendation
Heavy or painful periods from any cause can benefit from a plant-based diet alongside medical treatment. Vitamin D levels need to be adequate as do iron levels. It is recommended these are checked as baseline. Ginger can help with painful and heavy periods and may be as effective as NSAIDs, offering an alternative to those who do not wish to take or can't tolerate these medications.

Menopause

Understanding menopause
Menopause is defined as the absence of periods for at least one year from the last menstrual period, with an average age of menopause at 51 years (45–55 years) all around the world. Ovarian follicular depletion below a critical level results in a marked decrease in oestrogen levels and raised follicle stimulating hormone levels. Low levels of oestrogen are thought to trigger menopausal symptoms. Approximately 85% of women experience hot flushes during perimenopause and early menopause, however, only 25% ever seek intervention, the reasons for this low number are unclear.[35]

The perimenopause is the lead up to menopause and usually lasts four years (2–8 years) with an average age of 47 years (39–51 years). It is defined as the transition from normal ovulatory menstrual cycles to cessation of ovulation and menstruation; usually a gradual change unless there is a surgical or medical menopause. The ovaries start to fail, and hormonal fluctuations can cause perimenopausal symptoms and menstrual irregularities until the periods finally stop.

Symptoms of the menopause
The most common symptoms of menopause are hot flushes. Other troublesome symptoms include night sweats, sleep disturbances, mood swings, fatigue, depression, memory loss, osteoporosis, urinary and bowel symptoms, reduced sex drive

and vaginal dryness. Symptoms can last longer than expected with 50% of all women reporting vasomotor symptoms four years after the final menstrual period, and 10% still suffering as far as 12 years later.[37]

Menopausal symptoms appear to be significantly less common in Asia, a difference that is possibly attributed to lifestyle factors, including diet. A high-fat, low-fibre animal-based diet in the West seems to negatively affect oestrogen levels. Risk factors that predict severity of menopausal symptoms include smoking, race, lower socioeconomic status, low calcium intake and BMI, with higher BMI's correlating with more severe symptoms.[38, 39, 40, 41]

Management of menopause
Medical treatment
While oestrogen is the most effective treatment available for relief of menopausal symptoms, not everyone wishes to take menopausal hormone therapy (MHT, MT, HRT). Some may have contraindications to taking hormone replacement, including a previous history of cancer or thrombosis.

Lifestyle advice
Lifestyle measures have significant benefits and should be offered to all women, even if they choose MHT. The earlier these measures are put in place, the more noticeable the benefits, but it is never too late. Please refer to the detailed discussion on the six lifestyle pillars in Chapter 19.

Weight loss
In a study of more than 17,000 women with baseline vasomotor symptoms, those who lost 10% or more of their baseline weight were significantly more likely to experience elimination of their symptoms compared with women who did not lose weight. These women also had reductions in serum cholesterol, oestrogen levels and mammographic densities.[41] A beneficial effect of a low-fat diet on menopausal symptoms has not been established in large controlled clinical trials.

Plant-based diets in menopause
Whole plant food intake was associated with fewer menopausal symptoms in Chinese postmenopausal women with pre-hypertension or untreated hypertension.[42] Vegans reported less bothersome vasomotor and physical menopausal symptoms than omnivores. Eating a plant-based diet may be helpful for women in menopausal transition who prefer a natural means to manage their symptoms.[43] There appears to be a positive impact of vegetable and fruit intake on menopausal symptoms. In contrast, sweets, liquid oils, solid fats and ultra-processed snacks correlated to an increased risk of these symptoms.[44]

A small but significant RCT over a 12-week period by Barnard et al. in 2021 found the combination of a low-fat, vegan diet and whole soyabeans was associated with reduced frequency and severity of hot flashes and improved quality of life in vasomotor, psychosocial, physical, and sexual domains in postmenopausal women.[45]

Phytoestrogens are plant substances that have weak but similar effects to oestrogens in some tissues and blocking effects in others (selective estrogen receptor modulators, or SERM effect). Phytoestrogens appear to reduce the frequency of hot flushes in menopausal women, without serious side-effects.[46]

The most important groups are called isoflavones and lignans. The major isoflavones genistein and daidzein, found in soya beans, chickpeas, red clover, legumes, and beans help with bone health and menopausal symptoms. The major lignans enterolactone and enterodiol, found in flaxseed, whole cereals, fruit, and cereal bran help with lowering breast cancer risk in postmenopausal women.[47, 48]

The role of soya in menopause
Southeast Asian women report a lower prevalence

(15% vs 85%) of hot flushes compared to their Western counterparts. This has been attributed to the higher consumption of soya, although cultural influences, social status often increasing with age, and positive attitudes about menopause and aging may be other factors.[49] Almost all studies have used isolated soya isoflavones which is why there is a wide variation in results in animal in vitro versus epidemiologic studies.[50] The amount of genistein (a main soya isoflavone) appeared as a critical variable in these results.[51] Despite these limitations, the evidence favours the use of isoflavones due to their safety profile and benefit to overall health.[52] Soya foods should not be considered as endocrine disruptors as detailed in a technical review of the available observational and clinical data.[53]

Soya products should be included due to their cardiovascular benefits and potential efficacy for treating certain menopausal symptoms. A meta-analysis of controlled clinical trials in non-Asian women supplemented with soya isoflavones found significant reductions in body weight, fasting glucose, and fasting insulin when compared with placebo.[54]

Whole or minimally processed soya foods should be recommended over isolated soya isoflavones where possible, as these natural soya foods are a composite of intricate biologically active molecules. Minimally processed products such as edamame, tempeh, tofu and soya milk are to be preferred over processed soya foods. Soya is an excellent substitute for animal sources of protein, with all nine essential amino acids being in a similar proportion to egg white.

As part of a varied and diverse plant-based diet, two to four portions of minimally processed soya are recommended, unless one is allergic. A handful (80 g) of tofu, tempeh, edamame beans or a cup (200 mls) of soya milk counts as one portion. The benefits of soya appear to relate to traditional soya products and not to concentrated soya proteins, as soya protein isolates may increase insulin-like growth factor-1 (IGF-1) similar to animal protein.[55]

Soya is not a contraindication in those with thyroid problems but a gap of a couple of hours between soya intake and thyroid medications is recommended. Ensuring adequate iodine intake is also important for all (150 mcg daily) as British diets are generally lacking in iodine. If taking a supplement, this should be in the form of potassium iodate or iodide and not kelp derived, due to the potentially high iodine content in some seaweeds.

Alternative medicine
Red clover (*Trifolium pretense*) contains isoflavones and has been shown in a systematic review and meta-analysis to help with hot flushes.[56] Based on available evidence and lack of standardisation, other natural supplements and bioidentical hormones are not recommended. Hypnosis for hot flushes[57] and cognitive behavioural therapy for insomnia has shown some benefit.[58]

Recommendation
To help with menopausal symptoms, women should be encouraged to incorporate a healthy plant-based diet with regular soya intake from an early age when possible. The importance of maintaining a healthy body weight, a good sleep routine and regular strength exercises should be stressed for managing menopause (see Chapter 19).

Polycystic ovary syndrome (PCOS)

What is PCOS?
PCOS is a complex condition that affects the way the ovaries' function, resulting in a wide range of reproductive, metabolic, and psychological symptoms. The exact cause of PCOS is unknown, although insulin resistance is considered to be responsible for many of the symptoms. Genetic and environmental factors interact with each

other, resulting in a heterogeneous condition that presents with diverse clinical manifestations.[59]

PCOS is the most common endocrine condition affecting women of reproductive age and is a significant public health issue. At least 1 in 10 of women all over the world have the clinical condition of PCOS, with up to 70% of affected women remaining undiagnosed.[60] Presentation varies by ethnicity, and in high-risk populations prevalence and complications are higher.[61] There is a familial link with PCOS.[62]

PCOS is affected by lifestyle factors and diet, which in turn influence body weight, insulin resistance, inflammation, oxidative stress and androgen activity.[63] PCOS is a chronic condition so while there is no 'cure', making positive lifestyle changes especially through nutrition and exercise can go a very long way in managing PCOS and its symptoms, both in the short term and longer term. Lifestyle management helps by making tissues sensitive to the action of insulin again, so insulin levels drop and as a result androgen levels drop too. Even where weight loss is not needed, lifestyle modifications help by improving insulin resistance.[64]

Symptoms of PCOS
PCOS often starts in the teenage years and has long-term effects beyond the menopause, increasing risks of type 2 diabetes, metabolic syndrome, endometrial cancer and heart disease, especially in the presence of excess weight. While PCOS is the most common cause of infertility in women, PCOS has many consequences for women that go beyond this.[65]

Anovulatory menstrual irregularities such as infrequent or missed periods are the most common symptoms, while signs of androgen excess such as hirsutism, alopecia and adult acne tend to be the most distressing as well unwanted weight gain. Sleep disturbances, mood disorders, acanthosis nigricans and disordered eating are some of the less recognised symptoms of the condition.[66] Miscarriage, gestational diabetes and adverse pregnancy outcomes are associated with PCOS.[67]

Medical management of PCOS
Women with PCOS present with a wide range of symptoms that span many health disciplines, resulting in fragmented and disjointed medical advice and treatment. Diagnosis and treatment of PCOS remains controversial with several challenges. Lifestyle intervention for prevention or management of excess weight, education, self-empowerment and multidisciplinary care are important.[65]

Diagnosis is based on clinical history, biochemical tests and a pelvic ultrasound scan using the tightened 2003 Rotterdam PCOS criteria.[68]

Management options for PCOS, apart from dietary advice, include the use of hormonal medications, insulin-sensitising agents, fertility treatment and laparoscopic ovarian drilling. Treatment must be individualised and monitored carefully.

Lifestyle advice in PCOS
Lifestyle changes should be the first line of treatment to manage PCOS and its symptoms, both in the short term and longer term. Alongside dietary recommendations, it is important to include lifestyle interventions such as behavioural strategies. Addressing the other lifestyle pillars will help with successful management of the condition (see Chapter 19).

Weight loss
Lifestyle changes can help to reduce insulin resistance, the main driver of PCOS in 50–70% of cases and can restore hormonal balance. Weight loss where indicated, through diet, exercise and behavioural changes should be the first line of therapy and can help with all symptoms of PCOS. Losing as little as 5%–10% of body weight can see a return in normal ovulatory cycles and improved pregnancy rates. Weight loss results in a decrease

in serum androgen concentrations, increases in sex hormone binding globulin (SHBG) and, in some, improvements in hirsutism. Responsiveness to weight loss in women with PCOS who are overweight or obese varies considerably and more than one third of women may achieve full recovery.[64]

Benefits of a whole food plant-based diet in PCOS

Given that there is agreement that insulin resistance is the main driver behind PCOS and in the absence of clear-cut evidence and guidance for a particular diet strategy for the successful management of PCOS, it would be prudent and sensible to advise women to focus on a predominantly whole food plant-based way of eating, with or without weight loss intentions. This way of eating is healthy and can help achieve sustainable long-term weight loss where needed.[69, 70]

This fibre rich diet helps promote healthy gut bacteria, lowers inflammatory markers and oxidative stress, encourages excretion of excess circulating oestrogen, improves lipid profiles and normalises blood sugars. By reducing insulin resistance, androgen levels are lowered with an improvement in symptoms. Increased fibre and reduced trans fatty acid intake are primary predictors of metabolic improvement in women with PCOS who are overweight.[71]

Eating a varied diet with regular soya intake has been shown to lead to significant decreases in body weight, waist circumference, insulin, insulin resistance, blood sugar, and triglycerides. It also helps counteract hormone disruption.[72]

Women with PCOS also tend to have higher levels of AGEs (advanced glycation end products or glycotoxins) and AGE receptors in the ovaries. High AGE levels have been found in lean women with PCOS as well.[73] Diets low in AGEs reduce inflammation and insulin resistance in women with PCOS with examples of low AGE foods including whole grains, legumes, vegetables, mushrooms and fruits. High AGE foods include meat, chicken, cheese, butter, cream cheese, and processed snack foods. Cigarette smoking increases harmful glycotoxins. Dietary AGE intake can be decreased by changing the method of cooking from high temperature dry cooking to low heat, higher humidity methods.

Medical nutrition therapy

As there is a higher risk of eating disorders and disordered eating in people with PCOS, restrictive diets such as low carbohydrate diets or low-fat diets potentially can be triggering for some, even if they achieve the weight loss goal. Even a plant-based way of eating, if not explained correctly may hinder management if underlying mental health issues and eating disorders are not explored or addressed. Proper medical nutrition planning by qualified dietitians and nutritionists with a special interest in PCOS can be invaluable. Medical nutrition therapy (MNT) can help women with PCOS make and maintain the lifestyle changes needed to help reduce symptoms and prevent complications.

The role of supplements in women with PCOS

Vitamin D deficiency is common in women with PCOS, and there is some evidence that vitamin D supplementation after an initial blood test to measure levels, may improve reproductive function and insulin sensitivity.

A dietary supplement with at least the minimum intake of the trace mineral chromium (RDA 25 mcg/day) may be helpful in improving the chances of ovulation and reduce hirsutism.[70]

One of the key ingredients in a diet that emphasises whole grain intake, legumes and nuts in place of refined carbohydrates is inositol hexaphosphate. In clinical trials, inositol has been shown to improve insulin action, decrease androgen levels, and improve ovulatory function in both lean and obese women with PCOS.

The benefits of metformin in PCOS appear at

least partly due to increasing inositol availability. Myoinositol with folic acid for 3–6 months has shown some promising results in helping women ovulate and is thought to work by reducing testosterone/insulin levels, although it cannot yet be routinely recommended.[65]

Based on current evidence, omega-3 fatty acid supplementation may be recommended for the treatment of PCOS with insulin resistance, as well as high total cholesterol (especially LDL-cholesterol) and triglycerides.[74] Long term benefits beyond six months of treatment remain unknown. As previously mentioned, walnuts, chia, hemp, and flax seed powder contain good amounts of omega-3, but conversion rate to the active compounds may vary.

Recommendation
Management and treatment are based on individual patient needs, and combines lifestyle changes and advice, with or without medications. A nutrient dense, whole food plant-based diet rich in fibre and low in AGE's can be particularly beneficial for all symptoms of PCOS.

Men's health

Male-specific health problems, especially those relating to sexual function, are not as widely discussed as women's health, and sadly this leads to many men suffering in silence, with likely negative consequences on relationships and mental health. This section will discuss erectile dysfunction and how plant-based diets and lifestyle modifications can be used both as a preventative measure and as a key part of treatment.

Erectile dysfunction

What is erectile dysfunction (ED)?
ED is the inability to achieve or maintain an erection sufficient for 'satisfactory sexual intercourse'. It most commonly occurs between the ages of 40–70, with increased age predicting increased occurrence.[75]

ED is frequently a warning sign for atherosclerotic cardiovascular disease (CVD), typically manifesting 3–5 years before a CVD event,[75] and as such it has been labelled 'a symptom and not a disease'.[76] A prospective cohort study (n=1913), of men aged 40–79 in Europe, looking at the interrelationships between sex steroids and sexual symptoms with all-cause mortality, found that men with ED had a 1.4 times increased risk of mortality.[77]

Can diet and lifestyle modifications reduce risk factors?
There are a number of modifiable lifestyle risk factors, including poor diets, stress, lack of physical activity, smoking, and excessive alcohol consumption, and it is vital that positive changes are made to prevent chronic disease burden. However, although ED may be the first signs of impending CV disease, unlike CV where lifestyle interventions are known to lower risk, it is currently unclear whether such interventions are associated with a reduced risk of ED.[78] Nevertheless, as ED can signal an increased risk of future atherosclerotic CV events, it makes sense for the focus to be on lifestyle interventions, including positive dietary changes, to improve outcomes.

Nitric oxide (NO) plays a key role in the relaxation/erection of penile smooth muscle, and exerts antioxidant, anti-inflammatory and vasodilatory effects on vessel walls.[75] Consuming a plant-based diet high in nitrates provides a source of NO, with foods such as berries, pomegranates, oranges, walnuts, and leafy greens being among the best sources. Other vegetables also contain nitrates, and if eaten regularly, can make useful contributions. The body loses its ability to both produce and utilise NO as it ages, so it is beneficial to try and include regular plant-bases sources of nitrates as early as possible.[79]

The bioavailability of NO has been shown to increase with the consumption of plant-based foods high in polyphenolic compounds, and that by consuming more plant-based foods, the number of endothelial progenitor cells may increase, thereby exerting positive effects on endothelial, cardiovascular and erectile function. In addition, due to their high levels of antioxidants, plant-based foods are protective against reactive oxygen species (ROS), and by consuming these plants, the bioavailability of NO remains consistent. In contrast, the consumption of animal products promotes ROS via the inflammatory effects of compounds including haem-iron, AGEs, and animal-derived nitrates, thereby worsening erectile function. This is due to ROS reducing the bioavailability of NO and reducing endothelial cell function.[80, 81]

A large cross-sectional study looking at men with diabetes, just over a quarter of whom had already been diagnosed with ED, or were symptomatic, found that each daily serving of fruits or vegetables was associated with a 10% reduced self-reported incidence of ED.[82] Furthermore, data from a prospective cohort study (n=25,096) supported a link between dietary components and ED, with those consuming higher fruit intakes having a 14% reduction in risk of ED. The authors suggested this was due to the anthocyanin and flavone content of the fruit.[83]

Esposito et al. conducted an RCT, looking at the effects of a Mediterranean-style diet (rich in wholegrains, fruit, vegetables, legumes, walnuts and olive oil) on men with metabolic syndrome.[84] Endothelial function and inflammatory markers improved in the group following the diet, whereas there was no change in the control group. Furthermore, 11 men from the intervention group regained normal sexual function, compared to only two in the intervention group. Although these results are encouraging, larger, high quality RCT's are needed to determine the effects of dietary patterns on preventing or treating ED. Until that data is available, men should be advised that they are at higher risk of developing ED if they have a low adherence to healthy dietary patterns than men who adhere.[78]

A 14-week RCT looking at the effects of 60 g/day mixed nut supplementation, alongside a typical Western-style diet on erectile and sexual function, found a significant increase in the orgasmic function and sexual desire of men in the intervention group, compared with those who did not consume nuts, however, there was no significant difference in erectile function.[85] Limitations of the study included the healthy, fertile subjects, and that 60 g nuts alone may not have been sufficient to overcome the potential negative effects of a Western diet on erectile function.

There have been concerns raised about the potential feminising effects of soya. However, a 2010 meta-analysis found that neither isoflavone supplements nor soya foods alter free or circulating testosterone concentrations or have any effects on SHBG or free androgen index in men.[86] A more recent meta-analysis also found that regardless of dose and study duration, neither soya protein nor isoflavone exposure affects hormone levels in men.[87]

The role of the gut microbiome
Unlike animal products, plant-based foods provide fibre, and this is essential to promote a healthy, diverse gut microbiome through the production of short-chain fatty acids, such as butyrate and acetate. They also increase the growth of anti-inflammatory species while suppressing inflammatory species. In contrast, animal proteins such as red meat, dairy, and eggs, contain the amino acid, L-carnitine, and choline, both of which result in the gut bacterial production of trimethylamine N-oxide (TMAO). Increased TMAO is associated with an increased risk of vascular and peripheral artery disease, therefore it can be surmised that it also increases the risk of ED.[88]

Recommendation

Although there have been no published clinical trials to determine whether a WFPBD can help with erectile dysfunction, current data suggests that for healthy weight men, a mostly plant-based, Mediterranean-style diet should be encouraged. Recent research where the authors looked at participants from the National Health and Nutrition Examination Survey to evaluate the association between plant-based diets and ED gives strength to this, with a healthful plant-based diet index (hPDI) being associated with a reduced risk of ED.[89] The authors observed a dose-response relationship, where with every unit increase in hPDI there was a decrease in the risk of ED.

For men who are overweight/obese, a reduced calorie diet, alongside significant intakes of fruit and vegetables, and including legumes, nuts and fish has been shown to reduce risk. However, a clinical trial has been approved to look specifically at the effects of a WFPBD on sexual function, and the results are much anticipated.[75]

Male and female fertility

When it comes to discussing fertility, it is vital to include both partners, if that is applicable, in the conversation. This section discusses key nutrients needed for both men and women in order to optimise egg and sperm quality, and support implantation.

What is infertility?

The World Health Organization (WHO) defines infertility as 'a disease of the reproductive system defined by the failure to achieve a clinical pregnancy after 12 months or more of regular, unprotected sexual intercourse'. Infertility affects up to one in seven couples in the UK, and it is imperative that health care professionals (HCPs) understand the importance of implementing positive diet and lifestyle changes during the preconception period in order to improve chances of conception. As male infertility affects up to one third of couples, it is vital that both partners optimise their nutritional status prior to conception.

How can plant-based diets help to optimise fertility?

The ever-growing awareness of the importance of nutrition on preconception health is reflected in the growing academic literature, with *The Lancet* publishing a series of papers in 2018 suggesting context-specific interventions for pre-conception health.[90] These detail and recommend the role of HCPs in promoting pre-conception interventions, including supplementation and food fortification, to improve both parental nutritional status and long-term outcomes for mother and baby.

Fats

There is evidence to suggest that women who consume diets higher in monounsaturated fat have higher fertility rates.[91] In addition, higher intakes of plant proteins and non-haem iron are associated with lower rates of ovulation infertility (OI).[92] For men, diets rich in anti-inflammatory omega-3 fatty acids have been shown to improve sperm health, quality and motility, whereas high intakes of saturated and trans fats adversely affect sperm quality.[93]

There is a body of evidence suggesting that eating more plant sources of protein and less animal sources may help improve ovulatory infertility. An observational study of 18,555 women observed that intakes of plant protein reduced risk of OI by 50%,[92] and a systematic review found that whilst poorly-planned vegan and vegetarian diets carry an increased risk of vitamin and mineral deficiencies, well-planned, plant-based diets are protective against poor pregnancy outcomes and pre-term delivery.[94]

Vitamin D
Accumulating data suggests that vitamin D may be important for fertility, with receptors located in the ovaries, placenta and endometrium, as well as in testicles and sperm, with a recent meta-analysis concluding that adequate serum vitamin D levels are associated with more positive pregnancy tests, clinical pregnancies and live births in women undergoing artificial reproductive technology (ART). However, there is no association between miscarriage and vitamin D status.[95] There is a gap in the current literature for more RCT's specifically designed to assess vitamin D status and outcomes of ART. In men, vitamin D deficiency has been shown in observational studies to be associated with low serum testosterone concentrations and poor semen quality, including reduced sperm number, movement and morphology. However, RCT's have not shown improvements following supplementation.[96]

Folate and folic acid
The link between folate deficiency in women and the risk of neural tube defects (NTDs) is well documented. The guidelines for women who are trying to conceive are a daily supplement of 400 mcg of folic acid, although some women who are at an increased risk of having a pregnancy affected by neural tube defects (e.g., diabetes, previous neural tube defects in pregnancy) may benefit from a higher dose of 5 mg.[97]

Folate is also an important nutrient in terms of male fertility as it is needed for the synthesis of DNA in sperm.[98] When consuming a varied, plant-based diet, folate intakes will be high. However, this does not negate the need for a folic acid supplement, as factors such as morning sickness, variable folate content of fruit and vegetables, and cooking methods may mean that folate intakes are not sufficient to help prevent NTDs.

Zinc
Zinc is important for male and female fertility, in men as it is required for spermatogenesis and motility and in women as it plays a role in hormone balance and ovulation.[99] Dietary sources include wholegrains, nuts, seeds, especially sesame seeds, and beans. As men lose zinc in each ejaculate, their requirements are slightly higher than women (9.5 mg vs 7 mg) and they should be encouraged to consume adequate sources daily.

Iodine
Iodine is essential in the production of thyroid hormones which are vital for adequate brain and neurological development. Iodine is seen as a key nutrient for the first 1000 days of life: from conception to just before the child's second birthday, and deficiency or excess may lead to thyroid disorders which then impact further on fertility.

In men, thyroid hormones affect reproductive function by altering serum testosterone levels and the regulation components of semen such as calcium, zinc and magnesium. Low or deficient iodine levels have been associated with lower semen concentration and longer duration of time to pregnancy compared to men with optimum levels. Additionally, excessive intakes have also been linked to decreasing semen quality parameters.[100]

In women, it is important that iodine stores are sufficient prior to conception due to the role of iodine in egg maturation. In addition, the foetus is reliant on maternal iodine stores until around week 18 of pregnancy. There are currently no specific recommendations for the preconception period, with general iodine requirements for adults being 150 mcg daily. During pregnancy and lactation this increases to 200 mcg daily. It may be difficult to achieve adequate iodine levels on a plant-based diet, especially as seaweed is not a recommended regular source, due to its fluctuating iodine content. Therefore, it is sensible to take a daily non-kelp derived iodine supplement of no more than 150 mcg during the pre-conception period.

Advanced glycation end products (AGEs) and fertility

AGEs are compounds that form inside the body when sugars attach to protein molecules, and there are receptors for AGEs (RAGEs) in the uterus and ovaries. In overweight women, an accumulation of AGEs in the uterine tissue can have a negative impact on fertility. Not only does it take longer to conceive, but the uterus becomes inflamed by the accumulation of AGEs and inhibits the implantation of a fertilised egg into the endometrial tissue.[101]

Women with PCOS have also been shown to have high circulating levels of AGEs[102] and there is evidence that the accumulation of AGEs at the level of the ovarian follicle could trigger early ovarian aging.[103] The biggest dietary sources of AGEs are foods high in protein and fat, specifically meat and animal products, whereas carbohydrate-rich foods such as fruit, vegetables and wholegrains, contain low amounts.[104]

In men, high consumption of dietary AGEs doesn't seem to have an effect on sperm motility, but they do cause a reduction in the quality of the DNA within the sperm.[105]

Recommendation
Health professionals working with families considering pregnancy or undergoing a fertility journey, should promote a varied, balanced plant-based diet, alongside other important lifestyle interventions, such as stress reduction, increased physical activity, and restorative sleep. The importance of addressing the diet and lifestyle of both partners, not just the person who will carry the child should be highlighted and encouraging partners to participate in dietary counselling will offer benefits and improved conception outcomes. Every family's' fertility journey will look different, and positive dietary changes for non-biological parents or other family members offers benefits for family health as well as role modelling opportunities beyond the conception period.

Conclusion

It is clear that following a plant-predominant diet and making positive lifestyle changes can benefit women-specific health conditions in numerous ways. However, it is important to highlight that men can also benefit from such changes, not only in terms of their general health but also in targeting male-specific health conditions such as erectile dysfunction and infertility. Health care professionals should be aware of the importance of including plant-based nutrition and positive lifestyle advice within their consultations to enable a holistic approach with patients, which in turn will optimise care and health outcomes.

References

1. Parasar P, Ozcan P, Terry KL. Endometriosis: Epidemiology, Diagnosis and Clinical Management. *Curr Obstet Gynecol Rep* 2017; 6(1): 34-41. doi: 10.1007/s13669-017-0187-1
2. Cano-Sancho G, Ploteau S, Matta K, Adoamnei E, Louis GB, Mendiola J, et al. Human epidemiological evidence about the associations between exposure to organochlorine chemicals and endometriosis: Systematic review and meta-analysis. *Environment International* 2019; 123: 209-223. doi: 10.1016/j.envint.2018.11.065
3. Soave I, Occhiali T, Wenger JM, Pluchino N, Caserta D, Marci R. Endometriosis and food habits: Can diet make the difference? *Journal of Endometriosis and Pelvic Pain Disorders* 2018; 10(2): 59-71. doi: 10.1177/2284026518773212
4. Harris HR, Eke AC, Chavarro JE, Missmer SA. Fruit and vegetable consumption and risk of endometriosis. *Hum Reprod* 2018; 33(4): 715-727. doi: 10.1093/humrep/dey014

5. Parazzini F, Chiaffarino F, Surace M, Chatenoud L, Cipriani S, Chiantera V, et al. Selected food intake and risk of endometriosis. *Hum Reprod* 2004; 19(8): 1755-1759.
doi: 10.1093/humrep/deh395
6. Vallée A, Lecarpentier Y. Curcumin and endometriosis. *International Journal of Molecular Sciences* 2020; 21(7): 2440.
doi: 10.3390/ijms21072440
7. Signorile PG, Viceconte R, Baldi A. Novel dietary supplement association reduces symptoms in endometriosis patients. *J Cell Physiol* 2018; 233(8): 5920-5925. doi: 10.1002/jcp.26401
8. Tsuchiya M, Miura T, Hanaoka T, Iwasaki M, Sasaki H, Tanaka T, et al. Effect of soy isoflavones on endometriosis: Interaction with estrogen receptor 2 gene polymorphism. *Epidemiology* 2007; 18(3): 402-408.
doi: 10.1097/01.ede.0000257571.01358.f9
9. Hansen SO, Knudsen UB. Endometriosis, dysmenorrhoea and diet. *European Journal of Obstetrics and Gynecology and Reproductive Biology* 2013; 169(2): 162-171.
doi: 10.1016/j.ejogrb.2013.03.028
10. Yamamoto A, Harris HR, Vitonis AF, Chavarro JE, Missmer SA. A prospective cohort study of meat and fish consumption and endometriosis risk. *Am J Obstet Gynecol* 2018; 219(2): 178.e1-178.e10. doi: 10.1016/j.ajog.2018.05.034
11. Parazzini F, Cipriani S, Bravi F, Pelucchi C, Chiaffarino F, Ricci E, et al. A metaanalysis on alcohol consumption and risk of endometriosis. *Am J Obstet Gynecol* 2013; 209(2): 106.e1-10.
doi: 10.1016/j.ajog.2013.05.039
12. Nodler JL, Harris HR, Chavarro JE, Frazier AL, Missmer SA. Dairy consumption during adolescence and endometriosis risk. *American Journal of Obstetrics and Gynecology* 2020; 222(3): 257.e1-257.e16. doi: 10.1016/j.ajog.2019.09.010
13. Trabert B, Peters U, De Roos AJ, Scholes D, Holt VL. Diet and risk of endometriosis in a population-based case-control study. *Br J Nutr* 2011; 105(3): 459-467.
doi: 10.1017/S0007114510003661
14. Ilhan M, Güraǧaç Dereli FT, Akkol EK. Novel Drug Targets with Traditional Herbal Medicines for Overcoming Endometriosis. *Curr Drug Deliv* 2018; 16(5): 386-399.
doi: 10.2174/1567201816666181227112421
15. Vennberg Karlsson J, Patel H, Premberg A. Experiences of health after dietary changes in endometriosis: A qualitative interview study. *BMJ Open* 2020; 10(2): e032321.
doi: 10.1136/bmjopen-2019-032321
16. Simmen RCM, Kelley AS. Seeing red: diet and endometriosis risk. *Ann Transl Med* 2018; 6(S2): S119. doi: 10.21037/atm.2018.12.14
17. Boynton-Jarrett R, Rich-Edwards JW, Jun HJ, Hibert EN, Wright RJ. Abuse in childhood and risk of uterine leiomyoma: The role of emotional support in biologic resilience. *Epidemiology* 2011; 22(1): 6-14. doi: 10.1097/EDE.0b013e3181ffb172
18. Chiaffarino F, Parazzini F, La Vecchia C, Chatenoud L, Di Cintio E, Marsico S. Diet and uterine myomas. *Obstet Gynecol* 1999; 94(3): 395-398. doi: 10.1016/s0029-7844(99)00305-1
19. Wise LA, Radin RG, Palmer JR, Kumanyika SK, Boggs DA, Rosenberg L. Intake of fruit, vegetables, and carotenoids in relation to risk of uterine leiomyomata. *Am J Clin Nutr* 2011; 94(6): 1620-1631. doi: 10.3945/ajcn.111.016600
20. Brasky TM, Bethea TN, Wesselink AK, Wegienka GR, Baird DD, Wise LA. Dietary Fat Intake and Risk of Uterine Leiomyomata: A Prospective Ultrasound Study. *Am J Epidemiol* 2020; 189(12): 1538–1546. doi: 10.1093/aje/kwaa097
21. Roshdy E, Rajaratnam V, Maitra S, Sabry M, Ait Allah AS, Al-Hendy A. Treatment of symptomatic Uterine fibroids with green tea extract: A pilot randomized controlled clinical study. *Int J Womens Health* 2013;5(1): 477-486.
doi: 10.2147/IJWH.S41021
22. Dalton-Brewer N. The Role of Complementary and Alternative Medicine for the Management of Fibroids and Associated Symptomatology. *Curr Obstet Gynecol Rep* 2016; 5: 110-118.
doi: 10.1007/s13669-016-0156-0
23. Baird DD, Hill MC, Schectman JM, Hollis BW. Vitamin D and the risk of uterine fibroids. *Epidemiology* 2013; 24(3): 447-453.
doi: 10.1097/EDE.0b013e31828acca0
24. Ciebiera M, Ali M, Zgliczyńska M, Skrzypczak M, Al-Hendy A. Vitamins and uterine fibroids: Current data on pathophysiology and possible clinical relevance. *International Journal of Molecular Sciences* 2020; 21(15): 5528.

doi: 10.3390/ijms21155528

25. Wise LA, Palmer JR, Harlow BL, Spiegelman D, Stewart EA, Adams-Campbell LL, et al. Risk of uterine leiomyomata in relation to tobacco, alcohol and caffeine consumption in the Black Women's Health Study. *Hum Reprod* 2004; 19(8): 1746-1754. doi: 10.1093/humrep/deh309

26. Schoep ME, Adang EMM, Maas JWM, De Bie B, Aarts JWM, Nieboer TE. Productivity loss due to menstruation-related symptoms: A nationwide cross-sectional survey among 32 748 women. *BMJ Open* 2019; 9(6): e026186. doi: 10.1136/bmjopen-2018-026186

27. Barnard ND, Scialli AR, Hurlock D, Bertron P. Diet and sex-hormone binding globulin, dysmenorrhea, and premenstrual symptoms. *Obstet Gynecol* 2000; 95(2): 245-250. doi: 10.1016/s0029-7844(99)00525-6

28. Lasco A, Catalano A, Benvenga S. Improvement of primary dysmenorrhea caused by a single oral dose of vitamin D: Results of a randomized, double-blind, placebo-controlled study. *Arch Intern Med* 2012; 172(4): 366-367. doi: 10.1001/archinternmed.2011.715

29. Daily JW, Zhang X, Kim DS, Park S. Efficacy of Ginger for Alleviating the Symptoms of Primary Dysmenorrhea: A Systematic Review and Meta-analysis of Randomized Clinical Trials. *Pain Med (United States)* 2015; 16(12): 2243-2255. doi: 10.1111/pme.12853

30. Rahnama P, Montazeri A, Huseini HF, Kianbakht S, Naseri M. Effect of Zingiber officinale R. Rhizomes (ginger) on pain relief in primary dysmenorrhea: A placebo randomized trial. *BMC Complement Altern Med* 2012; 12: 92. doi: 10.1186/1472-6882-12-92

31. Javan R, Yousefi M, Nazari SM, Amiri P, Mosavi-Jarrahi A, Modiramani P, et al. Herbal Medicines in Idiopathic Heavy Menstrual Bleeding: A Systematic Review. *Phytotherapy Research* 2016; 30(10): 1584-1591. doi: 10.1002/ptr.5675

32. Khalesi ZB, Beiranvand SP, Bokaie M. Efficacy of chamomile in the treatment of premenstrual syndrome: A systematic review. *J Pharmacopuncture* 2019; 22(4): 204-209. doi: 10.3831/KPI.2019.22.028

33. Pattanittum P, Kunyanone N, Brown J, Sangkomkamhang US, Barnes J, Seyfoddin V, et al. Dietary supplements for dysmenorrhoea. *Cochrane Database of Systematic Reviews* 2016; 3(3): CD002124. doi: 10.1002/14651858.CD002124.pub2

34. Proctor M, Murphy PA. Herbal and dietary therapies for primary and secondary dysmenorrhoea. *Cochrane Database Syst Rev* 2001; (3): CD002124. doi: 10.1002/14651858.CD002124

35. Artymuk N V., Tachkova OA, Marochko TY. Modern approaches to the management of menopause. *Gynecology* 2021; 23(2): 137-143. doi: 10.26442/20795696.2021.2.200691

36. Office of National Statistics. Leading causes of death, UK: 2001 to 2018.

37. Politi MC, Schleinitz MD, Col NF. Revisiting the duration of vasomotor symptoms of menopause: A meta-analysis. *Journal of General Internal Medicine* 2008; 23(9): 1507-1513. doi: 10.1007/s11606-008-0655-4

38. Yim G, Ahn Y, Chang Y, Ryu S, Lim JY, Kang D, et al. Prevalence and severity of menopause symptoms and associated factors across menopause status in Korean women. *Menopause* 2015; 22(10): 1108-1116. doi: 10.1097/GME.0000000000000438

39. Gold EB, Colvin A, Avis N, Bromberger J, Greendale GA, Powell L, et al. Longitudinal analysis of the association between vasomotor symptoms and race/ethnicity across the menopausal transition: Study of women's health across the nation. *Am J Public Health* 2006; 96(7): 1226-1235. doi: 10.2105/AJPH.2005.066936

40. Thurston RC, Joffe H. Vasomotor Symptoms and Menopause: Findings from the Study of Women's Health across the Nation. *Obstetrics and Gynecology Clinics of North America* 2011; 38(3): 489-501. doi: 10.1016/j.ogc.2011.05.006

41. Kroenke CH, Caan BJ, Stefanick ML, Anderson G, Brzyski R, Johnson KC, et al. Effects of a dietary intervention and weight change on vasomotor symptoms in the Women's Health Initiative. *Menopause* 2012; 19(9): 980-988. doi: 10.1097/gme.0b013e31824f606e

42. Liu ZM, Ho SC, Xie YJ, Woo J. Whole plant foods intake is associated with fewer menopausal symptoms in Chinese postmenopausal women with prehypertension or untreated hypertension.

Menopause 2015; 22(5): 496-504. doi: 10.1097/GME.0000000000000349

43. Beezhold B, Radnitz C, McGrath RE, Feldman A. Vegans report less bothersome vasomotor and physical menopausal symptoms than omnivores. *Maturitas* 2018; 112: 12-17. doi: 10.1016/j.maturitas.2018.03.009

44. Soleymani M, Siassi F, Qorbani M, Khosravi S, Aslany Z, Abshirini M, et al. Dietary patterns and their association with menopausal symptoms: A cross-sectional study. *Menopause* 2019; 26(4): 365-372. doi: 10.1097/GME.0000000000001245

45. Barnard ND, Kahleova H, Holtz DN, Del Aguila F, Neola M, Crosby LM, et al. The Women's Study for the Alleviation of Vasomotor Symptoms (WAVS): a randomized, controlled trial of a plant-based diet and whole soybeans for postmenopausal women. *Menopause* 2021; 28(10): 1150-1156. doi: 10.1097/GME.0000000000001812

46. Chen MN, Lin CC, Liu CF. Efficacy of phytoestrogens for menopausal symptoms: A meta-analysis and systematic review. *Climacteric* 2015; 18(2): 260-269. doi: 10.3109/13697137.2014.966241

47. Rodriguez-Leyva D, Weighell W, Edel AL, Lavallee R, Dibrov E, Pinneker R, et al. Potent antihypertensive action of dietary flaxseed in hypertensive patients. *Hypertension* 2013; 62(6): 1081-1089. doi: 10.1161/HYPERTENSIONAHA.113.02094

48. Calado A, Neves PM, Santos T, Ravasco P. The Effect of Flaxseed in Breast Cancer: A Literature Review. *Frontiers in Nutrition* 2018; 5: 4. doi: 10.3389/fnut.2018.00004

49. im E ok, Lee SH, Chee W. Subethnic Differences in the Menopausal Symptom Experience of Asian American Midlife Women. *J Transcult Nurs* 2010; 21(2): 123-133. doi: 10.1177/1043659609357639

50. Lethaby A, Marjoribanks J, Kronenberg F, Roberts H, Eden J, Brown J. Phytoestrogens for menopausal vasomotor symptoms. *Cochrane Database of Systematic Reviews* 2013; (12): CD001395. doi: 10.1002/14651858.CD001395.pub4

51. Taku K, Melby MK, Kronenberg F, Kurzer MS, Messina M. Extracted or synthesized soybean isoflavones reduce menopausal hot flash frequency and severity. *Menopause* 2012; 19(7): 776-790. doi: 10.1097/gme.0b013e3182410159

52. Chen LR, Ko NY, Chen KH. Isoflavone supplements for menopausal women: A systematic review. *Nutrients* 2019; 11(11): 2649. doi: 10.3390/nu11112649

53. Messina M, Mejia SB, Cassidy A, Duncan A, Kurzer M, Nagato C, et al. Neither soyfoods nor isoflavones warrant classification as endocrine disruptors: a technical review of the observational and clinical data. *Critical Reviews in Food Science and Nutrition* 2021; 1-57. doi: 10.1080/10408398.2021.1895054

54. Zhang YB, Chen WH, Guo JJ, Fu ZH, Yi C, Zhang M, et al. Soy isoflavone supplementation could reduce body weight and improve glucose metabolism in non-Asian postmenopausal women-A meta-analysis. *Nutrition* 2013; 29(1): 8-14. doi: 10.1016/j.nut.2012.03.019

55. Messina M, Magee P. Does soy protein affect circulating levels of unbound IGF-1? *European Journal of Nutrition* 2018; 57(2): 423-432. doi: 10.1007/s00394-017-1459-2

56. Ghazanfarpour M, Sadeghi R, Roudsari RL, Khorsand I, Khadivzadeh T, Muoio B. Red clover for treatment of hot flashes and menopausal symptoms: A systematic review and meta-analysis. *Journal of Obstetrics and Gynaecology* 2016; 36(3): 301-311. doi: 10.3109/01443615.2015.1049249

57. Elkins GR, Fisher WI, Johnson AK, Carpenter JS, Keith TZ. Clinical hypnosis in the treatment of postmenopausal hot flashes: A randomized controlled trial. *Menopause* 2013; 20(3): 291-298. doi: 10.1097/gme.0b013e31826ce3ed

58. Drake CL, Kalmbach DA, Arnedt JT, Cheng P, Tonnu C V., Cuamatzi-Castelan A, et al. Treating chronic insomnia in postmenopausal women: A randomized clinical trial comparing cognitive-behavioral therapy for insomnia, sleep restriction therapy, and sleep hygiene education. *Sleep* 2019; 42(2): zsy217. doi: 10.1093/sleep/zsy217

59. Waterworth DM, Bennett ST, Gharani N, McCarthy MI, Hague S, Batty S, et al. Linkage and association of insulin gene VNTR regulatory polymorphism with polycystic ovary syndrome. *Lancet* 1997; 349(9057): 986-990. doi: 10.1016/S0140-6736(96)08368-7

60. March WA, Moore VM, Willson KJ, Phillips DIW, Norman RJ, Davies MJ. The prevalence of polycystic ovary syndrome in a community sample assessed under contrasting diagnostic criteria. *Hum Reprod* 2010; 25(2): 544-551. doi: 10.1093/humrep/dep399
61. Wolf WM, Wattick RA, Kinkade ON, Olfert MD. Geographical prevalence of polycystic ovary syndrome as determined by region and race/ethnicity. *International Journal of Environmental Research and Public Health* 2018; 15(11): 2589. doi: 10.3390/ijerph15112589
62. Vink JM, Sadrzadeh S, Lambalk CB, Boomsma DI. Heritability of polycystic ovary syndrome in a Dutch twin-family study. *J Clin Endocrinol Metab* 2006; 91(6): 2100-2104. doi: 10.1210/jc.2005-1494
63. Murri M, Luque-ramírez M, Insenser M, Ojeda-ojeda M, Escobar-morreale HF. Circulating markers of oxidative stress and polycystic ovary syndrome (pcos): A systematic review and meta-analysis. *Hum Reprod Update* 2013; 19(3): 268-288. doi: 10.1093/humupd/dms059
64. Lim SS, Hutchison SK, Van Ryswyk E, Norman RJ, Teede HJ, Moran LJ. Lifestyle changes in women with polycystic ovary syndrome. *Cochrane Database of Systematic Reviews* 2019; 2019(3): CD007506. doi: 10.1002/14651858.CD007506.pub4
65. Moran LJ, Tassone EC, Boyle J, Brennan L, Harrison CL, Hirschberg AL, et al. Evidence summaries and recommendations from the international evidence-based guideline for the assessment and management of polycystic ovary syndrome: Lifestyle management. *Obesity Reviews* 2020; 21(10): e13046. doi: 10.1111/obr.13046
66. Himelein MJ, Thatcher SS. Polycystic ovary syndrome and mental health: A review. *Obstetrical and Gynecological Survey* 2006; 61(11): 723-732. doi: 10.1097/01.ogx.0000243772.33357.84
67. Roos N, Kieler H, Sahlin L, Ekman-Ordeberg G, Falconer H, Stephansson O. Risk of adverse pregnancy outcomes in women with polycystic ovary syndrome: Population based cohort study. *BMJ* 2011; 343(7828): d6309. doi: 10.1136/bmj.d6309
68. Fauser BC, Tarlatzis BC, Rebar RW, Legro RS, Balen AH, Lobo R, et al. Consensus on women's health aspects of polycystic ovary syndrome (PCOS): The Amsterdam ESHRE/ASRM-Sponsored 3rd PCOS Consensus Workshop Group. *Fertil Steril* 2012; 97(1): 28-38.e25. doi: 10.1016/j.fertnstert.2011.09.024
69. Wright N, Wilson L, Smith M, Duncan B, McHugh P. The BROAD study: A randomised controlled trial using a whole food plant-based diet in the community for obesity, ischaemic heart disease or diabetes. *Nutr Diabetes* 2017; 7(3): e256. doi: 10.1038/nutd.2017.3
70. Faghfoori Z, Fazelian S, Shadnoush M, Goodarzi R. Nutritional management in women with polycystic ovary syndrome: A review study. *Diabetes and Metabolic Syndrome: Clinical Research and Reviews* 2017; 1: S429-S432. doi: 10.1016/j.dsx.2017.03.030
71. Nybacka Å, Hellström PM, Hirschberg AL. Increased fibre and reduced trans fatty acid intake are primary predictors of metabolic improvement in overweight polycystic ovary syndrome—Substudy of randomized trial between diet, exercise and diet plus exercise for weight control. *Clin Endocrinol (Oxf)* 2017; 87(6): 680-688. doi: 10.1111/cen.13427
72. Karamali M, Kashanian M, Alaeinasab S, Asemi Z. The effect of dietary soy intake on weight loss, glycaemic control, lipid profiles and biomarkers of inflammation and oxidative stress in women with polycystic ovary syndrome: a randomised clinical trial. *J Hum Nutr Diet* 2018; 31(4): 533-543. doi: 10.1111/jhn.12545
73. Tantalaki E, Piperi C, Livadas S, Kollias A, Adamopoulos C, Koulouri A, et al. Impact of dietary modification of advanced glycation end products (AGEs) on the hormonal and metabolic profile of women with polycystic ovary syndrome (PCOS). *Hormones* 2014; 13(1): 65-73. doi: 10.1007/BF03401321
74. Yang K, Zeng L, Bao T, Ge J. Effectiveness of Omega-3 fatty acid for polycystic ovary syndrome: A systematic review and meta-analysis. *Reproductive Biology and Endocrinology* 2018; 16(1): 27. doi: 10.1186/s12958-018-0346-x
75. Ostfeld RJ, Allen KE, Aspry K, Brandt EJ, Spitz A, Liberman J, et al. Vasculogenic Erectile Dysfunction: The Impact of Diet and Lifestyle. *American Journal of Medicine* 2021; 134(3):

310-316. doi: 10.1016/j.amjmed.2020.09.033
76. Salonia A, Bettocchi C, Boeri L, Capogrosso P, Carvalho J, Cilesiz NC, et al. European Association of Urology Guidelines on Sexual and Reproductive Health—2021 Update: Male Sexual Dysfunction. *European Urology* 2021; 80(3): 333-357. doi: 10.1016/j.eururo.2021.06.007
77. A L, D M, Frederick W, Al E. Sexual symptoms predict all-cause mortality independent of sex steroids in aging men. *Endocr Abstr* 2020; 71: 006. doi: 10.1530/endoabs.71.006
78. Bauer SR, Breyer BN, Stampfer MJ, Rimm EB, Giovannucci EL, Kenfield SA. Association of Diet with Erectile Dysfunction among Men in the Health Professionals Follow-up Study. *JAMA Netw Open* 2020; 3(11): e2021701.
doi: 10.1001/jamanetworkopen.2020.21701
79. Torregrossa AC, Aranke M, Bryan NS. Nitric oxide and geriatrics: Implications in diagnostics and treatment of the elderly. *Journal of Geriatric Cardiology* 2011; 8(4): 230-242.
doi: 10.3724/SP.J.1263.2011.00230
80. Mano R, Ishida A, Ohya Y, Todoriki H, Takishita S. Dietary intervention with Okinawan vegetables increased circulating endothelial progenitor cells in healthy young women. *Atherosclerosis* 2009; 204(2): 544-548.
doi: 10.1016/j.atherosclerosis.2008.09.035
81. Montezano AC, Touyz RM. Reactive oxygen species and endothelial function - Role of nitric oxide synthase uncoupling and nox family nicotinamide adenine dinucleotide phosphate oxidases. *Basic and Clinical Pharmacology and Toxicology* 2012; 110(1): 87-94.
doi: 10.1111/j.1742-7843.2011.00785.x
82. Wang F, Dai S, Wang M, Morrison H. Erectile dysfunction and fruit/vegetable consumption among diabetic Canadian men. *Urology* 2013; 82(6): 1330-1335.
doi: 10.1016/j.urology.2013.07.061
83. Cassidy A, Franz M, Rimm EB. Dietary flavonoid intake and incidence of erectile dysfunction. *Am J Clin Nutr* 2016; 103(2): 534-541.
doi: 10.3945/ajcn.115.122010
84. Esposito K, Ciotola M, Giugliano F, De Sio M, Giugliano G, D'Armiento M, et al. Mediterranean diet improves erectile function in subjects with the metabolic syndrome. *Int J Impot Res* 2006; 18(4): 405-410. doi: 10.1038/sj.ijir.3901447
85. Huetos AS, Muralidharan J, Galiè S, Salas-Salvadó J, Bulló M. Effect of nut consumption on erectile and sexual function in healthy males: A Secondary outcome analysis of the fertinuts randomized controlled trial. *Nutrients* 2019; 11(6): 1372. doi: 10.3390/nu11061372
86. Hamilton-Reeves JM, Vazquez G, Duval SJ, Phipps WR, Kurzer MS, Messina MJ. Clinical studies show no effects of soy protein or isoflavones on reproductive hormones in men: Results of a meta-analysis. *Fertil Steril* 2010; 94(3): 997-1007.
doi: 10.1016/j.fertnstert.2009.04.038
87. Reed KE, Camargo J, Hamilton-Reeves J, Kurzer M, Messina M. Neither soy nor isoflavone intake affects male reproductive hormones: An expanded and updated meta-analysis of clinical studies. *Reproductive Toxicology* 2021; 100: 60-67. doi: 10.1016/j.reprotox.2020.12.019
88. Senthong V, Wang Z, Li XS, Fan Y, Wu Y, Tang WHW, et al. Intestinal microbiota-generated metabolite Trimethylamine-N-oxide and 5-year mortality risk in stable coronary artery disease: The contributory role of intestinal microbiota in a COURAGE-like patient cohort. *J Am Heart Assoc* 2016; 5(6): e002816.
doi: 10.1161/JAHA.115.002816
89. Carto C, Pagalavan M, Nackeeran S, Blachman-Braun R, Kresch E, Kuchakulla M, et al. Consumption of a Healthy Plant-based Diet is Associated With a Decreased Risk of Erectile Dysfunction: A Cross- sectional Study of the National Health and Nutrition Examination Survey. *Urology* 2022; 161: 76-82.
doi: 10.1016/j.urology.2021.12.021
90. Barker M, Dombrowski SU, Colbourn T, Fall CHD, Kriznik NM, Lawrence WT, et al. Intervention strategies to improve nutrition and health behaviours before conception. *The Lancet* 2018; 391(10132): 1853-1864.
doi: 10.1016/S0140-6736(18)30313-1
91. Chavarro JE, Rich-Edwards JW, Rosner BA, Willett WC. Diet and lifestyle in the prevention of ovulatory disorder infertility. *Obstet Gynecol* 2007; 110(5): 1050-1058.
doi: 10.1097/01.AOG.0000287293.25465.e1
92. Chavarro JE, Rich-Edwards JW, Rosner BA,

Willett WC. Protein intake and ovulatory infertility. *Am J Obstet Gynecol* 2008; 198(2): 210.e1-7. doi: 10.1016/j.ajog.2007.06.057
93. Esmaeili V, Shahverdi AH, Moghadasian MH, Alizadeh AR. Dietary fatty acids affect semen quality: A review. *Andrology* 2015; 3(3): 450-461. doi: 10.1111/andr.12024
94. Sebastiani G, Barbero AH, Borrás-Novel C, Casanova MA, Aldecoa-Bilbao V, Andreu-Fernández V, et al. The effects of vegetarian and vegan diet during pregnancy on the health of mothers and offspring. *Nutrients* 2019; 11(3): 557. doi: 10.3390/nu11030557
95. Grzechocinska B, Dabrowski FA, Cyganek A, Wielgos M. The role of vitamin D in impaired fertility treatment. *Neuroendocrinology Letters* 2013; 34(8): 756-762.
96. The Scientific Advisory Committee on Nutrition. Vitamin D and Health. 2016.
97. Chitayat D, Matsui D, Amitai Y, Kennedy D, Vohra S, Rieder M, et al. Folic acid supplementation for pregnant women and those planning pregnancy: 2015 update. *Journal of Clinical Pharmacology* 2016; 56(2): 170-175. doi: 10.1002/jcph.616
98. Wong WY, Merkus HMWM, Thomas CMG, Menkveld R, Zielhuis GA, Steegers-Theunissen RPM. Effects of folic acid and zinc sulfate on male factor subfertility: A double-blind, randomized, placebo-controlled trial. *Fertil Steril* 2002; 77(3): 491-498. doi: 10.1016/s0015-0282(01)03229-0
99. Ebisch IMW, Thomas CMG, Peters WHM, Braat DDM, Steegers-Theunissen RPM. The importance of folate, zinc and antioxidants in the pathogenesis and prevention of subfertility. *Human Reproduction Update* 2007; 13(2): 163-174. doi: 10.1093/humupd/dml054
100. Sun Y, Chen C, Liu GG, Wang M, Shi C, Yu G, et al. The association between iodine intake and semen quality among fertile men in China. *BMC Public Health* 2020; 20(1): 461. doi: 10.1186/s12889-020-08547-2
101. Hutchison JC, Truong TT, Salamonsen LA, Gardner DK, Evans J. Advanced glycation end products present in the obese uterine environment compromise preimplantation embryo development. *Reprod Biomed Online* 2020; 41(5): 757-766. doi: 10.1016/j.rbmo.2020.07.026
102. Merhi Z. Advanced glycation end products and their relevance in female reproduction. *Human Reproduction* 2014; 29(1): 135-145. doi: 10.1093/humrep/det383
103. Tatone C, Amicarelli F. The aging ovary - The poor granulosa cells. *Fertility and Sterility* 2013; 99(1): 12-17. doi: 10.1016/j.fertnstert.2012.11.029
104. Uribarri J, Woodruff S, Goodman S, Cai W, Chen X, Pyzik R, et al. Advanced Glycation End Products in Foods and a Practical Guide to Their Reduction in the Diet. *J Am Diet Assoc* 2010; 110(6): 911-16.e12. doi: 10.1016/j.jada.2010.03.018
105. Mallidis C, Agbaje IM, Rogers DA, Glenn J V., Pringle R, Atkinson AB, et al. Advanced glycation end products accumulate in the reproductive tract of men with diabetes. *Int J Androl* 2009; 32(4): 295-305. doi: 10.1111/j.1365-2605.2007.00849.x

Chapter 13
Plant-based nutrition and Alzheimer's prevention

Ayesha Sherzai, Sophia Sherzai, Shireen Kassam, Dean Sherzai

Introduction

Dementia is a rising global problem, impacting quality of life and adding to the rising cost and burden of healthcare. Currently more than 55 million people live with dementia worldwide, and there are nearly 10 million new cases every year. In 2019, the estimated total global societal cost of dementia was US$1.3 trillion, and these costs are expected to surpass US$2.8 trillion by 2030 as both the number of people living with dementia and care costs increase.[1]

Dementia is an umbrella term for a number of different conditions in which an individual has difficulties with memory, language, problem-solving and other cognitive domains.[2] The most common type is Alzheimer's disease (AD), which constitutes 60-80% of all dementias, with vascular dementia being the second most common type. There can also be an overlap of the two, with vascular injury occurring more frequently in people with AD than without.[2] In their 2017 report, the Lancet Commission reported that 35% of cases could be prevented through modifiable lifestyle risk factors.[3] The latest studies have indicated that implementation of a healthy lifestyle can reduce up to 60% of cases of dementia.[4] The lifestyle factors include a healthy dietary pattern, physical activity, cognitive activity, social engagement, management of vascular risk factors, tobacco abstinence and, recently, alcohol abstinence[4,5,6,7] This chapter will discuss the role of nutrition, specifically plant-based nutrition, for prevention of AD.

Pathogenic mechanism underlying the development of AD

The hallmark pathologies of AD are the accumulation of beta-amyloid protein extracellularly, also referred to as 'plaques', and twisted strands of the intracellular protein tau, known as tau tangles. These changes are accompanied by neurodegenerative changes and cerebral atrophy. Mutations in the amyloid precursor protein (APP), presenilin 1 (PSEN1), and presenilin 2 (PSEN2) genes can cause early-onset AD, although this accounts for only 3-5% of cases, with the majority of cases occurring sporadically due to the interplay between genes and lifestyle.[1,8]

The central drivers of late-onset AD, which accounts for more than 90% of all cases, are glucose or energy dysregulation, lipid dysregulation, inflammation and oxidation as a result of poorly managed vascular risk factors and unhealthy lifestyle, which include smoking, alcohol abuse, poor nutrition, lack of exercise, stress, sleep disorders such as sleep apnoea, and lack of cognitive reserve.[4,7] Combined, we believe, more than 90% of risk factors ascribed to AD are due to these factors.

The driving force of any case depends on the primary risk factor contributing to the pathological process. There are patients who have a history of chronic insulin resistance or diabetes, and in these cases, insulin resistance primarily drives the disease,[9] and yet chronic inflammation may be the main driving force behind the inception and propagation of the disease in other cases, such as chronic traumatic encephalitis (CTE).[10] Lipid dysregulation, as driven by Apo e4 or other pathways, can serve as a driver of neurovascular and neurodegenerative disease as well. And finally, oxidative stress can be a major driver of neurodegeneration as a result of free radical formation, damaging neural architecture and vasculature.[11]

Vascular risk factors and AD

Dementia shares many similar risk factors to cardiovascular disease. Those with high blood pressure, high cholesterol, type 2 diabetes, and excess body weight are at significantly increased risk of developing dementia later in life. Addressing cardiovascular risk factors through a healthy lifestyle approach is a very effective way to prevent dementia.[7] An analysis from the Whitehall study of UK British civil servants included data from 7899 participants and reported the association of cardiovascular health at age 50 with the incidence of dementia using the Life Simple 7 cardiovascular health score devised by the American Heart Association.[12] After a median follow-up of 25 years, the results demonstrated that the better the cardiovascular health score at age 50 years, the lower the risk of dementia. For each 1-point increment in the score (14 points in total) there was a 11% reduction in the risk of dementia demonstrating that control of cardiovascular risk factors provides a powerful tool for prevention of dementia in later life.

A further analysis from the Whitehall study cohort assessed the association between underlying chronic conditions, termed multi-morbidity, and the risk of dementia after 32 years of follow up. The presence of two or more chronic conditions was associated with a 2.4-fold increase in risk of dementia. The younger the onset of the chronic conditions, the higher the risk of dementia, with the strongest association at age 55 years. The most common chronic conditions impacting risk were hypertension, depression, coronary heart disease and diabetes.[13] Unsurprisingly, people with two or more of these chronic conditions also had a higher risk of death during the follow up period: up to 4.8 times the risk of those without chronic conditions.[13]

Dietary patterns and AD

When looking at data coming to us from a variety of studies, there is a common theme: an unprocessed, plant-predominant diet rich in fibre, phytonutrients and polyunsaturated fats, especially omega-3 fatty acids; with or without fish; low in saturated fats derived from meats and dairy products, and low in processed foods. Processed foods are predominantly high in refined carbohydrates, saturated fats, trans fatty acids, salt, and sugar and have been associated with higher risk of AD and all-cause dementia.

There is strong evidence from a dietary perspective that a Mediterranean diet (MD) is associated with reduced risk of AD. Multiple observational studies have indicated that higher adherence to a MD is associated with reduced risk of AD and slower rates of cognitive decline.[15, 16, 17] In the PREDIMED (Prevención con Dieta

Mediterránea) study, MD supplemented with nuts or olive oil produced improved cognitive function.[18]

Another dietary approach called the Dietary Approach to Stop Hypertension (DASH) has been found to be strongly associated with improved cognitive outcomes.[18] Both MD and DASH dietary patterns have similar components, emphasising a plant-predominant diet while limiting the consumption of red meat and other sources of saturated fats. MD is a cultural diet that specifically highlights daily intake of greens, beans, whole grains, herbs, extra-virgin olive oil (monounsaturated fat), potatoes and fish, along with some moderate consumption of wine, while DASH restricts intake of sodium, processed sweets, and saturated fat.

The MIND diet, which stands for Mediterranean-DASH Intervention for Neurodegenerative Delay (MIND) is a hybrid of the MD and DASH diets, and was created by Martha Morris at Rush University, based on their population-based data.[19] This dietary pattern highlights nutrient-dense foods, such as green leafy vegetables, berries and other vegetables. Green leafy vegetables were especially highlighted, as their consumption seems to have been associated with lower risk of Alzheimer's incidence. In the Rush Memory and Aging Project, the rate of decline among those who consumed 1-2 servings of greens per day was the equivalent of being 11 years younger in age compared with those who rarely or never consumed green leafy vegetables.[20] Among fruits, the Nurses' Health Study revealed that only berries have been associated with slowing cognitive decline.[21] Other foods highlighted in the MIND diet are extra-virgin olive oil, nuts, whole grains, and low-fat sources of protein, such as legumes, and poultry on rare occasions. Nevertheless, certain foods included in DASH and MD are not included in the MIND diet due to lack of evidence for their importance in brain health, including high consumption of fruit (3-4 servings in both DASH and MD), dairy (DASH), potatoes and high fish consumption (2 servings per day and 6 fish meals per week in DASH and MD, respectively). The MIND diet also recommends no more than 1-2 fish meals per week as sufficient to lower dementia risk, with no additional benefit from higher numbers of servings. There is also evidence that the benefits of fish, often highlighted in MD, may be related to the higher concentration of omega-3 fats, which may be found in fish or plant-based sources such as algae, quinoa, flax seed, hemp seeds, and even nuts like walnuts.

A recent meta-analysis of nine studies encompassing 31,104 participants looked at the relationship between nutrition and cognitive impairment as well as dementia. The meta-analysis revealed that increased consumption of fruit and vegetables was associated with a 20% significant reduction in the risk for cognitive impairment and dementia. Further analysis demonstrated that a dose-response effect was seen with stepped increase in consumption of 100 g per day of fruit and vegetables, resulting in a 13% reduction in cognitive impairment and dementia risk.[22]

There are limited data on plant-based or plant-exclusive diets (vegetarian and vegan) and risk of dementia. The only study we had for a while was a preliminary report from the Adventist Health Study suggesting that meat eaters had a significantly higher risk of developing dementia compared with vegetarians.[23] A recent publication analysed data from the prospective Tzu Chi Vegetarian Study. It included data from 5710 participants who were aged 50 years or older at the time of recruitment in 2005 and followed till 2014.[24] The participants were all Buddhist volunteers: 3154 were non-vegetarian and 1737 were vegetarian. Vegetarians were classified based on not eating meat, fish or poultry for at least a year prior to recruitment. The vegetarians were less likely to consume alcohol and smoke tobacco and had significantly less diabetes, cerebrovascular disease and substance use disorder compared with the non-vegetarians.

During the average follow up of 9.2 years there were 121 cases of dementia (37 vegetarians and 84 non-vegetarians) identified, and vegetarians had a 33% reduction in the risk of dementia. Subgroup analysis found that vegetarians were specifically protected against dementia under the age of 75 years. However, the results were not statistically significant due to low case numbers, which in part is likely to be due to the fact that researchers only considered cases of dementia that required medical attention. These data are reassuring given the concerns about lack of fish in the diet and brain health. The reasons for the benefit of a vegetarian diet are likely to include the lower prevalence of comorbidities and the ability to address the key drivers of dementia – namely, dyslipidaemia, glucose dysregulation, oxidative stress, inflam-mation and abnormal gut microbiome.

In 2019, the World Health Organization published guidelines for the prevention of dementia.[25] For a healthy diet, the following recommendation were made:

- Eat a diet rich in fruit, vegetables, legumes (e.g. lentils and beans), nuts and whole grains (e.g. unprocessed maize, millet, oats, wheat and brown rice).
- Eat at least 400 g (i.e. five portions) of fruit and vegetables per day.
- Consume less than 10% of total energy from sugars, which is equivalent to 50 g (or about 12 level teaspoons) for a person of healthy body weight consuming about 2000 calories per day.
- Consume less than 30% of total energy intake from fats, choosing unsaturated fats rather than saturated fats and industrialised trans-fats (found in baked and fried foods, and pre-packaged snacks and foods, such as frozen pizza, pies, cookies, biscuits and wafers, and cooking oils and spreads) and ruminant trans-fats (found in meat and dairy foods from ruminant animals, such as cows, sheep, goats and camels). Keep saturated fat intake to less than 10% of total energy intake.
- Eat less than 5 g of salt (equivalent to about one teaspoon) per day.

Specific foods and nutrients

Saturated fats

Higher intake of saturated fat is associated with an increased risk of dementia.[26] Saturated fat in the diet comes predominantly from animal foods, and, in particular, the consumption of processed red meat seems to significantly increase the risk of dementia.[27] Diets high in refined sugars and carbohydrates also appear to impair cognitive function both in the short term[28] and long term,[29] the latter in part due to the ability of sugar to increase inflammation and the risk of cardiovascular disease.

Vegetables and fruit

Vegetables and fruit high in phytonutrients have a salutary effect on brain health.[30] When compared, green leafy vegetables appear to be more important than fruit in protecting against dementia, with the exception of berry consumption, which appears highly protective against cognitive decline.[31] A recent study highlighted the importance of eating fruit and vegetables early in life to prevent later cognitive impairment.[32] This study recruited more than 3000 participants in the United States aged 18-30 years in the 1980s and followed them for 25 years, regularly documenting their dietary intake. It found that those consuming the most fruit and vegetables in younger life had the best cognitive function later in life. Vegetable consumption had a greater effect than fruit, with nutrients such as lycopene from tomatoes/red vegetables and beta-carotene from yellow/orange vegetables having the best effect.[32] Overall, it seemed that it was the fibre intake that was responsible for much of this beneficial effect on brain health.

Consuming fruit and vegetables that are high in flavonoids may be of particular benefit.[30] Flavonoids are a class of polyphenols representing more than 5000 bioactive compounds that are found in a variety of fruit and vegetables, including grapes, berries and apples, and in tea. Several studies have reported a beneficial effect of flavonoids for preventing cognitive decline, reducing the risk by around 20%.[30] To further support the role of dietary flavonoids and polyphenols in general, an analysis of the prospective three-city cohort study in Europe, including 842 participants with a median age of around 75 years and followed for 12 years, showed that a higher intake of fruit, vegetables and plant-based foods providing polyphenols and other bioactive compounds was associated with the generation of beneficial compounds from the gut microbiota.[33] These gut-derived compounds detected in the blood were associated with a reduced risk of cognitive decline.

Fibre

Fibre intake is correlated with lower risk of many chronic diseases that increase the risk of dementia, such as cardiovascular disease, type 2 diabetes and elevated blood lipids. Fibre also benefits gut bacteria, which then can make short-chain fatty acids needed for brain hormone production and for reducing inflammation. In a Japanese cohort of 3739 individuals, dietary fibre intake was inversely associated with risk of dementia. Those consuming the most, particularly soluble fibre, had a 26% reduction in the risk of developing dementia over the almost 20-year follow up.[34]

Polyunsaturated fats including omega-3 fatty acids

DHA (docosahexaenoic acid, a long-chain omega-3 fatty acid) is very important for the developing brain and has also been shown to be important in protecting the aging brain. The brain is composed of around 50-60% fat and has a particularly high content of DHA. Regular consumption of fish appears to reduce the risk of dementia and it is thought that this is due to the high DHA content in fish.[35] Interestingly, supplementation with DHA does not seem to consistently reduce the risk of dementia so it may be that fish consumption is a reflection of a healthier diet where fish is replacing harmful foods such as processed and unprocessed red meat.[36]

Those on a plant-exclusive diet mainly derive their short-chain omega-3 fatty acids from nuts and seeds in the form of alpha-linolenic acid (ALA), which is then converted to DHA. There is currently no evidence to suggest a lack of fish in the diet is detrimental to brain health when the diet is otherwise composed of healthy, minimally processed plant foods. Long-chain omega-3 fatty acids can be obtained from algae supplements if required.[37] In addition, recent evidence suggests that vegetarians may have a reduced risk of developing dementia compared with non-vegetarians, suggesting that fish is not required for optimal brain health.

Vitamin supplementation

Clinical trials on nutritional supplements for the prevention of AD have remained inconclusive so far. However, replacement of B vitamins and DHA have been associated with lower rates of AD and cognitive decline. Low B vitamin levels, particularly vitamin B12, and a consequent increase in homocysteine are associated with cognitive impairment, and its replacement results in improved function.[38, 39]

Alcohol

Chronic alcohol use has been associated with lower brain volume and cortical thickness compared with healthy controls.[40] However, in the recent years, it has become evident that the brain is quite vulnerable to the neurotoxic effects of any alcohol use, and the previous notion that moderate drinking had any salutary effect on the brain has been disregarded.[41] An analysis of data from 36,678 adults from the UK Biobank found that light-to-moderate alcohol consumption was associated with reductions in overall brain volume.[42] Their analysis added that the negative association between alcohol intake and brain structure was evident in those who consumed one to two alcohol units per day, and the aging of the brain increased exponentially as alcohol consumption increased. As an illustration, a change from one to two units per day was equivalent to the effect of aging two years, and an increase from two to three units per day resulted in aging of the brain by three and a half years. Therefore, it is safe to say that, with the current evidence at hand, no amount of alcohol can be deemed harmless for the brain.

Lifestyle intervention and dementia prevention

Combining a plant-based diet with healthy lifestyle habits is an effective way to protect brain health and prevent a significant proportion of dementias. This was demonstrated in the Finnish Geriatric Intervention Study to Prevent Cognitive Impairment and Disability,[7] which examined the effects of a two-year comprehensive lifestyle intervention in 1269 adults (aged 60-77 years old) at risk of developing dementia. One group received the following intervention: a diet intervention based on the Finnish Nutrition Recommendations (emphasises whole, plant foods and minimises animal-derived and processed foods), regular aerobic exercise and resistance training, cognitively challenging computer programmes, and intensive management of metabolic and vascular risk factors. The second group received standard care (simply advice to eat healthily and exercise). After two years, the intervention group had a significantly higher score in overall cognitive performance. Currently, a large national study in the USA, which is an adaptation of the FINGER study, aims to test whether a multi-domain lifestyle intervention focused on physical and cognitive activity, nutrition and risk-factor management reduces the risk of cognitive decline in a heterogeneous population of older adults.[43]

Conclusion

There is an overwhelming number of studies that support the significant role of lifestyle intervention, and a plant-based diet in particular, in maintaining cognitive health and prevention of dementia. A planned, unprocessed plant-based diet low in saturated fats and processed simple carbohydrates and high in fruit and vegetables not only reduces the underlying chronic risk factors, but also addresses the downstream pathologic mechanisms involved in the development of dementias like Alzheimer's.

Given the fact that there are currently no effective pharmaceutical treatments for AD, global efforts should be aimed at addressing modifiable risk factors to prevent or delay AD in the first place.

References

1. Andrews SJ, Fulton-Howard B, O'Reilly P, Marcora E, Goate AM, collaborators of the Alzheimer's Disease Genetics Consortium, Farrer LA, Haines JL, Mayeux R, Naj AC, Pericak-Vance MA. Causal associations between modifiable risk factors and the Alzheimer's phenome. *Annals of Neurology* 2021; 89(1): 54-65.
2. Alzheimer's Association. 2022 Alzheimer's Disease Facts and Figures. *Alzheimers Dement* 2022; 18(4): 700-789. doi: 10.1002/alz.12638
3. Livingston G, Sommerlad A, Orgeta V, Costafreda SG, Huntley J, Ames D, Ballard C,

Banerjee S, Burns A, Cohen-Mansfield J, Cooper C. Dementia prevention, intervention, and care. *Lancet* 2017; 390(10113): 2673-2734.

4. Dhana K, Barnes LL, Liu X, Agarwal P, Desai P, Krueger KR, Holland TM, Halloway S, Aggarwal NT, Evans DA, Rajan KB. Genetic risk, adherence to a healthy lifestyle, and cognitive decline in African Americans and European Americans. *Alzheimer's & Dementia* 2022; 18(4): 572-580.

5. Licher S, Ahmad S, Karamujić-Čomić H, Voortman T, Leening MJ, Ikram MA, Ikram MK. Genetic predisposition, modifiable-risk-factor profile and long-term dementia risk in the general population. *Nature Medicine* 2019; 25(9): 1364-1369.

6. Dhana K, Barnes LL, Liu X, Agarwal P, Desai P, Krueger KR, Holland TM, Halloway S, Aggarwal NT, Evans DA, Rajan KB. Genetic risk, adherence to a healthy lifestyle, and cognitive decline in African Americans and European Americans. *Alzheimer's & Dementia* 2022; 18(4): 572-580.

7. Ngandu T, Lehtisalo J, Solomon A, et al. A 2 year multidomain intervention of diet, exercise, cognitive training, and vascular risk monitoring versus control to prevent cognitive decline in at-risk elderly people (FINGER): a randomised controlled trial. *Lancet* 2015; 385: 2255-2263. doi:10.1016/S0140- 6736(15)60461-5

8. Bateman RJ, Aisen PS, De Strooper B, Fox NC, Lemere CA, Ringman JM, Salloway S, Sperling RA, Windisch M, Xiong C. Autosomal-dominant Alzheimer's disease: a review and proposal for the prevention of Alzheimer's disease. *Alzheimer's Research & Therapy* 2011; 3(1): 1-3.

9. Sherzai D, Sherzai A, Lui K, Pan D, Chiou D, Bazargan M, Shaheen M. The association between diabetes and dementia among elderly individuals: a nationwide inpatient sample analysis. *Journal of Geriatric Psychiatry and Neurology* 2016; 29(3): 120-125.

10. Turner RC, Lucke-Wold BP, Robson MJ, Lee JM, Bailes JE. Alzheimer's disease and chronic traumatic encephalopathy: Distinct but possibly overlapping disease entities. *Brain Injury* 2016; 30(11): 1279-1292.

11. Feringa FM, Van der Kant R. Cholesterol and Alzheimer's disease; from risk genes to pathological effects. *Frontiers in Aging Neuroscience* 2021; 13: 333.

12. Sabia S, Fayosse A, Dumurgier J, Schnitzler A, Empana JP, Ebmeier KP, Dugravot A, Kivimäki M, Singh-Manoux A. Association of ideal cardiovascular health at age 50 with incidence of dementia: 25 year follow-up of Whitehall II cohort study. *Br Med J* 2019; 366: I4414. doi: 10.1136/bmj.l4414

13. Hassen CB, Fayosse A, Landré B, Raggi M, Bloomberg M, Sabia S, Singh-Manoux A. Association between age at onset of multimorbidity and incidence of dementia: 30 year follow-up in Whitehall II prospective cohort study. *Br Med J* 2022; 376: e068005. doi: 10.1136/bmj-2021-068005

14. Singh B, Parsaik AK, Mielke MM, Erwin PJ, Knopman DS, Petersen RC, Roberts RO. Association of mediterranean diet with mild cognitive impairment and Alzheimer's disease: a systematic review and meta-analysis. *Journal of Alzheimer's Disease* 2014; 39(2): 271-282.

15. Lourida I, Soni M, Thompson-Coon J, Purandare N, Lang IA, Ukoumunne OC, Llewellyn DJ. Mediterranean diet, cognitive function, and dementia: a systematic review. *Epidemiology* 2013; 24(4): 479-489. doi: 10.1097/EDE.0b013e3182944410

16. Scarmeas N, Stern Y, Tang MX, Mayeux R, Luchsinger JA. Mediterranean diet and risk for Alzheimer's disease. *Annals of Neurology* 2006; 59(6): 912-921.

17. Martínez-Lapiscina EH, Clavero P, Toledo E, Estruch R, Salas-Salvadó J, San Julián B, Sanchez-Tainta A, Ros E, Valls-Pedret C, Martinez-Gonzalez MÁ. Mediterranean diet improves cognition: the PREDIMED-NAVARRA randomised trial. *Journal of Neurology, Neurosurgery & Psychiatry* 2013; 84(12): 1318-1325.

18. Berendsen AA, Kang JH, van de Rest O, Feskens EJ, de Groot LC, Grodstein F. The dietary approaches to stop hypertension diet, cognitive function, and cognitive decline in American older women. *Journal of the American Medical Directors Association* 2017; 18(5): 427-432.

19. Morris MC, Tangney CC, Wang Y, Sacks FM, Barnes LL, Bennett DA, Aggarwal NT. MIND diet slows cognitive decline with aging. *Alzheimer's &*

Dementia 2015; 11(9): 1015-1022.
20. Morris MC, Wang Y, Barnes LL, Bennett DA, Dawson-Hughes B, Booth SL. Nutrients and bioactives in green leafy vegetables and cognitive decline: Prospective study. *Neurology* 2018; 90(3): e214-e222.
21. Morris MC, Tangney CC, Wang Y, Sacks FM, Bennett DA, Aggarwal NT. MIND diet associated with reduced incidence of Alzheimer's disease. *Alzheimer's & Dementia* 2015; 11(9): 1007-1014.
22. Jiang X, Huang J, Song D, Deng R, Wei J, Zhang Z. Increased consumption of fruit and vegetables is related to a reduced risk of cognitive impairment and dementia: Meta-analysis. *Frontiers in Aging Neuroscience* 2017; 9: 18.
23. Giem P, Beeson WL, Fraser GE. The incidence of dementia and intake of animal products: preliminary findings from the Adventist Health Study. *Neuroepidemiology* 1993; 12(1): 28-36.
24. Tsai JH, Huang CF, Lin MN, Chang CE, Chang CC, Lin CL. Taiwanese vegetarians are associated with lower dementia risk: A prospective cohort study. *Nutrients* 2022; 14(3): 588.
25. World Health Organization. *Risk reduction of cognitive decline and dementia: WHO guidelines.* WHO 1 Jan 2019. www.who.int/publications/i/item/9789241550543
26. Ruan Y, Tang J, Guo X, Li K, Li D. Dietary fat intake and risk of Alzheimer's disease and dementia: a meta-analysis of cohort studies. *Current Alzheimer Research* 2018; 15(9): 869-876.
27. Zhang H, Greenwood DC, Risch HA, Bunce D, Hardie LJ, Cade JE. Meat consumption and risk of incident dementia: cohort study of 493,888 UK Biobank participants. *American Journal of Clinical Nutrition* 2021; 114(1): 175-184.
28. Ginieis R, Franz EA, Oey I, Peng M. The "sweet" effect: comparative assessments of dietary sugars on cognitive performance. *Physiology & Behavior* 2018; 184: 242-247.
29. Gentreau M, Chuy V, Féart C, Samieri C, Ritchie K, Raymond M, Berticat C, Artero S. Refined carbohydrate-rich diet is associated with long-term risk of dementia and Alzheimer's disease in apolipoprotein E ε4 allele carriers. *Alzheimer's & Dementia* 2020; 16(7): 1043-1053.
30. Yeh TS, Yuan C, Ascherio A, Rosner BA, Willett WC, Blacker D. Long-term dietary flavonoid intake and subjective cognitive decline in US men and women. *Neurology* 2021; 97(10): e1041-e1056.
31. Hein S, Whyte AR, Wood E, Rodriguez-Mateos A, Williams CM. Systematic review of the effects of blueberry on cognitive performance as we age. *The Journals of Gerontology: Series A* 2019; 74(7): 984-995.
32. Mao X, Chen C, Xun P, Daviglus ML, Steffen LM, Jacobs Jr DR, Van Horn L, Sidney S, Zhu N, Qin B, He K. Intake of vegetables and fruits through young adulthood is associated with better cognitive function in midlife in the US general population. *Journal of Nutrition* 2019; 149(8): 1424-1433.
33. González-Domínguez R, Castellano-Escuder P, Carmona F, Lefèvre-Arbogast S, Low DY, Du Preez A, Ruigrok SR, Manach C, Urpi-Sarda M, Korosi A, Lucassen PJ. Food and Microbiota Metabolites Associate with Cognitive Decline in Older Subjects: A 12-Year Prospective Study. *Molecular Nutrition & Food Research* 2021; 65(23): 2100606.
34. Yamagishi K, Maruyama K, Ikeda A, Nagao M, Noda H, Umesawa M, Hayama-Terada M, Muraki I, Okada C, Tanaka M, Kishida R. Dietary fiber intake and risk of incident disabling dementia: the Circulatory Risk in Communities Study. *Nutritional Neuroscience* 2022:1-8. doi: 10.1080/1028415X.2022.2027592
35. González-Domínguez R, Castellano-Escuder P, Carmona F, Lefèvre-Arbogast S, Low DY, Du Preez A, Ruigrok SR, Manach C, Urpi-Sarda M, Korosi A, Lucassen PJ. Food and Microbiota Metabolites Associate with Cognitive Decline in Older Subjects: A 12-Year Prospective Study. *Molecular Nutrition & Food Research* 2021; 65(23): 2100606.
36. Bakre AT, Chen R, Khutan R, Wei L, Smith T, Qin G, Danat IM, Zhou W, Schofield P, Clifford A, Wang J. Association between fish consumption and risk of dementia: a new study from China and a systematic literature review and meta-analysis. *Public Health Nutrition* 2018; 21(10): 1921-1932.
37. Dangour AD, Andreeva VA, Sydenham E, Uauy R. Omega 3 fatty acids and cognitive health in older people. *British Journal of Nutrition* 2012; 107(S2): S152-S158.

38. Smith AD, Smith SM, De Jager CA, Whitbread P, Johnston C, Agacinski G, Oulhaj A, Bradley KM, Jacoby R, Refsum H. Homocysteine-lowering by B vitamins slows the rate of accelerated brain atrophy in mild cognitive impairment: a randomized controlled trial. *PloS One* 2010; 5(9): e12244.
39. Douaud G, Refsum H, de Jager CA, Jacoby R, Nichols TE, Smith SM, Smith AD. Preventing Alzheimer's disease-related gray matter atrophy by B-vitamin treatment. *Proceedings of the National Academy of Sciences* 2013; 110(23): 9523-9528.
40. Mackey S, Allgaier N, Chaarani B, Spechler P, Orr C, Bunn J, Allen NB, Alia-Klein N, Batalla A, Blaine S, Brooks S. Mega-analysis of gray matter volume in substance dependence: general and substance-specific regional effects. *American Journal of Psychiatry* 2019; 176(2): 119-128.
41. Demirakca T, Ende G, Kämmerer N, Welzel-Marquez H, Hermann D, Heinz A, Mann K. Effects of alcoholism and continued abstinence on brain volumes in both genders. *Alcoholism: Clinical and Experimental Research* 2011; 35(9): 1678-1685.
42. Daviet R, Aydogan G, Jagannathan K, Spilka N, Koellinger PD, Kranzler HR, Nave G, Wetherill RR. Associations between alcohol consumption and gray and white matter volumes in the UK Biobank. *Nature Communications* 2022; 13(1): 1-1.
43. Baker LD, Espeland MA, Kivipelto M, Whitmer RA, Snyder HM, Carrillo MC, Antkowiak S, Chavin M, Cleveland M, Day CE, Desai P. US POINTER (USA) World-Wide FINGERS network: The first global network of multidomain dementia prevention trials. *Alzheimer's & Dementia* 2020; 16: e046951.

Chapter 14
Plant-based nutrition for autoimmunity and chronic inflammation

Despina Marselou

Introduction

Developed societies have witnessed an increase in autoimmune diseases over the past years, with significant effects on mortality and morbidity. Yet, despite enormous advances in the diagnosis and the treatment of autoimmune diseases, there is still a lack of data on the aetiological events that lead to clinical pathology. Increasing evidence has shown that abnormal inflammatory response is closely associated with many chronic diseases, especially autoimmune diseases, and that understanding the mechanism on how to manage inflammation will lead to significant clinical benefits for the prevention and treatment of autoimmune diseases.[1]

It is well-accepted that inflammation underlies a wide variety of physiological and pathological processes. The fire-starters of inflammation, infection and tissue injury are responsible for initiating most adverse conditions that induce inflammation, and can trigger the recruitment of leukocytes and plasma proteins to the affected tissue site. Tissue stress or malfunction similarly induces an adaptive response, which is usually referred to as low-grade inflammation, or para-inflammation.[2] Para-inflammation is possibly responsible for the majority of inflammatory conditions with usual examples being diabetes mellitus (DM), obesity and degenerative diseases. A common characteristic of all inflammatory disease is premature accelerated atherosclerosis, and common features include increased number of macrophages and inflammatory cytokine such as IL-1 and TNF-a.[2]

Macrophages play an important role in the maintenance of tissue homeostasis by eliminating invading pathogens, while the gut microbiome, a regulator of the local intestinal immune system, also has a profound influence on systemic immune responses. The production of short-chain fatty acids (SCFAs) and gram-negative bacterial lipopolysaccharides (LPS), exert anti-inflammatory or pro-inflammatory effects by acting on macrophages.[3] Disturbance of the gut microbiome due to environmental factors, such as method of childbirth delivery (C-section), stress, application of antibiotics and changes in diet towards a more Westernised style can result in chronic inflammation and inflammatory diseases. Inflammatory diseases are usually linked with cancer, fibrosis, degeneration and autoimmunity, and are closely linked with oxidative stress.[4]

In terms of diet, microbiome and inflammation, it has been suggested that high-fibre plant-based diets can alter the composition of gut bacteria and increase bacterial diversity, and such actions can reduce markers of inflammation. Additionally, bioactive compounds occurring in plant foods, primarily carotenoids, phenolic acids and flavonoids seem to modulate inflammatory as well as immunological processes.[5]

There is convincing evidence that plant foods and non-nutritive constituents associated with these foods modulate immunological and inflammatory processes. Referring to the evidence-base, this chapter will therefore discuss how a plant-based diet and certain food and food components of such a diet can prevent and/or combat inflammation and thus autoimmunity through the establishment of improved gut microbiome and regulation of oxidative stress.

Epidemiology

The overall prevalence of autoimmunity is approximately 7–9% in the general population and encompasses nearly 100 distinct autoimmune diseases; some of which are organ specific and some of which involve multiple organs. Some of the most common autoimmune conditions in Europe and the UK, according to latest European data, include coeliac disease, inflammatory bowel disease, systemic lupus erythematosus (SLE), Sjogren disease, systemic vasculitis, rheumatoid arthritis, psoriasis, psoriatic arthritis, myasthenia gravis, polymyalgia, diabetes, Graves' disease, Hashimoto disease, Addison's disease and multiple sclerosis.[6]

Environmental influences on autoimmune diseases

Genetic predisposing has been identified, yet environmental factors make up a significant part of the risk in disease initiation and propagation, and their identification has critical importance for understanding individual susceptibility. These environmental factors include nutrition, microbiome changes, infectious processes and xenobiotics, such as tobacco, pharmaceutical agents, hormones, ultraviolet light, silica solvents and heavy metals. Numerous other infectious agents have been suggested but not proven to have a dominant role, including bacteria, other viruses (herpes simplex virus and cytomegalovirus), parasites and fungi.[7]

Environmental factors and infectious agents are potential triggers to an individual's predisposition and initiation of autoimmunity via altering the equilibrium of the gut microbiome and reducing gut microbial diversity (dysbiosis).[7] It is worth mentioning that one of the most ubiquitous environmental factors for autoimmunity is the pandemic of a Westernised diet which consists of high intakes of high-fat foods, high-sugar desserts and drinks, high intakes of red meat, refined grains, and high-fat dairy products.[4] Another important characteristic is the inadequate consumption of fruits and vegetables which, according to the WHO in 2017, was responsible for an estimated 3.9 million deaths worldwide.[8]

A Western-style diet is responsible for the upregulation of cell metabolism, including the release or expression of pro-inflammatory molecules, leading to low-grade systemic inflammation. It also results in dysbiotic gut microbiota which consequently alters intestinal immunity.[4,9] Researchers have conducted intensive investigation, revealing a direct influence of Western diets on immune homeostasis, immune regulatory processes and on bacterial communities colonising the gut microbiome.[9] Disruption of the microbiome to such an extent may also result in excessive bioavailability of reactive oxygen species (ROS) and contribute to increased levels of oxidative stress.[10]

The role of nutrition and the microbiome in autoimmunity and chronic inflammation

The number of genes in our microbiome far exceed those of human genes, making us genetically 1% human and 99% bacteria, with the human colon having the largest population of bacteria in the body.[11] Gut bacteria play a major role in numerous body functions including immunity, digestion and protection against disease.[9, 11] Dysbiosis has been characterised as a pathological imbalance in the intestinal microbiota.[4, 9] It can trigger several types of inflammatory and autoimmune diseases through an imbalance between T helper cells (Th1, Th2 and Th17) that are activated in case of inflammation, and regulatory T cells (Tregs). The latter are a specialised subpopulation of T cells responsible for immune response suppression.[12]

Possible reasons for dysbiosis

These include recurrent infections and inflammation, obesity, a diet high in saturated fat, animal protein, refined sugar and prepared processed foods, micronutrient deficiencies and micronutrient excesses.[13, 14] One example of the latter is that dietary iron has been found to be a major driver of the microbial community structure.[15] As such, dietary iron excess and or/supplementation can adversely alter gut microbiota composition.[15, 16] High iron body stores are correlated with increased markers of chronic inflammation and risk factors of diabetes and metabolic syndrome.[16] It has been observed that increased serum ferritin and transferrin levels in pregnant women are associated with lower *Bifidobacteriaceae* strains and increased *Eschericia coli* strains.[17] In two double-blind randomised controlled trials in 115 6-month-old Kenyan infants, iron fortification was correlated with high prevalence of pathogens, including *Salmonella*, *Clostridium difficile*, *Clostridium perfringens* and *E. coli*, causing intestinal inflammation.[18]

The above points are supported by a recent review conducted by Paoli et al. in order to evaluate the ketogenic diet. This is a very popular high-protein, (animal derived) dietary approach to autoimmunity and is used by many health professionals, despite the fact that most ketogenic studies have small number of participants and controversial findings. The authors concluded that a ketogenic diet reduces bacteria taxa, richness and diversity, and in order to avoid all the aforementioned detrimental effects to the microbiome and preserve good gut health, plant proteins such as pea protein and the introduction of probiotics and prebiotics with emphasis on water kefir, kimchi and fermented vegetables is necessary.[19]

With regards to oxidative stress and body oxidation, high intakes of haem iron and saturated fat, which can easily be achieved by following a Westernised diet, can cause mitochondrial dysfunction and increased ROS production through adverse effects on the mitochondrial life cycle. This can trigger an immunological response through high levels of oxidative and inflammatory damage and contribute to the pathology of autoimmunity. Severe mitochondrial dysfunction triggers an increased level of oxidative and inflammatory damage, impairs tissue function, and promotes chronic intestinal inflammation and age-related disease.[20]

When it comes to systemic autoimmune diseases, several studies have shown that patients with SLE are characterised by increased oxidative stress, resulting in immune system dysregulation, abnormal activation and processing of cell-death signals, and autoantibody production.[21]

Although meat cannot be considered a highly oxidised matrix, due to its relatively low polyunsaturated fatty acid (PUFA) content, meat and meat products undergo radical oxidative changes during storage, processing, digestion, and metabolism, which make them a potential cause of oxidative stress. A high haem iron intake through diet can promote ROS formation at the gastrointestinal tract and act as a nitrosating agent after being metabolised by intestinal bacteria. N-nitroso compounds are then generated, which are capable of causing DNA damage. Other proposed mechanisms of inflammatory-promoting effects of meat involve mutagens generation by high temperature grilling, high dietary intake of salt and saturated fat, pro-oxidant effects of haem iron, and production of trimethylamine N-oxide (TMAO) by the gut microbiome.[22]

Plant-based/vegan diet gut profile

It is well established that microbiota metabolise resistant starches and dietary fibre through fermentation and decomposition, which leads to the production of short chain fatty acids (SCFAs) in the host, creating a slightly acidic environment with values between pH 5.5 and 6.5. This pH does not support the growth of pathogenic bacteria. The major SCFAs are acetate, propionate and butyrate and pentanoate. Studies have suggested that SCFAs contribute to a wide range of functions, from immune regulation (regulation of T cell polarisation and induction), to metabolism in a variety of tissues and organs.[23] The production of SCFAs is thought to be altered by a high-fat diet, shown by decreased levels of butyrate which seem to play a role in maintaining intestinal homeostasis.[24]

Few studies include vegan subjects as a predominant group, yet when vegan diets are directly compared to vegetarian and Westernised omnivorous diets, a pattern of protective health benefits emerges. A study by De Filippo et al.[25] compared European children following a Western diet to children in Burkina Faso in Africa who followed a high-fibre, vegetarian diet (fibre: 10–14 g per day). The nutritional regime included mainly cereals and grains (millet, sorghum), legumes (black-eyed peas), vegetables and herbs. The results showed that the African microbiome is dominated by the *Prevotella* enterotype, with an overall enrichment in Gram-positive bacteria and increased production of SCFAs. The African microbiome is also characterised by a higher microbial richness and diversity, and a comparatively lower prevalence of pathogenic strain.

In a Slovenian Study with 31 participants (11 lacto-ovo vegetarians and 20 vegans), *Bacteroides-Prevotella* (Gram positive bacteria) have been shown to increase in abundance with a vegetarian or vegan diet.[26]

A large sample study by Zimmer et al.[27] that included volunteers attending the World Vegetarian and Vegan Congress, showed reduced *E. coli* and *Enterobacteriaceae* (pathogenic bacteria responsible for triggering low grade inflammation) in vegetarians and vegans compared to omnivores.

Plant-based diets and effectiveness in autoimmunity

When exploring the connection between diet and certain autoimmune diseases, a vegan diet can be preventive and possibly effective in modulating specific inflammatory markers, either by causing beneficial changes to the gut or due to its antioxidant and anti-inflammatory profile. Such a diet contains higher amounts of fibre, folic acid, vitamin C and E, potassium, magnesium, and has enhanced amounts of phytochemicals. In the following analysis, several studies supporting the accumulating scientific evidence and beneficial impact of vegan diets in autoimmunity and inflammation will be reviewed.

Autoimmune thyroid disease

Hashimoto disease and Graves' disease are characterised by an autoimmune reaction against thyroid autoantigens. The role of a vegan diet in relation to thyroid disorders has been explored by the Seventh Day Adventists study, which suggests that a vegan diet may be protective of thyroid disorders. The study, whereby 97,000 church members were asked about their dietary habits and health conditions, reported that people who followed a vegan diet were less likely to develop hypothyroidism, compared to those following the standard American diet. Those who followed a lacto-ovo (dairy and egg) vegetarian diet were more likely to develop hypothyroidism, compared to those following the standard American diet.[28]

In a cross sectional study, findings showed that frequent consumption of animal fats and butter is associated with positive plasma thyroid peroxidase antibody (TPO-Ab) and/or thyroglobulin antibody (Tg-Ab), while frequent consumption of vegetables (root, leafy and flower vegetables), as well as diets with high consumption of dried fruit, nuts, and muesli are associated with negative findings of TPO-Ab and/or Tg-Ab. Participants that had undergone thyroid surgery or were taking medication were excluded. The suggested theory underlying the results is that frequent consumption of animal fats and butter can result in a low dietary ratio of n-3 fatty acids, which have anti-inflammatory properties, to n-6 fatty acids, which promote inflammation. Phytosterols, a collective term for plant-derived sterols and stanols, which play an important role in the regulation of cardiovascular diseases and also exhibit anti-cancer properties, and PUFAs, are involved in the regulation of pro-inflammatory cytokines and act as anti-inflammatory mediators.[29]

Another study worth mentioning is by Eleutheriou et al., which concluded that patients with Hashimoto disease *and* anti-TPO positive samples had anti N-Glycolylneuraminic acid (Neu5Gc) antibody concentrations higher than the mean value of the general population. This direct relationship raised the concept of a probable association between anti-Neu5Gc antibody development and autoimmune hypothyroidism. According to research, Neu5Gc is widely expressed on most mammalian tissues and is found in foods and additives derived from animal origin, with major sources being lamb, pork and beef, and to a lesser extent milk and dairy products.[30]

Systemic lupus erythematosus (SLE)

A case study by Goldner (2019)[31] suggested a possible correlation between a raw plant-based food diet, combined with fasting and improved symptoms of SLE, while another study found that increased intakes of polyphenols in the diet, derived from apples, oranges, asparagus, white beans and walnuts were associated with faecal levels of beneficial bacteria (*lactobacillus Blautia* and *bifidobacterium*) in SLE patients.[32]

Multiple sclerosis (MS)

With reference to MS, the risk association between the disease and diets high in saturated fat and animal protein has been observed in multiple studies.[33, 34] Additionally, it has been observed that the risk of MS is increased when there is less consumption of vegetable protein (nuts, legumes), less fibre (all unrefined plants), less vitamin C and potassium (fresh fruits and vegetables).[35]

A low saturated fat diet seems to be the most effective treatment according to literature reviews, with emphasis on increased consumption of fruits and vegetables. For example, the HOLISM study[36] showed that higher intakes of fruits and vegetables were associated with reduced levels of disease activity and disability according to several patients' reports. Similarly, a recent large cross-sectional survey with 7,639 participants in the North American Research Committee on MS suggested that patients with high diet quality scores, which indicated higher consumption of fruits and vegetables, legumes and whole grains and less foods with added sugars and red/processed meat had lower odds of disability and symptom severity.[37]

Another significant multicentre study in 2019, with paediatric patients, investigating the relationship between saturated fat and increased risk of MS, showed that for each 10% increase in saturated fat consumption, there was an associated 237% increased risk of relapse. Conversely, each cup of vegetables was associated with a 50% decreased risk of relapse.[38]

Finally, a randomised controlled, blinded, one-year study, with 61 participants with MS were assigned to a low-fat, plant-based diet. The nutritional protocol, which is widely known as the McDougall diet, was based entirely on foods like beans, breads, corn, pastas, potatoes, sweet potatoes, and rice, with the addition of fruits and non-starchy vegetables.[39] There were no significant differences in clinical relapse rates or disability. However, the participants showed significant improvements in measures of fatigue, BMI and metabolic biomarkers such as LDL, an important finding since recent studies have suggested that cholesterol level and markers of cholesterol turnover in the peripheral blood may be associated with adverse clinical outcomes in MS.[40]

Rheumatoid arthritis (RA)

RA is a systemic, chronic inflammatory autoimmune disorder, with an altered intestinal microbiota being implicated in the etiopathogenesis. Patients generally complain of gastrointestinal tract problems, particularly dyspepsia (bloating, postprandial fullness, nausea, early satiety, epigastric pain), mucosal ulceration, and altered bowel habits (constipation/diarrhoea).[41] Multiple studies have shown that patients with RA may benefit from following diets rich in fibre, thereby increasing bacterial diversity. Such diets have high antioxidant capacity and can therefore help to reduce pain and inflammation in RA patients.

Nenonen et al. demonstrated that a raw vegan diet rich in *lactobacilli* and fibre decreased symptoms of RA, suggesting that the probiotic *lactobacilli*, among other anti-inflammatory components, such as berries, fruits, vegetables and roots, nuts, germinated seeds and sprouts may be helpful for RA patients.[42] A recent, randomised controlled crossover trial, assigned 50 patients to either an anti-inflammatory diet, referred to as the 'fibre diet' (fruits, whole-grain cereals, pomegranate and blueberries, nuts, and juice shots with probiotics, salmon), or to a control group, referred to as the 'protein group' (meat or chicken, and refined grains daily, protein bar or quark for snacks, and breakfasts based on white bread with either a butter-based spread or cheese). The results showed significant improvements in disease activity during the intervention period, using unadjusted analysis.[43]

Peltonel et al. randomly assigned 43 RA patients to either a raw vegan diet rich in *lactobacilli*, or an omnivorous diet. There was a significant change in the faecal flora after a month of the 18 patients in the vegan diet group, while no change was reported in the omnivore control group. More importantly, the vegan diet also induced a decrease in disease activity in some of the RA patients.[44] Kjeldsen-Kragh et al. followed their lead with a controlled, single-blind trial of patients with rheumatoid arthritis. These patients were advised to follow a fasting diet, followed by three and a half months of a vegan diet, followed by a 9-month lactovegetarian diet. Subjects in the vegan/vegetarian diet group improved significantly in terms of their clinical symptoms and faecal composition compared to those who maintained an omnivorous diet.[45]

Benefits from following a mostly plant-based

diet can also be shown without remarkable effects on the intestinal flora. Such findings were established in several studies, for example, Michalsen et al. assigned participants with RA to a mostly vegetarian-modified, whole grain, Mediterranean diet, or to a supervised, modified fast of eight days with partial nutrient intake of vegetable broth, herbal teas, parsley, garlic, and decoction of potatoes, including juice extracts from carrots, beets, and celery.[46] Fasting participants showed better clinical outcomes and symptom-relief despite no reported changes to the faecal flora.

A single-blind dietary intervention study evaluated the influence of a four week, very low-fat (approximately 10% of energy from fat) vegan diet and found that rheumatoid factor was decreased by 10 % and C-reactive protein (CRP) by 16%.[47]

Another randomised clinical trial showed that a vegan diet, free of gluten improved signs and symptoms of patients with active RA and decreased a pro-inflammatory antibody (immunoglobulin), which is often elevated in RA patients.[48]

Despite the fact that no effect on the intestinal flora was noticed, these studies showed significant decreases in swollen and tender joints, pain, morning stiffness and CRP. These outcomes suggest that certain food antigens found in the gastrointestinal tract might play a role in the pathology of RA, since improvements in disease activity were evident as soon as diet was changed, with such antigens originating from the omnivorous diet being eliminated. Additionally, regular consumption of fresh fruits packed with important phytochemicals can reduce oxidative stress and inflammation, both contributors to autoimmunity, and cohort studies have reported that regular and high consumption is associated with downregulation of disease activity and may also provide protective effects against RA and polyarthritis.[49, 50]

Indeed, bioactive compounds occurring in fruits and vegetables, primarily carotenoids and flavonoids, seem to regulate inflammatory as well as immunological responses according to research. Looking more closely to specific fruits and vegetables that have anti-inflammatory and antioxidant properties, one study suggested that consumption of tomato-based products or lycopene supplements led to a significant reduction in the serum concentrations of low-density lipoprotein cholesterol, and inflammatory markers such as interleukin (IL)-6, as well as C-reactive protein (CRP).[51]

In another randomised controlled trial including 42 volunteers undergoing peritoneal dialysis, 26 of them were shown to have significant reductions in CRP concentrations (-71.4%) and IL-6 (-51.7%) after the consumption of 400 mg of standardised garlic allium twice a day for two months.[52]

Supporting the anti-inflammatory effect of fruits and vegetables, a study evaluated the impact of anthocyanin-rich fruit, including the type and amount of fruit, as well as the processing methods, on inflammatory and oxidative stress markers. They described significant changes in IL-6, TNF-α, hs-CRP, IL-1 receptor antagonist (IL-1ra), and IL-10 levels as markers of inflammation, and changes in malondialdehyde (MDA) and protein carbonyls levels as markers of oxidative stress. Blackcurrants, tart cherries, and blueberries showed the highest anti-inflammatory effect, while acai and tart cherries showed the highest antioxidant effect.[53]

Additionally, an in vivo controlled study reported improvements in inflammatory markers such as CRP and TNF-α after the intake of 30 g/day of broccoli sprouts for 10 weeks respectively, in relation to inflammation and endothelial function.[54]

Finally, a unique compound under investigation is anatabine, a naturally occurring alkaloid found in *Solanaceae* family plants and nightshade vegetables, such as peppers, potatoes, tomatoes, and eggplant. According to an internet-based study, the compound has been suggested to reduce the level of inflammation and pain caused by musculoskeletal disorders. Participants that took part in the study had a medical diagnosis of osteoarthritis (20%) while others had no diagnosis for their joint pains, but had experienced pain across their joints, including wrists, knees, fingers and hands for more than seven years. 82% of the survey respondents reported that anatabine supplementation was helpful for joint pain or stiffness relief within a period of four weeks to two months, while 138 of 232 of individuals reported that they had cut back on the use of pain relief or other medications for joint pain or stiffness while using anatabine.[55]

Despite the fact the results showed a remarkable improvement in joint pain and stiffness, controlled studies are necessary to investigate the above results, with the focus being on the consumption of naturally occurring anatabine from nightshades vegetables instead of supplementation.

Conclusion

There is currently a satisfactory evidence-base supporting the benefits of a plant-based diet against chronic inflammatory diseases and autoimmune disease. Most studies are focused on:
- the anti-inflammatory properties of such a diet
- the unique gut profile of those eating a predominantly plant-based diet
- the low-fat, low-cholesterol, high fibre, antioxidant content, pure characteristics of a mostly plant-based diet.

More research is required to determine the strength of the association between a vegan diet, microbiota profile, degrees of inflammation, and autoimmune response, with the highest level of evidence based on the results of well-designed, large, long-term RCTs. Similar methodologies are necessary in order to minimise controversial interpretation, and observation of contrasting effects between vegan diets, lacto-ovo vegetarian and Mediterranean diets is essential. Research needs to address the importance of following a long-term vegan diet, as this may reveal alternative enterotype states beneficial for the gut microbiota. Furthermore, the quantity and quality of fibre, diet, and dietary components might need attention in certain autoimmune conditions.

It is also important to analyse the dose of fruits and vegetables' bioactive compounds to achieve the maximum benefit of antioxidant capacity. Finally taking a closer look at agricultural science, it seems that the polyphenol, phytochemical, and flavonoid effect of several crops, including night shade vegetables, seem to be significant. Possible culinary combinations that take into consideration the ratios of hydrophilic and lipophilic phytochemicals of each combination, in order to create stronger synergistic antioxidant and anti-inflammatory effects, might be the key to reducing inflammation effectively.

References

1. Duan L, Rao X, Sigdel KR. Regulation of Inflammation in Autoimmune Disease. *J Immunol Res* 2019; 2019: 7403796. doi:10.1155/2019/7403796
2. Biswas SK. Does the Interdependence between Oxidative Stress and Inflammation Explain the Antioxidant Paradox?. *Oxid Med Cell Longev* 2016; 2016: 5698931. doi:10.1155/2016/5698931
3. Vinolo MA, Rodrigues HG, Nachbar RT, Curi R. Regulation of inflammation by short chain fatty acids. *Nutrients* 2011; 3(10): 858-876. doi:10.3390/nu3100858
4. Martinez KB, Leone V, Chang EB. Western diets, gut dysbiosis, and metabolic diseases: Are they linked? *Gut Microbes* 2017; 8(2): 130-142. doi: 10.1080/19490976.2016.1270811
5. Liu RH. Health-promoting components of fruits

and vegetables in the diet. *Adv Nutr* 2013; 4(3): 384S-392S. doi:10.3945/an.112.003517
6. Cooper GS, Bynum ML, Somers EC. Recent insights in the epidemiology of autoimmune diseases: improved prevalence estimates and understanding of clustering of diseases. *J Autoimmun* 2009; 33(3-4): 197-207. doi:10.1016/j.jaut.2009.09.008
7. Wang L, Wang F-S, Gershwin ME. Human autoimmune diseases: a comprehensive update. *J Intern Med* 2015; 278: 369–395. doi: 10.1111/joim.12395
8. World Health Organization. Increasing Fruit and Vegetable Consumption to Reduce the Risk of Noncommunicable Diseases. www.who.int/elena/titles/fruit_vegetables_ncds/en/ (accessed on 24 April 2021).
9. Brown K, DeCoffe D, Molcan E, Gibson DL. Diet-induced dysbiosis of the intestinal microbiota and the effects on immunity and disease. Nutrients 2012; 4(11): 1552-1553. *Nutrients* 2012; 4(8): 1095-1119. doi:10.3390/nu4081095
10. Bhattacharyya A, Chattopadhyay R, Mitra S, Crowe SE. Oxidative stress: an essential factor in the pathogenesis of gastrointestinal mucosal diseases. *Physiol Rev* 2014; 94(2): 329-354. doi:10.1152/physrev.00040.2012
11. Sender R, Fuchs S, Milo R. Revised Estimates for the Number of Human and Bacteria Cells in the Body. *PLoS Biol* 2016; 14(8): e1002533. doi: 10.1371/journal.pbio.1002533
12. Pott J, Stockinger S. Type I and III Interferon in the Gut: Tight Balance between Host Protection and Immunopathology. *Front Immunol* 2017; 8: 258. doi: 10.3389/fimmu.2017.00258
13. Hawrelak JA, Myers SP. The causes of intestinal dysbiosis: a review. *Altern Med Rev* 2004; 9(2): 180-197.
14. Hibberd MC, Wu M, Rodionov DA, Li X, Cheng J, et al. The effects of micronutrient deficiencies on bacterial species from the human gut microbiota. *Sci Transl Med* 2017; 9(390): eaal4069. doi: 10.1126/scitranslmed.aal4069
15. Kortman GA, Raffatellu M, Swinkels DW, Tjalsma H. Nutritional iron turned inside out: intestinal stress from a gut microbial perspective. *FEMS Microbiol Rev* 2014; 38(6): 1202-1234. doi: 10.1111/1574-6976.12086

16. Rajpathak SN, Crandall JP, Wylie-Rosett J, Kabat GC, Rohan TE, Hu FB. The role of iron in type 2 diabetes in humans. *Biochim Biophys Acta* 2009; 1790(7): 671-681. doi: 10.1016/j.bbagen.2008.04.005
17. Santacruz A, Collado MC, García-Valdés L, et al. Gut microbiota composition is associated with body weight, weight gain and biochemical parameters in pregnant women. *Br J Nutr* 2010; 104(1): 83-92. doi: 10.1017/S0007114510000176
18. Jaeggi T, Kortman GA, Moretti D, et al. Iron fortification adversely affects the gut microbiome, increases pathogen abundance and induces intestinal inflammation in Kenyan infants. *Gut* 2015; 64(5): 731-742. doi: 10.1136/gutjnl-2014-307720
19. Paoli A, Mancin L, Bianco A, et al. Ketogenic Diet and Microbiota: Friends or Enemies? *Genes (Basel)* 2019; 10(7): 534. doi: 10.3390/genes10070534
20. Liesa M, Shirihai OS. Mitochondrial dynamics in the regulation of nutrient utilization and energy expenditure. *Cell Metab* 2013; 17(4): 491-506. doi: 10.1016/j.cmet.2013.03.002
21. Gergely P Jr, Niland B, Gonchoroff N, et al. Persistent mitochondrial hyperpolarization, increased reactive oxygen intermediate production, and cytoplasmic alkalinization characterize altered IL-10 signaling in patients with systemic lupus erythematosus. *J Immunol* 2002; 169(2): 1092-1101. doi: 10.4049/jimmunol.169.2.1092
22. Macho-González A, Garcimartín A, López-Oliva ME, et al. Can Meat and Meat-Products Induce Oxidative Stress?. *Antioxidants (Basel)* 2020; 9(7): 638. doi:10.3390/antiox9070638
23. Luu M, Pautz S, Kohl V, et al. The short-chain fatty acid pentanoate suppresses autoimmunity by modulating the metabolic-epigenetic crosstalk in lymphocytes. *Nat Commun* 2019; 10(1): 760. doi: 10.1038/s41467-019-08711-2
24. Coppola S, Avagliano C, Calignano A, Berni Canani R. The Protective Role of Butyrate against Obesity and Obesity-Related Diseases. *Molecules* 2021; 26: 682. doi: 10.3390/molecules26030682
25. De Filippo C, Cavalieri D, Paola M, et al. (2010). Impact of diet in shaping gut microbiota revealed by a comparative study in children from Europe

and rural Africa. *Proceedings of the National Academy of Sciences* 2010; 107(33): 14691-14696. doi: 10.1073/pnas.1005963107
26. Matijašić BB, Obermajer T, Lipoglavšek L, et al. Association of dietary type with fecal microbiota in vegetarians and omnivores in Slovenia. *Eur J Nutr* 2014; 53(4): 1051-1064. doi: 10.1007/s00394-013-0607-6
27. Zimmer J, Lange B, Frick JS, Sauer H, Zimmermann K, Schwiertz A, Rusch K, Klosterhalfen S, Enck P. A vegan or vegetarian diet substantially alters the human colonic faecal microbiota. *Eur J Clin Nutr* 2012; 66(1): 53-60. doi: 10.1038/ejcn.2011.141
28. Tonstad S, Nathan E, Oda K, Fraser GE. Prevalence of hyperthyroidism according to type of vegetarian diet. *Public Health Nutr* 2015; 18(8): 1482-1487. doi: 10.1017/S1368980014002183
29. Matana A, Torlak V, Brdar D, et al. Dietary Factors Associated with Plasma Thyroid Peroxidase and Thyroglobulin Antibodies. *Nutrients* 2017; 9(11): 1186. doi:10.3390/nu9111186
30. Eleftheriou P, Kynigopoulos S, Giovou A, et al. Prevalence of Anti-Neu5Gc Antibodies in Patients with Hypothyroidism. *BioMed Research International* 2014; 2014: 963230. doi: 10.1155/2014/963230
31. Goldner B. Six Week Raw Vegan Nutrition Protocol Rapidly Reverses Lupus Nephritis: A Case Series. *International Journal of Disease Reversal and Prevention* 2019; 1(1). doi: 10.22230/ijdrp.2019v1n1a47
32. Cuervo A, Hevia A, López P, et al. Association of polyphenols from oranges and apples with specific intestinal microorganisms in systemic lupus erythematosus patients. *Nutrients* 2015; 7(2): 1301-1317. doi:10.3390/nu7021301
33. Katz Sand I. The Role of Diet in Multiple Sclerosis: Mechanistic Connections and Current Evidence. *Curr Nutr Rep* 2018; 7(3): 150-160. doi:10.1007/s13668-018-0236-z
34. Esparza ML, Sasaki S, Kesteloot H. Nutrition, latitude, and multiple sclerosis mortality: an ecologic study. *Am J Epidemiol* 1995; 142(7): 733-737. PMID: 7572944.
35. Ghadirian P, Jain M, Ducic S, Shatenstein B, Morisset R. Nutritional factors in the aetiology of multiple sclerosis: a case-control study in Montreal, Canada. *Int J Epidemiol* 1998; 27(5): 845-852. doi: 10.1093/ije/27.5.845
36. Hadgkiss EJ, Jelinek GA, Weiland TJ, et al. The association of diet with quality of life, disability, and relapse rate in an international sample of people with multiple sclerosis. *Nutr Neurosci* 2015; 18(3): 125-136. doi:10.1179/1476830514Y.0000000117
37. Fitzgerald KC, Tyry T, Salter A, Cofield SS, Cutter G, Fox R, Marrie RA. Diet quality is associated with disability and symptom severity in multiple sclerosis. *Neurology* 2018; 90(1): e1-e11. doi: 10.1212/WNL.0000000000004768
38. Azary S, Schreiner T, Graves J, et al. Contribution of dietary intake to relapse rate in early paediatric multiple sclerosis. *J Neurol Neurosurg Psychiatry* 2018; 89(1): 28-33. doi: 10.1136/jnnp-2017-315936
39. Yadav V, Marracci G, Kim E, Spain R, Cameron M, Overs S, Riddehough A, Li DK, McDougall J, Lovera J, Murchison C, Bourdette D. Low-fat, plant-based diet in multiple sclerosis: A randomized controlled trial. *Mult Scler Relat Disord* 2016; 9: 80-90. doi: 10.1016/j.msard.2016.07.001
40. Zhornitsky S, McKay KA, Metz LM, Teunissen CE, Rangachari M. Cholesterol and markers of cholesterol turnover in multiple sclerosis: relationship with disease outcomes. *Mult Scler Relat Disord* 2016; 5: 53-65. doi: 10.1016/j.msard.2015.10.005
41. Gul'neva MIu, Noskov SM. Colonic microbial biocenosis in rheumatoid arthritis. *Klin Med (Mosk)* 2011; 89(4): 45-48. PMID: 21932563.
42. Nenonen MT, Helve TA, Rauma AL, Hänninen OO. Uncooked, lactobacilli-rich, vegan food and rheumatoid arthritis. *Br J Rheumatol* 1998; 37(3): 274-281. doi: 10.1093/rheumatology/37.3.274
43. Vadell AKE, Bärebring L, Hulander E, Gjertsson I, Lindqvist HM, Winkvist A. Anti-inflammatory Diet In Rheumatoid Arthritis (ADIRA)-a randomized, controlled crossover trial indicating effects on disease activity. *Am J Clin Nutr* 2020; 111(6): 1203-1213. doi:10.1093/ajcn/nqaa019
44. Peltonen R, Nenonen M, Helve T et al. Faecal microbial flora and disease activity in rheumatoid arthritis during a vegan diet. *Br J Rheumatol* 1997; 36(1): 64-68. doi: 10.1093/rheumatology/36.1.64

45. Kjeldsen-Kragh J. Rheumatoid arthritis treated with vegetarian diets. *Am J Clin Nutr* 1999; 70(3 Suppl): 594S-600S. doi: 10.1093/ajcn/70.3.594s
46. Michalsen A, Riegert M, Lüdtke R, Bäcker M, Langhorst J, Schwickert M, Dobos GJ. Mediterranean diet or extended fasting's influence on changing the intestinal microflora, immunoglobulin A secretion and clinical outcome in patients with rheumatoid arthritis and fibromyalgia: an observational study. *BMC Complement Altern Med* 2005; 5: 22. doi: 10.1186/1472-6882-5-22
47. McDougall J, Bruce B, Spiller G, Westerdahl J, McDougall M. Effects of a very low-fat, vegan diet in subjects with rheumatoid arthritis. *J Altern Complement Med* 2002; 8(1): 71-75. doi: 10.1089/107555302753507195
48. Hafström I, Ringertz B, Spångberg A, von Zweigbergk L, Brannemark S, Nylander I, Rönnelid J, Laasonen L, Klareskog L. A vegan diet free of gluten improves the signs and symptoms of rheumatoid arthritis: the effects on arthritis correlate with a reduction in antibodies to food antigens. *Rheumatology (Oxford)* 2001; 40(10): 1175-1179. doi: 10.1093/rheumatology/40.10.1175
49. Islam MA, Alam F, Solayman M, et al. Dietary Phytochemicals: Natural Swords Combating Inflammation and Oxidation-Mediated Degenerative Diseases. *Oxid Med Cell Longev* 2016; 2016: 5137431. doi: 10.1155/2016/5137431
50. Pattison DJ, Silman AJ, Goodson NJ, et al. Vitamin C and the risk of developing inflammatory polyarthritis: prospective nested case-control study. *Ann Rheum Dis* 2004; 63(7): 843-847. doi: 10.1136/ard.2003.016097
51. Cheng HM, Koutsidis G, Lodge JK, Ashor AW, Siervo M, Lara J. Lycopene and tomato and risk of cardiovascular diseases: A systematic review and meta-analysis of epidemiological evidence. *Crit Rev Food Sci Nutr* 2019; 59(1): 141-158. doi: 10.1080/10408398.2017.1362630
52. Zare E, Alirezaei A, Bakhtiyari M, Mansouri A. Evaluating the effect of garlic extract on serum inflammatory markers of peritoneal dialysis patients: a randomized double-blind clinical trial study. *BMC Nephrol* 2019; 20(1) :26. doi: 10.1186/s12882-019-1204-6
53. Bloedon TK, Braithwaite RE, Carson IA, et al. Impact of anthocyanin-rich whole fruit consumption on exercise-induced oxidative stress and inflammation: a systematic review and meta-analysis. *Nutr Rev* 2019; nuz018. doi: 10.1093/nutrit/nuz018
54. López-Chillón MT, Carazo-Díaz C, Prieto-Merino D, et al. Effects of long-term consumption of broccoli sprouts on inflammatory markers in overweight subjects. *Clin Nutr* 2019; 38(2): 745-752. doi: 10.1016/j.clnu.2018.03.006
55. Lanier RK, Gibson KD, Cohen AE, Varga M. Effects of dietary supplementation with the solanaceae plant alkaloid anatabine on joint pain and stiffness: results from an internet-based survey study. *Clin Med Insights Arthritis Musculoskelet Disord* 2013; 6: 73-84. doi: 10.4137/CMAMD.S13001

Chapter 15
Plant-based nutrition and bone health

Rajiv Bajekal and Lisa Simon

Introduction

While the beneficial effects of a plant-based diet have been demonstrated in relation to many common chronic conditions, its role in supporting a more 'mechanical' framework, such as the skeleton, has been called into question and some concerns have been raised by sceptics in relation to studies like the EPIC-Oxford study.[1] This has certainly increased the focus on obtaining nutrients of concern in an exclusively whole food plant-based (WFPB) diet, such as vitamin B12 from supplementation, and having a body mass index (BMI) in the healthy range from an increase in muscle mass as a result of resistance training. Exclusively plant-based diets are undoubtedly becoming more popular, and this chapter will review the available evidence to see whether a well-planned WFPB diet, with appropriate supplements, can be nutritionally adequate to sustain bone health and prevent fractures.

Studies of bone health in vegans and vegetarians

The EPIC-Oxford study was a well-designed, epidemiological study with a sizeable vegan group. A previous report from the same group in 2007 had self-reported fracture data but this time it was from hospital-collected data which is considered more reliable. While some of the statistical methods and categorisations have been criticised, there is little doubt that lessons should be learned from this study as there was shown to be an overall 231% higher incidence of hip fractures in vegans compared to meat eaters. In real terms this equated to 19 more fractures in every 1000 patients over a ten-year period. Vegans in this study had lower than recommended intakes of calcium and a lower use of hormone replacement therapy in women compared with meat-eaters, factors that are relevant to the risk of bone fractures. The mean calcium intake for vegans was around 600 mg/day, so not meeting UK recommendations for 700 mg/day. Non-meat eaters also had a lower protein intake than meat-eaters, which appeared to be contributing to the risk of fractures in the analysis. In this study a

BMI below 22.5, especially in women, seemed to correlate with a much higher rate of fracture incidence, and leaner vegans seemed to suffer fractures more readily. However, as discussed throughout this book, those consuming plant-based diets have a reduced risk of chronic illnesses so a sensible approach may be to build BMI from an increase in muscle and strength-building activities, which correlates well with bone strength.

The study had a major limitation in that it did not consider vitamin D levels or correlate this with fractures, and as discussed later in the chapter, vitamin D is an important factor in bone health. It is well known from a previous report of the EPIC-Oxford study that only 50% of vegans were supplementing vitamin D and B12. This is relevant as at that time (the 1990s), when this data was being collected, the evidence base showing how essential these nutrients are to good bone health was not as strong as it is today.

The other large cohort study is a report from the Adventist Health Study 2,[2] which includes more than 96,000 Adventists from North America, followed since 2002. The study showed that vegans have a 55% increased risk of developing a hip fracture compared to omnivores. Again, this figure sounds alarming, but in absolute terms amounts to 1.5 extra hip fractures per 1000 vegans per year. Again, the increased risk was only seen in women, not men, and this time the risk completely disappeared in vegans taking both calcium and vitamin D supplements.

What is osteoporosis?

Osteoporosis is a quantitative reduction in bone mass due to an imbalance between bone formation (osteoblasts) and bone resorption (osteoclasts), which is part of the remodelling process and prevents microfractures from becoming macrofractures.[3] These two processes are normally in balance, and our skeleton, which stores 99% of calcium in our bodies, is replaced every 10 years. Bone stock is maximal at age 30–35 years, although 90% of bone mass has already been accumulated by age 18, showing us how essential this early phase of life is in building 'reserve'.[4] After this time, we steadily lose bone mass and strength, with maximal loss of 3–4% occurring in the one year around the age of menopause in women due to the loss of the bone protective effect of oestrogen.

Hip and spinal fractures caused by osteoporosis are becoming more common in the aging populations around the world, especially in Western societies, and according to the International Osteoporosis Foundation, one in three women and one in five men will experience an osteoporotic fracture in their lifetime.

Primary osteoporosis, where there is no identified cause, is often due to lifestyle factors. Thus, prevention and treatment should primarily be focused on lifestyle approaches. If there is a history of a fragility fracture (fall from ground height), then due consideration must be given to starting medication such as a bisphosphonate. Discussion of medication is outside the remit of this chapter.

Secondary osteoporosis is when there is a known underlying cause. This could be one of several disorders, such as hyperthyroidism, or neoplastic conditions such as multiple myeloma, and the management focus should be to identify and treat the cause.

Primary osteoporosis is of two main types. Type I involutional affects mainly post-menopausal women. The effects are seen primarily in cancellous or trabecular bone. Type II involutional is also called senile osteoporosis and affects mainly cortical bone.[3]

Genetic factors

Primary osteoporosis, like many other disorders, can be linked to multiple genes, but healthy lifestyle factors can still significantly reduce this risk, and like many other conditions, optimising lifestyle often overcomes a poor deal from the genetic angle.

Hip fracture and associated mortality

Osteoporosis is not a painful condition unless one sustains a fracture, and even these may not be painful in the spine in 60% of patients. However, there is a real concern that osteoporosis can result in a hip fracture, which is often associated with an extremely high mortality. Data from the International Osteoporosis Foundation reveals mortality rates up to 20–24% in the first year after a hip fracture, and a greater risk of dying may persist for at least five years afterwards. Loss of function and independence among survivors is profound, with 40% unable to walk independently and 60% requiring assistance a year later. Consequently, a third of these patients are totally dependent or in a nursing home in the year following a hip fracture. Often these fractures occur in those with several chronic degenerative diseases, which cause general ill health and persistent inflammatory states. This is further worsened by lack of mobility, social isolation, malnutrition, and often cognitive impairment.

The skeletal framework

Osteoporosis was virtually unknown until the 20th century, despite having been described 250 years ago. It may be that the higher incidence is linked to the agricultural and industrial revolutions, which have contributed to our lifestyles becoming more sedentary.[5]

The skeleton provides a mechanical framework for the body and there is no doubt that mechanical factors, and in particular weight bearing or resistance exercises, will play a major role in the strengthening of our skeletal framework, in addition to the nutrients that play such an important role. Historically, Julius Wolff, a German anatomist and surgeon described 'Wolff's Law', which states that bones will adapt based on the stress or demands placed on them.[5] When the muscles are worked, they put stress on the bones and in response the bone tissue remodels and becomes stronger.[6]

It is also important to understand that bone stock and volume increases during growth and reaches a maximum at age 25 to 35. Little changes over the next 10 years, but after this time there are major periods of decrease in bone stock, especially in women around menopause.

Assessment of bone strength

The most popular and accessible method of assessing bone strength is quantitative and depends on a DEXA scan. This is, however, an aerial measurement rather than a true measure of 'density' and comes with its own inaccuracies, especially in younger patients, with poor standardisation and a degree of operator dependence. In the absence of qualitative measurement of strength, however, which would necessarily have to look at microarchitecture of bone, a DEXA scan is still the cornerstone of diagnosis.

Factors that influence bone health

While all the pillars of lifestyle medicine will impact on bone health and strength, we will place particular emphasis on a WFPB diet, as a diet rich in whole plant foods and minimal in refined and processed foods, works to create an ideal environment for bone formation. We will also allude to exercise and its role too.

Macronutrients

Protein

Plant sources of proteins, including vegetables and legumes, seeds and whole grains contain all nine essential amino acids. However, soya and quinoa have a similar biological profile to egg white, which is regarded by many as the 'gold standard'. In general, though, most plant-based diets will usually combine a whole grain with a legume or lentil, and this combination ensures the appropriate amino acid balance. It must be remembered however that the body has a pool of amino acids and can synthesise a huge number of proteins without needing to have the much-peddled 'complete' protein at each meal.

Plant protein has a lower potential renal acid load (PRAL)[7] as it has a lower content of sulphur-containing amino acids compared to animal sources of protein.[8] This has led to the theory that as these amino acids (methionine and cysteine) produce sulphuric acid during their metabolism, acid levels are increased in the blood which prompts calcium to act as a buffer to neutralise the acid. This then leads to increased calcium excretion in the urine,[9] resulting in a calcium deficit. This theory has not yet been proven so we cannot say that diets high in animal protein result in impaired calcium balance. What is more likely is that high protein intakes increase the excretion of calcium in the urine due to increased calcium absorption from the gut rather than due to resorption from the bone. Soya products, such as tempeh, or calcium-set tofu, which are rich in phytonutrients, are excellent for promoting bone health and strength.[10] This is not only due to their calcium content but also the essential amino acids and phytoestrogens daidzein, genistein and glycitein, which exert strengthening oestrogenic effects on the bones.

Protein is a major component of the matrix and collagen in bone (25% of the dry weight) and is necessary for the integrity of bone. Given the fact that muscle size and strength is what subjects our bones to regular loading, it stands to reason that protein is important in the diet. In older patients who are more prone to the debilitating effects of sarcopenia, the reference nutrient intake (RNI) rises to 1.2 g/kg and in athletes involved in muscle building or endurance sport, the requirement may be as high as 1.8 g/kg.[10]

Proteins are present in varying quantities in all plant foods, including non-starchy vegetables and fruit. Given that most adults require around 0.8 g of protein per kg body weight, this can be easily met in a plant-based diet which incorporates a variety of the principal food groups, namely whole grains, fruit, vegetables, and legumes, with some nuts and seeds. Legumes (beans) are the richest source of protein in a plant-based diet and although soya is a richer source of protein than several other legumes, all contain other nutrients which help with bone strength too. Soya also has a high digestibility and a higher proportion of the protein in it is available for absorption.[11]

Fat

Saturated fat consumption has been shown to be inversely linked to bone mineral density (BMD). It is thought that saturated fats make the cells of the intestinal brush border stiff, and this decreases absorption of calcium. Saturated fats also have an inhibitory effect on osteoblasts, and oxidised fats have an inductive effect on osteoclastic activity.[8]

Conversely, polyunsaturated fatty acids (PUFA's) are positively associated with bone mineral density (BMD) at the hip and lumbar spine in normal and osteopenic women.[12] PUFAs, including omega-3 fatty acids, are essential for bone formation, although the interaction is complex,[13] and plant-based sources such as ground flax, chia seeds, hemp seeds and walnuts should be a daily part of the diet. They also promote a positive calcium balance by increasing its absorption through the gut and lowering renal excretion.[8] Grinding seeds rather than eating in their whole form improves bioavailability and absorption. Conversely, the omega-6 fatty acids, found in many plant-based foods, including vegetable oils and processed foods, tend to increase bone loss.[14] It is therefore important to achieve a balance of omega-3 and omega-6-containing foods.

Extra virgin olive oil too seems to have a positive impact on bone health, with omega-3 PUFAs and flavonoids contained therein, as well as monounsaturated fatty acids (MUFAs) and other multiple antioxidants and phytonutrients, all of which provide an anti-inflammatory benefit.[15]

Carbohydrates

Fruit and vegetables have been widely recognised as healthful components of our diet in terms of treating and preventing most chronic diseases. The acid-base hypothesis postulates that the acid load, especially in protein of animal origin, is in part buffered by bone tissue which is alkaline, leading to bone resorption and reduced bone density. Fruit and vegetables are a good source of alkaline precursors and could effectively neutralise the calciuric effects of acids derived from the diet. This was shown in a large meta-analysis,[16] which included high quality cohort studies and randomised controlled trials in people over the age of 50. The authors felt that the anti-inflammatory nature of fruit and vegetables, and the redox potential provided by the nutrients and antioxidants in fruit and vegetables, possibly contributed to the healing of microfractures and improved the remodelling of bone.

In a population-based cross-sectional study from China,[17] fruit and vegetable consumption and fruit consumption seemed to have a linear relation to bone mineral density in middle-aged and elderly Chinese subjects, who had a BMI less than 24, with fruit being of greater benefit than vegetables. The authors felt that the way vegetables were cooked in China, with high heat and with high salt, may have caused them to lose some of their nutrients, and increased urinary calcium losses.

Vitamin C, vitamin K, and phytochemicals contribute to the formation of healthier bone. Vitamin C may affect bone mass in the hydroxylation of lysine and proline, which are needed for the formation of stable collagen triple helixes. Vitamin K2, present in fermented foods such as kimchi, sauerkraut and natto, may play a protective role against age-related bone loss via vitamin K-dependent γ-carboxylation of osteocalcin. Antioxidative nutrients and phytochemicals, such as vitamin C, β-carotene, and other carotenoids found in fruit and vegetables, may improve bone health by scavenging oxygen radicals and lowering the risk of inflammation posed by free radicals. These were useful conclusions from the Guangzhou cross sectional study.[17]

Both the above studies were in people following omnivorous diets, but a cross sectional study that spanned a year by Knurick et al.[18] showed no detrimental effect on BMD in vegans, even though their protein consumption was on an average 30% less, possibly for the reasons stated above.

Similarly, a longitudinal cohort study in postmenopausal Vietnamese women over a two-year period found no detrimental effect on BMD and bone turnover markers in the vegan group compared to the omnivore group.[19]

Dietary fibre

Fibre, being an important constituent of plant-based foods, has generated interest in relation to whether there are effects on bone metabolism and health. The Framingham offspring study[20] looked at this aspect in a cohort study and drew some interesting conclusions. By improving the gut microbiome through a diverse, fibre-rich diet, it may be that minerals such as calcium are absorbed better. However, it did not seem to alter bone markers sufficiently to draw any meaningful conclusions, other than the fact that men had less bone loss around the hips if they consumed more fibre rich foods, and women less bone loss from the spine. By consuming more prebiotic fibre, and thereby increasing production of short chain fatty acids and signalling molecules, there may be positive effects on bone and improved absorption of many minerals.

A cross sectional study from Scotland in a large group of women, showed that a healthier pattern of eating a fibre-rich diet was associated with better bone density and markers of bone health than a nutrient-poor, processed food diet.[21]

Inositol
This is a carbohydrate found in fruit such as cantaloupe and prunes and is essential for bone formation. Prunes are also rich in phenolics and vitamin K and have been seen to be particularly beneficial in postmenopausal women in preserving bone.[33] They are also a good source of fibre, which helps with constipation and are easier to consume for older women struggling to meet the recommended fruit and vegetable requirements. The high vitamin K content may also help with calcium balance.

Body composition

Maintaining a BMI in the ideal range is important for maintaining good bone strength, and there is good evidence to suggest that muscle mass is much more important than fat. Obesity, by virtue of its inflammatory effects, has a negative impact on bone microstructure and quality.[4] Obesity may benefit from treatment with vitamin D, but there is some evidence that fat can sequester vitamin D and result in secondary hyperparathyroidism, which has a harmful effect on bone.[22] Obesity and overweight have a complex relationship with bone strength, as obesity promotes sarcopenia, which is linked to osteoporosis. There is also a higher incidence of falls and although the extra adipose tissue offers some cushioning benefit in falls, the overall risks of suffering a fracture are greater because of obesity.[22]

Excessive visceral fat (central obesity) and metabolically unhealthy obesity seems to correlate with osteoporosis and a high waist to hip ratio is a reasonably reliable indicator of this type of fat.[23]

Sarcopenia (loss of muscle strength) is a more recently recognised condition leading to frailty and is intimately related to osteoporosis. Muscle loss and weakness undoubtedly also contribute to a propensity to falls and therefore the likelihood of sustaining fractures. It is now recognised that muscles and bones communicate by several paracrine and endocrine molecules. Numerous studies support the concept of a bone–muscle unit, where constant cross-talking between the two tissues takes place, involving molecules released by the skeletal muscle secretome. This affects bone, and osteokines secreted by the osteoblasts and osteocytes, in turn, impact muscle cells.[24]

Important micronutrients

Vitamins

Vitamin A
Plant-based diets are rich in carotenoids and lycopene, which by virtue of their antioxidant effect are bone protective, with an inverse relationship with bone resorption markers. Higher carotenoid intake and lycopene intakes from vegetables and fruit, correlate directly with a reduced fracture risk.[13] To enhance absorption, carotenoid-rich vegetables, such as carrots, butternut squash, sweet potato, and tomatoes should be cooked, rather than eaten raw, and a portion-controlled source of unsaturated fat eaten alongside.

Vitamin D
Vitamin D helps the body absorb calcium in our

diet from the gastrointestinal tract and prevents excessive loss in urine. It is mostly made from the action of sunlight on our skin and is more like an evolutionary hormone. As the UVB rays are not strong enough to enable this between the months of October–March in the UK, a daily 10 mcg (400 IU) supplement is required for the general population during the winter, although some groups are advised to take supplements all year round. These include pregnant and breast-feeding women, those over 65 years of age, babies and young children, those with darker skin and those who spend a lot of their time indoors. Mushrooms exposed to UVB rays are a source of vitamin D2,[25] as are fortified foods such as soya milk.

As the margin for toxicity of vitamin D is quite high, if in doubt, especially in latitudes higher than 30 degrees, it is better to supplement vitamin D, especially over the winter months with a minimum of 400 international units a day. Vitamin D also has a role in muscles and is involved in making type 2 muscle fibres, which are recruited first to prevent falls.[26]

Vitamin B12
This needs to be supplemented in all vegans and anyone above the age of 50. It has a role in preserving bone density by its action on homocysteine metabolism, and its main role is to prevent neurological damage and therefore falls and fractures as a result. Vitamin B12's direct role in bone strength is unclear but it may be that by reducing homocysteine levels it preserves bone strength.[27] Fortified foods include non-organic plant milks and yoghurts, nutritional yeast and Marmite. Because B12 is not found in plant sources and is made by bacteria in the soil, vegans must supplement their vitamin B12 levels (omnivores are also recommended a supplementation if above 50 years of age). It is best to seek advice and chose an appropriate supplement rather than an excessively high, or 'combination' supplement, which are sometimes counterproductive. In the Nurses' health study,[27] post-menopausal participants who took a high dose B6 and B12 supplement together, seemed to have a higher incidence of hip fractures (even though both these vitamins are water soluble and therefore one would have thought the excess would pass in the urine), and the incidence was even greater if they were at a lower BMI. We would urge caution against reductionism of this kind.

Vitamin C
Vitamin C is an antioxidant and is inhibitory to osteoclasts, while being a cofactor in osteoblast differentiation, and a cofactor in collagen synthesis and the formation of stable triple helices through hydroxyproline and hydroxylysine.[28] The RNI is 40 mg daily, and this can be achieved with the consumption of a single orange, which contains about 70 mg. All citrus fruit, strawberries, blueberries, kiwi fruit, bell peppers, and green leafy vegetables are good sources of vitamin C and should be consumed in some form at every meal. This also aids non-haem iron absorption.

Vitamin K
This is required to make the proteins involved in forming and strengthening bone, and phylloquinone (vitamin K1) is a cofactor in the carboxylation of osteocalcin.[29] There appears to be a clear link to a higher incidence of fractures but a less clear link with bone density in the group that consumed least amounts of phylloquinone. Adult requirements are 1 mcg/kg/body-weight per day, and this can be achieved easily by consuming dietary sources, rather than relying on a supplement. Good sources include dark green leafy vegetables such as spinach, kale, Brussel sprouts, broccoli and cauliflower, kiwi, blueberries, and parsley.

Vitamin K2
This is produced in the gut by bacteria in the fibre contained in green leafy vegetables. Vitamin K2 seems to have a role in calcification of bone matrix and regulates calcium metabolism by preventing calcification of blood vessels, especially when

calcium is in excess as supplements.[30] It may also increase bone strength without increasing bone density. A plant-based source is sauerkraut and natto (fermented soya bean). Currently there is no consensus on vitamin K2 requirements.

Important minerals

Calcium

Bone and teeth are the main storehouses of calcium, and it is intuitive to think of calcium as being the 'vital mineral' for bone health. Blood calcium levels are kept within a very narrow range, with many hormones and vitamin D working in harmony to fine tune this. Calcium has a vital role in muscle and nerve function in addition to being of structural importance in bone.

Despite the dairy industry overemphasising the importance of milk as an essential source of calcium, there are plenty of plant sources of calcium, which are devoid of the potential negative impacts of dairy consumption. The consumption of cow's milk and dairy does not correlate with bone health, and in fact countries that consume the most dairy, such as Sweden, have some of the highest rates of hip fracture, although these are epidemiological studies that show association rather than causation. Calcium is best obtained from the diet rather than supplementation in tablet form, as this can result in high levels of elemental blood calcium, which can disrupt calcium homeostasis. The RNI is 700 mg per day.

The absorption of calcium in dairy is roughly 33%, and this can be compared to leafy greens, including kale, spring greens, pak choi, broccoli, rocket and watercress, calcium-fortified plant milks and yoghurts, and calcium-set tofu, all of which have an absorption of between 35–60% Moderate absorption of between 20–30% comes from legumes and beans, tempeh, chia and sesame seeds, almonds, oranges, figs and aromatic herbs. Greens such as spinach and swiss chard have poor absorption due to their high oxalate content, which binds with the calcium and reduces absorption to as little as 5–10%.[10] Soya foods on the other hand, despite being high in phytates and oxalates, allow for a high percentage of calcium absorption.[11]

Calcium supplementation alone has been shown to predispose to renal stones and coronary heart disease due to deposition in atherosclerotic plaques, with an incidence of 30% in a meta-analysis of randomised controlled trials totalling 12,000 participants.[31] A reappraisal of the women's health initiative study, which allowed for a low-dose vitamin D along with calcium supplement showed that the vitamin D was not protective of cardiac complications owing to patients supplementing non-protocolled doses of calcium.[32] Calcium supplements, which were thought to reduce incidence of hypertension, obesity and diabetes in some epidemiological studies, have in fact shown an increased cardiac risk from myocardial infarctions in a prospective cohort in Germany (EPIC Heidelberg cohort).[30]

Phosphorus

Along with calcium, phosphorus is the most abundant mineral in the body, with approximately 85% residing in bone. This mineral works with calcium to build and maintain bones and is regulated in part by vitamin D. Adult requirements are 550 mg/day and good sources include beans, chickpeas, lentils, soya, nuts and pumpkin seeds. The ratio of phosphorus to calcium is thought to be more important, with a ratio of 0.5–1.5 being optimum.[28]

Magnesium

Magnesium is present in bone and teeth and therefore plays an important role in bone health. It plays a vital role in preventing endothelial dysfunction and it has a mitogenic effect on osteoblasts, with a deficiency resulting in osteoporosis.

The RNI for men is 300 mg/day, and for women 270 mg. Magnesium is abundant in fruit and vegetables, whole grains, nuts and beans.

Zinc
Zinc stimulates the formation of bone osteoblasts and inhibits osteoclastic activity. It is a structural component of bone matrix and a cofactor of alkaline phosphatase which mineralises bone. Although zinc is important for bone health, it is only required in small amounts and needs are easily met via a balanced PBD. Sources include whole grains, nuts, seeds, and legumes, and absorption can be increased by soaking and sprouting such foods.

Silicon
Silicon is important for bone formation and although there is no RNI in the UK, epidemiological studies show that intakes of more than 40 mg/day are associated with increased BMD.[28] It is found in green beans, carrots, nuts and seeds, whole grains, and cereals. It is also found in beer, likely due to the processing of hops and barley, and men seem to find it easier to achieve the recommended quantities than women. However, this cannot be a recommended source of silicon.

Copper and manganese
Similarly to zinc, these nutrients are only needed in small amounts and should be consumed via the diet, rather than a supplement. This is due to them being a pro-oxidant, and excessive intakes of manganese have been associated with cognitive disorders and Parkinsons disease.[34] Sources include asparagus, avocados, beans, dried fruit, dark chocolate, nuts and seeds.

Boron
Boron seems to extend the half-life of vitamin D and oestrogens, and the small amount needed is easily obtained from plant sources such as prunes, raisins, dried apricots and avocados.[28]

Specific phytonutrients

Special mention must be made of mounting evidence that soya isoflavones seem to have a beneficial effect on bone health. While there are no randomised controlled trials, as in many other areas of nutrition, there is certainly good quality evidence to suggest that genistein, by virtue of its SERM (selective (o)estrogen receptor modulation) effect, modulates the positive action on bone by acting on beta oestrogenic receptors (exerts a third of the potency of oestradiol), while having weak effects (a thousandth as effective as oestradiol 1) on the alpha receptors. It does not therefore cause some of the undesirable oestrogenic side effects.[35] Bone turnover studies and longitudinal cohort studies certainly seem to point towards favourable results from consumption of one to two portions daily of the less-processed soya products such as soya milk, soya yoghurt, tofu and tempeh. Equol producers (generally more common in southeast Asian populations) have a microbiome that can get more out of the isoflavones by virtue of this, and therefore it enhances the effects of isoflavones even more. In general, 1 g of soya protein is associated with 3.5 mg of isoflavones in traditional soya foods and these two together seem to be bone protective.[11]

Fortified soya foods
Calcium-set tofu is a rich source of calcium (the average content being 350 mg per 100 g) and isoflavones, as is tempeh, although the calcium content is lower than tofu. Commercially available soya milk in the UK is often fortified (with the exception being organic brands) with vitamin D, B2 and B12, in addition to calcium.

Soya has beneficial effects on muscle building, and we know this would have a benefit on bone health too. Soya also has a much lower amount of carbohydrates compared to other legumes, and this may be of a greater advantage in diabetes.

The main carbohydrate in it is stachyose, an oligosaccharide that forms an especially useful prebiotic for beneficial gut bacteria such as bifidobacteria. Soya is also a good source of both omega-3 and omega-6 PUFA.[11] Two large prospective cohort studies from Asia suggest a 30% lowering of fracture rates in postmenopausal women with higher consumption of traditional soya foods.[35, 36]

'Calcium thieves'

Certain dietary and lifestyle factors result in calcium losses and are referred to as 'calcium thieves'. These factors are more prevalent in Western societies, contributing to the higher RNI of calcium. Smoking, alcohol consumption, coffee (more than 3–4 cups a day), sugar-sweetened beverages and fizzy drinks; especially cola drinks[37] that contain caffeine as well as phosphoric acid, result in calcium loss. A Chinese study suggested that all fizzy drinks cause osteoporosis, a finding that was attributed to the high sugar, salt and phosphoric acid content.[38]

In moderate amounts (three cups or less a day), coffee has been found to be helpful for bone health, a finding reflected in a study looking at men and premenopausal women in the Taiwanese populations.[39]

Excess salt in food has deleterious effects on bone health, with a gram of extra sodium per day (the main source being processed foods) having the potential to result in loss of 1% of bone stock per year. This is largely due to sodium and calcium appearing to compete for the same transport system in the proximal renal tubule.[40]

A meta-analysis in 2019 looked at alcohol and found it to adversely affect bone health in a dose-related manner, even though some historical studies suggest moderate consumption improves bone strength.[41]

Exercise

The focus on calcium consumption has taken away the importance of regular, daily exercise and activity, which is vital for bone health. Osteoporosis is predominantly a disease of our sedentary modern-day lifestyle and is far more prominent now than a few centuries ago. Even continually active people tend to focus on one form of exercise rather than doing a variety of different cardio and strength exercises. It is recommended that all adults undertake at least 150 minutes per week of moderately vigorous physical activity. Walking maintains bone density but does not help to increase it unless one wears weighted jackets, or wrist and ankle weighted bands to increase the joint reaction force. Multicomponent exercises, especially including some form of resistance training at least three times a week are recommended. Impact exercises such as jogging, skipping, star jumps, and stair climbing are all helpful. Whole body vibration plates are also helpful in increasing bone strength and density, as well as reducing falls risk through muscle strengthening and improvement of balance. Even in post-menopausal women there is some evidence of improvement in bone density.[42]

Conclusion

1. Consider a predominantly whole food plant-based diet rich in fruit, vegetables, whole grains, legumes, with smaller quantities of nuts and seeds.
2. Consume two portions of minimally processed soya every day.
3. Supplement vitamin B12.
4. Supplement vitamin D, especially in the winter and autumn months, and in some racial groups throughout the year, with blood tests if available to check vitamin D levels.

5. Ensure an adequate intake of calcium via dietary sources. Whole foods are preferred but fortified foods can make useful contributions. Isolated calcium supplements are not recommended.
6. Combination of exercises are good for bone strength, especially weight bearing exercises and strength training, and resistance exercises to improve muscle strength and coordination.
7. Avoid substances that increase calcium loss such as smoking, coffee in excess, sugar sweetened beverages (especially cola drinks), alcohol, and excess salt.

References

1. Tong TYN, Appleby PN, Armstrong MEG, Fensom GK, Knuppel A, Papier K, et al. Vegetarian and vegan diets and risks of total and site-specific fractures: results from the prospective EPIC-Oxford study. *BMC Medicine* 2020; 18(1): 353. doi: 10.1186/s12916-020-01815-3
2. Thorpe DL, Beeson WL, Knutsen R, Fraser GE, Knutsen SF. Dietary patterns and hip fracture in the Adventist Health Study 2: combined vitamin D and calcium supplementation mitigate increased hip fracture risk among vegans. *American Journal of Clinical Nutrition* 2021; 114(2): 488-495. doi: 10.1093/ajcn/nqab095
3. Sozen T, Ozisik L, Calik Basaran N. An overview and management of osteoporosis. *European Journal of Rheumatology* 2017; 4(1): 46-56. doi: 10.5152/eurjrheum.2016.048
4. Bierhals IO, dos Santos Vaz J, Bielemann RM, de Mola CL, Barros FC, Gonçalves H, et al. Associations between body mass index, body composition and bone density in young adults: Findings from a southern Brazilian cohort. *BMC Musculoskeletal Disorders* 2019; 20(1): 322. doi: 10.1186/s12891-019-2656-3
5. Curate F. Osteoporosis and paleopathology: A review. *Journal of Anthropological Sciences* 2014; 92: 119-146. doi: 10.4436/JASS.92003
6. Gómez-Cabello A, Ara I, González-Agüero A, Casajús JA, Vicente-Rodríguez G. Effects of training on bone mass in older adults: A systematic review. *Sports Medicine* 2012;42(4): 301-325. doi: 10.2165/11597670-000000000-00000
7. Barzel US, Massey LK. Excess dietary protein may can adversely affect bone. *Journal of Nutrition* 1998; 128(6): 1051-1053. doi: 10.1093/jn/128.6.1051
8. Hejazi J, Davoodi A, Khosravi M, Sedaghat M, Abedi V, Hosseinverdi S, et al. Nutrition and osteoporosis prevention and treatment. *Biomedical Research and Therapy* 2020; 7(4): 3709-3720. doi: 10.15419/bmrat.v7i4.598
9. Delimaris I. Adverse Effects Associated with Protein Intake above the Recommended Dietary Allowance for Adults. *ISRN Nutrition* 2013; 2013: 126929. doi: 10.5402/2013/126929
10. Melina BD and V. Becoming Vegan - the Complete Guide to Plant-Based Nutrition. 2014th ed. US: Book Publishing Company; 2014.
11. Messina M. Soy and health update: Evaluation of the clinical and epidemiologic literature. *Nutrients* 2016; 8(12): 754. doi: 10.3390/nu8120754
12. Lavado-García J, Roncero-Martin R, Moran JM, Pedrera-Canal M, Aliaga I, Leal-Hernandez O, et al. Long-chain omega-3 polyunsaturated fatty acid dietary intake is positively associated with bone mineral density in normal and osteopenic Spanish women. *PLoS One* 2018; 13(1): e0190539. doi: 10.1371/journal.pone.0190539
13. Sahni S, Mangano KM, McLean RR, Hannan MT, Kiel DP. Dietary Approaches for Bone Health: Lessons from the Framingham Osteoporosis Study. *Current Osteoporosis Reports* 2015; 13(4): 245-255. doi: 10.1007/s11914-015-0272-1
14. Griel AE, Kris-Etherton PM, Hilpert KF, Zhao G, West SG, Corwin RL. An increase in dietary n-3 fatty acids decreases a marker of bone resorption in humans. *Nutrition Journal* 2007; 6: 2. doi: 10.1186/1475-2891-6-2
15. Martínez-Ramírez MJ, Palma S, Martínez-González MA, Delgado-Martínez AD, de la Fuente C, Delgado-Rodríguez M. Dietary fat intake and the risk of osteoporotic fractures in the elderly. *European Journal of Clinical Nutrition* 2007; 61(9): 1114-1120. doi: 10.1038/sj.ejcn.1602624

16. Brondani JE, Comim F v., Flores LM, Martini LA, Premaor MO. Fruit and vegetable intake and bones: A systematic review and meta-analysis. *PLoS One* 2019; 14(5): e0217223. doi: 10.1371/journal.pone.0217223
17. Qiu R, Cao WT, Tian HY, He J, Chen GD, Chen YM. Greater intake of fruit and vegetables is associated with greater bone mineral density and lower osteoporosis risk in middle-aged and elderly adults. *PLoS One* 2017; 12(1): e0168906. doi: 10.1371/journal.pone.0168906
18. Knurick JR, Johnston CS, Wherry SJ, Aguayo I. Comparison of correlates of bone mineral density in individuals adhering to lacto-ovo, vegan, or omnivore diets: A cross-sectional investigation. *Nutrients* 2015; 7(5): 3416-3426. doi: 10.3390/nu7053416
19. Ho-Pham LT, Vu BQ, Lai TQ, Nguyen ND, Nguyen TV. Vegetarianism, bone loss, fracture and vitamin D: A longitudinal study in Asian vegans and non-vegans. *European Journal of Clinical Nutrition* 2012; 66(1): 75-82. doi: 10.1038/ejcn.2011.131
20. Dai Z, Zhang Y, Lu N, Felson DT, Kiel DP, Sahni S. Association Between Dietary Fiber Intake and Bone Loss in the Framingham Offspring Study. *Journal of Bone and Mineral Research* 2018; 33(2): 241-249. doi: 10.1002/jbmr.3308
21. Hardcastle AC, Aucott L, Fraser WD, Reid DM, MacDonald HM. Dietary patterns, bone resorption and bone mineral density in early post-menopausal Scottish women. *European Journal of Clinical Nutrition* 2011; 65(3): 378-385. doi: 10.1038/ejcn.2010.264
22. Hou J, He C, He W, Yang M, Luo X, Li C. Obesity and Bone Health: A Complex Link. *Frontiers in Cell and Developmental Biology* 2020; 8: 600181. doi: 10.3389/fcell.2020.600181
23. Shapses SA, Sukumar D. Bone metabolism in obesity and weight loss. *Annual Review of Nutrition* 2012; 32: 287-309. doi: 10.1146/annurev.nutr.012809.104655
24. Reginster JY, Beaudart C, Buckinx F, Bruyère O. Osteoporosis and sarcopenia: Two diseases or one? *Current Opinion in Clinical Nutrition and Metabolic Care* 2016; 19(1): 31-36. doi: 10.1097/MCO.0000000000000230
25. Cardwell G, Bornman JF, James AP, Black LJ. A review of mushrooms as a potential source of dietary vitamin D. *Nutrients* 2018; 10(10): 1498. doi: 10.3390/nu10101498
26. Laird E, Ward M, McSorley E, Strain JJ, Wallace J. Vitamin D and bone health; Potential mechanisms. *Nutrients* 2010; 2(7): 693-724. doi: 10.3390/nu2070693
27. Meyer HE, Willett WC, Fung TT, Holvik K, Feskanich D. Association of High Intakes of Vitamins B6 and B12 From Food and Supplements With Risk of Hip Fracture Among Postmenopausal Women in the Nurses' Health Study. *JAMA network open* 2019; 2(5): e193591. doi: 10.1001/jamanetworkopen.2019.3591
28. Price CT, Langford JR, Liporace FA. Essential Nutrients for Bone Health and a Review of their Availability in the Average North American Diet. *The Open Orthopaedics Journal* 2012; 6: 143-149. doi: 10.2174/1874325001206010143
29. Schwalfenberg GK. Vitamins K1 and K2: The Emerging Group of Vitamins Required for Human Health. *Journal of Nutrition and Metabolism* 2017; 2017: 6254836. doi: 10.1155/2017/6254836
30. Li K, Kaaks R, Linseisen J, Rohrmann S. Associations of dietary calcium intake and calcium supplementation with myocardial infarction and stroke risk and overall cardiovascular mortality in the Heidelberg cohort of the European Prospective Investigation into Cancer and Nutrition study (EPIC-Heidelberg). *Heart* 2012; 98(12): 920-925. doi: 10.1136/heartjnl-2011-301345
31. Bolland MJ, Avenell A, Baron JA, Grey A, MacLennan GS, Gamble GD, et al. Effect of calcium supplements on risk of myocardial infarction and cardiovascular events: Meta-analysis. *BMJ* 2010; 341(7767): c3691. doi: 10.1136/bmj.c3691
32. Bolland MJ, Grey A, Avenell A, Gamble GD, Reid IR. Calcium supplements with or without vitamin D and risk of cardiovascular events: Reanalysis of the Women's Health Initiative limited access dataset and meta-analysis. *BMJ* 2011; 342(7804): d2040. doi: 10.1136/bmj.d2040
33. Wallace TC. Dried plums, prunes and bone health: A comprehensive review. *Nutrients* 2017; 9(4): 401. doi: 10.3390/nu9040401

34. Powers KM, Smith-Weller T, Franklin GM, Longstreth WT, Swanson PD, Checkoway H. Parkinson's disease risks associated with dietary iron, manganese, and other nutrient intakes. *Neurology* 2003; 60(11): 1761-1766. doi: 10.1212/01.wnl.0000068021.13945.7f
35. Zhang X, Shu XO, Li H, Yang G, Li Q, Gao YT, et al. Prospective cohort study of soy food consumption and risk of bone fracture among postmenopausal women. *Archives of Internal Medicine* 2005; 165(16): 1890-1895. doi: 10.1001/archinte.165.16.1890
36. Koh WP, Wu AH, Wang R, Ang LW, Heng D, Yuan JM, et al. Gender-specific associations between soy and risk of hip fracture in the singapore chinese health study. *American Journal of Epidemiology* 2009; 170(7): 901-909. doi: 10.1093/aje/kwp220
37. Tucker KL, Morita K, Qiao N, Hannan MT, Cupples LA, Kiel DP. Colas, but not other carbonated beverages, are associated with low bone mineral density in older women: The Framingham osteoporosis study. *American Journal of Clinical Nutrition* 2006; 84(4): 936-942. doi: 10.1093/ajcn/84.4.936
38. Chen L, Liu R, Zhao Y, Shi Z. High consumption of soft drinks is associated with an increased risk of fracture: A 7-year follow-up study. *Nutrients* 2020; 12(2): 530. doi: 10.3390/nu12020530
39. Chang HC, Hsieh CF, Lin YC, Tantoh DM, Ko PC, Kung YY, et al. Does coffee drinking have beneficial effects on bone health of Taiwanese adults? A longitudinal study. *BMC Public Health* 2018; 18(1): 1273. doi: 10.1186/s12889-018-6168-0
40. Nordin BEC, Need AG, Morris HA, Horowitz M. The nature and significance of the relationship between urinary sodium and urinary calcium in women. *Journal of Nutrition* 1993; 123(9): 1615-1622. doi: 10.1093/jn/123.9.1615
41. Cheraghi Z, Doosti-Irani A, Almasi-Hashiani A, Baigi V, Mansournia N, Etminan M, et al. The effect of alcohol on osteoporosis: A systematic review and meta-analysis. *Drug and Alcohol Dependence* 2019; 197: 197-202. doi: 10.1016/j.drugalcdep.2019.01.025
42. Benedetti MG, Furlini G, Zati A, Mauro GL. The Effectiveness of Physical Exercise on Bone Density in Osteoporotic Patients. *BioMed Research International* 2018; 2018: 4840531. doi: 10.1155/2018/4840531

Chapter 16
Plant-based nutrition and dermatological conditions

Niyati Sharma

Introduction

Skin diseases like other systems, are a myriad of complex interplay between the immune system, the skin microbiome and the environment resulting in breakdown of the skin barrier. As cutaneous diseases can be visible and cause cosmetic concerns, it is not uncommon for patients to ask if their skin disease is related to any foods they have been eating. Although not always the case, the more prevalent skin diseases such as acne, eczema, rosacea, psoriasis, and urticaria have a dietary link, the evidence for which is discussed in this chapter.

Even though these studies are in small numbers they demonstrate that cutaneous diseases are not just skin deep but go beyond just what we expose our skin to. Emerging studies are demonstrating the link between the gut and skin microbiome and when a component in the diet is eliminated or reduced, often the patient reports disease improvement and sometimes complete resolution.

With increasing demand from patients for alternative treatment to the conventional therapies, nutritional advice that is based on nutritional evidence-based medicine can be very effective in providing a holistic care to patients. The field of nutrition is complex and requires ongoing research in each of the topics explored in dermatology. It is exciting times and even though challenging, the longer-term impact of diet intervention leaves both the patient and dermatologist immensely satisfied.

Acne

Acne vulgaris is a common chronic dermatological condition, affecting 9.4% of individuals worldwide and the incidence is on the rise.[1,2] It is a multifactorial disorder characterised by inflammation of the pilosebaceous unit, and is driven by hormonal, immunological, bacterial, and genetic factors. It has a high psychosocial impact, associated with lower quality of life, anxiety, depression and body dissatisfaction.[2] Lifestyle factors, particularly diet, are commonly cited by patients as contributing to acne, and there is increasing evidence that these factors play an important role in its pathogenesis.[3] In populations that are not influenced by Western culture, like the indigenous subpopulations of

Papua New Guinea and Paraguay, no signs of acne have been seen, strengthening the dietary link.[2]

The Western diet is high in glycaemic index, dairy and red meat which enhances insulin and insulin-like growth factor-1 (IGF-1) production.[4] This then promotes the FOX01 signal transduction increasing mTOR activation and thereby resulting in increased keratinocyte desquamation and sebaceous lipogenesis, driving the pathogenesis of acne vulgaris.[5] IGF-1 also stimulates 5α-reductase in the adrenal glands and gonads, promotes androgen synthesis, and activates the androgen receptor signal transduction.[6] By also inhibiting the hepatic synthesis of sex hormone binding globulin (SHBG) that is known to reduce free testosterone in the serum, IGF-1 further plays a role in acne formation.[6, 7, 8]

The IGF-1 theory in acne can also be supported by patients that have Laron syndrome, where patients are born with a rare recessive disease that leads to severe IGF-1 deficiency. In these patients there is no evidence of acne until they are treated with recombinant IGF-1 (r-IGF-1).[2] Similarly in acromegaly, where there is an increase in IGF-1 production, all patients tend to display signs of hyperandrogenism and acne.

Dairy contains proteins such as casein which stimulates IGF-1 and whey which is predominantly responsible for the insulinotropic effects of milk.[9] Two meta-analyses demonstrated statistically significant associations between dairy consumption and an increased risk of acne across large patient samples.[10, 11] Observational studies published more recently show similar associations.[12, 13] Across both meta-analyses, greater quantities and frequencies of milk intake correlated with a higher risk of acne. Interestingly, those patients who were lactose intolerant had a 50% lower incidence of acne than otherwise.[14] It is thought that mammalian milk is more than just food but rather a signalling system for mechanistic target of rapamycin complex 1 (mTORC1), which further accentuates insulin signalling, lipogenesis and androgen hormone secretion leading to acne formation.[14]

Acne is most pronounced with the intake of skimmed milk which contains larger amounts of whey protein to make it appear 'creamier'.[5] Whey protein supplements are increasingly used to augment muscle bulk and strength, with nearly half of recently-surveyed Australian adolescent boys reporting current protein powder use.[15] A variety of whey protein constituents (namely insulin, IGF-1 and leucine) have been implicated in the pathogenesis of acne, and several case series and observational studies have reported an increased incidence of truncal and facial acne amongst protein supplement users, who predominantly consist of young males.[16, 17, 18, 19, 20] Although further prospective studies assessing this relationship are needed, studies have shown the discontinuing whey protein supplements resulted in improvement within two weeks and the effects were long-lasting.[18] Interestingly, fermented dairy products (such as yoghurt and cheese) are not as acnegenic, possibly due to a reduction in IGF-1 levels following fermentation by probiotic bacteria.[21]

The protein complex mTORC1 is also stimulated by leucine, a branched chain amino acid found to be in high amounts in dairy and red meat, but also in eggs and soya protein isolate.[5, 17] Leucine is an important precursor for sebaceous lipogenesis and also plays a role in T cell activation and function, causing inflammation in acne pathogenesis.[17] Although plants such as apples contain leucine, the amounts are significantly lower than with consumption of an animal meat and dairy protein-based diet thus suggesting why acne incidence is much lower in vegetarians and vegans.[9]

The protein complex mTORC1 is also synergistically stimulated by high glycaemic-load diets and has been shown to increase the risk of acne, in addition to contributing to insulin resistance.

Across two randomised controlled trials, a low-glycaemic diet significantly decreased acne lesion counts in male participants.[22, 23] In another randomised interventional study, males who received a low-glycaemic diet and metformin therapy experienced significantly greater acne improvement, compared to those who used symptomatic treatment alone.[24] This suggests a possible synergistic benefit from combined dietary and medical hypoglycaemic interventions, although a comparison with dietary modification alone has not been studied. Observational studies have also demonstrated an increased risk or severity of acne in association with high glycaemic-load diets.[25, 26, 27] Although weight loss has been flagged as a potential confounder in this association, there was no consistent correlation between body mass index and acne risk.

Micronutrient intake generally does not seem to influence acne risk.[28] However, there have been case reports of vitamin B12-induced acne, which typically affects females and presents as a monomorphic inflammatory acneiform eruption on the face and upper trunk.[29, 30, 31] The eruption develops acutely and then rapidly disappears with the cessation of B12 injections.

Although there is plenty of evidence to demonstrate the link between nutrition and acne, larger studies are still required. It is important to recognise the mTORC1 signalling pathway that is triggered by diet for acne pathogenesis and to educate and initiate dietary measures in correcting the overstimulation of mTORC1 signalling through simple changes as follows.

Recommendations for management

(a) Reduce foods with high mean glycaemic index.
(b) Reduce intake of dairy products. Check for hidden dairy in products including milk solids, casein or whey protein, often found in milk chocolate.
(c) Discontinue use of whey protein.
(d) Reduce foods high in leucine (dairy and red meat).
(e) If your patient is plant-based and still producing acne, check the serum vitamin B12 levels and reduce supplementation.

Treating acne is more than skin deep and the effects of targeting dietary changes can not only improve the appearance but as we know can impact greater systemic changes, as explored elsewhere in the book.

Rosacea

Rosacea, another common dermatosis, affects up to 15% of the population worldwide and is frequently exacerbated by environmental triggers such as diet.[32] There are four different subtypes of rosacea including erythematotelangiectatic (ETR), papulopustular, phymatous, and ocular. The papulopustular subtype has common dietary triggers as seen in acne but the ETR subtype is more complex. Usually, the patient experiences initially intermittent flushing but with time permanent erythema and telangiectasia with or without the flushing occurs. Treatment of rosacea continues to be sub-optimal and hence lifestyle adjunct therapy is required and sought by patients to reduce disease severity.

Although dermatologists frequently counsel rosacea patients on avoidance of dietary triggers, the exact pathogenesis is unknown thereby making management often difficult.[32] Rosacea is likely a combination of immune dysregulation, abnormal vascular and neurological signalling, dysbiosis of both the skin and gut microbiome and skin inflammation.[32] The aetiopathogenesis is still unknown, however, one potential link is with the transient receptor potential (TRP) channels.[33] These channels are ubiquitously expressed all over the body, on both neuronal and non-neuronal tissues, and are responsible for inflammation and vasodilation.[34] There are TRP channels including vanilloid 1 (TRPV1) and ankyrin 1 (TRPA1) and these are implicated in triggering vasodilation and hence flushing via various stimuli in the diet.[34] TRPV1 is usually triggered by capsaicin and TRPA1 by mustard oil and cinnamaldehyde.[32]

Dietary triggers are commonly reported by patients suffering with rosacea and in a survey conducted by the National Rosacea Society of over 400 patients, 78% had altered their diet due to rosacea with 95% of patients reporting an improvement in their disease.[35] Generally patients tend to avoid certain spices, alcohol and hot beverages. Capsaicin-related spices trigger rosacea in 75% of patients and include foods that contain cayenne pepper and red pepper.[35] Cinnamaldehyde containing foods include cinnamon, tomatoes, chocolate and citrus fruits and are responsible for triggering rosacea in up to 1/3 of patients.[35] Alcohol, especially wine, triggers rosacea in 52% of patients and is likely due to triggering peripheral vasodilation.[35] Hot beverages such as hot coffee and tea trigger vasodilation and sympathetic activation resulting in flushing in rosacea and is responsible as a trigger in 30%.[35] There is still insufficient evidence to suggest caffeine plays a role in rosacea aetiology.[36] Niacin-containing foods such as peanuts, salmon, chicken breast, tuna, and liver acts on niacin G-protein-coupled-receptors in Langerhans cells that results in prostaglandin release and hence erythema and flushing in rosacea patients, and should maybe be avoided in those with refractory rosacea.[36] Histamine-releasing foods may also exacerbate symptoms of rosacea and are further discussed in the 'urticaria' section of this chapter.[36]

Increasingly, research is demonstrating the link between rosacea and the gut microbiome. Studies have linked rosacea with coeliac disease, *Helicobacter pylori (H. pylori)* infection, small intestinal bacterial overgrowth (SIBO), Crohn's disease and irritable bowel syndrome.[32, 37] The strongest link, however, has been with inflammatory bowel disease (IBD) and rosacea, with numerous studies replicating the same link.[32] It is likely because they share the same genetic link to the histocompatibility complex class II gene HLA DRB1*03:01.[32] Even though the data is limited, treatment of gut diseases has provided a therapeutic avenue to treat rosacea. In one research study, sustained response was obtained in 100% of the patients who had treatment for their SIBO, for up to the 3-year follow-up mark.[32] Other treatments include high-fibre intervention for SIBO treatment, and for promoting a healthy gut microbiome.[32] Another link to the gut and rosacea is shown through studies done by Manzhalii et al. and Fortuna et al. with the use of probiotics.[38, 39] In both studies, patients on the probiotics improved their skin condition compared with the control arm, thus further strengthening the skin gut microbiome link hypothesis.[38, 39]

Recommendations for management

(a) Investigate for gut disease including *H. pylori* and SIBO that are non-invasive tests.
(b) Implementation of gut health by encouraging patients to eat fibre rich (prebiotic) diet.
(c) Avoidance of certain foods including those containing capsaicin, cinnamaldehydes, niacin-rich foods, alcohol, and hot beverages.
(d) If your patient has ocular rosacea, consider omega-3 supplementation with 325 mg of eicosapentaenoic acid (EPA) and 175 mg of docosahexaenoic acid (DHA) twice daily, as it has been shown to be of benefit.[32]

Eczema

Eczema or atopic dermatitis (AD) is a complex and multifactorial disease that forms part of the atopic triad which includes asthma and allergic rhinitis. It is a chronic relapsing skin disease that results in skin barrier dysfunction, inflammation and chronic pruritus which affects sleep and patients' quality of life.[40] It is a growing public health problem, with prevalence of up to 35% in children.[40] Interestingly, food allergy is commonly associated with AD and it is estimated that a third of those with AD have food allergies and 10% of adults with food allergies also have AD.[41, 42] This showcases the importance of a link between diet, food allergies and perhaps the development of AD, however this association is still not completely understood.

Although a complex genetic disorder, AD shows a predominant maternal influence. Mothers with the disease are more likely to pass it on to their offspring rather than fathers with atopy.[43] Therefore, the epigenetics of the disease starts with maternal diet exposure in the uterus. It is known that maternal dietary antigens cross the placenta.[44] However, there are many studies such as those reported by Kramer et al. that show maternal dietary antigen avoidance did not decrease the incidence of eczema in the offspring.[44] A systematic review also did not show any evidence of maternal dietary exposure and infantile eczema as well as a meta-analysis done by Beckhaus et al.[45, 46] This is because not only can diet vary even in one individual but the modification of diet through preparation such as cooking can also affect the nutrients of the food. Especially in eczema, it is important to review articles that assess dietary patterns common within a population such as the research done by Zulyniak et al.[47] They found that when reviewing the diet of populations, a plant-based diet (which included dairy) showed an overall reduction in eczema incidence at one year of age.[47]

Tanaka et al. also found that eating a vegetarian diet showed similar clinical effectiveness to cyclosporin-A, an immunosuppressive therapy used in AD patients.[48] They found there was a reduction in the total number of neutrophils, eosinophils and LDH5 levels that tend to be higher in those with AD.[48] They also demonstrated the inhibition of interleukin-5 production and a reduction in synthesis of IFN-γ and peripheral natural killer (NK) cell activity and PGE2 secretion by monocytes; all contributing to a decrease in disease activity.[48]

Maternal dietary link

Maternal dietary protein consumption can affect the offspring through various mechanisms such as gut microbiome alteration and immune development, and through DNA methylation via amino acids such as methionine and serine.[49] Higher maternal meat intake during pregnancy is significantly associated with an increased risk of AD in the offspring.[50] This is likely due to the carcinogenic compounds found in red meat such as heterocyclic amines and nitroso compounds elevated with cooking meat at high temperatures that affect the foetal immune system.[50, 51] Maternal poultry meat consumption is also strongly associated with development of AD in infants, even more so than red meat.[49]

Dairy and dairy products consumption by mothers in one study demonstrated higher rates of eczema in the offspring.[52] However, egg consumption during pregnancy didn't seem to increase the risk of AD in the offspring.[49, 52] Egg-avoidance during breastfeeding however, did significantly reduce the incidence of AD in infants.[53] A study by Saito et al. found no relationship between intake of maternal fish and eczema in their Japanese female patients, however a study by Zeng et al. found a greater incidence of AD in infants whose mothers consumed a higher intake of freshwater fish in the postpartum period.[49, 50] The beneficial effects of fish may be offset by foetal exposure to mercury and other toxic substances and should be taken into account when making such recommendations.[51]

Components in the maternal diet that may provide protection against AD include higher antioxidant consumption and dietary fibre.[40] Dietary fibre comprises both insoluble and soluble fibre as well as prebiotics and resistant starch.[54] Although research into the role of fibre in immune development is limited, mothers who predominantly ate a Western diet, which is low in dietary fibre, had slightly higher rates of eczema in their infants.[54] Further interventional studies are required to establish this link.

A meta-analysis and systematic review by Garcia-Larsen et al. found that supplementation of mothers (rather than infants) with probiotic supplements such as *Lactobacillus rhamnosus*, did reduce the risk of infantile eczema, even though previously no strong link was established.[55]

Children and adult dietary link

As the neonate enters infancy, with a naïve immune system, food allergies start to emerge in some infants with AD. Interestingly, in an infant with a positive family history of food allergies, the incidence of egg allergy is high and should warrant investigating the infant for such via IgE mediated tests.[42] Furthermore, children with AD and egg allergy are also more likely to have cow's milk and wheat allergy.[42] Cow's milk allergy is present in up to 7.5% of the population and also increases the incidence of AD as seen through higher levels of serum IgE level compared with infants with no allergies.[56] This subgroup of patients have then subsequently benefited from elimination diets.[42, 56, 57]

A large intervention trial of 17,000 breastfed infants, found an overall lower incidence of AD at 1 year follow up thus further promoting the beneficial effects of breast milk.[58]

Adult eczema is also associated with increased odds of diabetes, hypertension, hypercholesterolemia, and obesity, and therefore is an independent risk factor for the development of cardiovascular disease.[59] Patients with eczema also tend to have chronic inflammation, itch and sleep deprivation and these also contribute to increased risk, thus there is a need for greater clinical and public health interventions for cardiovascular risk modification in patients with AD.[59]

Obesity is linked with more severe eczema and plausible mechanisms include the release of inflammatory chemokines and cytokines by adipocytes, or higher consumption of fast food that contains high levels of saturated fats, trans fatty acids, sodium, simple carbohydrates, sugar and preservatives.[60, 61, 62] These components contribute to further inflammation through either direct mechanisms such as triggering the release of more inflammatory cytokines or indirectly via obesity.

Recommendations for management

(a) Pregnant women to avoid meat and poultry and reduce dairy and dairy product consumption.
(b) Pregnant woman to consider adding probiotics to their diet.
(c) Breastfeeding women to decrease egg consumption.
(d) Infants with AD: check for egg, milk and wheat allergy and consider elimination diet if positive on allergy testing.
(e) Adults with AD need to be further educated on improving their overall cardiovascular health.

Overall recommendations

(a) Eat a high-fibre diet, high in antioxidants.
(b) Consider vitamin D supplementation as it has been shown to improve AD

(c) Avoid foods high in trans-fat such as in fast food.
(d) Plant-based diets should be encouraged given that they may be just as effective as immunosuppression.

Psoriasis

Psoriasis is a chronic inflammatory skin disease, with genetic, immune and environmental factors contributing to its complex pathogenesis, and can affect not only the skin but the joints and nails too.[64] The incidence of psoriasis over the last 30 years has increased by 100% and this increase is largely attributed to the lifestyle factors such as diet rather than its genetic component that is relatively stable.[64] One reason for this is that psoriasis is commonly associated with other diseases that are commonly associated with a Western diet such as cardiovascular diseases, dyslipidaemia, obesity and diabetes.[65]

Obesity increases the risk of psoriasis as large scale studies have shown that adipocytes are involved in the upregulation of T-Helper (Th) 17 cells that result in secretion of interleukin-17 which plays a pivotal role in psoriasis pathogenesis and one that is targeted by anti-IL17 biological therapies.[64] Furthermore, leptin and visfatin, molecules derived from adipocytes also promote 'antimicrobial peptides, human b-defensin-2/3 or chemokines and CXCL8/10, CCL20 in epidermal keratinocytes'.[66] It is no wonder that weight-loss strategies always result in improvement of psoriasis and its counterpart, psoriatic arthritis.[65] The initial link between weight loss and diet was seen in a study of eight out of 13 Dutch men with psoriasis in Japanese concentration camps that had near total resolution of their psoriasis. More recently a study reported an improvement in PASI (psoriasis area and severity index) scores in patients during Ramadan fasting.[67, 68]

Diving deeper into the nutritional aspects of psoriasis, certain components of the diet are more likely to exacerbate psoriasis while others seem to be useful in improving its appearance. In a study by Kanda et al., the main contributor to psoriasis was a diet high in saturated fatty acids (SFAs), simple sugars, red meat and alcohol.[65] These components collectively activate a cascade of inflammatory cytokines, reactive oxygen species and promote gut dysbiosis.[65] SFAs are commonly found in meat and dairy and exacerbate psoriasis via stimulating the dendritic cells in the epidermis and promoting Th17 response.[66] Red meat contains not only SFAs but also sulphur that can promote gut dysbiosis, leading to bacteria reaching the epithelium and resulting in activation of Toll like receptors and NFκB inflammation.[66] Red meat is also a significant source of advanced glycation end products (AGEs), along with dairy and highly processed foods that are implicated in the pathogenesis of psoriasis, resulting in increased production of free oxygen radicals leading to oxidative stress and damage and release of inflammatory cytokines.[69]

Alcohol plays a key role in initiation and exacerbation of psoriasis. Alcohol at a molecular level releases many pro-inflammatory mediators such as TNF-α that are directly related to the formation of psoriasis as well as creating gut dysbiosis. Gut dysbiosis can lead to an increase in pathogenic bacteria thereby resulting in increased gut permeability and contributing to endotoxaemia and resulting in increased systemic inflammation.[70]

A number of studies have also linked gluten with psoriasis. The link was first established when patients with both coeliac disease and psoriasis improved after the patients went gluten-free. It is likely that both diseases mediate a Th-1 phenotype and generate cytokines interferon-γ and IL-2 in response to gluten.[71] A few studies have observed the significant elevation of serum anti-transglutaminase and anti-gliadin antibodies (AGA) levels in up to 16% of patients with psoriasis and observed that a gluten-free diet (GFD) for three to six months resulted in significant improvement despite not being treated with any systemic therapies.[72] The same authors also found that there was significant recurrence of psoriasis if a conventional gluten diet was consumed and a larger study found that those who responded to a GFD didn't necessarily need to have any gluten insensitivity, symptom wise.[73] It is thought that a GFD contributes to a reduction in Ki67+ cells in the dermis that are responsible for cellular proliferation in both affected and unaffected skin on histology, thereby suggesting a systemic improvement.[74] However, there are many studies that do not link a GFD to improvement in psoriasis and thus further research needs to be done.

Improvement in psoriasis is also observed in those consuming certain components of the diet that include complex carbohydrates from beans and legumes. Soya beans contain an isoflavone called genistein, that has been shown in studies to be a potent, anti-psoriatic agent and in a small study by Smolińska et al., demonstrated the positive impact of this isoflavone at a genetic level for a small group of patients and overall improved the disease burden.[75] Potential mechanisms include suppressing the hyperproliferation of keratinocytes, and reduction in inflammatory cytokines such as TNF-α, interleukin (IL) 1β, IL-6 and ILK-8.[66] Furthermore, polyunsaturated fatty acids (PUFAs), found in fish result in formation of resolvin E1 and D1 which decrease inflammation in psoriasis.[66] Eating fish, however, has some negative health implications, including concerns about pollutants, microplastics and the saturated fat content so it is important to obtain PUFAs in the diet via plant-based omega-3 sources such as flaxseeds, chia seeds and hemp seeds.[76, 77]

Vitamins such as A, D, B12, selenium and zinc tend to be lower in patients with psoriasis and many studies have shown the benefits for vitamin supplementation.[67]

Recommendations for management

(a) Reduce the pro-inflammatory components of their diet such as those listed above, reducing the intake of alcohol, simple sugars, and red meat.
(b) Reduce SFAs and increase PUFAs in the form of omega-3 intake through diet or supplementation.[78]
(c) Supplement with vitamin D, selenium, and 75–100 mg of genistein.
(d) Adopt a gluten-free diet if screening has detected serum IgA and IgG for AGA in moderate to severe psoriasis.
(e) Promote improvement in the associated comorbidities including diabetes, obesity, hypertension and dyslipidaemia.

Hidradenitis suppurativa

Hidradenitis suppurativa (HS) is also known as acne inversa and affects 0.4 to 4% of the population worldwide.[79, 80] The disease results initially in abscesses and nodules in the skin folds such as axilla and groin and can lead to purulent sinus tracts or fistulas and significant scarring leading to poor quality of life. Despite the significant impact on individuals the aetiology remains unknown, but it is likely a complex interaction of genes, inflammation and lifestyle factors.

HS is commonly associated with other conditions such as metabolic syndrome, atherosclerosis, spondyloarthritis and inflammatory bowel disease and central obesity which is found in over 60% of patients.[79] To date, drug therapy has not been effective with only partial improvement with Adalimumab or Infliximab, anti-TNF-α biological agents, immunosuppressive therapies like cyclosporin or long-term antibiotics, thereby emphasising the need to improve disease outcomes through more sustainable options like lifestyle interventions.[81]

Not only does obesity result in larger skin folds, it is well known that adipocytes generate pro-inflammatory cytokines including interleukin-1β and TNF-α.[79] These cytokines are known to recruit different immune cells such neutrophilic granulocytes, monocytes, and different subtypes of T-helper cells that generate permeability of the basement membrane around the hair follicle to different bacteria.[79] The bacteria along with the inflammatory cytokines, further perpetuates the inflammatory reactions and leads to the rupture of the hair follicle resulting in the phenotype typical to that of HS. Furthermore, obesity contributes to insulin resistance and dyslipidaemia that contribute to the aetiopathogenesis of HS.[79] Weight-loss strategies are imperative to treatment of this disease and a study on weight loss due to bariatric surgery resulted in decrease in severity of HS.[80] A high glycaemic index food diet, with high simple carbohydrate meals have been shown to play a role in the 'phosphoinositol 3/kinase/Akt/Fox01' pathway and is likely to contribute to disease severity.[80]

A well-established link between acne and dairy exists as discussed earlier in this chapter and it is likely the same mechanisms contribute to HS. Dairy contains whey, casein and natural androgens from the cow that are not broken down in the pasteurisation process and can impact the pathogenesis of rupture of the follicular sebaceous cysts.[80] The casein in dairy is also linked to increase in IGF-1 whereas whey promotes hyperinsulaemia.[80] Both IGF-1 and hyperinsulaemia lead to an increase in susceptibility of androgen receptors to both endogenous and exogenous hormones, further contributing to HS pathogenesis.[80, 82]

Wheat and brewer's yeast are also implicated in the disease progression and considered a plausible link, similar to Crohn's disease. Yeast contains *Saccharomyces cerevisiae* and these antibodies are often found in chronic inflammatory conditions like Crohn's disease and its associated condition, HS.[80, 83] Even though the studies are limited, Cannistrá et al. found that even in their small cohort of 12 patients, there was long-term improvement of the disease and improvement in quality of life for all their patients, and immediate recurrence of disease 24–48 hours post ingestion of yeast.[81] Aboud et al. looked at over 185 patients and found a 70% improvement in HS with 87% of their patients having a recurrence after consuming yeast containing food or beverage, again supporting the yeast hypothesis in HS pathogenesis.[83]

Lastly, a recent publication in 2021 by Barrea et al. showed that HS patients tend to have higher circulating levels of trimethylamine N-oxide (TMAO).[84] TMAO is a pro-inflammatory compound generated from choline, betaine and carnitine via gut microbial metabolism which are mainly sourced from animal products such as meat, fish, poultry, dairy and egg.[85] This research is the first of its kind and will require more research to establish the link between animal products and HS. However, it does provide insight that perhaps HS is also linked with gut dysbiosis, as are its associated diseases.[84]

Interestingly, there is usually a lower level of vitamin D, B12 and zinc in patients with HS and supplementation of these nutrients has resulted in some clinical improvement of the disease.[86, 87] Overall it is difficult to conclude that dietary interventions alone provide complete disease resolution but they certainly are helpful in improving disease score and patient quality of life, are safe and healthy and provide an adjuvant therapy to conventional treatment in HS.

Recommendations for management

(a) Follow a low-glycaemic index food diet with reduction in the amount of sugary beverages and food, as well as simple

carbohydrates such as processed white bread, pasta and sweets.[88]
(b) Eliminate dairy and yeast-containing products.[80]
(c) Supplement with zinc, vitamin D, and vitamin B12.[86]

Urticaria

Chronic urticaria (CU) is often difficult to manage as the aetiology remains mainly unknown. The underlying pathogenesis of CU is mast cell activation and the release of histamine and other pro-inflammatory mediators such as tumour necrosis factors (TNFs).[89] This results in tissue vasodilation and extravasation of plasma, leading to dermal oedema and wheals.[89] There is now increasing evidence to suggest that there are a few immunological and non-immunological triggers for mast cell activation in the diet that affect disease outcome.[89]

Even though true immunological food allergies in CU are very rare, emerging research shows that individuals that are bitten by ticks, are more likely to become allergic to galactose-α-1,3-galactose (α-gal) representing a meat allergy or those individuals that eat raw, marinated or smoked fish may develop an *Anisakis simplex (A. simplex)* allergy.[89]

The oligosaccharide α-gal is transmitted to humans by ticks via a bite. This results in development of IgE-mediated allergy to α-gal antigen, which is also common in mammalian meat such as beef, lamb, and pork.[90] Usually, it can take 2–4 hours post ingestion of meat for symptoms to occur, thereby making the link to diet usually difficult and often results in the misdiagnosis of idiopathic CU. In a small study by Pollack et al., 69% of their patients had detectable IgE antibodies to α-gal out of which 45% had complete symptom resolution after avoiding mammalian meat or mammalian-derived products, including dairy.[90]

Anisakiasis is a parasitic disease caused by an anisakid nematode and can occur in individuals who consume undercooked or raw fish. Hypersensitivity can occur to allergens in *Anisakis simplex* and 50% of these patients have a positive skin prick allergy. A few studies have shown that in these patients, excluding marinated and raw fish, resulted in complete resolution of CU in 77% of patients.[89] There are a few more studies that didn't show consistent results but with more research, the link will likely be more firmly established in time.

Additional considerations in patients with CU

(a) Ensure patients do not have coeliac disease where dietary avoidance of gluten is advisable.
(b) Short-term avoidance of pseudo allergens such as tomatoes, common food additives, herbs and wine.[91]
(c) Avoidance of certain foods that contain high levels of histamine including seafood, and fermented foods such as aged cheeses, dry sausage and fermented soya.[89]
(d) Check your patient's vitamin D level as this is often low and early interventional studies have shown promising results in symptomatic improvement of CU.[89]

Conclusion

This chapter provides a brief overview of the link between diet and cutaneous diseases that tend to be highly prevalent. Research in skin and nutrition is limited and can be difficult to navigate through the confounding factors and selective reporting bias. Research in the field of nutritional dermatology is ongoing, including growing evidence on the link between the gut microbiome and its effect on skin health regulation, the gut-skin axis. Patients are always keen to seek a link between what they eat and the health of their skin. Even though counselling patients on diet can be difficult, when patients do make that change, the effects can be long-lasting.

References

1. Vos T, Flaxman AD, Naghavi M, Lozano R, Michaud C, Ezzati M, et al. Years lived with disability (YLDs) for 1160 sequelae of 289 diseases and injuries 1990–2010: a systematic analysis for the Global Burden of Disease Study 2010. *The Lancet* 2012; 380(9859): 2163-2196.
2. Tan JK, Bhate K. A global perspective on the epidemiology of acne. *Br J Dermatol* 2015; 172(Suppl 1): 3-12.
3. Tan JKL, Vasey K, Fung KY. Beliefs and perceptions of patients with acne. *Journal of the American Academy of Dermatology* 2001; 44(3): 439-445.
4. Dall'Oglio F, Nasca MR, Fiorentini F, Micali G. Diet and acne: review of the evidence from 2009 to 2020. *Int J Dermatol* 2021; 60(6): 672-685. doi: 10.1111/ijd.15390
5. Maarouf M, Platto JF, Shi VY. The role of nutrition in inflammatory pilosebaceous disorders: Implication of the skin-gut axis. *Australas J Dermatol* 2019; 60(2): e90-e8. doi: 10.1111/ajd.12909
6. Kucharska A, Szmurło A, Sińska B. Significance of diet in treated and untreated acne vulgaris. *Postepy Dermatol Alergol* 2016; 33(2): 81-86. doi: 10.5114/ada.2016.59146
7. Rahaman SMA, De D, Handa S, Pal A, Sachdeva N, Ghosh T, et al. Association of insulin-like growth factor (IGF)-1 gene polymorphisms with plasma levels of IGF-1 and acne severity. *Journal of the American Academy of Dermatology* 2016; 75(4): 768-773. doi: 10.1016/j.jaad.2016.05.019
8. Melnik BC, Schmitz G. Role of insulin, insulin-like growth factor-1, hyperglycaemic food and milk consumption in the pathogenesis of acne vulgaris. *Experimental Dermatology* 2009; 18(10): 833-841. doi: 10.1111/j.1600-0625.2009.00924.x
9. Baldwin H, Tan J. Effects of Diet on Acne and Its Response to Treatment. *Am J Clin Dermatol* 2021; 22(1): 55-65. doi: 10.1007/s40257-020-00542-y
10. Juhl C, Bergholdt H, Miller I, Jemec G, Kanters J, Ellervik C. Dairy Intake and Acne Vulgaris: A Systematic Review and Meta-Analysis of 78,529 Children, Adolescents, and Young Adults. *Nutrients* 2018; 10(8): 1049. doi: 10.3390/nu10081049
11. Dai R, Hua W, Chen W, Xiong L, Li L. The effect of milk consumption on acne: a meta-analysis of observational studies. *Journal of the European Academy of Dermatology and Venereology* 2018; 32(12): 2244-2253. doi: 10.1111/jdv.15204
12. Chen H. Dairy consumption and acne: a case control study in Kabul, Afghanistan. *Clinical, Cosmetic and Investigational Dermatology* 2019; 12: 481-487. doi: 10.2147/CCID.S195191
13. Suppiah TSS, Sundram TKM, Tan ESS, Lee CK, Bustami NA, Tan CK. Acne vulgaris and its association with dietary intake: A Malaysian perspective. *Asia Pacific Journal of Clinical Nutrition* 2018; 27(5): 1141-1145. doi: 10.6133/apjcn.072018.01
14. Melnik BC. Lifetime Impact of Cow's Milk on Overactivation of mTORC1: From Fetal to Childhood Overgrowth, Acne, Diabetes, Cancers, and Neurodegeneration. *Biomolecules* 2021; 11(3): 404. doi: 10.3390/biom11030404
15. Yager Z, McLean S. Muscle building supplement use in Australian adolescent boys: relationships with body image, weight lifting, and sports engagement. *BMC Pediatrics* 2020; 20(1): 1-9. doi: 10.1186/s12887-020-1993-6
16. Simonart T. Acne and Whey Protein Supplementation among Bodybuilders. *Dermatology* 2013; 225(3): 256-258. doi: 10.1159/000345102
17. Melnik B. Dietary intervention in acne: Attenuation of increased mTORC1 signaling promoted by Western diet. *Dermato-Endocrinology* 2012; 4(1): 20-32. doi: 10.4161/derm.19828
18. Silverberg NB. Whey protein precipitating moderate to severe acne flares in 5 teenaged athletes. *Cutis* 2012; 90(2): 70-72.
19. Cengiz FP, Cevirgen Cemil B, Emiroglu N, Gulsel Bahali A, Onsun N. Acne located on the trunk, whey protein supplementation: Is there any

association? Health Promot Perspect. 2017; 7(2): 106-108. doi: 10.15171/hpp.2017.19
20. Pontes TdC, Fernandes Filho GMC, Trindade AdSP, Sobral Filho JF. Incidence of acne vulgaris in young adult users of protein-calorie supplements in the city of João Pessoa--PB. *Anais brasileiros de dermatologia* 2013; 88(6): 907-912. doi: 10.1590/abd1806-4841.20132024
21. Kang SH, Kim JU, Imm JY, Oh S, Kim SH. The Effects of Dairy Processes and Storage on Insulin-Like Growth Factor-I (IGF-I) Content in Milk and in Model IGF-I–Fortified Dairy Products. *Journal of Dairy Science* 2006; 89(2): 402-409. doi: 10.3168/jds.S0022-0302(06)72104-X
22. Smith RN, Mann NJ, Braue A, Makelainen H, Varigos GA. The effect of a high-protein, low glycemic-load diet versus a conventional, high glycemic-load diet on biochemical parameters associated with acne vulgaris: A randomized, investigator-masked, controlled trial. *Journal of the American Academy of Dermatology* 2007; 57(2): 247-256. doi: 10.1016/j.jaad.2007.01.046
23. Kwon HH, Yoon JY, Hong JS, Jung JY, Park MS, Suh DH. Clinical and histological effect of a low glycaemic load diet in treatment of acne vulgaris in Korean patients: a randomized, controlled trial. *Acta Derm Venereol* 2012; 92(3): 241-246. doi: 10.2340/00015555-1346
24. Fabbrocini G, Izzo R, Faggiano A, Del Prete M, Donnarumma M, Marasca C, et al. Low glycaemic diet and metformin therapy: a new approach in male subjects with acne resistant to common treatments. *Clinical and Experimental Dermatology* 2016; 41(1): 38-42. doi: 10.1111/ced.12673
25. Çerman AA, Aktaş E, Altunay İK, Arıcı JE, Tulunay A, Ozturk FY. Dietary glycemic factors, insulin resistance, and adiponectin levels in acne vulgaris. *Journal of the American Academy of Dermatology* 2016; 75(1): 155-162. doi: 10.1016/j.jaad.2016.02.1220
26. Ismail N, Manaf Z, Azizan N. High glycemic load diet, milk and ice cream consumption are related to acne vulgaris in Malaysian young adults: a case control study. *BMC Dermatology* 2012; 12(1): 13. doi: 10.1186/1471-5945-12-13
27. Burris J, Rietkerk W, Shikany JM, Woolf K. Differences in Dietary Glycemic Load and Hormones in New York City Adults with No and Moderate/Severe Acne. *Journal of the Academy of Nutrition and Dietetics* 2017; 117(9): 1375-1383. doi: 10.1016/j.jand.2017.03.024
28. Heng AHS, Chew FT. Systematic review of the epidemiology of acne vulgaris. *Scientific Reports* 2020; 10(1): 5754. doi: 10.1038/s41598-020-62715-3
29. Dupré A, Albarel N, Bonafe JL, Christol B, Lassere J. Vitamin B-12 induced acnes. *Cutis* 1979; 24(2): 210-211.
30. Balta I, Ozuguz P. Vitamin B12-induced acneiform eruption. *Cutaneous and Ocular Toxicology* 2014; 33(2): 94-95. doi: 10.3109/15569527.2013.808657
31. Kang D, Shi B, Erfe MC, Craft N, Li H. Vitamin B12 modulates the transcriptome of the skin microbiota in acne pathogenesis. *Science translational medicine* 2015; 7(293): 293ra103. doi: 10.1126/scitranslmed.aab2009
32. Weiss E, Katta R. Diet and rosacea: the role of dietary change in the management of rosacea. *Dermatol Pract Concept* 2017; 7(4): 31-37. doi: 10.5826/dpc.0704a08
33. Schwab VD, Sulk M, Seeliger S, Nowak P, Aubert J, Mess C, et al. Neurovascular and Neuroimmune Aspects in the Pathophysiology of Rosacea. *J Investig Dermatol Symp Proc* 2011; 15(1): 53-62. doi: 10.1038/jidsymp.2011.6
34. Aubdool AA, Brain SD. Neurovascular Aspects of Skin Neurogenic Inflammation. *J Investig Dermatol Symp Proc* 2011; 15(1): 33-39. doi: 10.1038/jidsymp.2011.8
35. Drake L. Hot sauce watcf-u, survey finds, 2005. https://www.rosacea.org/ rr/2005/fall/article_3.php.
36. Searle T, Ali F, Carolides S, Al-Niaimi F. Rosacea and Diet: What is New in 2021? *Journal of Clinical and Aesthetic Dermatology* 2021; 14: 49-54.
37. Daou H, Paradiso M, Hennessy K, Seminario-Vidal L. Rosacea and the Microbiome: A Systematic Review. *Dermatology and Therapy* 2021; 11(1): 1-12. doi: 10.1007/s13555-020-00460-1
38. Manzhalii E, Hornuss D, Stremmel W. Intestinal-borne dermatoses significantly improved by oral application of Escherichia coli Nissle 1917. *World Journal of Gastroenterology* 2016; 22(23):

5415-5421. doi: 10.3748/wjg.v22.i23.5415
39. Fortuna MC, Garelli V, Pranteda G, Romaniello F, Cardone M, Carlesimo M, et al. A case of Scalp Rosacea treated with low dose doxycycline and probiotic therapy and literature review on therapeutic options. *Dermatologic Therapy* 2016; 29(4): 249-251. doi: 10.1111/dth.12355
40. Milewska-Wróbel D, Lis-Święty A. Does antioxidant-rich diet during pregnancy protect against atopic multimorbidity in children? *Explore (NY)* 2022; 18(1): 96-99. doi: 10.1016/j.explore.2020.11.001
41. Yu HS, Tu HP, Hong CH, Lee CH. Lifetime Increased Risk of Adult Onset Atopic Dermatitis in Adolescent and Adult Patients with Food Allergy. *Int J Mol Sci* 2016; 18(1): 42. doi: 10.3390/ijms18010042
42. Salehi T, Pourpak Z, Karkon S, Shoormasti RS, Sabzevari SK, Movahedi M, et al. The study of egg allergy in children with atopic dermatitis. *World Allergy Organ J* 2009; 2(7): 123-127. doi: 10.1097/WOX.0b013e3181abe7cb
43. Sehgal VN, Khurana A, Mendiratta V, Saxena D, Srivastava G, Aggarwal AK. Atopic Dermatitis; Etio-Pathogenesis, An Overview. *Indian J Dermatol* 2015; 60(4): 327-331. doi: 10.4103/0019-5154.160474
44. Kramer MS, Kakuma R. Maternal dietary antigen avoidance during pregnancy or lactation, or both, for preventing or treating atopic disease in the child. *Cochrane Database Syst Rev* 2012; 2012(9): CD000133-CD. doi: 10.1002/14651858.CD000133.pub3
45. Venter C, Agostoni C, Arshad SH, Ben-Abdallah M, Du Toit G, Fleischer DM, et al. Dietary factors during pregnancy and atopic outcomes in childhood: A systematic review from the European Academy of Allergy and Clinical Immunology. *Pediatric Allergy and Immunology* 2020; 31(8): 889-912. doi: 10.1111/pai.13303
46. Beckhaus AA, Garcia-Marcos L, Forno E, Pacheco-Gonzalez RM, Celedón JC, Castro-Rodriguez JA. Maternal nutrition during pregnancy and risk of asthma, wheeze, and atopic diseases during childhood: a systematic review and meta-analysis. *Allergy* 2015; 70(12): 1588-1604. doi: 10.1111/all.12729
47. Zulyniak MA, de Souza RJ, Shaikh M, Ramasundarahettige C, Tam K, Williams N, et al. Ethnic differences in maternal diet in pregnancy and infant eczema. *PLoS One* 2020; 15(5): e0232170. doi: 10.1371/journal.pone.0232170
48. Tanaka T, Kouda K, Kotani M, Takeuchi A, Tabei T, Masamoto Y, et al. Vegetarian diet ameliorates symptoms of atopic dermatitis through reduction of the number of peripheral eosinophils and of PGE2 synthesis by monocytes. *J Physiol Anthropol Appl Human Sci* 2001; 20(6): 353-361. doi: 10.2114/jpa.20.353
49. Zeng J, Wu W, Chen Y, Jing J, Cai L. Maternal dietary protein patterns during pregnancy and the risk of infant eczema: a cohort study. *Frontiers in nutrition* 2021; 8:608972. doi: 10.3389/fnut.2021.608972
50. Saito K, Yokoyama T, Miyake Y, Sasaki S, Tanaka K, Ohya Y, et al. Maternal meat and fat consumption during pregnancy and suspected atopic eczema in Japanese infants aged 3-4 months: the Osaka Maternal and Child Health Study. *Pediatr Allergy Immunol* 2010; 21(1 Pt 1): 38-46. doi: 10.1111/j.1399-3038.2009.00897.x
51. Baïz N, Just J, Chastang J, Forhan A, de Lauzon-Guillain B, Magnier A-M, et al. Maternal diet before and during pregnancy and risk of asthma and allergic rhinitis in children. *Allergy, Asthma & Clinical Immunology* 2019; 15(1): 40. doi: 10.1186/s13223-019-0353-2
52. Gao X, Yan Y, Zeng G, Sha T, Liu S, He Q, et al. Influence of prenatal and early-life exposures on food allergy and eczema in infancy: a birth cohort study. *BMC Pediatrics* 2019; 19(1): 239. doi: 10.1186/s12887-019-1623-3
53. Nurani N, Prawirohartono E, Wahab A. Effect of egg avoidance diet by nursing mothers on the incidence of atopic dermatitis in infants. *Paediatrica Indonesiana* 2008; 48(2). doi: 10.14238/pi48.2.2008.71-5
54. Pretorius RA, Bodinier M, Prescott SL, Palmer DJ. Maternal Fiber Dietary Intakes during Pregnancy and Infant Allergic Disease. *Nutrients* 2019; 11(8): 1767. doi: 10.3390/nu11081767
55. Garcia-Larsen V, Ierodiakonou D, Jarrold K, Cunha S, Chivinge J, Robinson Z, et al. Diet during pregnancy and infancy and risk of allergic or autoimmune disease: A systematic review and meta-analysis. *PLoS Med* 2018; 15(2): e1002507.

doi: 10.1371/journal.pmed.1002507
56. Pourpak Z, Farhoudi A, Mahmoudi M, Movahedi M, Ghargozlou M, Kazemnejad A et al. The role of cow milk allergy in increasing the severity of atopic dermatitis. *Immunol Invest* 2004; 33(1): 69-79. doi: 10.1081/imm-120027686
57. Lever R, MacDonald C, Waugh P, Aitchison T. Randomised controlled trial of advice on an egg exclusion diet in young children with atopic eczema and sensitivity to eggs. *Pediatr Allergy Immunol* 1998; 9(1): 13-19.
doi: 10.1111/j.1399-3038.1998.tb00294.x
58. Kramer MS, Chalmers B, Hodnett ED, Sevkovskaya Z, Dzikovich I, Shapiro S, et al. Promotion of Breastfeeding Intervention Trial (PROBIT): a randomized trial in the Republic of Belarus. *JAMA* 2001; 285(4): 413-420.
doi: 10.1001/jama.285.4.413
59. Silverberg JI, Greenland P. Eczema and cardiovascular risk factors in 2 US adult population studies. *J Allergy Clin Immunol* 2015; 135(3): 721-8.e6. doi: 10.1016/j.jaci.2014.11.023
60. Wang CS, Wang J, Zhang X, Zhang L, Zhang HP, Wang L, et al. Is the consumption of fast foods associated with asthma or other allergic diseases? *Respirology* 2018; 23(10): 901-913.
doi: 10.1111/resp.13339
61. Ellwood P, Asher MI, García-Marcos L, Williams H, Keil U, Robertson C, et al. Do fast foods cause asthma, rhinoconjunctivitis and eczema? Global findings from the International Study of Asthma and Allergies in Childhood (ISAAC) Phase Three. *Thorax* 2013; 68(4): 351-360.
doi: 10.1136/thoraxjnl-2012-202285
62. Cho SI, Lee H, Lee DH, Kim K-H. Association of frequent intake of fast foods, energy drinks, or convenience food with atopic dermatitis in adolescents. *European Journal of Nutrition* 2020; 59(7): 3171-3182.
doi: 10.1007/s00394-019-02157-4
63. Nosrati A, Afifi L, Danesh MJ, Lee K, Yan D, Beroukhim K, et al. Dietary modifications in atopic dermatitis: patient-reported outcomes. *J Dermatolog Treat*. 2017;28(6):523-38.
64. Jensen P, Skov L. Psoriasis and Obesity. *Dermatology* 2017; 232(6): 633-639.
doi: 10.1080/09546634.2016.1278071
65. Kanda N, Hoashi T, Saeki H. Nutrition and Psoriasis. *International Journal of Molecular Sciences* 2020; 21(15): 5405.
doi: 10.3390/ijms21155405
66. Yamashita H, Morita T, Ito M, Okazaki S, Koto M, Ichikawa Y, et al. Dietary habits in Japanese patients with psoriasis and psoriatic arthritis: Low intake of meat in psoriasis and high intake of vitamin A in psoriatic arthritis. *The Journal of Dermatology* 2019; 46(9): 759-769.
doi: 10.1111/1346-8138.15032
67. Amin SS, Adil M, Alam M. Role of dietary intervention in psoriasis: A review. *IJCD* 2018; 1(01): 13.
68. Damiani G, Watad A, Bridgewood C, Pigatto PDM, Pacifico A, Malagoli P, et al. The Impact of Ramadan Fasting on the Reduction of PASI Score, in Moderate-To-Severe Psoriatic Patients: A Real-Life Multicenter Study. *Nutrients* 2019; 11(2): 277.
doi: 10.3390/nu11020277
69. Papagrigoraki A, Maurelli M, Del Giglio M, Gisondi P, Girolomoni G. Advanced glycation end products in the pathogenesis of psoriasis. *Int J Mol Sci* 2017; 18(11): 2471.
doi: 10.3390/ijms18112471
70. Engen PA, Green SJ, Voigt RM, Forsyth CB, Keshavarzian A. The Gastrointestinal Microbiome: Alcohol Effects on the Composition of Intestinal Microbiota. *Alcohol Res* 2015; 37(2): 223-236.
71. Dhattarwal N, Mahajan VK, Mehta KS, Chauhan PS, Yadav RS, Sharma SB, et al. The association of anti-gliadin and anti-transglutaminase antibodies and chronic plaque psoriasis in Indian patients: Preliminary results of a descriptive cross-sectional study. *Australas J Dermatol* 2020; 61(4): e378-e382. doi: 10.1111/ajd.13308
72. Michaëlsson G, Gerdén B, Hagforsen E, Nilsson B, Pihl-Lundin I, Kraaz W, et al. Psoriasis patients with antibodies to gliadin can be improved by a gluten-free diet. *British Journal of Dermatology* 2000; 142(1): 44-51.
doi: 10.1046/j.1365-2133.2000.03240.x
73. Kolchak NA, Tetarnikova MK, Theodoropoulou MS, Michalopoulou AP, Theodoropoulos DS. Prevalence of antigliadin IgA antibodies in psoriasis vulgaris and response of seropositive patients to a gluten-free diet. *J Multidiscip Healthc* 2017; 11: 13-19. doi: 10.2147/JMDH.S122256

74. Michaëlsson G, Ahs S, Hammarström I, Lundin IP, Hagforsen E. Gluten-free diet in psoriasis patients with antibodies to gliadin results in decreased expression of tissue transglutaminase and fewer Ki67+ cells in the dermis. *Acta Derm Venereol* 2003; 83(6): 425-429. doi: 10.1080/00015550310015022
75. Smolinska E, Wegrzyn G, Gabig-Ciminska M. Genistein modulates gene activity in psoriatic patients. *Acta biochimica polonica* 2019; 66(1): 101-110. doi: 10.18388/abp.2018_2772
76. Van Cauwenberghe L, Janssen CR. Microplastics in bivalves cultured for human consumption. *Environ Pollut*.2014; 193: 65-70. doi: 10.1016/j.envpol.2014.06.010
77. Kris-Etherton PM, Harris WS, Appel LJ. Fish consumption, fish oil, omega-3 fatty acids, and cardiovascular disease. *Arterioscler Thromb Vasc Biol* 2003; 23(2): e20-30. doi: 10.1161/01.atv.0000038493.65177.94
78. Garbicz J, Całyniuk B, Górski M, Buczkowska M, Piecuch M, Kulik A, et al. Nutritional Therapy in Persons Suffering from Psoriasis. *Nutrients* 2022; 14(1): 119. doi: 10.3390/nu14010119
79. Wolk K, Join-Lambert O, Sabat R. Aetiology and pathogenesis of hidradenitis suppurativa. *British Journal of Dermatology* 2020; 183(6): 999-1010. doi: 10.1111/bjd.19556
80. Silfvast-Kaiser A, Youssef R, Paek SY. Diet in hidradenitis suppurativa: a review of published and lay literature. *Int J Dermatol* 2019; 58(11): 1225-1230. doi: 10.1111/ijd.14465
81. Cannistrà CMDP, Finocchi VMD, Trivisonno AMD, Tambasco DMD. New perspectives in the treatment of hidradenitis suppurativa: Surgery and brewer's yeast–exclusion diet. *Surgery* 2013; 154(5): 1126-1130. doi: 10.1016/j.surg.2013.04.018
82. Danby FWMD. Diet in the prevention of hidradenitis suppurativa (acne inversa). *J Am Acad Dermatol* 2015; 73(5): S52-S54. doi: 10.1016/j.jaad.2015.07.042
83. Aboud C, Zamaria N, Cannistrà C. Treatment of hidradenitis suppurativa: Surgery and yeast (Saccharomyces cerevisiae)–exclusion diet. Results after 6 years. *Surgery* 2020; 167(6): 1012-1015. doi: 10.1016/j.surg.2019.12.015
84. Barrea L, Muscogiuri G, Pugliese G, de Alteriis G, Maisto M, Donnarumma M, et al. Association of Trimethylamine N-Oxide (TMAO) with the Clinical Severity of Hidradenitis Suppurativa (Acne Inversa). *Nutrients* 2021; 13(6): 1997. doi: 10.3390/nu13061997
85. Janeiro MH, Ramírez MJ, Milagro FI, Martínez JA, Solas M. Implication of Trimethylamine N-Oxide (TMAO) in Disease: Potential Biomarker or New Therapeutic Target. *Nutrients* 2018; 10(10): 1398. doi: 10.3390/nu10101398
86. Choi F, Lehmer L, Ekelem C, Mesinkovska NA. Dietary and metabolic factors in the pathogenesis of hidradenitis suppurativa: a systematic review. *International Journal of Dermatology* 2020; 59(2): 143-153. doi: 10.1111/ijd.14691
87. Hendricks AJ, Hirt PA, Sekhon S, Vaughn AR, Lev-Tov HA, Hsiao JL, et al. Non-pharmacologic approaches for hidradenitis suppurativa - a systematic review. *J Dermatolog Treat* 2021; 32(1): 11-18. doi: 10.1080/09546634.2019.1621981
88. Eiken HC, Holm JG, Thomsen SF. Studies on the role of diet in the management of hidradenitis suppurativa are needed. *Journal of the American Academy of Dermatology* 2020; 82(4): e137-8. doi: 10.1016/j.jaad.2019.10.137
89. Jaros J, Shi VY, Katta R. Diet and Chronic Urticaria: Dietary Modification as a Treatment Strategy. *Dermatology practical & conceptual* 2019; 10(1): e2020004. doi: 10.5826/dpc.1001a04
90. Pollack K, Zlotoff BJ, Borish LC, Commins SP, Platts-Mills TAE, Wilson JM. α-Gal Syndrome vs Chronic Urticaria. *JAMA Dermatol* 2019; 155(1): 115-116. doi: 10.1001/jamadermatol.2018.3970
91. Zuberbier T, Pfrommer C, Specht K, Vieths S, Bastl-Borrmann R, Worm M, et al. Aromatic components of food as novel eliciting factors of pseudoallergic reactions in chronic urticaria. *J Allergy Clin Immunol* 2002; 109(2): 343-348. doi: 10.1067/mai.2002.121309

Chapter 17
Plant-based nutrition for athletes

Leila Dehghan-Zaklaki

Introduction

The movie *Game Changers* (2018) attracted a growing number of athletes and hobby exercisers to the idea of eliminating animal products from their diet, and instead adopting a plant-based diet in the hope of enhancing their athletic performance. This is neither surprising nor new – when we look at the history of sports, we encounter countless vegetarian or vegan athletes who have excelled at their chosen sport and inspired others to follow suit.

A healthy baseline is key for athletes, and that is what a plant-based diet promises. A plant-based diet has proven to mitigate the risk for many lifestyle diseases. It lowers fat and optimises body composition. It also reduces blood viscosity and therefore improves the blood flow and oxygen delivery to the working muscles. In addition, there is a strong, anecdotal evidence that a plant-based diet shortens recovery time after training and competition.

However, the two misconceptions that, on the one hand, protein is the most important macronutrient in an athlete's diet, and on the other hand, plant protein is incomplete, have created a great deal of concern for those who are seriously contemplating a plant-based diet. It is therefore critical to debunk the common myths surrounding the link between this particular diet and athletic performance by providing evidence-based guidance to plant-based athletes.

This chapter will examine athletes' nutritional requirements and outline how to meet these needs with a plant-based diet. The chapter begins by laying out the energy requirements of athletes independent of their diet. Next, it focuses on the three macronutrients and their role in the athlete's diet, before turning to a discussion of hydration for optimal athletic performance. Finally, this chapter provides an overview of the vitamins and minerals of concern in an athlete's plant-based diet and discusses the evidence for ergogenic aids.

Energy requirements of athletes

Energy expenditure

Energy expenditure refers to the amount of energy required to carry out physical functions. Plant-based healthcare professionals often say that as long as we consume enough calories, we obtain enough protein. This is often cited to assure athletes that a plant-based diet can meet their protein needs. However, the first part of that sentence draws attention to a vital fact, namely that athletes who push beyond their boundaries require a higher caloric intake to fuel the increased activity level. Meeting this increased energy requirement should be high priority for athletes. Inadequate caloric intake results in poor intake of essential nutrients, which can put the athlete's health at risk and affect their athletic performance.

Given that plant foods tend to be lower in energy density, obtaining adequate calories can be more challenging for plant-based athletes, and without appropriate planning, athletes may struggle to take in an adequate number of calories. Additionally, athletes have varying energy requirements depending on their sports event. To illustrate this point, the energy necessities of athletes competing in different disciplines can be compared, as outlined in Table 17.1. The energy requirements depend not only on sex, age and body composition, but also on the training programme, thus fluctuating from training to non-training days. Nevertheless, many athletes, especially hobby exercisers, tend to consume insufficient calories on their rest days, which can ultimately have a negative impact on their performance.[1]

Low energy intake can suppress the immune system, increase the risk of various diseases, bring about hypotension and arrhythmias, and lead to iron deficiency. Female athletes with inadequate energy may suffer from hormonal dysfunction and menstrual disturbances.[2] While the lack of menstrual cycle is often brushed off as part of a normal, hard training regimen, it is important to note that low oestrogen levels are associated with low bone mineral density, and this, in turn, can put one at risk of stress fractures and overuse injury.[1] The effects of low energy consumption are less researched in male athletes, but it is to be expected that they too suffer from impaired bone health and increased probability of injuries.

Table 17.1 Calorie requirements of different athletes

Sport	Energy expenditure (kcal/day)
Lightweight female rower	3957±1219
Male elite soccer player	3566 ± 585
Male college wrestler	4283±590
Male ultra-marathon runner	6095–6550
Elite female distance runner	2826±312

For all the above reasons, it is paramount for athletes to be able to calculate their own daily energy requirements, also known as the total energy expenditure (TEE). This is done by first establishing the basal metabolic rate (BMR), often referred to as resting energy expenditure (REE). BMR is the amount of energy needed to maintain normal body functions at rest, such as breathing, heart and brain function. By multiplying the BMR with a factor that reflects the physical activity level (PAL), the daily energy requirement can be determined. The American College of Sport Medicine recommends using two equations to estimate BMR: the Harris-Benedict equation, or the Cunningham equation (see Table 17.2),[4] and PAL can range from 1.2 to 2.1, depending on the extent of the activity (see Table 17.3).[5]

Table 17.2 Equations to calculate BMR[4]

Source	Equation
Cunningham	RMR (kcal/24 h) = 500 + 22 X FFM (kg)
Harris-Benedict	Females: RMR (kcal/24 h) = 655.96 + 1.850 X H (cm) + 9.563 X BW (kg) – 4.676 X A (years) Males: RMR (kcal/24 h) = 66.473 + 5.003 X H (cm) + 13.752 X BW (kg) – 6.755 X A (years)

Table 17.3 Physical activity factor to calculate energy requirements[5]

Activity level	Description	Activity factor
Sedentary	Little or no exercise, seated and standing activities	1.2–1.3
Lightly active	Light exercise, 30 min, 1–3 days per week	1.5–1.6
Moderately active	Moderate exercise, 30–60 min, 3–4 days per week	1.6–1.7
Extremely active	Vigorous activity, full-time athletes, 6–7 days per week	1.9–2.1

Athletes may find it easier to consume more frequent meals and snacks throughout the day to meet their high caloric needs. Plant-based athletes who strive to eat only whole foods must include in their diet more calorie-dense foods such as nuts, seeds, nut butters, dried fruits and avocados. Consuming a small amount of refined carbohydrates on occasions is acceptable.

One of the widely debated areas in nutrition is the optimal ratio of the macronutrients in the human diet. However, we know that all three macronutrients (carbohydrates, protein and fat) are equally important for the various body functions and our wellbeing. A better appreciation of how the breakdown of these macronutrients produce energy may aid the clarification of the current dietary recommendations for athletes. These energy systems will be addressed next.

Energy systems

There are three pathways to break down macronutrients and generate energy in form of adenosine triphosphate (ATP). ATP is a high-energy compound that cannot be stored within the tissues and needs to be synthesised during exercise. The type of exercise and its associated intensity, duration and oxygen availability determine which of the three energy systems is utilised to produce ATP.

Short bursts of high-intensity activities require huge amounts of instantaneous energy. This is provided by the so-called phosphocreatine energy system, which is anaerobic and does not depend on oxygen. ATP is produced from creatine phosphate (CrP) stored in skeletal muscle, although because of the limited availability of CrP, the energy will only sustain activities lasting 5–8 seconds, as seen in sprinting or jumping.

High-intensity activities that last longer than 10 seconds necessitate ATP to be produced quickly. This is done via glycolysis, a process that converts glycogen (the stored form of carbohydrates) to glucose and produces ATP. Glycolysis can occur anaerobically in the absence of oxygen, which has the advantage of producing ATP during high intensity exercise when the circulatory system is not yet able to deliver enough oxygen. The disadvantage, however, is that lactic acid is made as a by-product. High lactate levels reduce a muscle's ability to work, which in turn makes anaerobic activities self-limiting. The anaerobic glycolysis provides energy for about two minutes.

Longer activities are fuelled by the aerobic (in presence of oxygen) glycolysis that results in larger amounts of ATP. The downside is that this reliance on oxygen renders the aerobic energy system limited as it is contingent on the maximum amount of oxygen the body can utilise during exercise (known as VO2 max). The aerobic energy system is engaged during moderate- to high-intensity activities and makes use of a mixture of carbohydrates and fats.

Most sports involve energy from a mixture of aerobic and anaerobic metabolisms. The discussion so far demonstrates the significance of carbohydrates as fuel during exercise. Carbohydrates are also necessary for fat metabolism to avoid the creation of ketones. In brief, protein is not the fuel of choice for energy production; instead, it is only used as a last resort when carbohydrates are depleted, and fat stores are minimal. With this in mind, the next section will discuss carbohydrates in more detail.

Carbohydrates

Carbohydrates are the primary source of energy for the working muscles and brain. After ingestion, carbohydrates are broken down to glucose, which either becomes fuel for the production of ATP energy or is stored in liver and muscles as glycogen. Depending on body mass and diet, the body can contain 350–400 g of muscle glycogen and about 100 g of liver glycogen.[6] There is an additional 12 g of glucose in blood and extracellular space. Since muscle lacks glucose-6-phosphatase, the enzyme necessary to convert glycogen to free glucose, the glycogen stored in muscles is only utilised locally to provide energy for the exercising muscle. It is the liver glycogen that contributes to blood glucose homeostasis and maintains the blood glucose levels within a normal range (4.0 and 5.5 mmol/l).

The higher the intensity of an activity, the more we depend on carbohydrates as a fuel. Without adequate replenishment the glycogen stores become depleted. Low or insufficient glycogen stores lead to what many endurance athletes refer to as 'hitting the wall' or 'bonking'. This happens when the body switches to fat metabolism, which is not as efficient or rapid as carbohydrates. Breaking down fat for energy production requires more energy, and this will inevitably slow down the athlete.

Low glycogen reserves will also have an adverse effect on the brain. To emphasise, glucose is the primary fuel for our nervous system. When glycogen stores are exhausted, the liver deploys non-carbohydrate substances such as fatty acids and proteins to produce glucose and stabilise the blood glucose levels. This process, called gluconeogenesis, is slow and can lead to temporary hypoglycaemia, which manifests itself as lethargy, lightheadedness and general fatigue. Though 'hitting the wall' is an expression familiar to endurance athletes, the sudden loss of energy can happen in all sports, especially in team sports that involve intense intermittent activities.

The benefits of carbohydrates are also backed by the existing research. For example, a 2013 cross-over study[7] investigated the relationship between carbohydrate intake and the distance 22 male football players could cover during a match. After a diet high in carbohydrates, they ran further than when consuming a low carbohydrate diet. Similarly, an earlier small-scale study in 1999[8] analysed the pre-game muscle glycogen concentration in six male football players during a 90-minute game on two occasions. A 33% improvement to the athletes' performance was reported after the high carbohydrate diet. We can thus surmise that a high carbohydrate diet improves athletic performance in intermittent sports that involve short bouts of high activity like football, volleyball, softball and tennis.

For optimal performance, the pre-workout concentration of glycogen stores is key. Therefore, athletes need to ensure appropriate carbohydrate intake pre- and post-workout to replenish their spent glycogen stores.[6]

Carbohydrate recommendations for athletes range from 5 to 10 g per kg body weight per day (g/kg/day). Carbohydrate needs depend on the athlete's gender and body size, and their training intensity and duration. On days when athletes engage in lighter or shorter training sessions, less carbohydrates are necessary to restore glycogen stores. Other factors such as extreme cold temperatures and high altitudes may also affect the carbohydrate consumption. Consumption of 5–7 g/kg/day is believed to be sufficient for general training, and 7–10 g/kg/day for endurance athletes. Higher intensity activities may raise the athlete's carbohydrate needs up to 12 g/kg/day.[9]

Athletes have the option of consuming either a large meal with 3–4 g of carbohydrate per kg body weight 3–4 hours pre-workout, or a carbohydrate-rich snack of 1–2 g/kg 1–2 hours before their training. The research remains inconclusive as to which of these two options produce better results. When engaging in training sessions lasting more than one hour, we need to consume 30–60 g of carbohydrates per hour. Activities longer than 2.5 hours call for 90 g of carbohydrates per hour.[3]

Post-exercise carbohydrate intake depends on whether the athlete will be training later that same day. If they are, then 1–1.2 g of carbohydrate per kg per hour is recommended in the first four hours after their first exercise session.

One last point to address is the common practice of carbohydrate loading or glycogen supercompensation by endurance athletes prior to an event in an attempt to boost their muscle glycogen above normal levels. There is no set protocol on how to achieve above-normal muscle glycogen levels. Earlier studies suggested emptying the glycogen stores by intense training sessions followed by high carbohydrate intakes of 12 g per kg body weight per day a few days before an event. However, this practice is not supported by recent research which recommends gradual tapering of training and carb-loading two days prior to the event.[9] Most athletes develop and follow a tailored protocol that works best for them.

One of the central gains from a plant-based diet is that it is naturally high in carbohydrates, which covers the high intake of carbohydrates for efficient athletic performance. Considering that complex, unprocessed carbohydrates provide more nutrients, athletes should choose those over processed, refined carbohydrates. Nevertheless, the latter can on occasion be included in the athlete's diet to assist them in meeting their high caloric requirements. Another macronutrient essential for an athlete's daily energy needs are fats, which will be discussed next.

Fat

Fats supply vital nutrients and contribute to the absorption and transport of fat-soluble vitamins A, D, E and K, as well as fat-soluble phytonutrients (e.g., carotenoids and lycopene). One gram of fat yields nine calories, more than double that provided by carbohydrates and protein. That is why fats play an invaluable role in delivering high energy to athletes.

Since even the leanest athletes carry more fat stores than glycogen stores, it is crucial to study how to efficiently metabolise fats and conserve their glycogen reserves for high-intensity activities. During exercise, fat is primarily sourced from subcutaneous adipose tissues and muscle fat stores. Peripheral fat from adipose tissues is transported on the protein albumin in the blood, to the muscle cells and mitochondria, the ATP-generating organelle within cells. As a result, fat oxidation cannot provide rapid fuel for high-intensity activities, but it supplies the main fuel for light to moderate activities. Light activities performed at 25% of maximal oxygen consumption (VO2 max) employ fat from adipose tissue while muscle fat stores power activities that are moderate and use 65% of VO2 max. Recent research[10] indicates that the intramuscular triglyceride is to some degree used alongside glycogen to fuel intense exercises at 85% VO2 max. Additionally, the longer the duration of an activity, the more muscle fat can be metabolised if sufficient amounts are available.

Studies suggest that post-exercise foods with fat content of about 35% can help to top-up the muscle fat reserves in endurance athletes more than a low-fat diet with 10% fat content.[11, 12] For this reason, fat intakes below 10%, as advised by some plant-based doctors for patients with coronary atherosclerosis, are not suitable for athletes. In fact, fat consumption below 15% can compromise the immune system and bring about menstrual disorders in female athletes. It is recommended that fat comprises 20%–35% of the daily energy intakes of athletes.[3]

The source of fat is another important consideration. While saturated fats are mainly found in animal foods, tropical oils such as coconut oil, as used in most vegan cheese alternatives and other vegan processed foods, contain a high percentage of saturated fat, and their consumption is better limited. The current UK health guidelines endorse a daily intake of saturated fat below 11% of total dietary energy to lower the risk for vascular diseases. Athletes are encouraged to obtain their fat from unsaturated fat sources. Nuts, avocado and olive oils are rich sources of monounsaturated fats that reduce the blood levels of ('bad') LDL cholesterol.

Polyunsaturated fats are divided into omega-6 and omega-3 fatty acids, and these essential fats need to be obtained from the diet. Omega-6 fatty acids are plentiful in plant foods like leafy green vegetables, grains, nuts and seeds. The most common omega-3 fats in our diets are the short-chain fatty acids α-linolenic acid (ALA), which can be found in soybeans, flaxseeds, walnuts, chia seeds and canola oils. ALA can be converted to the long-chain omega-3 fatty acids, eicosapentaenoic acid (EPA) and docosahexaenoic acid (DHA). It is noteworthy that omega-6 fats compete with the omega-3 fats for the same pathway, which can affect the conversion rate of omega-3 fats into their bioavailable forms. To guarantee adequate omega-3 intake, a ratio of omega-6 to omega-3 of 3:1 is proposed.[15]

Omega-3 fats contribute to the reduction of exercise-induced inflammation and boost recovery time in athletes. They also lessen blood viscosity and aid the delivery of oxygen and nutrients to working muscles. This, in turn, leads to better aerobic metabolism. Two tablespoons of flaxseeds or chia seeds, or three to four walnuts, are good ways to cover athletes' needs for daily omega-3 fats.

Protein

This section will review the most controversial macronutrient in a plant-based diet: protein.

Protein is regarded as one of the most important macronutrients in the fitness industry. Protein offers amino acids (AA) which are the building blocks for structural components of our body, such as muscle, tissue, tendon, hair, enzymes and hormones. In the absence of carbohydrates and fats, the body can turn to AA as a fuel source during prolonged activities and starvation. There are 20 amino acids; however, only nine of them are essential to our diet (histidine, isoleucine, leucine, lysine, methionine, phenylalanine, threonine, tryptophan, and valine).

Single plant protein sources tend to contain

insufficient amounts of some of the essential AA. For example: grains and nuts are low in lysine, maize is low in tryptophan, pea protein – while it contains all essential AA – is low in methionine, and legumes (except soya) are low in methionine. This has created the myth that to obtain all nine essential AA on a plant-based diet, one must combine different protein sources in the same meal (e.g., rice with legumes, bread with peanut butter). Many fitness professionals and authors still argue for protein-combining even though this belief has been convincingly disputed in literature since 1990s.[13] Correspondingly, the Academy of Nutrition and Dietetics updated their recommendation in their 2016 position statement to now advise those adhering to a plant-based diet to consume a variety of different plant protein sources in a day, not at a single meal.[14] The reference nutrient intake (RNI) for protein is at 0.75 g/kg/day for adults according to the British Nutrition Foundation.

Whether physical activity increases our protein intake depends on the training programme. Hobby exercisers who work out a few times per week do not need to increase their protein intake above the recommended RNI for the general population. However, athletes training more than eight hours per week have higher protein requirements because muscle fibres sustain micro-tears during exercise and need additional AA to repair the damage. Besides, AA are necessary to stimulate muscle protein synthesis and replace the protein lost in urine and sweat.

In a joint statement, the Academy of Nutrition and Dietetics, Dietitians of Canada, and the American College of Sports Medicine recommends 1.2–2 g of protein per kg body weight per day for athletes.[3] Some argue that the protein requirement of plant-based athletes is 10% higher than omnivorous athletes because of the lower digestibility of plant proteins. This viewpoint, however, has been rejected by the Food and Nutrition Board of the National Academy of Sciences Institute of Medicine, which does not approve a higher intake as long as a variety of different plant proteins are consumed.[15]

It is worth stressing that high-protein diets can have potential negative health effects. Excess protein will either become fuel or fat. When protein is broken down to be used as an energy source, the nitrogen in the AA molecule is removed and excreted together with water. This can increase the risk of dehydration in athletes. Evidence also suggests that excess protein is associated with increased calcium loss in urine and the ensuing risk for kidney stones and bone loss. The detrimental effects have been observed with excess animal proteins; however, protein intakes higher than the RNI do not carry any extra benefit to athletes. A systemic review and a meta-analysis of 49 studies confirm that protein intakes higher than 1.62 g/kg/day do not offer any additional advantage to resistance exercise training.[16] Protein certainly plays an invaluable role in muscle synthesis, but without the right training the extra dietary protein will not produce any boost in strength or endurance performance.

As previously noted, protein will turn into an energy source in the absence of carbohydrates and fats. In that state, AA will not be used to build new muscle tissue. For this reason, consuming adequate amounts of calories should be an athlete's priority before considering the ratio of macronutrients in their diet. Similarly, post-exercise protein consumption will only aid muscle recovery in the presence of sufficient carbohydrate intake.

The current evidence-base does not support the claim that protein consumption before or during exercise boosts athletic performance. In fact, pre-workout protein intake can upset the gastrointestinal tract.[3] Recent evidence suggests that protein consumed in smaller amounts of 20–30 g during the day may be more effective at stimulating protein synthesis than large protein portions consumed in fewer meals.[16]

Any discussion on protein would not be complete without reviewing the use of protein supplements, which will be examined later as part of the ergogenic aids section.

Micronutrients

Micronutrients are essential vitamins and minerals. They may not be a source of fuel but are important to metabolise macronutrients and maintain optimal tissue function.

It is thought that athletes require more vitamins and minerals to protect the body against free radicals released during exercise and to aid recovery from exercise-induced muscle damage and the resulting inflammation. To ensure satisfactory intake of antioxidants, athletes may resort to multivitamin and mineral supplements. Many also hold the view that if something is good then more is better and turning to supplements will enhance their performance. However, just as an overconsumption of calories can impair athletic performance, an excess intake of micronutrients can cause toxicity and create imbalances. This not only compromises athletic performance but also puts the athlete's health at risk.

A plant-based diet is rich in antioxidants and anti-inflammatory compounds. By and large, higher caloric consumption also means an increase in the number of micronutrients in an athlete's diet. Nevertheless, there are a few micronutrients that deserve extra attention.

Vitamin B12

Vitamin B12 is essential for DNA synthesis, red blood cell formation, a healthy nervous system, fatty acid synthesis and bone health. Since vitamin B12 cannot be found in plant foods, all those following a plant-based diet, including athletes, must take regular supplementation. B12 deficiency symptoms develop late, and as deficiency can cause irreversible neurological damage, it is advised to have annual blood tests. Older athletes in particular must monitor their levels as B12 absorption in the gut reduces with age.

Vitamin D

Vitamin D is vital for optimal bone health, and immune system and muscular function. Vitamin D is made in our skin after sun exposure. However, there are factors that impair vitamin D production and put athletes at risk of deficiency, such as those with darker skin living in the northern hemisphere, those with insufficient sun exposure during winter or because of indoor training, and those using excessive sunscreens. Poor vitamin D intake leads to decreased calcium absorption which can increase the risk of stress fractures in athletes.[17]

Public Health England recommends everyone in the UK over the age of 5 to take a vitamin D supplement from October to March. At-risk groups should consider year-round supplementation. The recommended daily intake is 400 IU (equal to 10 mcg). Plant-based athletes should take vitamin D3 supplements derived from lichen, which evidence suggests is more effective at increasing the vitamin D status.[18]

Calcium

Calcium plays a role in muscle and nerve function, blood clotting and bone formation. Maintaining adequate calcium intake in childhood and adolescence is associated with better bone mineral density later in life.[19]

In the UK, the RNI for calcium is set at 700 mg per day for adults over 19 years. Higher intakes are advised during childhood, lactation, menopause, and for those suffering from gastrointestinal diseases. Exercise does not necessarily increase the calcium requirements;[20] however, athletes are advised to pay special attention to their calcium intake because poor dietary calcium consumption reduces bone mineral density and increases the risk for stress fractures.[21]

Obtaining enough calcium in a plant-based diet is easy as long as the total calorie intake is not restricted. Plant sources of calcium include green leafy vegetables low in oxalate (e.g., kale, pak choy, broccoli), tahini, legumes, blackstrap molasses and calcium-set tofu.

Athletes can reach the optimal calcium levels through diet, and there is no official recommendation for additional supplementation. However, if they wish to do so, athletes should supplement with both calcium and vitamin D, as vitamin D is essential for calcium absorption.[22] Furthermore, calcium is not the sole nutrient necessary for optimal bone health; other key nutrients such as magnesium and vitamin K are also essential.

Iron

Iron is an essential mineral that plays a role in energy production, oxygen transport and in the synthesis of DNA and neurotransmitters. Approximately 70% of iron is found in our red blood cells as haemoglobin, and in our muscles as myoglobin. Haemoglobin transports the oxygen from lungs to muscles and tissues and eliminates the by-products of carbohydrate and fat metabolism during exercise. Myoglobin is an oxygen reservoir that provides oxygen to the exercising muscles.

Iron is predominantly stored in the protein ferritin. Some ferritin is also present in blood, which is used to assess the iron status. However, ferritin levels do not offer an accurate reflection of iron stores in athletes because they can rise with inflammation, whether from exercise or illness.[23]

Athletes have higher iron requirements due to increased iron loss. They can lose iron in urine (haematuria), sweat, and via gastrointestinal bleeding and the destruction of red blood cells (haemolysis). The blood in urine originates from either haemolysis, or from intense training causing micro-tears in muscles and the release of myoglobin. Iron loss through sweat is minimal, but the longer the training duration, the more is lost.[24] Iron loss via gastrointestinal bleeding is thought to be due to regular use of anti-inflammatory medication by athletes.[25] Lastly, intravascular haemolysis, also referred to as 'foot-strike' haemolysis, is caused by running on hard surfaces in endurance athletes, and the increased pressure of blood cells flowing through the vessels during intense muscle training.[26]

In severe cases the above-mentioned iron losses could result in anaemia. However, most cases of low haemoglobin in athletes are due to sports anaemia, or dilution pseudo-anaemia. This is not a true anaemia but happens when increased blood volume in athletes leads to dilution of the blood components. Since no blood cells have been lost, the blood's oxygen-carrying function is not affected. This phenomenon is common at the beginning of hard training periods and persists for up to five days post-exercise. True iron deficiency anaemia in athletes can be determined with lower mean cell volume and lower ferritin levels.

In the UK, there is no official guidance for athletes to aim for higher intakes, and the recommended intake for the general population is 8.7 mg for male adults and 14.8 mg for female adults. A number of scientists suspect that athletes, especially female athletes, are an at-risk group and propose that female endurance athletes increase their intake by 70%, which would be an additional 10 mg.[27] Some sports dietitians in the US recommend a daily intake of 15–18 mg iron for athletes.[28]

Plant-based athletes can obtain their daily requirements via diet, but like other athletes, they are advised to monitor their iron status. Iron supplements are not recommended routinely and should only be consumed if low iron status has been confirmed.

Iodine

Iodine is a key component of thyroid hormones. It is involved in many biochemical reactions, such as protein synthesis, and is crucial for foetal brain development. Because of the high prevalence of iodine deficiency worldwide, many countries have iodised salt.[29] This strategy, however, has not been implemented in the UK.

The iodine content in plant foods can vary, making it a nutrient of concern for those following a plant-based diet. As athletes require more sodium, they can meet their daily recommended intake of 150 mcg of iodine by consuming 3 g of iodised salt (half a teaspoon). Alternatively, they can include sea vegetables in their diet or take an iodine supplement.

Zinc

Zinc, an essential component of many enzymes, is a nutrient of concern for athletes in general, especially plant-based athletes, as low zinc levels hinder athletes in their training.[14] Low zinc may be caused by an inadequate diet or increased losses in sweat.[30] In the UK, the RNI for zinc is 11 mg for male and 8 mg for female adults. Plant-based athletes can reach the optimal daily intake by including legumes, whole grains, nuts and soya products in their diet. Studies examining the role of zinc supplementation in athletic performance have failed to demonstrate any benefit.[31]

Hydration

Two of the most significant factors for top athletic performance are optimal glucose levels and adequate hydration.

When the body metabolises macronutrients to produce ATP, heat is generated. The large volume of energy required for training produces a large amount of heat which is then dissipated via increased sweat. Subsequently the body cools. The fluid lost must be replaced to avoid dehydration and electrolyte imbalance.

Our hydration status alters our urine colour. A dilute urine suggests a state of hyperhydration, whereas a concentrated urine is a sign of dehydration. A clear urine suggests good hydration which athletes can use to test their hydration status.

Depending on the workout intensity, athletes can lose up to 2.5 litres of sweat per hour. If this fluid loss is not replaced, there is a risk of dehydration. Sweat has also high concentrations of sodium and chloride, and the body can lose about 3 g of sodium chloride in each litre of sweat. To maintain a good state of hydration, athletes need to start hydrating 24 hours or more before the event. It is sensible to drink half a litre of fluid 1 to 1.5 hours before training, and then have half a cup every 10 minutes before the workout. During training, drinking should continue in order to cool the body. Mixing in a source of carbohydrates and electrolytes proves more advantageous than drinking water.[32] Post-training, athletes should drink half a litre of fluid containing carbohydrates and sodium, and then continue to drink 0.25 litres every 15 minutes over three hours.

Ergogenic aids

Many athletes choose to ingest performance-enhancing drugs, ergogenic aids. However, there are some who do not make use of any ergogenic aids, with some even questioning whether performance-enhancing substances are in the spirit of true athleticism.[33] For now, the decision to use supplements is at each athlete's discretion.

A multitude of supplements claim to give athletes a winning edge; however, the following will focus solely on the most common ones.

Protein supplements

Protein supplements are often purchased in the hope of promoting muscle building. On the contrary, evidence suggests that protein supplements only help meet an athlete's high caloric requirements. Moreover, studies have demonstrated that we can only anabolically utilise protein intakes of 1.66 g/kg.[34] Anything above this threshold is likely to be stored as fat or turned into fuel. As previously mentioned, it is preferable to distribute the protein intake in smaller and more frequent amounts throughout the day rather than large amounts less frequently. What is more, an independent study by Clean Label Project in 2018, examining over 100 popular protein powders (including plant-based and organic protein powders) concluded that a significant number of them were contaminated with above-healthy levels of heavy metals such as lead, mercury and arsenic. Athletes should therefore aim to obtain their protein needs from whole plant foods.

Creatine

Creatine is naturally found in our skeletal muscles as creatine phosphate, which is utilised in ATP production. It has been shown that supplementing with oral creatine can increase the creatine stores in our muscles and subsequently improve short, high-intensity physical activities. Studies also suggest that creatine supplements can boost muscle gains in strength training.[35] Since creatine is missing in plant foods, plant-based athletes may benefit the most from creatine supplementation.[36] Athletes without a history of kidney problems can take creatine supplements of 3–5 g per day but only for short periods, because the long-term health effects of creatine supplementation (beyond four years) remain unresearched.[33, 37]

Carnitine

Carnitine is another amino acid found only in small amounts in plant foods. It is involved in fat metabolism and often marketed for weight loss. However, there is no evidence that carnitine supplements promote weight loss,[38] nor that supplementation can enhance low-intensity activities. Caution is advised when supplementing with carnitine because its safety beyond six months has not been tested.

Caffeine

Caffeine is an easily available supplement due to its ubiquity in coffee, tea, chocolate and some beverages. Caffeine is said to improve performance by stimulating the central nervous system and reducing fatigue.[39] Doses of 3–6 mg/kg shortly before or during an event are believed to boost endurance performance.[40] There are opposing views on whether habitual caffeine consumption reduces its effect on exercise. Athletes should make a decision based on their own response to caffeine.[40]

Nitrate

Nitrates are naturally found in beetroot juice. They improve blood flow and oxygen delivery to the working muscles. Drinking beetroot juice has proven to be more effective than nitrate supplementation.[41] Recent evidence supports consuming half a litre of beetroot juice two hours prior to an event to boost performance.[42] Including nitrate-rich vegetables in the diet is an easy way for plant-based athletes to optimise their performance.

Conclusion

A plant-based diet does not have any adverse effects on athletes' performance. On the contrary, plant-based athletes may enhance their progress as long as they meet their high caloric needs and monitor micronutrients of concern. Further studies are required to establish the specific benefits of a plant-based diet for athletic performance.

References

1. Mountjoy M, Sundgot-Borgen J, Burke L et al. International Olympic Committee (IOC) Consensus Statement on Relative Energy Deficiency in Sport (RED-S): 2018 Update. *International Journal of Sport Nutrition and Exercise Metabolism* 2018; 28(4): 316-331. doi: 10.1123/ijsnem.2018-0136
2. Manore M, Kam L, Loucks A. The female athlete triad: Components, nutrition issues, and health consequences. *Journal of Sports Sciences* 2007; 25(sup1): S61-S71. doi: 10.1080/02640410701607320
3. Thomas D, Erdman K, Burke L. Position of the Academy of Nutrition and Dietetics, Dietitians of Canada, and the American College of Sports Medicine: Nutrition and Athletic Performance. *Journal of the Academy of Nutrition and Dietetics* 2016; 116(3): 501-528. doi: 10.1016/j.jand.2015.12.006
4. Thompson J, Manore M. Predicted and Measured Resting Metabolic Rate of Male and Female Endurance Athletes. *Journal of the American Dietetic Association* 1996; 96(1): 30-34. doi: 10.1016/S0002-8223(96)00010-7
5. National Academy of Sports Medicine, Sutton BG. Nasm Essentials of Personal Fitness Training. 4th ed. Lippincott Williams & Wilkins; 2012.
6. Knuiman P, Hopman M, Mensink M. Glycogen availability and skeletal muscle adaptations with endurance and resistance exercise. *Nutrition & Metabolism* 2015; 12(1). doi: 10.1186/s12986-015-0055-9
7. Souglis A, Chryssanthopoulos C, Travlos A, Zorzou A, Gissis I, Papadopoulos C, et al. The Effect of High vs. Low Carbohydrate Diets on Distances Covered in Soccer. *Journal of Strength and Conditioning Research* 2013; 27(8): 2235-2247. doi: 10.1519/JSC.0b013e3182792147
8. Balsom P, Wood K, Olsson P, Ekblom B. Carbohydrate Intake and Multiple Sprint Sports: With Special Reference to Football (Soccer). *International Journal of Sports Medicine* 1999; 20(01): 48-52. doi: 10.1055/s-2007-971091
9. Burke L, Hawley J, Wong S, Jeukendrup A. Carbohydrates for training and competition. *Journal of Sports Sciences* 2011; 29(sup1): S17-S27. doi: 10.1080/02640414.2011.585473
10. Romijn J, Coyle E, Sidossis L, et al. Regulation of endogenous fat and carbohydrate metabolism in relation to exercise intensity and duration. *American Journal of Physiology-Endocrinology and Metabolism* 1993; 265(3): E380-E391. doi: 10.1152/ajpendo.1993.265.3.E380
11. Larson-Meyer D, Borkhsenious O, Gullett J, et al. Effect of Dietary Fat on Serum and Intramyocellular Lipids and Running Performance. *Medicine & Science in Sports & Exercise* 2008; 40(5): 892-902. doi: 10.1249/MSS.0b013e318164cb33
12. Larson-Meyer D, Newcomer B, Hunter G. Influence of endurance running and recovery diet on intramyocellular lipid content in women: a 1H NMR study. *American Journal of Physiology-Endocrinology and Metabolism* 2002; 282(1): E95-E106. doi: 10.1152/ajpendo.2002.282.1.e95
13. Young V, Pellett P. Plant proteins in relation to human protein and amino acid nutrition. *The American Journal of Clinical Nutrition* 1994; 59(5): 1203S-1212S. doi: 10.1093/ajcn/59.5.1203S
14. Melina V, Craig W, Levin S. Position of the Academy of Nutrition and Dietetics: Vegetarian Diets. *Journal of the Academy of Nutrition and Dietetics* 2016; 116(12): 1970-1980. doi: 10.1016/j.jand.2016.09.025
15. Otten JJ, Hellwig JP, Meyers LD, editors. Dietary reference intakes: The essential guide to nutrient requirements. Washington, D.C., DC: National Academies Press; 2006.
16. Morton R, Murphy K, McKellar S et al. A systematic review, meta-analysis and meta-regression of the effect of protein supplementation on resistance training-induced gains in muscle mass and strength in healthy adults. *British Journal of Sports Medicine* 2017; 52(6): 376-384. doi: 10.1136/bjsports-2017-097608
17. Heaney R, Dowell M, Hale C, Bendich A. Calcium Absorption Varies within the Reference Range for Serum 25-Hydroxyvitamin D. *Journal of the American College of Nutrition* 2003; 22(2): 142-146. doi: 10.1080/07315724.2003.10719287
18. Tripkovic L, Lambert H, Hart K et al. Comparison of vitamin D2 and vitamin D3 supplementation

in raising serum 25-hydroxyvitamin D status: a systematic review and meta-analysis. *The American Journal of Clinical Nutrition* 2012; 95(6): 1357-1364. doi: 10.3945/ajcn.111.031070

19. Johnston C, Miller J, Slemenda C et al. Calcium Supplementation and Increases in Bone Mineral Density in Children. *New England Journal of Medicine* 1992; 327(2): 82-87. doi: 10.1056/NEJM199207093270204

20. Kunstel K. Calcium Requirements for the Athlete. *Current Sports Medicine Reports* 2005; 4(4): 203-206. doi: 10.1097/01.CSMR.0000306208.56939.01

21. Tenforde A, Sayres L, Sainani K, Fredericson M. Evaluating the Relationship of Calcium and Vitamin D in the Prevention of Stress Fracture Injuries in the Young Athlete: A Review of the Literature. *PM&R* 2010; 2(10): 945-949. doi: 10.1016/j.pmrj.2010.05.006

22. Weaver C, Gordon C, Janz K et al. The National Osteoporosis Foundation's position statement on peak bone mass development and lifestyle factors: a systematic review and implementation recommendations. *Osteoporosis International* 2016; 27(4): 1281-1386. doi: 10.1007/s00198-015-3440-3

23. Hinton P. Iron and the endurance athlete. *Applied Physiology, Nutrition, and Metabolism* 2014; 39(9): 1012-1018. doi: 10.1139/apnm-2014-0147

24. Waller MF, Haymes EM. The effects of heat and exercise on sweat iron loss. *Med Sci Sports Exerc* 1996; 28(2): 197–203. doi: 10.1097/00005768-199602000-00007

25. Moses F, Baska R, Graeber G et al. Gastrointestinal bleeding during an ultramarathon. *Medicine and Science in Sports and Exercise* 1980; 21(Supplement): S78. doi: 10.1007/BF01536777

26. Robinson Y, Cristancho E, Boening D. Intravascular Hemolysis and Mean Red BloodCell Age in Athletes. *Medicine & Science in Sports & Exercise* 2006; 38(3): 480-483. doi: 10.1249/01.mss.0000188448.40218.4c

27. Alaunyte I, Stojceska V, Plunkett A. Iron and the female athlete: a review of dietary treatment methods for improving iron status and exercise performance. *Journal of the International Society of Sports Nutrition* 2015; 12(1): 38. doi: 10.1186/s12970-015-0099-2

28. Benardot D. Advanced Sports Nutrition. 3rd ed. Champaign, IL: Human Kinetics; 2020

29. de Benoist B, Andersson M, Takkouche B, Egli I. Prevalence of iodine deficiency worldwide. *Lancet* 2003; 362(9398): 1859–1860. doi: 10.1016/S0140-6736(03)14920-3

30. Brun JF, Dieu-Cambrezy C, Charpiat A et al. Serum zinc in highly trained adolescent gymnasts. *Biol Trace Elem Res* 1995; 47(1–3): 273–278. doi.org/10.1007/BF02790127

31. Wilborn CD, Kerksick CM, Campbell BI et al. Effects of zinc magnesium aspartate (ZMA) supplementation on training adaptations and markers of anabolism and catabolism. *J Int Soc Sports Nutr* 2004; 1(2): 12–20. doi: 10.1186/1550-2783-1-2-12

32. Mitchell JB, Costill DL, Houmard JA et al. Influence of carbohydrate dosage on exercise performance and glycogen metabolism. *J Appl Physiol* 1989; 67(5): 1843–1849. doi: 10.1152/jappl.1989.67.5.1843

33. Terjung R, Clarkson P, Eichner R, et al. Physiological and health effects of oral creatine supplementation. *Med Sci Sports Exerc* 2000; 32(3): 706–717.

34. Tarnopolsky MA, MacDougall JD, Atkinson SA. Influence of protein intake and training status on nitrogen balance and lean body mass. *J Appl Physiol* 1988; 64(1): 187–193. doi: 10.1152/jappl.1988.64.1.187

35. Becque MD, Lochmann JD, Melrose DR. Effects of oral creatine supplementation on muscular strength and body composition. *Med Sci Sports Exerc* 2000; 32(3): 654–658. doi: 10.1097/00005768-200003000-00016

36. Shomrat A, Weinstein Y, Katz A. Effect of creatine feeding on maximal exercise performance in vegetarians. *Eur J Appl Physiol* 2000; 82(4): 321–325. doi: 10.1007/s004210000222

37. Stone MH, Sanborn K, Smith LL et al. Effects of in-season (5 weeks) creatine and pyruvate supplementation on anaerobic performance and body composition in American football players. *Int J Sport Nutr* 1999; 9(2): 146–165. doi: 10.1123/ijsn.9.2.146

38. Villani RG, Gannon J, Self M, Rich PA. L-Carnitine supplementation combined with aerobic training does not promote weight loss in

moderately obese women. *Int J Sport Nutr Exerc Metab* 2000; 10(2): 199–207.
doi: 10.1123/ijsnem.10.2.199

39. Peeling P, Binnie MJ, Goods PSR et al. Evidence-based supplements for the enhancement of athletic performance. *Int J Sport Nutr Exerc Metab* 2018; 28(2): 178–187.
doi: 10.1123/ijsnem.2017-0343

40. Yarnell AM, Deuster PA. Caffeine and performance. *J Spec Oper Med* 2016; 16(4): 64–70. PMID: 28088820.

41. Clifford T, Howatson G, West DJ, Stevenson EJ. Beetroot juice is more beneficial than sodium nitrate for attenuating muscle pain after strenuous eccentric-bias exercise. *Appl Physiol Nutr Metab* 2017; 42(11): 1185–1191.
doi: 10.1139/apnm-2017-0238

42. Maughan RJ, Burke LM, Dvorak J, Larson-Meyer DE, Peeling P, Phillips SM, et al. IOC consensus statement: dietary supplements and the high-performance athlete. *Br J Sports Med* 2018; 52(7): 439–455. doi: 10.1136/bjsports-2018-099027

Chapter 18
Barriers and strategies to adopting a plant-based diet

Trent Grassian and Arvind Kaur Maheru

Introduction

The ability of practitioners to support patients to sustainably transition to a healthy, plant-based diet can have significant benefits for their patients' long-term health. This process can be best supported through an understanding of what may help (and hinder) this process and the strategies that may most effectively support a long-term change. This chapter is written in three parts, with the aim of providing an overview of existing research and practical insights for healthcare practitioners and those involved in research, advocacy and policy-making processes.

First, this chapter will provide an overview of some of the theoretical frameworks that can be used to understand the barriers to and facilitators for the promotion of plant-based diets (PBDs). It also provides insights into the 'Behaviour Change Wheel' – a comprehensive framework that may be useful for those who are designing interventions or involved in the policy-making process. Next, we provide an overview of existing research into the barriers and facilitators in achieving a successful transition. The concluding section builds on this research to provide some practical strategies, tips and sample dialogues from real practitioners, using motivational interviewing strategies.

Theoretical frameworks underpinning dietary change

There are a variety of theoretical frameworks that practitioners and advocates can use to understand the nature of transition and the strategies that might be most effective in achieving successful, sustained dietary change. Behaviour change theories and interventions provide a common framework for understanding dietary transition and tend to focus exclusively on the individual as the locus of change. One of the most widely used models amongst medical practitioners and much of behaviour change research is the 'Transtheoretical Model' (TTM), also known as the 'Stages of Change' model.[1,2] The TTM focuses on the individual's transition through a series of stages (see Figure 18.1): first becoming aware of the need to change their behaviour, then deciding to change (or not), before maintaining this new behaviour.[3]

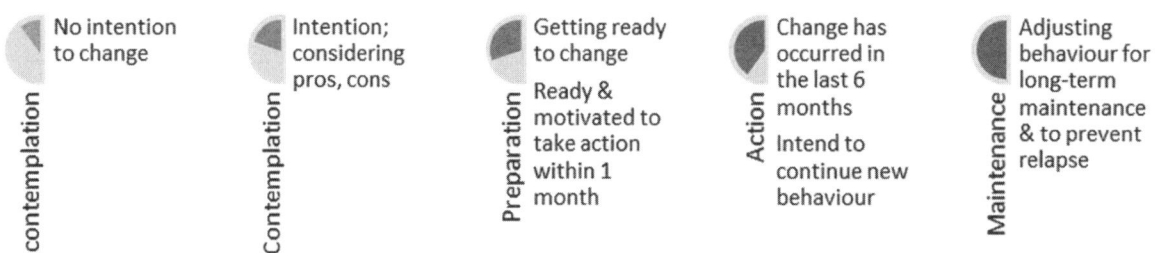

Figure 18.1 Transtheoretical model

The TTM can help practitioners identify the types of information that are likely to be most useful for an individual (e.g., assistance with planning the transition process for those in the contemplation stage or motivational materials for those in the pre-contemplation stage). However, the framework's reliance on motivation as the sole driver for change, despite the reality that behaviour does not always (or even often) follow beliefs, limits its usefulness to clinicians.[4] It is also important for practitioners to consider external factors, such as the influence of social norms and structural restraints within the modern food system.[5]

A framework that accounts for the influence of external factors (e.g., cultural or financial) can not only help practitioners provide relevant advice and support, but can also help provide alignment across practitioners and those working to change policy or design interventions supporting PBDs. The Behaviour Change Wheel – described as the first comprehensive behaviour change model, was created following a comprehensive examination of all behaviour change models and research to date.[1]

As can be seen in Figure 18.2, the Behaviour Change Wheel, designed by Susan Michie and colleagues, includes three components. The inner circle is derived from their COM-B (capability, opportunity, motivation and behaviour) system, which seeks to identify the specific components underlying any behaviour, including: *who* will be performing it, *when* it will occur, *where*, *with whom*, *how often* and *what* they may need to do differently.[1] The middle section of the wheel links these behavioural components (e.g., taste, cost or habits) directly to strategies to target these areas (e.g., an education-based strategy or the providing of incentives).

Intervention functions are the methods that practitioners can use in supporting dietary change. For instance, to help develop physical skills (e.g., the ability to cook plant-based dishes), patients may need training or enablement.[1] The outer ring of the Behaviour Change Wheel then connects these interventions to types of policy. For instance, to support patients in developing the skills necessary to cook plant-based dishes, Michie et al. outline three types of interventions that could be used: education, training and enablement. These, in turn, are each linked to different types of policy (e.g., supporting education through clear food labelling).

Thus, practitioners can use the Behaviour Change Wheel to identify a target behaviour and then link it directly to strategies for their own practice and policies to support more widespread change. Michie et al.'s book *The Behaviour Change Wheel: A Guide to Designing Interventions* provides more detailed guidance. The first step for practitioners in understanding why behaviour occurs and how to change it, is to identify the factors enabling its maintenance. The

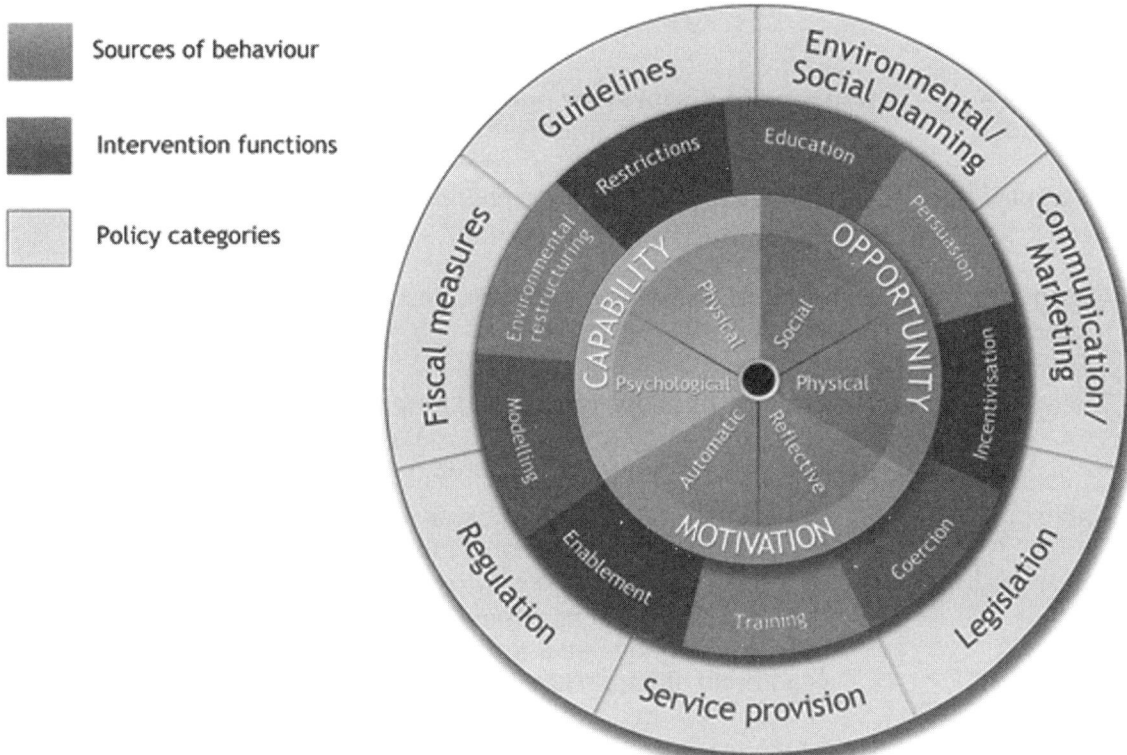

Figure 18.2 The behaviour change wheel[1]

Behaviour Change Wheel delineates behavioural components into three bifurcated areas (capability – physical and psychological; opportunity – physical and social; and motivation – reflective and automatic).

Barriers to adopting a plant-based diet

Dietary transition is a complex process that involves a wide variety of internal and external factors, ranging from an individual's habits to their ability to access plant-based foods and their underlying motives to change the way they eat. Here we review three main factors: motivation, capability and opportunity.

Motivation: the desire to follow a plant-based diet at the present (or relevant) time

In order to change their diet, an individual needs to know why this change would benefit them (and/or others) and be motivated to do so. These factors are summarised in Table 18.1. Reflective motivation is an essential component of successfully following a PBD. Research has found that those planning to reduce their meat consumption or become vegetarian or vegan are most likely to be motivated by the environment/climate change, health and/or animal welfare.[6, 13] Other commonly cited motivators include: saving money, religion, food safety and social justice/global food security. Health motives may be short- or long-term

Table 18.1 Motivation

Reflective motivation	**Reasons to perform (or not perform) a behaviour, involving conscious planning and assessments**
Awareness	Knowledge and support for reasons to follow a plant-based diet
Automatic motivation	**Habituated, impulsive instincts and actions involving desires, needs and reflexive responses**
Taste	• Thinking of oneself as a meat and/or (dairy) cheese lover • Believing that plant-based foods are boring • Preferring certain food textures
Habits	• One's daily, regular eating behaviours and routines that generally supersede 'rational', fully-informed decisions
Identity	• Thinking of oneself as a meat eater • Believing negative stigmas associated with plant-based, vegetarian or vegan identities

and may be based on personal or social factors, such as lowering one's blood pressure or avoiding familial illnesses.

Motivating factors can also include instinctive, unconscious elements, such as one's habits, taste preferences or personal identities. Taste has repeatedly been identified by researchers as a key barrier to transitioning to a PBD.[7] Taste preferences are developed from a young age and fostered through habituated dietary habits formed over an entire lifetime. Not being exposed to many types of plant-based foods or textures and/or experiencing such foods as bland or boring (e.g., only eating plain, boiled vegetables as a 'side' to the 'main' meat) can make a plant-based diet unappealing to life-long meat eaters.

Modern foods use concentrated amounts of chemicals that enhance taste and pleasure. Frequently eating highly-processed, sugary, salty and high-fat foods, what Lisle and Goldhamer refer to as 'magic foods' in their book *The Pleasure Trap*,[8] can desensitise taste nerves to the pleasure of natural whole foods (see Figure 18.3). Over time, more and more of these foods will be craved as 'neuroadaptation' leads to tolerance. A temporary taste sacrifice can also occur, as evidence suggests that it may take 30 to 90 days to re-sensitise taste preferences to natural foods and flavours.[8 (p. 89)]

Consumers may also have an intrinsic sense of self as a meat eater, fostered by common stigmas associated with those following a PBD. In many countries meat is commonly seen as a source of strength and vitality closely linked to masculinity.[9] Research has found that men who do not eat meat can be considered less masculine.[10] Over time, particularly if positive associations are being created with one's new dietary lifestyle, following a PBD can, instead, become part of one's identity.

As vegetarianism and veganism have become more prominent amongst high-income, high meat-eating countries, some of the negative stigmas associated with these identities may be dissipating. However, recent research suggests that consumers still may view vegans in a negative

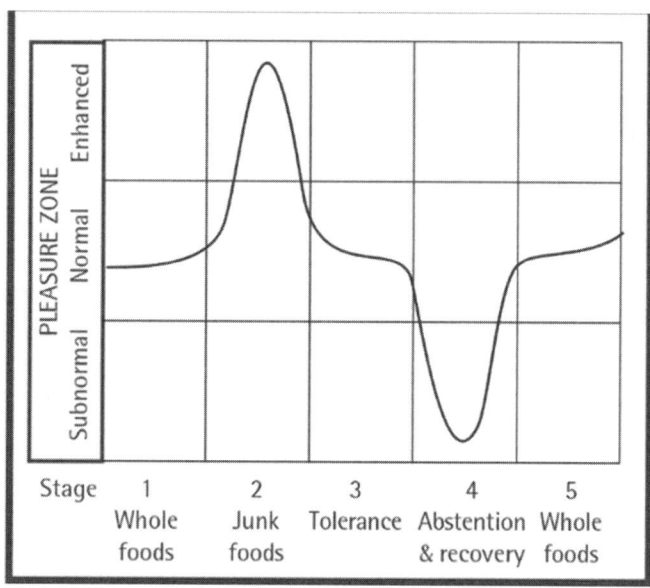

Figure 18.3 The pleasure trap

light, including seeing those following a PBD as 'fussy', 'extreme', 'awkward' 'hippies' or 'privileged'.[6, 11, 12, 13]

Capability: the physical ability and cognitive skills required to eat a plant-based diet

Capabilities pertain to one's physical and cognitive abilities and skills that will support (or hinder) their transition to a PBD as described in Table 18.2. While health-based motivating factors, such as a desire to lower one's cholesterol or treat a medical condition, can help foster motivation to learn more about PBDs, health misinformation has been found to be a key barrier, particularly amongst those following a meat-heavy diet. Individuals may believe that meat (or other animal-derived foods) are essential components of a healthy diet or that a PBD is inherently lacking in certain nutrients.[13, 14]

Individuals need to be able to identify what foods are plant-based and know how to prepare them. Plant-based foods may be seen as too difficult or time-consuming to cook or individuals may not know how to find recipes that they like.[5] For instance, they may struggle to maintain habits if they cannot identify suitable plant-based options with familiar tastes and textures. Those who are lacking in skills (or motivation) to cook may experience their new diet as a dramatic change. These new behaviours may not fit into their daily routine and instead require conscious planning to overcome unconscious, habituated behaviours – e.g., no longer being able to quickly grab the foods one is used to and/or needing to shop more often to access fresh fruits and vegetables.[15]

Research has found that, while psychological capabilities can be key inhibitors in the transition to a PBD, it is also an area where there can be significant improvements in a relatively short period of time, particularly for those following a fully PBD.[6] However, it is worth mentioning that some, especially disabled or elderly people, may have challenges related to physical capabilities (e.g., the

Table 18.2 Capability

Psychological capability	Strength and endurance to engage in essential mental processes and the underlying knowledge and psychological skills
Health perceptions	• Believing that the consumption of animal food products is essential • Not knowing how to eat a healthy, plant-based diet, including concerns about specific health risks (e.g., protein or iron deficiencies)
Knowledge	• Not knowing how to prepare or find plant-based recipes and/or food
Physical capability	Endurance, strength and physical skills

ability to get to the store or chop vegetables) that may require additional training, modification or support.

Opportunity: the social and physical environment necessary to follow a plant-based diet

Opportunities pertain to the physical and social environment in which we select foods and seek them out, prepare them and, ultimately, eat them. These are summarised in Table 18.3. The transition to a PBD can be supported (or hindered) by three types of physical opportunities: availability and convenience, time and cost. While plant-based options are generally readily available in the form of whole plant foods (i.e., fruits, vegetables, grains, beans and legumes), some may not possess the skills, motivation or time to prepare these foods.

With the emphasis on convenience in many modern cultures, patients may seek out ready-made, affordable plant-based options. The number of plant-based options has increased dramatically in many high-income countries over the past five to ten years; for instance, nearly one in four of the UK's new food products in 2019 was plant-based.[16] Nonetheless, many of these new, heavily processed foods are likely to be less healthful, environmentally sustainable or affordable.

Disproportionate governmental support through marketing and subsidies has contributed to the maintenance of artificially-low prices for animal-derived foods.[17] Consumers may also perceive plant-based foods as more expensive than they actually are due to cultural beliefs that animal-based foods are inherently more 'valuable'.[18] In many cultures, a meal is considered to require or be centred around a central, meat component – the 'meat of the dish'.

Red meat, in particular, is generally prized as the most 'valuable' centrepiece to a meal.[18] For many in Britain, this has historically included the Sunday roast, a turkey at Christmas or a leg of lamb at Easter. Many cultures, including some throughout South Asia, Africa, the Caribbean and the Middle East place high importance on eating meat at a communal meal, especially for larger social gatherings. While South Asian diets are traditionally high in plant-based foods, they also

Table 18.3 Opportunity

Physical opportunity	That which is supported or allowed by the physical environment
Availability & convenience	• Availability of plant-based options in restaurants or stores • Convenience-focused culture emphasising fast, ready-made food
Time	• Time spent identifying, buying and preparing food
Cost	• External factors influencing the cost of food • Finances available to spend on food • Conceptions of animal-based foods as more 'valuable'
Social opportunity	Influence of relationships with others, cultural norms and social cues
Social	• Norms, pressure and perceptions of one's social networks and family • Access to others following a plant-based diet
Culture and tradition	• Ideas of what is or is not acceptable to eat, including cultural associations of foods (i.e., meat is highly esteemed, high-status or masculine) • A desire to be 'normal' • Cultural constructs of what makes a 'meal' (e.g., 'meat and two veg' in the UK)

tend to be high in dairy, refined grains, refined oils and added foods, such as clarified butter (ghee).

As norms of consumption are complex and culture-bound, so too are norms and beliefs around healthy eating. For instance, some South Asian patients can hold a prevalent fatalistic and religious belief called '*kismet*' or destiny, considering their lives/health to be preordained by chance, fate or a higher power.[19] Similarly, the cultural norm whereby 'family needs come first' can hinder dietary change when individuals feel that they must put the health and dietary needs of family members above their own. Such norms and beliefs of consumption can derive from and be reinforced by social and familial ties.

Social opportunities, including cultural norms and the influence of family and friends, have been found to be a powerful barrier, particularly amongst those newly-transitioned or transitioning to a PBD.[6, 13] Each eating occurrence cannot be disentangled from the social and cultural factors in which it is both constructed and consumed. Social norms determining how and when one should eat can be so powerful that to follow a PBD can be perceived as disruptive of one's societal, familial and social identities.

For those living with, dependent upon or preparing food for others, the transition can be particularly challenging, potentially requiring the preparation of different meals and social pressure from the people one eats with. Having access to others who are following a similar diet through one's social circles or online communities can be a significant source of support and counter feelings that one is 'odd' or 'difficult', while increasing opportunities to access new information, skills and tips.

Strategies for practitioners

At the societal level, policy, research and interventions can facilitate the adoption of PBDs. Yet much of the effort happens at the individual practitioner-patient level. Although PBDs are cost-effective, low-risk, evidence-based interventions in chronic disease management, they remain underused. Clearly the task of bringing PBDs into the arena of clinical practice is more complex than simply following the evidence.

In the remainder of this chapter, we will explore how the adoption of a PBD for health can be facilitated within clinical practice. The hope is that in years to come health promotion, disease prevention and treatment of chronic disease will each be directly informed by the knowledge and practice of plant-based nutrition. For practitioners, our key challenge is to understand and address the behavioural patterns and motives underlying our patients' daily dietary decisions (see Table 18.4 for more detailed strategies).

Practitioner factors

Although awareness of the many clinical benefits of PBDs is rising amongst healthcare practitioners (HCPs), substantial gaps remain in knowledge, practice and skills. Many clinicians currently practise medicine as if their patients' diets have little effect upon the diseases they are managing. Clinicians have both an actual and a perceived lack of competencies in the nutritional sciences, which can hinder their ability to discuss nutrition with patients.[20]

While plant-based nutrition courses are offered by some institutions (e.g., the University of Winchester and eCornell), there is currently no compulsory applied nutrition training within the medical Royal Colleges for doctors in the UK. The inclusion of nutrition competencies (including motivational interviewing skills) in all healthcare curricula, potentially including hands-on cooking experiences (so-called 'culinary medicine'), may support the development of this essential knowledge.

Practitioners need the skills and strategies to shift their focus from diagnosing and treating existing diseases to preventing them (a clinician-as-coach model). It can seem counterintuitive (both for HCPs and their patients) to, instead of prescribing something or performing a procedure, counsel patients to remove dietary excesses. Furthermore, clinicians' own personal attitudes and beliefs may influence their clinical practice, leading many practitioners to avoid discussions of PBDs (or dietary change in general) under the preconception that PBDs are unrealistic for patients, or that patients will wholly reject such a change.[21] Failed prior attempts to influence patient dietary behaviour may also contribute to a sense that such efforts are wasted, as patients will not follow their advice.

Even when a knowledgeable clinician has invested time and effort into guiding the patient towards a PBD, others involved in the patient's care may challenge the patient about the changes they have made. As clinicians we may need to support patients by increasing their own knowledge base, providing them with a portable summary of the evidence and rationale for PBDs, and by raising awareness with healthcare colleagues.

In routine practice, time constraints can be a barrier. Later in the chapter we will highlight some tailored gains from even the smallest segment of clinical contact time. A practical way to get more from the time with a patient is by asking them to fill a pre-visit or waiting room nutrition

Table 18.4 Strategies for practitioners to support behaviour change

Reflective motivation	Reasons to perform (or not perform) a behaviour, involving conscious planning and motives

- Identifying personal motives and use as a basis to set an action plan and clear process goals
- Support small, stepped changes (e.g., replace highly processed snacks with fruit)
- SMART goals (Specific, Measurable, Actionable, Realistic, and Time-bound)
- Help with food planning, such as creating a batch-cooking meal schedule, strategies for social gatherings

Automatic motivation	Habituated, impulsive instincts and actions involving desires, needs and reflexive responses

- Encourage to explore new tastes and cuisines, including using herbs and spices, build depth of flavours with aromatic vegetables and citrus to replace salt
- Help find ways to save time, including bulk buying, batch cooking and eating leftovers for lunch

Psychological capability	Strength and endurance to engage in essential mental processes and the underlying knowledge and psychological skills

- Give simple, concise advice and signpost to key resources:
  - Reliable whole food plant-based (WFPB) web sources and factsheets
  - WFPB books, recipes and cookbooks
  - Training in nutritional label reading and plant-based cooking
- Give suggestions for healthy plant-based snacks and how to plan a calorie-replete PBD meal
- Connect with a health coach or nutritional professional

Physical opportunity	That which is supported or allowed by the physical environment

- Purchase helpful kitchen aids, such as a pressure or slow cooker or air fryer
- Encourage to try local or 'ethnic' supermarkets
- Help to creat a supportive food environment at home, in the car and at work (e.g., replacing junk food with prepared 'snack packs')
- Help to identify local restaurants with healthy plant-based options

Social opportunity	Influence of relationships with others, cultural norms and social cues

- Help to foster family buy-in and participation (e.g., each choosing a meal to convert to a plant-based version and cook together)
- Encourage to increase family-members' own awareness/motivation (e.g., watching the movie Forks over Knives together)
- Invite partner/family to consultation
- Put in touch with an online WFPB group
- Encourage to prepare and bring food to social meals and events
- Share culturally relevant resources and information (e.g. www.sharon-india.org website)
- Prepare patients with proactive strategies for festivals, weddings and celebrations (e.g., Christmas, Ramadan or Diwali)

questionnaire. Organising group interventions is another novel time-efficient possibility that we explore later.

Patient factors: the importance of a strong 'why'

Some patients come to the practitioner fully-informed of the benefits of a PBD. They may have been motivated by a past experience or recent development of a chronic illness in themselves or a family member. What they are seeking, then, is further guidance on how to tailor the diet to their specific health needs. Others have never considered the link between recovering their health and switching to a PBD. By identifying the key barriers and motivators for a patient, clinicians can tailor approaches to meet their individual needs.

For patients to change their eating behaviours, they need a reason or reasons to do so (i.e., reflective motivation). Motivation comes from two broad sources: extrinsic and intrinsic. Extrinsic motivators (i.e. sources of reflective motivation) are external drivers such as rewards, praise, approval or avoiding undesirable consequences. These can include, for instance, improved health parameters or lowered health costs. For more sustained dietary change, patients also need intrinsic motivation – internal rewards related to personal interests, values, priorities, sense of purpose and hopes for the future. Intrinsic motivators (i.e. sources of automatic motivation) give a sense of inherent satisfaction and connection. These can include feeling energetic and healthy for family or relief from pain. Feeling healthy, energised, happy and fit continues to motivate patients towards following a PBD. Intrinsic motivation engenders persistence in spite of challenges and creative solutions to setbacks.

Focusing within the consultation on searching for deeply personal intrinsic motivators will pay dividends for both patient and practitioner. This is the vital motivational fuel that drives the change to a healthful PBD.

Enabling patients to change their eating behaviours: Motivational Interviewing strategies

It is not easy changing behaviours around eating; those of us who have transitioned from a standard Western diet to a PBD will have found our own solutions to the challenges. As clinicians, if we are to do the most good with our new-found knowledge of plant-based nutrition, then we need to learn and apply the essential skills of behaviour change counselling. Within the framework of the Behaviour Change Wheel, clinicians need strategies to work at the level of the inner circle (COM-B) with a patient – improving their capabilities, opportunities and motivation to adopt a PBD for health.

Traditional training in the medical and allied fields emphasises a disease model, diagnosis and problem finding and solving. But for managing chronic illness (so-called 'lifestyle diseases'), clinicians need to adopt a collaborative, person-centred coaching approach. Cajoling, persuading or advising patients to embrace dietary change is rarely fruitful. With a guiding mindset, we view the patient as a *person* who has strengths. Happily, coaching skills are learnable and can be integrated into existing consultation skills. The art is in gauging *when* and *how* to broach the topic of dietary change, even when the patient is not asking for this help, or when consultation time is short.

Key tasks of a behaviour change consultation:
- Build an empathic connection – a working partnership.
- Listen to the patient's own values, beliefs, agenda and interests whilst identifying *intrinsic motivators*.
- Enable them to find their own solutions and plan goal-directed changes.

- Arrange support and accountability (a follow-up plan).

Motivational Interviewing (MI) is an evidence-based intervention that guides the patient to take responsibility for their health behaviours. It is not coercive persuasion, rather a sophisticated conversation about change: 'MI is a collaborative, goal-oriented style of communication with particular attention to the language of change'.[22]

So how does MI work? It supports patients by enhancing their *intrinsic motivation* to change their behaviour by connecting it to what the patient most cares about. MI is about more than just motivating; it is about empowering, educating, supporting, informing and affirming. Equipped with new strategies, clinician wellbeing and efficiency also improves, as MI lifts the burden of solving the patient's problems. MI has generated over 1000 peer-reviewed research studies across cultures, 200 RCTs and over 20 meta-analyses in many settings, including primary, secondary and community care, with positive trials in the management of cardiovascular disease, diabetes, diet and hypertension.[23, 24] 'Motivational interviewing is a conversation about behaviour change, where the patient is in the driving seat, and you are in the passenger seat as an expert guide.'[25]

The underlying principles of MI are: (a) to support the patient's *self-efficacy* (i.e., the belief that they have the resources, skills and solutions within them and *can* change their diet) and (b) to maintain an equal partnership with them (i.e., asking permission before broaching the subject of diet). A unique component of MI is *evoking* the person's own strong reasons for change, their *why*.[25] Evoking will tease out their intrinsic motivations and relies on deeply exploring the patient's values, priorities, hopes and dreams.

So, even when faced with the importance of it, why don't people change their diet? As we've seen, there can be a variety of factors inhibiting dietary transition. In MI, we accept it is normal to simultaneously want and not want a change. In the past, we would say a patient is in denial, or resistant, but they are simply *ambivalent*.[25] In MI, we try to resolve this ambivalence by working with the patient's intrinsic motivations and teasing out the discrepancy between what the person holds most dear and their current behaviour. Then we elicit and recognise '*change talk*'.

Change talk is a concept unique to MI. It is any speech from the patient that favours a movement towards change. Examples include statements about **d**esire, **a**bility (e.g., 'I want to…, maybe I could eat fruit at snack times'), **r**easons, **n**eed or **c**ommitment to change (e.g., 'I will buy a plant-based cookbook'.) The acronym **darn-c** helps here.[25] Reflecting change talk for the patient is a key MI strategy (e.g., 'You want your life to be different').

So how can we integrate MI into our clinical practice? Before beginning an MI intervention, it is a good idea to consciously 'shift from an expert problem-solver mindset to that of a supportive guide'.[26] The foundation skill is *engagement*, getting to know who the person before us is, to be interested in their values and motivations, i.e., elicit what really matters to this person in their life. To build trust and understanding, *reflect back* what they have said. Put the patient in touch with their goals for their life and family and prepare them to adjust their actions to achieve those. The MI processes of *focusing, evoking* and *planning* follow from engagement (see Table 18.5).

In MI, we use micro-skills throughout the consultation to guide the patient. We can use the OARS acronym as our memory aid (see Table 18.6).[22]

MI encourages the clinician *to seek permission* to give advice, information or ideas. We start from a position of equals, rather than clinician as expert. A helpful statement can be 'You are the expert on your life, and I am the expert on what has worked for others. You can decide what to do next'.

Table 18.5 The four processes of Motivational Interviewing[25]

Engage (the Who)	Open-ended questions to build empathic engagement.
Focus (the What)	1. Open-ended questions and reflective listening to negotiate an agenda, ensuring the topic (diet change) matches the patient's sense of purpose at this time in their life (or it may be abandoned). 2. Seek permission to move into a directional conversation about change: 'Do you mind if we spend a few minutes talking about diet?' 'Can I check what you know about plant-based diets?' 'Are you interested in learning more about how a plant-based diet might help you?' 3. Provide with relevant materials, signpost to websites or move on to evoking.
Evoke (the Why)	4. Then, investigate and build on motivation: 'What is it that you want to stay healthy for in your life?' 'When you think ahead to [losing weight / not having angina], what would be the impact on you?' 'What would it look like for you?' 'Why might you do that?'
Plan (the How)	5. Brainstorm various ways to reach health goals so that the patient has options if one approach does not work. 'I wonder what you'll do next?' 'What might you do to give yourself the best chance?' 6. Ensure accountability e.g., self-monitoring of health parameters for review or a Change Plan check-in via phone/text.

Using the stages of change model to guide a consultation

The stages of change or transtheoretical model (TTM) (see Figure 18.1) is intended to provide a comprehensive conceptual model of how and why changes occur, whereas MI is a specific clinical method to enhance personal motivation for change. If we tune our ear to *change talk*, it is not necessary to assign people to a stage of change as part of (or in preparation for) MI, though it can be helpful. In practice, we can tailor strategies at each stage of change as suggested below (see Table 18.7). Sometimes clinicians believe that the patient must walk out of their consultation with a plan but change often happens outside the consultation.

Group consultations

Also called 'shared medical appointments' or 'group appointments', group consultations (GCs) are consultation-interventions delivered by a clinician and a non-medical facilitator to groups of patients with similar health issues.[27] They are distinct from self-help groups or patient education groups and are aimed at patients living with long term conditions (LTC) that are affected

Table 18.6 Core microskills in Motivational Interviewing

Open-ended questions	These enable collaboration. e.g., 'What concerns you most about your heart disease?' A typical day strategy: 'Tell me what you have to eat in a typical day, starting in the morning, so we can chat about any possible areas for change?'
Affirmations of strengths, efforts and past successes	These will build confidence and hope. Notice and appreciate any positive action towards change. e.g., 'You showed [strength, courage, determination] by doing that'.
Reflections	These convey understanding and are hypotheses about the meaning behind the patient's words. They invite the patient to give voice to the change process. e.g., 'I don't have time to cook' can be reflected as 'You would cook more if you could free up more minutes in your week'.
Summarising	A motivating summary of change talk can help patients move forward. e.g., 'This new diagnosis has you motivated to look after your health and to stay active in your older years and you believe that improving your diet now might pay off later'.

by lifestyle factors, including diet. It is hoped that they may replace one-to-one consultations for LTCs in the UK.[27] Successful GC schemes have been running for some years in both primary and secondary care in the USA and Australia. Group consultations can be run by specialists, nurses, GPs, pharmacists, dieticians or allied professionals. Although evidence is currently limited, especially in the UK, several pilot schemes are underway.

The group supports behaviour change through a range of strategies, including education, persuasion (e.g., using imagery showing fat in arteries), social incentivisation (using social comparison, displaying participants' monitored weight/cholesterol readings over time or showcasing successful participants), training (e.g., food label reading, adapting recipes or meal preparation and planning), modelling (e.g., graduates from the programme, showing videos or inviting spouses) and enablement (e.g., recipe cards, books or starter foods hampers).

Dr CB Esselstyn Jr has been running a 1-day in-person intensive group seminar for over 10 years (Cardiovascular Disease Prevention and Reversal: The Esselstyn Program) at the Cleveland Clinic and has had over 1000 participants.[28] He explains: 'a key component is obtaining a personal understanding of each patient's circumstances via a 20–30-minute pre-seminar telephone call between myself, the patient and most importantly, their significant other. I also insist on the spouse or family member attending on the day.' Hence, patient engagement, preparation and motivation begin before the seminar. The seminar covers how to shop, prepare and enjoy WFPB foods and includes a detailed explanation of the hazards and pitfalls of restaurant eating. A WFPB cook shares tips, and past participants will share their experiences. A WFPB buffet lunch is served. In addition

Table 18.7 Using the transtheoretical stages of change model to inform strategies within a consultation[1,2]

Pre-contemplation Simply ask patients to reflect on your discussions and book in a follow-up appointment to discuss further or provide informative materials. • asking patients to monitor current dietary behaviour (self-monitoring) can be an eye-opener.
Contemplation Here the patient may begin to show an interest and ask questions. MI is particularly useful here, as the person is undecided about switching their diet. We can provide encouragement, increase their confidence, discuss importance and enhance readiness to change. • write down why change would be beneficial (e.g. consequences of prediabetes) • brainstorm small, concrete steps to help get them ready to change (e.g. Meatless Monday)
Preparation Focus on concrete behavioural changes, anticipating barriers and how to overcome them. If... happens, then... Also schedule in accountability and review.
Action (active for <6 months) Prepare action plan with small manageable changes, anticipating barriers and how to overcome them. If... happens, then... Also schedule in accountability and review.
Maintenance Affirmations and phone/text contact if barriers need brainstorming and problem-solving. Discuss relapse triggers, coping strategies and brainstorm new approaches.

to a recording of the seminar, each participant receives a copy of Dr Esselstyn's book (outlining the scientific basis and practical guidance), a cookbook, eating out/ grocery shopping guidelines and recipe ideas.

The evidence-based Complete Health Improvement Program (CHIP) is an intensive lifestyle intervention targeting chronic disease.[29] It is delivered over 6 to 12 weeks in 18 group sessions of 1 to 1.5 hours each and advocates a mostly WFPB diet, along with training on managing stress, emotional health, overcoming barriers and developing strategies for maintaining behaviour changes.

Health coaching

Whilst MI is a useful communication tool to incorporate into routine clinical care, a health coach can help patients enact their change plan.[30] Health coaching is a relatively new field and usually involves coaching on many health behaviours over time. It can move beyond the initial single behavioural MI component to see the patient through the entire change process. In the USA, health coaches are becoming popular in lifestyle medicine settings and some primary care services in the UK fund access to health coaches for their patients. Professional bodies for health coaching include the International Coaching Federation (ICF), European Mentoring and Coaching Council (EMCC), Association of Coaching (AoC) and UK Health Coaches Association.

Conclusion

The tools and frameworks outlined in this chapter can help clinicians to identify each patient's individual set of barriers and facilitators in transitioning to a healthy PBD. The Behaviour Change Wheel is a valuable tool in identifying precisely which areas need to be addressed to achieve sustainable dietary transition, while enabling the identification of strategies for fostering essential skills and knowledge.

Guiding patients towards adopting a PBD will require clinicians to practise and develop new skills. Motivational Interviewing is a powerful tool that can enable clinicians to focus on the change talk in the consultation, picking out ingrained eating habits and concerns about changing one's habits. MI takes practice and requires self-awareness and discipline from the clinician.[22] The art of MI will be refined throughout a clinician's career and there are many practical MI courses available online and in-person.

As clinicians, it is a privilege to bear witness to the health transformations that we have nurtured. These experiences motivate us to refine our skills to help more people move to a life of abundant health. Plant based diets fuel this alchemy.

References

1. Michie S, Atkins L and West R. *The Behaviour Change Wheel: A Guide to Designing Interventions*. UK: Silverback Publishing; 2014.
2. Prochaska JO, Diclemente CC and Norcross JC. In Search of How People Change. *American Psychologist* 1992; 47(9): 1102–1114.
3. Blake J. Overcoming the 'value- action gap' in environmental policy: tensions between national policy and local experience. *Local Environment* 1999; 4(3): 257–278. doi: 10.1080/13549839908725599
4. Akenji L. Consumer scapegoatism and limits to green consumerism. *Journal of Cleaner Production* 2013; 63: 13–23. doi: 10.1016/j.jclepro.2013.05.022
5. Fehér, A, Gazdecki, M, Véha M, Szakály M and Szakály Z. A Comprehensive Review of the Benefits of and the Barriers to the Switch to a Plant-Based Diet. *Sustainability* 2020; 12(10): 1-18. doi: 10.3390/su12104136
6. Grassian T. *A New Way of Eating: Creating Meat Reducers, Vegetarians and Vegans*. Canterbury: University of Kent; 2019.
7. Dibb S, Fitzpatrick I. Let's talk about meat: changing dietary behaviour for the 21st century. Eating Better Alliance. 2014. www.eating-better.org/uploads/documents/Let'sTalkAboutMeat.pdf [Accessed 22nd July 2015].
8. Lisle D, Goldhamer D. *The Pleasure Trap*. USA: Healthy Living Publications; 2006.
9. Adams CJ. *The Sexual Politics of Meat*. Cambridge, UK: Polity Press; 1990.
10. Thomas MA. Are vegans the same as vegetarians? The effect of diet on perceptions of masculinity. *Appetite* 2016; 97: 79–86.
11. Greenebaum JB. Questioning the Concept of Vegan Privilege: A Commentary. *Humanity & Society* 2016; 4(3): 355–372. doi: 10.1177/0160597616640308
12. Markowski KL and Roxburgh S. "If I became a vegan, my family and friends would hate me": Anticipating vegan stigma as a barrier to plant-based diets. *Appetite* 2019; 135: 1–9. doi: 10.1016/j.appet.2018.12.040
13. Twine R. Vegan Killjoys at the Table—Contesting

Happiness and Negotiating Relationships with Food Practices. *Societies* 2014; 4(4): 623–639. doi: 10.3390/soc4040623

14. Macdiarmid JI, Douglas F and Campbell J. Eating like there's no tomorrow: Public awareness of the environmental impact of food and reluctance to eat less meat as part of a sustainable diet. *Appetite* 2016; 96: 487–493.
doi: 10.1016/j.appet.2015.10.011

15. Southerton D. Habits, routines and temporalities of consumption: From individual behaviours to the reproduction of everyday practices. *Time & Society* 2013; 22(3): 335–355.
doi: 10.1177/0961463X12464228

16. Press Association. Almost one in four food products launched in UK in 2019 labelled vegan. Weblog. www.theguardian.com/food/2020/jan/17/almost-one-in-four-food-products-launched-in-uk-in-2019-labelled-vegan [Accessed 10th May 2020].

17. Nestle M. *Food Politics: How the Food Industry Influences Nutrition and Health*. Berkeley, CA, USA: University of California Press; 2002.

18. Twigg J. Food for thought: Purity and vegetarianism. *Religion* 1979; 9(1): 13–35. doi: 10.1016/0048-721X(79)90051-4

19. Vaja I, Umeh KF, Abayomi JC, Patel T, Newson L. A grounded theory of type 2 diabetes prevention and risk perception. *Br J Health Psychol* 2021; 26(3): 789-806. doi: 10.1111/bjhp.12503

20. Crowley J, Ball L, Hiddink G. Nutrition in medical education: a systematic review. *Lancet Planet Health* 2019; 3(9): e379-e389.
doi: 10.1016/S2542-5196(19)30171-8

21. Betz M, et al. Abstract #336 [Presentation]. National Kidney Foundation Spring Clinical Meetings (virtual meting). April 6-10 2021.

22. Miller WR, Rollnick S. Motivational Interviewing: Helping people to change (3rd Edition). New York: The Guilford Press; 2013.

23. Burke B, Arkowitz H, Menchola M. The efficacy of motivational interviewing: A meta-analysis of controlled clinical trials. *J Consulting and Clinical Psychology* 2003; 71(5): 843-861.
doi: 10.1037/0022-006X.71.5.843

24. Lundahl B, Moleni T, Burke BL, Butters R, Tollefson D, Butler C, Rollnick S. Motivational interviewing in medical care settings: a systematic review and meta-analysis of randomized controlled trials. *Patient Educ Couns* 2013; 93(2): 157-168. doi: 10.1016/j.pec.2013.07.012

25. Rollnick. Motivational Interviewing in Health Care. [Training course] Psychwire. 2020.

26. Rollnick S, Miller W, Butler C. *Motivational Interviewing in Health Care: Helping patients change behaviour*. New York, NY, USA: The Guilford Press; 2008.

27. Birrell F, Lawson R, Sumego M, Lewis J, Harden A, Taveira T, Stevens J, Manson A, Pepper L, Ickovics J. Virtual group consultations offer continuity of care globally during Covid-19. *Lifestyle Medicine* 2020; 1(2): E17.
doi: 10.1002/lim2.17

28. Esselstyn CB, Gendy G, Doyle J, Golubic M, Roizen MF. A way to reverse CAD? *The Journal of Family Practice* 2014; 63(7): 356-364b.

29. Wennehorst K, Mildenstein K, Saliger B, Tigges C, Diehl H, Keil T, Englert H. A Comprehensive Lifestyle Intervention to Prevent Type 2 Diabetes and Cardiovascular Diseases: the German CHIP Trial. *Prev Sci* 2016; 17(3): 386-397.
doi: 10.1007/s11121-015-0623-2

30. Frates EP, Bonnet J. Collaboration and Negotiation: The Key to Therapeutic Lifestyle Change. *American Journal of Lifestyle Medicine* 2016; 10(5): 302-312.
doi: 10.1177/1559827616638013

Chapter 19
Lifestyle Medicine in clinical practice

Laura Freeman

Introduction

Lifestyle Medicine is an exciting emerging specialty in medicine which offers a usefully different approach to patient care. However, as a healthcare concept it is not so new. Indeed, it is thought that Hippocrates identified the connection between lifestyle and health two and a half thousand years ago: 'In order to keep well, one should simply avoid too much food, too little toil'. Over the last decade or so, an abundance of relevant scientific research has been published and this evolving discipline has gained considerable momentum. This chapter will provide an introduction to the power and necessity of this fresh approach as well as an up-to-date briefing of the evidence crossing all six pillars of Lifestyle Medicine.

What is Lifestyle Medicine?

Lifestyle Medicine, as defined by the American College of Lifestyle Medicine is the use of evidence-based therapeutic interventions including a whole-food, plant-predominant eating pattern, regular physical activity, restorative sleep, stress management, avoidance of risky substances, and positive social connections. These six Lifestyle Medicine pillars should be used as the primary modality in order to prevent, treat, and in some cases, reverse chronic disease. Its goal, as Dr Saray Stancic describes in her book What's Missing From Medicine is to 'live an optimal existence, free of chronic disease and pain and suffering'. Indeed, a Lifestyle Medicine approach has been shown to extend life expectancy by a number of years – allowing people to live in better health, with less disability and improved quality of life.

Lifestyle Medicine interventions encompass the aforementioned six pillars of health, and a Lifestyle Medicine consultation should include an assessment of all these domains – with a thorough exploration into patients' habits, health goals, life priorities and environmental and social influences.

The Lifestyle Medicine approach can be practiced by many different members of the multidisciplinary team. It is a cross-cutting approach relevant to all areas of medicine and healthcare. Evidence supports its application in the prevention and treatment of many non-communicable diseases as well as its efficacy for all people, of all ages, genders and different social and cultural backgrounds. Lifestyle Medicine practitioners are able to effectively deal with the root cause of disease rather than simply managing patients' symptoms. By tackling the underlying causes, they are able to target the lifestyle-associated pathogenesis of the most common chronic diseases. Research has demonstrated that unhealthy lifestyles cause dysbiosis, epigenetic changes, cellular stress and injury. These processes perpetuate inflammation which in turn feeds back into this mechanistic pathway and contributes further to the development of many common chronic diseases such as obesity, type 2 diabetes, cardiovascular disease, and certain cancers. It is plain that lifestyle can be both the cause and cure of disease and so, by adopting a lifestyle-first approach, it is possible to interrupt these unhealthy processes and change the trajectory of our patients' health outcomes.

Lifestyle Medicine is neither alternative or complementary. It is an evidence-based approach which itself endorses the use of more conventional allopathic practices. Lifestyle Medicine practitioners support the appropriate use of medication, surgery and vaccinations, for example, but the emphasis is shifted by the practitioner largely onto the patient to make lifestyle changes as a means of first-line management. This is both a meaningful and rewarding shift in practice for both the clinician and the patient.

The burden of chronic disease and its connection with lifestyle habits

The prevalence of chronic disease is rapidly increasing worldwide, placing a heavy burden not only on the individuals affected but also on our health and social care systems. Chronic diseases are, presently, the leading cause of morbidity and mortality and also responsible for the majority of healthcare costs.[1]

Three in five global deaths are attributed to four major non-communicable diseases (NCDs) – cardiovascular disease, cancer, chronic lung diseases and diabetes.[2] And it is estimated that 80% of chronic diseases in high-income countries are themselves due to four lifestyle behaviours: an unhealthy diet; lack of physical activity; excess alcohol consumption; and tobacco smoking.[3]

It is interesting to think about the impacts of these behaviours from a Lifestyle Medicine perspective. Indeed, this was the viewpoint taken in one of the most important studies demonstrating the power of a Lifestyle Medicine approach. In an aptly-titled study 'Healthy living is the best revenge' 23,000 participants were followed for an eight-year period. The study evaluated compliance with four health lifestyle habits: not smoking, 30 minutes of exercise five days a week, maintaining a healthy weight (BMI <30) and eating a plant-predominant diet. Participants who adhered to all four healthy lifestyle factors had an overall 78% decreased risk of development of chronic disease even after adjusting for age, sex, educational and occupational status.[4] The study clearly demonstrated that lifestyle interventions can have a very significant impact on disease prevention. And this was not an isolated finding – other studies along with the World Health Organisation have reported similar outcomes: 80% of heart disease, stroke and type 2 diabetes and 40% of cancers could be prevented, primarily with improvements to diet and lifestyle.

Facilitating healthy change

In order to help the average person implement healthier lifestyle habits we need trained, certified and enthusiastic Lifestyle Medicine practitioners to embrace this challenge of tackling chronic disease. Although many healthcare professionals are already aware of the importance of counselling patients on such habit changes and the importance of healthy lifestyles, they often lack the time and confidence to do so. The majority do not always screen for unhealthy behaviours or provide the necessary recommendations to facilitate positive change.[5]

Healthcare professionals hold some of the most trusted positions in society and are viewed as credible sources of health information. As Lifestyle Medicine practitioners, we are placed perfectly to offer patient-centred, evidence-based dietary and other lifestyle interventions to help our patients make optimal choices in order to improve their health, as well as the health of the planet.

Wider societal changes alongside supportive government policies should play an important role in facilitating healthier choices. This, however, often takes time and so, the growing influence of Lifestyle Medicine and aligned practitioners taking immediate action with their patients is crucial. We need not rely on or wait until wider changes become commonplace before we move forward with our patients.

A more ethical approach

As healthcare professionals we are obliged to work with integrity, compassion and uphold a strong moral compass. This becomes relevant to the discussion of Lifestyle Medicine as the emerging research seeks to challenge current consensus around the most effective approach to treating chronic disease. For example, the American College of Lifestyle Medicine position paper on type 2 diabetes demonstrated that clinical remission of the disease is possible with adequate lifestyle management and that this, therefore, should be the end goal to strive for. Several years prior, the Counterpoint study detailed a whole food plant-based diet as the preferred dietary intervention for type 2 diabetes and stated 'diabetes reversal should be the goal in the management of type 2 diabetes'. This is crucially important as it redefines our current understanding of what 'chronic' disease means. It highlights the case that if we are not at least to offer our patients with type 2 diabetes this treatment, we could be considered to be practicing unethically. Maximillian Andreas Storz proposed exactly this and suggested that doctors should be offering plant-based diets to all those suffering with chronic conditions. By not advocating for this diet, we could cause harm to our patients as well as the health of the planet.[6]

Pillar 1: Plant-based nutrition

Unhealthy diets alone are the top cause of death and disability globally, accounting for 20% of all deaths.[7] Eating patterns high in meat, dairy and processed foods have fuelled our current global health crisis with rising rates of non-communicable diseases. These diseases include obesity, cardiovascular disease, type 2 diabetes, certain cancers and Alzheimer's dementia – all of which have been shown to be preventable, treatable and in some cases reversible with a whole food plant-based diet and healthy lifestyle changes. Whilst all six pillars of Lifestyle Medicine are relevant in the management of these conditions, plant-based diets are a crucial component in the treatment plan. Yet the pillar of nutrition is probably the most challenged and hotly debated area of Lifestyle Medicine. Nevertheless, there is an overwhelming amount of evidence which supports a whole food plant-based diet as one of the healthiest choices we can make in order to tackle the root cause of these diseases. It is also a low-risk and cost-effective approach. A whole food plant-based diet is nutrient dense and rich in phytochemicals and fibre and as such, has been shown to enhance immunity, lower inflammation and optimise the gut microbiome. It is key to any sustainable and effective Lifestyle Medicine intervention.

Although many misconceptions remain, major dietetic organisations around the world, including the British Dietetic Association in the UK have confirmed that a 100% plant-based diet can meet nutritional requirements for all stages of life from birth through to old age. Indeed, the impact of a whole food plant-based diet is so significant that national and international guidelines now recommend plant-based diets for prevention of cancer[8] and the treatment of type 2 diabetes.[9]

Whilst many doctors do not receive adequate nutrition education, the majority do agree on the importance of nutrition and health. Only a minority, however, are confident in counselling their patients on the subject.[10] Nevertheless, they are also in a strong position to interpret emerging scientific data on plant-based diets and translate this into the delivery of effective nutritional advice. Whilst doing so, it is imperative to tailor their advice to their patients' religious and cultural backgrounds and be considerate of any financial implications or issues with accessibility.

It is crucial for us to recognise the responsibility we hold as healthcare professionals to educate our patients about the evidence base linking our food choices, our physical health, and the health of our planet. Guiding our patients towards a plant-based lifestyle provides an opportunity to work in partnership with our patients and to empower them on their health journey. Lifestyle Medicine practitioners should be able to communicate clearly on the subject of dietary change whilst assessing patients for stages of behaviour change. By doing so, we can improve our patients' adherence to a healthier and more sustainable dietary pattern whilst improving the trajectory of their health.

Pillar 2: Exercise

The impact of physical activity

Exercise has a profound effect on all body systems. The beneficial impact of physical activity in terms of primary and secondary prevention for many chronic diseases is highly significant. Moreover, an increased level of physical fitness is known to reduce the risk of premature death from all causes.[11]

The converse is true whereby inadequate levels of exercise are well-established as a major risk factor for many chronic diseases and premature mortality. Indeed, it is recognised as the fourth risk factor for global mortality according to the World Health Organization.[12]

Physical activity assessments and exercise prescriptions should be regarded as a crucial component of any Lifestyle Medicine consultation. In times of increasing health expenditures, exercise is an important low-cost evidence-based intervention that can benefit those of all ages and genders, for those at any body weight and fitness levels. Health care spending is known to increase as patient activity levels decrease.

The number of medical conditions with evidence regarding the benefits of regular exercise are extensive. The common lifestyle conditions such as type 2 diabetes, cardiovascular disease and obesity may seem obvious inclusions but the conditions with recognised benefits extend far beyond those to also include other frequently seen conditions such as chronic fatigue, osteoporosis, low back pain, chronic pain and premenstrual syndrome, stress, depression and anxiety.[13]

Exercise also promotes restorative sleep, longevity and improved quality of life and has been associated with reduced risk of age-related cognitive decline and improved outcomes in cancer patients.[14]

Sedentary problems

Even though the research regarding the benefits of exercise are well-established and the mechanisms well-understood, the reality is that the majority of the population are not exercising routinely. In England only 21% of men and 18% of women aged 65–74 achieve the current national physical activity recommendations, dropping to 9% and 6% respectively for those aged 75 and over.[15]

Additionally, sedentary behaviours have been on the rise across many populations in the last few decades as many spend longer driving, sitting, watching TV and working at the computer. Recent estimations report a total number of 9–10 sitting hours per day in middle aged and older US adults.[16]

There is a growing body of evidence which confirms that these prolonged periods of sitting are detrimental to health. Sedentary behaviour is now considered an independent risk factor and contributes to an increased risk of all-cause mortality, cardiovascular disease, certain cancers, type 2 diabetes, depression, anxiety and perceived tiredness.

As we guide our patients with exercise recommendations we should also, therefore, be helping them to set intentions to break up extended sitting periods. Suggestions such as standing desks and short bursts of movements (such as climbing the stairs or walking lunch breaks) offer feasible and convenient strategies to increase movement through the day.

Exploring the barriers to exercise

In order to maximise the effectiveness of our counselling and guidance on exercise, we need to gently explore our patients' barriers to exercise. Helping our patients to identify these, with a compassionate and non-judgemental approach, can improve self-management and optimise compliance with exercise recommendations.

There are many perceived barriers to exercise which vary from patient to patient according to cultural backgrounds, socioeconomic status as well as baseline physical and emotional levels of wellbeing. Conversations around overcoming these barriers are an important part of any Lifestyle Medicine assessment.

Prescribing exercise

Developing an exercise prescription for patients is a valuable tool for any healthcare professional. Whilst all patients should be screened for contraindications to start exercising, the majority of patients are able to start at least with low levels of physical activity. These prescriptions should be tailored to age, personal preferences, cultural background, socioeconomic status and local facilities. They should also be reviewed regularly in order to ensure the prescription remains relevant, personalised, safe and clinically effective. Ideally, a multidisciplinary team should be involved wherever possible.

Pillar 3: Sleep

Sleep is a state of rest defined as a 'rapidly reversible state of immobility with greatly reduced sensory responsiveness'. It is a complex but necessary biological function for every creature in the animal kingdom. And although it is thought we spend up to a third of our lives sleeping, many remain apathetic, underestimating its importance and failing to prioritise healthy sleep habits into their lives.

Not so long ago, scientific explanations were lacking as to why we sleep. However, emerging research has shown, unequivocally, that healthy sleep is fundamental to our physical and emotional wellbeing as well as our ability to function optimally throughout the day. It has two dimensions: duration (quantity) and depth (quality) and both offer a crucial component to true health by mitigating the risk of a wide spectrum of morbidities.

Although the amount of sleep can vary across different stages of the life cycle, the amount of sleep needed for healthy adults, as recommended by the National Sleep Foundation, is 7–9 hours per night[43] Research confirms that inadequate sleep – of both duration and quality – is associated with serious health implications such as mood disorders, decreased cognition including memory, suppressed immune response, heart disease and fatigue-related accidents. Although a crucial component to health, it is typically underreported by patients in the medical setting.[17] Inquiries into sleep habits and daytime energy levels should, therefore, be included in all lifestyle consultations.

There is an abundance of evidence showing that the number of average sleep hours are declining, especially in Western societies. Increasing trends in sleep disorders such as insomnia have been well documented over the last few decades with psychological and physical health disorders contributing in almost equal proportions. Similar data is also emerging from low-income countries, reporting sleep problems being especially prevalent in women over the age of 50.[18] Insufficient sleep can be considered then, as a global and growing public health epidemic which will have significant social and economic implications.

The health consequences of insufficient sleep

Insufficient sleep has been shown to cause a 13% increased risk of premature mortality when comparing individuals who slept for less than six hours per night to those who achieved 7–9 hours per night.[19] This included all causes of death, including fatal car accidents, strokes, cancer and cardiovascular disease.

Unhealthy sleep has also been associated with an increased risk of cardiovascular disease,[20] type 2 diabetes,[21] weight gain and suppression of the immune system. Increased risk of cancer development has also been an important finding whereby insufficient sleep has been linked with a decreased response in natural killer cells, increased sympathetic nervous activity and levels of inflammation. These findings are robust enough for the World Health Organization to officially classify night-time shift work as a 'probable carcinogen'.

Emerging research has also shown that adequate sleep allows for the recently discovered 'glymphatic system' to clear toxic waste and replenish the brain. As such, insufficient sleep is now recognised as a key determinant of Alzheimer's dementia.

Insufficient sleep has also been linked with the development of certain mood disorders, increased frequency of migraines, clinical burnout, work accidents, personal injury as well as poor decision making and slow reaction times, low moral awareness and inattention.[22]

Sleep cycles

Understanding the sleep cycles can allow for important insights into patient sleep patterns as part of an overall sleep assessment.

Healthy sleep cycles last approximately 90 minutes and are characterised by two different types: NREM (non-rapid eye movement) and REM (rapid eye movement). There are three stages of NREM and one stage of REM and a healthy night of sleep will allow for 4–6 completions of these cycles with non-memorable short 1–2 minute periods of waking every couple of hours. Most sleep occurs in the NREM stages with REM sleep comprising only a quarter of total night's sleep, mostly occurring in the second half of the night.

Sleep assessment

A mini sleep assessment may include typical hours of sleep on weekdays and weekends, perceived sleep quality, frequency of daytime fatigue, frequency and type of sleep disturbance and attitude towards sleep. It is important to screen for any 'red flags' such as less than seven hours sleep, one or more hours weekday-weekend difference, shift work, poor sleep quality despite more than seven hours spent in bed or more than nine hours sleep.

A sleep diary is an important tool for both practitioner and patient. It can raise awareness of helpful or unhelpful behaviours and provide insight into the patients' routines. Details such as time to bed and waking, ease of falling asleep, number of waking periods, reasons for sleep disturbance and feelings when waking (e.g., refreshed, fatigued) should be recorded for seven nights in a row.

Recommendations

In order to achieve restorative sleep, attention must first be drawn to the other pillars of Lifestyle Medicine. Eating a healthy plant-based diet, exercising regularly, effectively managing stress and avoiding alcohol for example all have important consequences on the quality and quantity of sleep.

Additionally, the patient's sleep environment is of importance and should be kept cool, dark and as quiet as possible.

Patients should be encouraged to develop a consistent bedtime routine which may include relaxing rituals such as a warm bath, listening to soft music, breathing exercises or meditations. Other helpful sleep hygiene practices are shown below but will depend on patients' individual preferences.

Good sleep hygiene practices:
- avoiding eating too late
- avoid alcohol
- dim lights 1–2 hours before bedtime
- avoid screens (television, iPad or other devices) at least one hour before bed
- relaxing ritual 30 minutes before bed
- keep the bedroom for sleeping and sex only
- keep your sleep and wake times consistent seven days/week.

Pillar 4: Stress

Stress consists of behavioural and physiological responses that occur when we perceive a threat to our existence or wellbeing. Many report they are 'stressed' when in actual fact they are experiencing nervous tension. This is a common and important element of the stress experience, but it is possible to be stressed without feeling tension. Similarly, it is possible to feel tension without experiencing stress. In either respect stress can be regarded as a choreographed state of events and is not merely a psychological experience. Stress leads to the disruption of homeostasis and if chronic, leads to ongoing allostatic overload and consequently, creates a risk to health.

The harmful effects of stress on disease

Scientific research has firmly established the relationship between stress and disease with demonstrable effects on the cardiovascular, gastrointestinal and neurohormonal systems as well as a dampened immune response. These occur because of various changes such as elevated cortisol and norepinephrine levels, changes in serotonin levels and altered cytokine activity. Consequently, it can be understood that stress has an important impact on all systems of the body – albeit not in equal proportions.

Current technology allows for the analysis of the effect of stress on the body at the molecular level. Telomere caplets at the end of each chromosome assist in the regulation of appropriate genetic replication. Each time a cell divides, telomere base pairs shorten, resulting in a lessening of their effective regulation of normal cell replication. Chronic stress has been demonstrated to result in such 'shortening damage' of telomeres[23] which itself has been associated with a hastened pace of ageing, increased incidence of disease, malignancy and poor survival.[24]

Screening for stress

Actively creating opportunities within the Lifestyle Medicine consultation to screen for patient stress is of utmost importance. It is prudent to consider whether stress is influencing certain behaviours, for example the use of alcohol, drugs or interfering with relationships or occupation. The severity should be determined and individualised management options for effective stress management discussed in detail.

Stress-management techniques

Whilst acute stress in life is unavoidable, living with chronic stress can be actively managed. Helping our patients incorporate stress management techniques into their lifestyle often offers great benefits. It is true that there is a genetic component to pathological stress which can shape an individual's stress response but even the most resilient will benefit from effective stress-management techniques. Many stress management modalities are low-cost and low-risk and empower the patient to regain some control over their lives. Further, identifying stresses in patients' lives provides a useful opportunity to explore the connection between emotions and health.

That being said, it is important to help our patients realise that some stress can be considered useful. Indeed, when we recognise that it can help us achieve goals, meet deadlines and perform well in different scenarios, we can change our mindset around the stress experience. Our bodies do need some amount of stress in order to activate certain biological pathways. However, the benefits of this exists only up to a point after which excessive strain can quickly lead to reduced activity, fatigue, and ultimately poor health outcomes.

We can also encourage our patients to think specifically around their psychological, behavioural and physical signs associated with their stress response. When we help our patient tune in to these, they can develop awareness when stress starts to build and proactively turn to constructive approaches to managing stress.

Common stress-management techniques

Tai chi, meditation, mindfulness, progressive muscle relaxation, gratitude and journaling are all examples of helpful practices to manage stress.

Although these methods can all be beneficial, they are highly individualised with preference for different options often depending on age, gender, cultural backgrounds and spirituality. Other therapeutic techniques could include art therapy, music therapy, time in nature, knitting, reading, writing or any hobby as deemed by the patient to be stress reducing.

At times of stress, we should aim to continue to apply the other pillars of Lifestyle Medicine. In reality, however, stressful events can fuel risky health behaviours such as drinking or smoking and efforts to maintain healthy lifestyles often fall neglected. This makes it even more urgent that we work with our patients proactively. In order to effectively reduce stress, we should encourage them to make healthy decisions that will support their health.

Pillar 5: Risky substances

Smoking

The health risks of smoking cigarettes are very well known yet it remains a significant cause of morbidity and mortality and is responsible for 7 million deaths globally each year. In 2019, the UK office for national statistics reported a falling number of adult smokers as well as a decline in the average number of cigarettes smoked per day. Worryingly however, the highest proportion of smokers were reported in young adults aged 25–34.[25] Additionally, there was a 1% increase in the number of hospital admissions attributable to smoking and no improvements relating to the number of deaths.[26] As such, it remains a very real public health concern.

Adverse effects on health
Tobacco smoke is a complex mixture of thousands of toxic compounds many of which are carcinogenic.[27] Its use negatively affects every organ of the body and its detrimental effects on the cardiovascular and respiratory system are well known. The number of diseases known to be caused by tobacco use continues to increase and now also includes a wide range of ailments including: age-related macular degeneration, diabetes, colorectal cancer, liver cancer, adverse health outcomes in cancer patients and survivors, tuberculosis, erectile dysfunction, oro-facial clefts in infants, ectopic pregnancy, rheumatoid arthritis, inflammation, and impaired immune function.[28]

Exposure to second-hand smoke
The health effects of second-hand smoke are also considerable and as such, there is considered to be no risk-free level of second-hand smoke exposure with even periods of brief exposure being linked to detrimental health outcomes for infants, children and adults alike.[29]

Tobacco control efforts
It took a number of years for the medical community to embrace the scientific research linking cigarette smoking to adverse health outcomes. Nevertheless, education and smoking cessation campaigns as well as smoke-free policies and other legislative steps have allowed for some progress. The public image around smoking has certainly shifted since tobacco control efforts first emerged and in many countries, the majority of people do think unfavourably of smoking in public places.

Helping our patients quit
The benefits of stopping smoking are extensive and will be gained by all at any stage in the smoking history. The effects are, however, thought to be notable in younger smokers who have the most to gain from increased life expectancy following quitting. Short-term benefits of quitting include lower blood pressure levels and reduced risk of infection. Long-term health benefits are considerable and include reduced risk of cardiovascular disease, lung disease and various cancers.

Smoking is a major modifiable risk factor for disease and all healthcare professionals should be working to help our patients quit. Although increasing in popularity, e-cigarettes or 'vaping' lack evidence as an effective smoking cessation strategy and long-term safety effects are not known. Other smoking cessation therapies are better established and can take various forms – as guided by patient preference or other individualised factors – and may include brief interventions, counselling, nicotine replacement strategies, prescription medications or a combination. Extra effort should be made to target these groups including those of lower socioeconomic status, minority groups and those with a history of mental illness and/or substance use disorders. Whilst smoking cessation deserves our continued attention we should also, ideally, make every effort to focus on prevention and in turn, truly impact the burden of avoidable disease.

Alcohol

Whilst our patients are familiar with the negative effects of smoking, the impact and loss of health attributable to alcohol is less well appreciated. Indeed, alcohol is one of the most widely-used, socially-acceptable drugs consumed across the world. Although in the past, some studies have supported moderate health benefits to low alcohol consumption such as for ischaemic heart disease, the adverse effects of alcohol are becoming increasingly obvious and the original claims for any benefits have been called into question.[30] Instead, emerging evidence reports alcohol use as having a very significant effect on the burden of disease globally with more than 60 acute and chronic diseases being attributable to alcohol.

The most compelling data comes from the *Lancet* report published in 2018 which noted alcohol as the leading risk factor for premature death and disability for those aged 15–49 years with 10% of global deaths attributable to alcohol for this age group.[30] The message is clearly stated: the safest level of alcohol consumed is zero. It calls for a change in global policy to achieve lower alcohol consumption in order to protect the future health of the world's population.

Acutely, alcohol can reduce sleep latency and hasten sleep initiation, however, it will also adversely affect the quality and depth of sleep leading to fatigue and decreased productivity the next day. Alcohol is classified as a depressant and there is a strong relationship with injury, violence, domestic abuse, deliberate self-harm and risky sexual behaviours.

Chronic use and misuse of alcohol affects every system of the body with some of the most well-known health effects including fatty liver, cirrhosis, hypertension and pancreatitis as well as detrimental behavioural effects and social disadvantages.

A note on alcohol and cancer

There is strong scientific consensus that alcohol can cause many types of cancer and as such, it has been listed as a group 1 'known' human carcinogen. A report on the global burden of cancer worldwide confirmed 4.1% of cancer diagnoses were attributable to alcohol consumption.[31]

Its effects on the development of head and neck cancers, oesophageal cancer, gastric cancer, breast and colorectal cancer as well as other types of cancers are well-documented and its synergistic effect with cigarette smoking is also well established. Drinking any amount of alcohol, even in low levels[32] can increase cancer risk though the level of risk is linked with increasing consumption. Several biological mechanisms are thought to be involved – such as damage from acetaldehyde, altered hormone regulation and folate deficiency. Alcohol is also high in its energy content with 7 kcal/gram and as such, is associated with weight gain and obesity thus explaining its contribution to weight-related cancers.[33]

An alcohol history should feature in all Lifestyle Medicine consultations and screening tools – such as AUDIT C – can be used where concerns of misuse or addiction are raised. Patients should be supported in their efforts to reduce their alcohol intake with referrals being made to local support groups or specialist services where appropriate and possible. Any counselling should be patient-centred, delivered with compassion and without judgement.

Pillar 6: Social connections

Positive relationships and a strong support system are vital for both physical and emotional health.

Some of the most fascinating research on the impact of healthy lifestyles has come from those living in areas coined 'the Blue Zones'. These are five regions of the world – Okinawa, Japan; Sardinia, Italy; Nicoya, Costa Rica; Ikaria, Greece; and Loma Linda, California – where people are living the longest, healthiest lives – often beyond their 100th year and without disease. Inhabitants of these regions share in common several healthy lifestyle habits such as a plant-predominant diet and regular physical activity. Inhabitants also demonstrate how social behaviour has a positive impact on health. One of the key components of the Blue Zones is that they share a strong sense of community and close support groups. In this case, their social networks have a very positive influence on health. It is worth noting that the opposite effect is seen in other groups. For example, some social networks will have a negative effect on health by facilitating or normalising unhealthy behaviours such as smoking. Indeed, it has been shown that obese people were more likely to have social networks of family and friends who were also obese.[34]

As such, we increasingly recognise the importance of positive relationships and a strong social support system – they are significant determinants of health and vital for both physical and emotional wellbeing. Research supports this and has also documented its benefits for lowering inflammation[35] and improving metabolic health[36] as well as reducing incidence of acute myocardial infarction and stroke.[37]

Social interactions also have an important effect on brain health. They involve many complex cognitive processes such as face recognition, focus, attention and a variety of communication skills as well as emotional expression. They are thought therefore, to increase cognitive reserve and as such, have been associated with a reduced risk of dementia. Research has shown that social isolation can double your risk of dementia in later life.[38]

Loneliness

Loneliness is different from the physical state of social isolation. It is instead, a complex emotional state of which there have been various definitions including 'the negative perception of being alone and disconnected' and is much more to do with perceived isolation rather than objective isolation.[39] The impact of loneliness on health is irrefutable. People who are lonely use health care services more frequently yet are also more likely to suffer from – and find it more difficult to recover from – both acute and chronic illness.

Historical data on loneliness is negligible but there is plenty of evidence which now suggests levels of loneliness are increasing amongst many populations. Whilst commonly recognised in elderly people, loneliness is now more prevalent in younger populations across the world.[40]

Lifestyle Medicine can offer positive connections

It is well understood then that as humans, we desire acceptance and crave belonging. Studies have shown positive connections and strong sense of community favourably affects health outcomes and can drive healthy habits. In order to fully support our patients, we must screen for social aspects including loneliness. We can then work with them to understand this connection to their health and thereafter, try to increase their social engagement and facilitate quality connections.

Conclusion: The future of Lifestyle Medicine

One of the most important and useful approaches for rippling out a Lifestyle Medicine approach will be integrating Lifestyle Medicine into the medical school curricula. This is starting to gain momentum and certainly in the US, advances have been made with wide reporting of medical schools increasing their uptake of Lifestyle Medicine curricula as well as assessments and residency programmes for postgraduates. Active student interest groups are also forming within medical schools further driving the enthusiasm for the subject.

To date, research has confirmed that medical students, universally, receive inadequate training on nutrition with one study citing 70% of medics reporting less than two hours of training.[41] Similar research also confirms that a significant number of final year medical students remain unaware of the physical activity guidelines[42] with only 8.4% of students feeling adequately trained to give physical activity advice to the general population. However, 91.1% said they would like more formal training on physical activity.[43] This highlights both the need and desire for Lifestyle Medicine societies and colleges to work closely with medical schools.

Certainly, delivering Lifestyle Medicine in either virtual or in person format will make important strides in efforts to prevent and treat non-communicable disease with an effective, sustainable and scalable way to educate future physicians and indeed, all other healthcare professionals. Whilst curricula are being built, other effective strategies may include student interest groups, workshops, electives and specialist study modules.

In the meantime, the Lifestyle Medicine Global Alliance (LMGA) – founded by the American College of Lifestyle Medicine in 2015 – continues its mission to unite all Lifestyle Medicine professional associations. This international convergence of aligned healthcare professionals will spur on the movement of Lifestyle Medicine with the hope of eradicating lifestyle-related diseases. This united front – which spans low-, middle- and high-income countries – will allow for the much needed positive change in the medical system and in our patients' lives all around the world.

References

1. Bodai BI, Nakata TE, Wong WT, Clark DR, Lawenda S, Tsou C, Liu R, Shiue L, Cooper N, Rehbein M, Ha BP, Mckeirnan A, Misquitta R, Vij P, Klonecke A, Mejia CS, Dionysian E, Hashmi S, Greger M, Stoll S, Campbell TM. Lifestyle Medicine: A Brief Review of Its Dramatic Impact on Health and Survival. 2018; 22: 17-025. doi: 10.7812/TPP/17-025. PMID: 29035175; PMCID: PMC5638636
2. Wang H., Naghavi M., Allen C. Global, regional, and national life expectancy, all-cause mortality, and cause-specific mortality for 249 causes of death, 1980–2015: a systematic analysis for the Global Burden of Disease Study 2015. 2016; 388(10053): 1459–1544.
3. Schmidt H. Chronic Disease Prevention and Health Promotion. 2016 Apr 13. In: H. Barrett D, W. Ortmann L, Dawson A, et al., editors. . Cham (CH): Springer; 2016. Chapter 5. Available from: www.ncbi.nlm.nih.gov/books/NBK435779/ doi: 10.1007/978-3-319-23847-0_5
4. Ford ES, Bergmann MM, Kröger J, Schienkiewitz A, Weikert C, Boeing H. Healthy living is the best revenge: findings from the European Prospective Investigation Into Cancer and Nutrition-Potsdam study. *Arch Intern Med* 2009; 169(15): 1355-1362. doi: 10.1001/archinternmed.2009.237.
5. Flocke SA, Clark A, Schlessman K, Pomiecko G. Exercise, diet, and weight loss advice in the family medicine outpatient setting. *Family Medicine* 2005; 37(6): 415-421.
6. Maximilian Andreas Storz. Will the plant-based movement redefine physicians' understanding of chronic disease? *New Bioethics* 2020; 26(2): 141-157. doi.org/10.1080/20502877.2020.1767921
7. GBD 2017 Diet Collaborators. Health effects of dietary risks in 195 countries, 1990–2017: a systematic analysis for the Global Burden of Disease Study 2017. *Lancet* 2019; 393(10184): 1958-1972. doi: 10.1016/S0140-6736(19)30041-8
8. Rock CL, Thomson C, Gansler T, et al. American Cancer Society guideline for diet and physical activity for cancer prevention. *CA Cancer J Clin* 2020; 70(4): 245-271. doi: 10.3322/caac.21591
9. John Kelly, MD, MPH, Micaela Karlsen, PhD, MSPH, Gregory Steinke, MD, MPH. Type 2 Diabetes Remission and Lifestyle Medicine: A Position Statement From the American College of Lifestyle Medicine. *American Journal of Lifestyle Medicine* 2020; 14(4): 406-419. doi: 10.1177/1559827620930962.
10. Macaninch E, Buckner L, Amin P, Broadley I, Crocombe D, Herath D, Jaffee A, Carter H, Golubic R, Rajput-Ray M, Martyn K, Ray S. Time for nutrition in medical education. *BMJ Nutr Prev Health* 2020; 3(1): 40-48. doi: 10.1136/bmjnph-2019-000049
11. Warburton DE, Nicol CW, Bredin SS. Health benefits of physical activity: the evidence. *CMAJ* 2006; 174(6): 801-809. doi:10.1503/cmaj.051351
12. World Health Organization. 2010. Global Recommendations on Physical Activity for Health. Geneva. http://whqlibdoc.who.int/

publications/2010/9789241599979_eng.pdf
13. Brill P. ACSM's Exercise Management for Persons With Chronic Diseases and Disabilities, edited by J Larry Durstine, Geoffrey E Moore, Patricia L Painter, and Scott O Roberts. *Activities, Adaptation & Aging* 2012; 36:2, 182-183. doi: 10.1080/01924788.2012.677794
14. MacMillan Cancer Support. The importance of Physical Activity for People living with and beyond Cancer: A concise Evidence Review. https://be.macmillan.org.uk/Downloads/CancerInformation/LivingWithAndAfterCancer/

Chapter 20
An inclusively responsible food and agriculture system for planetary health

Laila Kassam and Amir Kassam

Introduction

Human society is degrading the Earth's natural systems at a terrifying rate. We are causing the 'sixth mass extinction', the only human-caused mass species extinction, so referred to by some as the 'first mass extermination'. Despite the central importance of biodiversity in sustaining life on the planet, it is declining faster than ever before. Much of this decline is due to deforestation which destroys habitats. We have cut down an estimated 46% of trees since the start of human civilisation[1] and destroyed about 17% of the Amazon rainforest over the past 50 years.[2] Nearly 20 years ago the Millennium Ecosystem Assessment, which estimated 89% of our ecosystems were degraded or severely degraded and only 11% were in reasonable condition, warned 'the ability of the planet's ecosystems to sustain future generations can no longer be taken for granted'.[3] A recent study estimated just under 3% of the Earth's land surface is ecologically intact.[4]

Alongside this ecological breakdown we also face climate breakdown. Both are closely connected and pose equally serious threats. At the current rate we will reach 1.5°C warming above the pre-industrial average in the early 2030s when 14% of the world's population will suffer severe heatwaves at least once every five years. At 2°C warming, this will increase to 37% of the population and the risk of extreme weather events, crop failure, poverty, displacement, and death for hundreds of millions of people will increase significantly.[5] The risks to health of temperature increases include 'increased dehydration and renal function loss, dermatological malignancies, tropical infections, adverse mental health outcomes, pregnancy complications, allergies, and cardiovascular and pulmonary morbidity and mortality'.[6] These risks disproportionately affect vulnerable populations such as children, older adults and those living in the Global South. Between 2030 and 2050 climate change is expected to lead to an additional 250,000 deaths a year due to heat, undernutrition and diarrhoeal disease and malaria.[7] The UCL-Lancet Commission on Managing the Health Effects of Climate Change stated that 'climate change is the biggest global health threat of the 21st century'.[8]

Of the nine planetary boundaries that regulate the Earth system, safe limits have been exceeded for four: climate change, biosphere integrity, land-system change and biochemical flows (nitrogen and phosphorus). Of these, climate change and biosphere integrity are 'core boundaries' due to their fundamental importance to the Earth system. When these core boundaries are significantly altered, they are likely to 'drive the Earth system into a new state', seriously affecting human wellbeing.[9] Given humans' significant impact on Earth, some have described the current geological epoch as the 'Anthropocene'. Others call it the 'Capitaloscene' to highlight destructive human activity linked to colonial capitalism as driving this impact, not humans or human nature.[10]

The health, wellbeing and quality of life of humans is deeply dependent on and connected to the health of the planet. The term 'planetary health' is being increasingly used to emphasise this connection and reflects the understanding that 'human health and human civilisation depend on flourishing natural systems and the wise stewardship of those natural systems'.[11] Planetary health has been defined as the 'health and wellbeing of humans and the natural environments we depend on'[12] and points to the need to regenerate and protect the health of the global ecosystem if we are to ensure human health and wellbeing. As the negative health impacts from ecological and climate breakdown are threatening the global health gains of the past several decades and are becoming more prevalent, all of us, especially healthcare professionals, must broaden our view of health beyond individual health, to the more holistic concept of planetary health.

The importance of these connections was highlighted by the 2019 Lancet Commission on Obesity which stated that the interacting 'pandemics of obesity, undernutrition, and climate change represent the paramount challenge for humans, the environment and our planet'. They called these three pandemics 'The Global Syndemic ….a synergy of pandemics that co-occur in time and place, interact with each other, and share common underlying societal drivers'. The underlying drivers identified include food systems which: 'not only drive the obesity and undernutrition pandemics but also generate 25–30% of greenhouse gas emissions (GHGs), and cattle production accounts for over half of those.'[12] In the same year the EAT-Lancet Commission also pointed to the global food and agriculture system as the main driver of climate and ecological breakdown: 'global food production threatens climate stability and ecosystem resilience and constitutes the single largest driver of environmental degradation and transgression of planetary boundaries. Taken together the outcome is dire. A radical transformation of the global food system is urgently needed.'[13] It is clear then that ecological and climate breakdown, environmental degradation, malnutrition and obesity are not separate issues. They are interconnected global crises, and the role of the food and agriculture system is central to them all.

In this chapter we look briefly at the history and key aspects of the dominant agriculture production paradigm and the corporate food regime which is needed to understand how and why the food and agriculture system is causing such negative environmental impacts. We then review some of the food and agriculture system's key impacts on planetary health. We go on to envision what a just, sustainable and healthy future food and agriculture system could look like using the framework of 'inclusive responsibility'[14] and end with some calls to action.

The dominant industrial agriculture paradigm

Since World War I the food and agriculture system has been increasingly driven by the corporate sector that developed and spread the now dominant industrial Green Revolution agriculture paradigm globally. The 'Green Revolution' refers to the global spread of new agriculture technologies between the 1940s and 1970s. These technologies included new high-yielding varieties of cereals that responded well to irrigation and chemical fertilisers and required pesticides, and new cultivation methods including mechanisation. These technologies replaced 'traditional' methods which were based on manual and animal-powered tillage, diversified cropping and animal integration as a source of power, manure, and food. After World War II the use of agrochemicals and intensive tillage became the norm and drove the expansion of industrial agriculture along with cheap oil, credit and new machinery.[15]

Industrial Green Revolution agriculture is now characterised by: large-scale production; emphasis on a few crops; genetic manipulation of germplasm; increasing use of chemical fertilisers, pesticides and fossil fuels; intensive tillage; and investment into farm machinery and equipment. Farming has lost much of its resilience which had been based upon low-intensity tillage, crop diversification, and maintenance of habitats. In the Green Revolution paradigm, loss of topsoil from intensive tillage is partially dealt with by increased use of chemical fertilisers. Pesticides and herbicides have allowed farmers to stop their traditional crop mixtures and rotations and other soil and water conservation practices and focus on short-term yields. As a result, industrial agriculture systems have very poor agricultural biodiversity and soil health and are ecologically unsustainable. They have suboptimal productivity and cannot deliver ecosystem services. They are large emitters of greenhouse gases (GHG) and contribute to rather than mitigate climate change.[14] The Green Revolution model is also characterised by industrial animal farming. The industrialisation of crop agriculture and the resulting grain surpluses reduced the price of animal feed which led to the industrialisation of animal farming and the massive increase in animal agriculture and 'meat' consumption worldwide. Since World War II global 'meat' production has increased by nearly five times and consumption per person has doubled.[16]

This industrial agriculture model, and the interconnected crises we are facing, are being driven by the capitalist economic system. This system is deeply rooted in European colonial history and the exploitation and oppression of marginalised humans and other animals and destruction of nature. Colonial capitalism views everything and everyone as a resource to exploit or a commodity to sell in order to maximise profit. It externalises its social and environmental costs, requires infinite and extractive growth, and concentrates power, wealth and resources into fewer and fewer corporate hands that are unaccountable to society or nature. The 30%–40% of food that is wasted along the value chain is just one symptom of the capitalist food system where contradictions such as overproduction and waste on the one hand and artificial scarcity on the other are inherent. The current organisation of global food production and circulation, characterised by the concentration of corporate power, is referred to as the 'corporate food regime'. This regime, supported and facilitated by governments and international institutions, perpetuates neo-colonial relations with countries in the Global South using free trade agreements, land grabbing and expropriation of labour, seeds and other resources, to force local food systems to integrate into the globalised food system and spread industrial, input intensive, monocultural, commodity production globally.[17]

Impacts of industrial agriculture on planetary health

The industrialisation of agriculture has had serious negative environmental, social and health impacts. Below we discuss some of these key impacts which will show in more detail why our food system is considered to be one of the main drivers of ecological and climate breakdown and the destruction of planetary health.

Land use change, deforestation and mass extinction

Today, half of the world's habitable land is used for agriculture compared to less than 4% 1000 years ago.[18] The benignly termed 'land use change' or 'land conversion', where natural and seminatural habitats such as forests are transformed into fields for crop production and plantations, and pastures for animal agriculture, is the strongest driver of our destruction of nature.[19] Forests provide many critical ecosystem services (e.g., carbon sequestration, climate stabilisation, water cycle maintenance and rainfall generation) and are home to both free living animals and humans.

Over half of the world's plant and animal species live in tropical forests.[20] Deforestation, occurring at a rate of 5 million hectares a year, is therefore one of the biggest extinction risks to many species. Agriculture is responsible for at least 75% of deforestation worldwide, of which animal agriculture, including animal feed production, is a significant driver.[21] In the Amazon, 70%–80% of deforested land has been converted into pasture for grazing, with much of the remaining land used to grow animal feed such as soya.[22, 23] Animal agriculture is the most significant driver of habitat loss on the planet[24] and one of the biggest drivers of biodiversity loss.[23] Globally, 44% of grain and 80% of soya is used to feed farmed animals.[25] This has led to significant shifts in agricultural land use. While both intensive (industrial) and extensive animal agriculture (including pasture for grazing, feed grains and fodder) currently takes up 83% of the world's agricultural land it only provides 18% of calories and 37% of protein.[26] These figures show what an inefficient use of resources animal agriculture is compared to crop agriculture which supplies the majority of the world's calories and protein on just a fifth of agricultural land.

Tillage agriculture, both industrial and traditional, is the main reason an estimated quarter of animal and plant species are under threat from extinction.[19] Of the 60% of wildlife populations we have destroyed since 1970, industrial agriculture is responsible for 60%.[27] The continuing decline of wildlife in countries such as the UK long after 'land conversion' is due to the excessive use of agrochemicals, large-scale production of monocrops, intensive tillage and destruction of habitats such as hedgerows, perennial grasslands, and wetlands caused by the increasing agricultural intensification over the last 70 years. Over 40% of all insect species are in decline and one-third threatened with extinction due mainly to industrial farming and heavy pesticide use which is five times higher than in 1950.[28]

Biodiversity

Agricultural biodiversity (including domesticated plants, animals and fishes) is also under threat from industrial agriculture. Since the 1900s, 75% of plant genetic diversity has been lost as farmers worldwide have left their local varieties for genetically uniform, high-yielding varieties. Despite the thousands of plant and animal species used for food, 75% of the world's food is generated from only 12 plant and five animal species.[29] This over-reliance on a handful of species, due to industrial crop and animal farming promoted by powerful corporations, makes food supplies more vulnerable to pests, diseases and climate change. This destruction of biodiversity is brought into stark relief when you consider that farmed chickens make up 70% of all birds on the planet, with just 30% being free-living, while 60% of all mammals are farmed animals, mostly cows and pigs, 36% are human animals and just 4% are free-living.[30]

Agrochemical use in industrial agriculture is also contributing to destruction of biodiversity. Pesticides are destroying many species including mammals, earthworms and important pollinators such as bees. Neonicotinoids, introduced in the early 1990s and the most widely used insecticides globally, are leading to a decline in wild and domesticated pollinators. Large-scale use of systemic insecticides represent a worldwide threat to biodiversity, ecosystems and ecosystem services such as pollination and nutrient cycling which are vital for food security.[31]

Greenhouse gas emissions and climate breakdown

The global food system, from production to consumption, is estimated to contribute between 26% and 34% of GHG emissions, of which animal agriculture is estimated to contribute 56%–58%. These estimates come from the largest meta-analysis of global food systems to date by Poore and Nemecek (2018) which analysed data on the environmental impact of different foods from over 38,000 farms in 119 countries.[26] This meta-analysis found that even the lowest-impact animal products have a greater impact than substitute vegetable proteins on GHG emissions, eutrophication, acidification and land use. This includes emissions from grass-fed ruminants in 'well-managed' grazing systems, often argued (mistakenly in our view) to be necessary for sustainable agriculture and carbon sequestration.

The GHG emissions from animal agriculture are due mainly to: 'land conversion' for feed production and grazing; methane emissions from ruminant farmed animals; nitrous oxide emissions from manure; and fossil fuel use in production and along the value chain.[23] While animal agriculture is often quoted as contributing at least 14.5% of GHG emissions based on studies by FAO,[23, 32] this is likely an underestimate for various reasons explored by Twine (2021) including outdated data and incomplete accounting of land use changes related to animal agriculture.[33] Twine argues the new minimum should be 16.5% but suggests it is likely to be significantly higher. Poore and Nemecek (2018) explored the impact of a global shift to a plant-based diet and calculated that 'the land no longer required for food production could remove ~8.1 billion metric tons of CO_2 from the atmosphere each year over 100 years as natural vegetation re-establishes and soil carbon re-accumulates'.[26] In an Erratum published later they clarified that this 'carbon uptake is additional to the 6.6 Gt yr–1 of avoided agricultural CO2eq emissions that the authors reported (which is a 49% reduction in the annual emissions of the food sector). In total, the "no animal products" scenario delivers a 28% reduction in global greenhouse gas emissions across all sectors of the economy relative to 2010 emissions'.[34]

There is a plethora of studies confirming that plant-based or vegan diets have significantly lower GHG emissions and other environmental impacts than vegetarian and omnivorous diets. For example, a 2019 systematic review comparing vegan, vegetarian and omnivorous diets found that a 100% plant-based or vegan diet has the least environmental impact in terms of GHG emissions, land and water use.[35] A 2020 study which analysed the environmental impacts of different dietary pattens in 140 countries found that a 100% plant-based or vegan diet reduced GHG emissions by an average of 70% compared with the baseline omnivorous diet.[36] While there is currently a lot of focus in public discourse on GHG emissions and climate change (though much less on animal agriculture's contribution to this), the indirect impacts of animal agriculture on climate breakdown through degrading and destroying the planet's natural carbon sinks such as forests and its role in driving mass species extinction are just as important.

However, in our view shifting to plant-based diets without changing the agricultural system that produces these plant-based diets, does not go far enough. Intensive tillage agriculture, producing both plants for human consumption and animal feed, makes a significant contribution to climate breakdown through GHG emissions from soil. The loss of soil organic matter caused by tillage has caused large-scale carbon dioxide emissions since the dawn of settled agriculture, intensifying since World War II.[37] The excessive use of fossil energy in manufacturing industrial agricultural production inputs such as agrochemicals and machinery and in intensive farm operations also contributes to climate breakdown.[38,39]

Soil degradation and erosion

We have lost half of the topsoil on the planet in the last 150 years[40] and are losing 24 billion tonnes every year.[41] While tillage-based agriculture has existed for centuries and has caused soil and land degradation, it is the intensification of agriculture and tillage, as well as the practice of keeping soils bare, that has resulted in the large-scale soil and land degradation and loss of soil health we are seeing today.[40] Conventional tillage-based industrial Green Revolution agriculture is responsible for 75% of the destruction of our soils. In the last 70 years it has led to the abandonment of approximately half a billion hectares of land due to soil erosion and degradation and loss of soil health and ecosystem functions.[40] As degraded land is abandoned, new land is converted and the destructive cycle continues.

Tillage-based agriculture destroys soil organic matter which is vital for soil aggregate formation and healthy soil function, including the cycling of nutrients and water that enable plant growth. The loss of soil organic matter also reduces the resilience of soils. For example, soils with a higher level of organic matter hold more water than soils where it has been depleted. Crops growing in healthier soils are thus more likely to withstand drought than those in more degraded soils. Also, urban and other areas adjacent to degraded areas of soils can be more susceptible to floods as the land tends to shed rather than hold water.

Ecosystem services

Ecosystems support plant and animal life and provide humans access to natural resources and processes that enable them to sustain their lives, livelihoods and habitats. These natural resources and processes are referred to as 'ecosystem services' and include: clean water; water storage and regulation; minimisation of runoff and soil erosion; enhancement of soil health and biodiversity; avoidance of soil and land degradation and environmental pollution; sustaining pollination; and minimisation of GHGs. The integrity of these services depends on how much natural ecosystem processes are negatively altered through human interference such as agriculture. This is because agriculture involves clearing the original vegetation, producing crops, altering water, carbon and nutrient cycles and stocks, changing the nature and speed of ecological processes and their interactions with other components of the ecosystem.

Agriculture is multifunctional due to its role in facilitating ecosystem, social and economic services beyond agricultural production. However, this multifunctionality is ignored by the industrial Green Revolution paradigm. As a result, industrial tillage-based agriculture is responsible for a significant loss of the ecosystem services that rely on healthy soils and landscapes.[15] This, to a lesser degree, also applies to tillage-based non-industrial or traditional agriculture in much of the low-income countries which still disrupts soil mediated ecosystem functions and destroys soil health and function.[42] As a result, there are huge economic and social costs to society which, in many cases cannot be adequately costed. Once degradation or loss of function or species has occurred, in some cases involving severe soil erosion or desertification, they can never be fully recovered. In some instances, the loss can be total, and the natural resource gone forever.[43]

Water and agrochemical use

Agriculture accounts for 70% of freshwater use worldwide.[44] Pumping groundwater for surface irrigation dries up aquifers and leads to negative environmental externalities including salinity, stream depletion and land subsidence. In addition, agriculture is a major source of pollution from agrochemicals and effluent from animal agriculture contaminating waterways, groundwater and the air. Erosion of topsoil in runoff water and wind carries agrochemicals and microorganisms, polluting water systems and the atmosphere. Nearly 89% of global ocean and freshwater eutrophication (the pollution of waterways with nutrient-rich pollutants) is caused by agriculture.[26] The runoff of chemical fertilisers and sewage from animal agriculture has created over 400 aquatic dead zones all over the world.[45] The overall excessive and continuous use of agrochemicals has also led to exceeding the planetary boundaries for nitrogen and phosphorus.[9]

Nonhuman animals

The industrialisation of animal agriculture has had devastating effects on farmed animals by significantly increasing the scale and intensity of the suffering we inflict on them. In 1961, we killed around 7 billion land animals for food, and we are currently killing approximately 70 billion land animals per year (not including male chicks killed in the egg industry).[46] We also kill an estimated 51 to 167 billion farmed fishes every year.[47] The use of growth hormones and antibiotics in animal agriculture, including dairy, has led to toxins accumulating up the food chain with disastrous effects. For example, all over India, the vulture population has been almost exterminated because of the high levels of antibiotic toxicity in dead cows, whom they scavenge upon.[43]

Life in the sea is also being destroyed by fishing. We kill an estimated 0.79 to 2.3 trillion free-living fishes every year for food.[48] Aside from the suffering this causes to the fishes themselves, this is causing major ecological damage including destruction of seabed habitats by trawling gear and plastic pollution from discarded fishing gear. For example, 46% of the plastic and nylon material in the Great Pacific Garbage Patch is from fishing nets.[49] A third of the world's fish stocks are now overexploited.[50]

Human health

Currently we produce enough food to feed 10 billion humans[42, 51] and yet an estimated 2 billion people remain hungry.[52] At the same time nearly 2 billion adults are overweight, over 650 million of whom are obese. Malnutrition including undernutrition, obesity, and other dietary risks for non-communicable diseases (NCDs) such as cancer, diabetes and heart disease, is the biggest cause (19%) of ill-health and premature death globally.[12]

Undernutrition is directly related to the corporate food regime which drives the inefficient and unjust use of land and other resources e.g. to the production of feed for animals, and vastly unequal distribution of food. The rise in obesity and NCDs is strongly related to Western diets, high in processed and animal-based foods and low in whole plant foods. This diet is spread globally by the corporate food regime. While these diseases are more prevalent among wealthier countries, the globalisation of animal-based Western diets has resulted in a worldwide pandemic of chronic diseases that are intimately related to lifestyle and dietary choices, as described in this book.

The food and agriculture system is also contributing to the increasing spread of zoonotic diseases. Animal agriculture, and the habitat destruction for feed production it drives, along with the wildlife trade, has led to the increasing spread of novel zoonotic diseases.[53] It is estimated that 60% of known infectious diseases and 75%

of emerging infectious diseases are zoonotic in origin and that globally, zoonoses are responsible for 2.5 billion cases of human illness and 2.7 million human deaths every year.[54] Factory farms are breeding grounds for infectious diseases and it is well-recognised that factory farming of animals is a major pandemic risk. The continuation of industrial animal agriculture means further pandemics are inevitable.

The link between animal agriculture and antibiotic resistance is also very strong. The WHO has identified antibiotic resistance as one of the greatest threats to global health, development and food security.[55] While overuse of antibiotics contributes to this resistance, approximately 70% to 80% of antibiotics globally are given to farmed animals.[56] Currently 700,000 people are estimated to die each year due to antibiotic-resistant diseases[55] which will only increase if no action is taken.

The use of agrochemicals in industrial agriculture also has negative impacts on public health. Increasing global nitrogen fertiliser use is linked with nitrate pollution of ground and surface water bodies. Nitrate pollution of freshwaters is now increasingly becoming a pervasive global public health problem.[57] Pesticides can pose serious health and safety risks.[58] While farmers are at risk of acute poisoning from exposure on the field, pesticides can also lead to longer-term health impacts for farmers, workers and those living nearby farms. For example organophosphate insecticides can affect brain function and have been found to be especially dangerous to children, even in utero.[59] Endocrine-disrupting pesticides have been linked to low birthweight, abnormal brain development, reduced fertility and prostate cancer among people who live in agricultural areas.[60] Glyphosate, a broad spectrum systemic herbicide and crop desiccant was classed as a 'probable carcinogenic' by the WHO in 2015.[61] Glyphosate is the most used herbicide globally and its use has increased significantly since the development of genetically modified crops that are resistant to it. Pesticides in the food supply are also an increasing health concern. Much of the produce available to buy, not just fruit and vegetables but also animal products and processed food, may have pesticide residues present. For example, on average, 30% of food bought in the UK contains pesticide residues.[62] While consumers are unlikely to suffer acute poisoning from pesticide residue found in food, the possible long-term consequences are of concern. Risk assessments by governments are done on single chemicals, not on the mixture of pesticides consumers are exposed to. As a result, scientists do not know the effects of these 'cocktails' on human health.[62]

An inclusively responsible food and agriculture system

Given that the current food and agriculture system is such a significant driver of the interconnected ecological, climate and planetary health crises, it is clear that food system transformation is central to addressing them all. In this section we discuss what we believe a just, sustainable and healthy future food and agriculture system could look like, following the framework of 'inclusive responsibility' developed in our book ,[14] in particular the concluding chapter on which the following section is based. We envision an 'inclusively responsible' food and agriculture system which would 'encourage society to focus on agroecological sustainability as an integral part of overall ecosystem sustainability based on planetary boundaries. Such a system would place importance on quality of life, pluralism, equity and justice for all. It would emphasise the health, wellbeing, sovereignty, dignity and rights of farmers, consumers and all other stakeholders, as well as of nonhuman animals and the natural world'.[14]

Inclusive responsibility

In our view, the multiple connected crises we are facing ultimately reflect a crisis of ethics and values. For example, our economic system, one of the key drivers of these crises, is based on the principles and ideologies of competition, individualism, colonisation, racism, patriarchy, extraction, materialism, injustice, exploitation and domination and commodification of humans, other animals and the Earth. If we want to find systemic solutions to the root causes, rather than technofixes that address symptoms while further entrenching the current system, we need to build systems that are underpinned by ethical frameworks aligned with universal human values, otherwise we will keep recreating the same problems.

Inclusive responsibility is an ethical framework based on universal human values of: inclusion, interdependence, pluralism, justice, equity, and care, which we suggest should guide our transformation of the food and agriculture system. Based on these values and informed by the destructive impact of the current food and agriculture system discussed above, we envision an inclusively responsible food and agriculture paradigm would be aligned with six principles. This system would:

1. Be ecologically sustainable and multifunctional
2. Be relevant for smallholders, their innovation and development strategies
3. Meet the increasing need for sustainable and healthy whole-food plant-based diets
4. Integrate into the wider social movements resisting the corporate food regime and fighting for local autonomy, food sovereignty, and land and seed justice
5. Respect and protect the rights of all sentient beings, both human and nonhuman, to live free from human oppression, exploitation and harm, and
6. Respect and protect the rights of nature based on a duty of care towards the Earth.

Inclusive responsibility offers an alternative guiding framework of principles and values to all stakeholders. We hope this framework can serve as a transformative force by helping to interrogate and inform decision-making at all levels, leading to mainstreaming a pluralistic food and agriculture system that is good for society, the natural world and all who depend on it.

The holistic nature of this framework reflects our view that transforming the current industrial agricultural production paradigm (principles 1 and 2) is necessary but not sufficient to transform our food system into one that is inclusively responsible, sustainable, and just for all (humans, other animals and the planet). Given the huge role of animal agriculture and animal-based diets in driving the ecological, climate and planetary health crises, we also need to shift to sustainable and healthy, whole food plant-based diets to not only tackle climate change and stay within planetary boundaries but also address the pandemic of diet related NCDs (principle 3).[13]

There is a wealth of empirical and clinical evidence showing that whole-food plant-based diets are the healthiest diet pattern for health and longevity. One of the most comprehensive analyses in this area is the 2019 Eat-Lancet Commission on Food, Planet and Health[13] which looked at what constitutes a healthy diet that would allow us to produce enough food for 10 billion people within planetary boundaries. It accounted for country-based differences in food accessibility and recommended a planetary health reference diet based predominantly on whole plant foods, and emphasised fruits, vegetables, whole grains, legumes, nuts, and seeds. In Europe and the US, following this diet pattern would require a huge reduction in the consumption of unhealthy foods, including at least halving the consumption of red meat, and more than doubling the consumption of whole plant foods. Whole food plant-based diets are not only healthier for humans, other animals and the planet, they are also cheaper than standard Western diets.[63]

Along with transforming the agriculture production paradigm and shifting to plant-based diets, we also need to transform the corporate food regime into one based on 'food sovereignty' (principle 3). The corporate food regime and the broader capitalist economic system are the underlying drivers of the increasingly destructive and irresponsible practices of industrial agriculture and our unhealthy and inequitable food system. Food sovereignty has been defined by the global peasant movement La Via Campesina as 'the right of peoples to healthy and culturally appropriate food produced through ecologically sound and sustainable methods, and their right to define their own food and agriculture systems. It puts the aspirations and needs of those who produce, distribute and consume food at the heart of food systems and policies rather than the demands of markets and corporations'.[64] Food sovereignty is based on six principles, it focuses on: food for people; values food providers; localises food systems; puts control locally; builds knowledge and skills; and works with nature. We need to do all these things while also protecting and respecting the rights of humans, other animals and the planet and coming back into right relationship with other animals, each other and the natural world (principles 5 and 6).

Discussing the details of all these different aspects of needed transformation is beyond the scope of this chapter (but explored in depth in *Rethinking Food and Agriculture*[14]). Below we focus on the heart of this transformation and the basis of an ecologically sustainable plant-based food system – the agricultural production paradigm of Conservation Agriculture (CA) as a plant-based regenerative alternative to the current destructive industrial Green Revolution agriculture production paradigm and traditional tillage-based production systems (principles 1 and 2).

Conservation Agriculture (CA)

CA is an ecosystem approach to regenerative sustainable agriculture and land management, the development of which has been driven and led by farmers in both the Global North and South[65] CA is based on the context-specific, locally adapted practical application of three interlinked principles of:
1. Continuous no or minimum mechanical soil disturbance (no-till seeding/planting and weeding, and minimum soil disturbance with all other farm operations, including harvesting)
2. Permanent maintenance of soil mulch cover (crop biomass, stubble, and cover crops), and
3. Diversification of cropping systems (economically, environmentally, and socially adapted rotations and/or sequences and/or associations involving annuals and/or perennials, including legumes and cover crops).

These principles are used along with complementary good agricultural practices of integrated crop, soil, water, nutrients, and pest management. They are the ecological underpinnings that enable production systems to mimic natural ecosystems and deliver biological products and ecosystem services in a regenerative way. CA is holistic in design and practice, optimising not just production and yield but all other multifunctional processes of the ecosystem. Thus, CA systems also have the ability to address ecosystem issues by harnessing the rehabilitation, regeneration, and other life-giving processes of nature. CA minimises the use of external inputs, including agrochemicals, seeds, animal manure, water, energy, time, and machinery, based on maximising input use efficiency and output factor productivity. CA systems maintain agroecosystem resilience by sustaining crop health and productivity, soil and landscape health and functions, and offer the best climate change adaptability and mitigation.[15]

In short, CA does the opposite of conventional tillage-based industrial Green Revolution agriculture. It enables farmers to use land sustainably and profitably while minimising agrochemical inputs and energy and enhancing ecosystem services. CA systems are: mitigators of climate change, have a much lower carbon footprint; sequester carbon; use less water; minimise soil degradation, erosion and runoff thus reducing waterlogging and flooding; reduce or minimise the use of agrochemicals; reduce machinery, energy, and labour use and costs; offer increased and more stable yields; reduce the risk of crop failure due to droughts, floods and heat stress; and rehabilitate and regenerate degraded lands and ecosystem services.[38, 39]

CA is being applied to all crops and its advantages apply to rainfed and irrigated annual systems (including rice-based systems and roots and tuber crops) and perennial systems (orchards, plantations, cropping with trees) and to organic and non-organic systems. Annual CA cropland covers 15% of global cropland (in all continents and agroecologies in different climates, altitudes, and soils) and is increasing at an annual rate of 10 million hectares. There is also extensive area under perennial CA systems in all continents and climates, but their area estimates are not available.

While CA is practiced both inorganically and organically or biologically, in our view we must move towards CA systems that are biological, either totally or mostly organic. CA systems are regenerative in the sense that they are restorative, self-protecting, self-repairing, and over time become increasingly self-sufficient, requiring lower levels of external inputs and intervention. Small- and large-scale organic or mainly biological CA systems already exist in all major environments and more CA farms will adopt organic or biological practices to enhance and manage soil health and productivity and to protect crops as such technologies become increasingly available and adoptable.

It is not possible to manage agricultural landscapes and watersheds for sustainable production and the delivery of ecosystem services based on tillage agricultural systems, including conventional organic farming. The only way to achieve this is through CA-based landscape management which enables multifunctional land use to be established, connecting ecological processes at the production field level to those at the landscape and watershed levels. There are many examples of landscape-based CA management e.g., for carbon sequestration in Alberta, Canada; watershed services in Parana basin, Brazil; and control of land degradation and erosion in Western Australia and Andalusia, Spain.[38, 39]

Use of animal inputs

CA is plant-based by default. It does not require the use or integration of domesticated animals or their inputs, whether practiced organically or nonorganically. Other alternative agriculture paradigms, including organic agriculture, rely heavily on animal manure for plant nutrients. However, biomass does not need to pass through the guts of farmed animals to become a source of plant nutrients. If crop biomass is left on the soil surface, as in natural ecosystems, earthworms ingest it and produce worm manure. This is what happens in those organic CA systems which rely on nature's own nutrient cycling process where farmed animals and/or their products are not used. Integration of domesticated animals is also not needed to emulate the diversity found in nature given the biodiversity that is generated below and above the ground in CA systems.

In recent years, rotational or mob grazing has become seen as an important or necessary component in some regenerative agriculture systems for the regeneration of grassland, soil health, and carbon sequestration, despite the lack of empirical evidence.[66, 67] On the contrary, evidence suggests the 'contribution of grazing ruminants to soil carbon sequestration is…substantially outweighed by the greenhouse gas emissions they generate'[68] unlike the carbon sequestration potential of arable CA systems.[14, 38, 39] In our view, grazing is not necessary for ecologically sustainable soil and nutrient management. Reforesting the 76% of global agricultural land that would be liberated if we shifted to plant-based diets[26] would make a much larger contribution not only to carbon sequestration but also to wildlife habitats and the reduction of nitrogen and phosphorus pollution (from both manure and chemical fertilisers applied to feed crops). After all, the vast majority of grazing land was originally forests that were cut down for agriculture and forests are much more effective than pasture and grassland at sequestering and storing carbon.

Conclusion: A call to action

The food and agriculture system is one of the biggest drivers of the multiple interconnected crises we are facing and its transformation into an 'inclusively responsible' system is vital for planetary health. We live in an interdependent world where the health, wellbeing and quality of life of humans are inextricably linked to the health of the planet and all her inhabitants. There is no individual health without planetary health, no healthy humans without a healthy planet. All of us, especially health professionals, need to recognise this interdependence. As Dr David Katz, a past president of the American College of Lifestyle Medicine, states: 'you cannot rightly call yourself a health professional any longer if you don't advocate frequently, and fervently, for the health of the planet.' But what kind of advocacy do we need?

There have been multiple 'calls to action' for health professionals to date including: the Sao Paulo Declaration from the Planetary Health Alliance; the 'Call for emergency action to limit global temperature increases, restore biodiversity, and protect health' editorial published in 233 health journals worldwide;[6] and the 'Climate, Health and Equity Policy Action Agenda'[69] signed by over 100 US health care organisations. As reflected in these calls to action, health professionals play multiple roles and must act not only as healthcare professionals but also as advocates and engaged citizens.[70]

Healthcare professionals must recognise the impact of climate and ecological breakdown on patient health and move towards the more holistic understanding of planetary health. Healthcare professionals have a responsibility to educate patients about the evidence base linking food choices, physical health, and the health of our planet and guide patients towards a plant-based diet for their own health and the health of the planet.

As advocates, healthcare professionals can focus on transforming the health system from their own contexts, for example by working with colleagues to: mainstream the concept and values of planetary health and incorporate them into curricula and professional codes of conduct; shift to more sustainable and healthful organisational practices e.g., reducing energy use and shifting towards whole-food plant-based diets; advocate for patient-centred policies that focus on planetary health; find ways to incorporate solutions and community services beyond the clinic; and collectively respond to the 'calls to action' noted above.

As engaged citizens healthcare professionals can change their own behaviours (e.g., by making more sustainable food and transport choices) and encourage others, including patients, to do the same. In addition, they can support official environmental activities and commitments through putting pressure on their local representatives, getting engaged in local politics, voting etc. More importantly however, to bring about the rapid, transformative, structural change we need to address these crises we need to build people powered social movements, which have been central to social change in the past. As engaged citizens we all need to reclaim our power to make change by taking action, whether that be participating in protests, non-violent civil disobedience or direct action or organising behind the scenes. We need to support those movements working not only to address the climate and ecological emergencies but also those working to change the food and agriculture system (the food and animal freedom movements) and the economic system. We also need to support farmers and their communities to become actively engaged in driving change. All of these issues are interconnected. Healthcare professionals are positioned at their intersection, and as such have a unique and vital role to play in bringing about the transformative change we need to address these crises and the destruction of planetary health, before it is too late.

References

1. Crowther T, Glick H, Covey K, Nature CB-, 2015 undefined. Mapping tree density at a global scale. 525; 201-205.
https://doi.org/10.1038/nature14967
2. Deforestation and Forest Degradation. Threats. WWF. [cited 2021 Dec 6]. Available from: www.worldwildlife.org/threats/deforestation-and-forest-degradation
3. Reid WV, Mooney HA, Cropper A, Capistrano D, Carpenter SR, Chopra K, et al. Ecosystems and human well-being - Synthesis: A Report of the Millennium Ecosystem Assessment. Washington DC: Island Press, 2005.
https://research.wur.nl/en/publications/ecosystems-and-human-well-being-synthesis-a-report-of-the-millenn
4. Plumptre AJ, Baisero D, Belote RT, Vázquez-Domínguez E, Faurby S, J'drzejewski W, et al. Where Might We Find Ecologically Intact Communities? 2021; 4: 626635. https://doi.org/10.3389/ffgc.2021.626635
5. AR6 Climate Change 2021: The Physical Science Basis — IPCC. [cited 2021 Dec 5]. Available from: https://www.ipcc.ch/report/sixth-assessment-report-working-group-i/
6. Atwoli L, Baqui AH, Benfield T, Bosurgi R, Godlee F, Hancocks S, et al. Call for emergency action to limit global temperature increases, restore biodiversity, and protect health. 2021; 374: n1734. doi: 10.1136/bmj.n1734
7. World Health Organization. Quantitative risk assessment of the effects of climate change on selected causes of death, 2030s and 2050s. 2014 [cited 2021 Dec 6].
https://apps.who.int/iris/bitstream/handle/10665/134014/9789241507691_eng.pdf
8. Costello A, Abbas M, Allen A, Ball S, Bell S, Bellamy R, et al. Managing the health effects of climate change: Lancet and University College London Institute for Global Health Commission. 2009; 373(9676): 1693–1733.
www.thelancet.com/article/S0140673609609351/fulltext
9. Steffen W, Richardson K, Rockström J, Cornell SE, Fetzer I, Bennett EM, et al. Planetary boundaries: Guiding human development on a changing planet. 2015; 347(6223).
www.science.org/doi/abs/10.1126/science.1259855
10. Moore JW. . USA: Verso Books; 2015.
11. Whitmee S, Haines A, Beyrer C, Boltz F, Capon AG, de Souza Dias BF, et al. Safeguarding human health in the Anthropocene epoch: Report of the Rockefeller Foundation-Lancet Commission on planetary health. 2015; 386(10007): 1973–2028.
www.thelancet.com/article/S0140673615609011/fulltext
12. Swinburn BA, Kraak VI, Allender S, Atkins VJ, Baker PI, Bogard JR, et al. The Global Syndemic of Obesity, Undernutrition, and Climate Change: The Lancet Commission report. 2019; 393(10173): 791–846.
www.thelancet.com/article/S0140673618328228/

fulltext
13. Willett W, Rockström J, Loken B, Springmann M, Lang T, Vermeulen S, et al. Food in the Anthropocene: the EAT–Lancet Commission on healthy diets from sustainable food systems. 2019; 393(10170): 447–492. doi: 10.1016/S0140-6736(18)31788-4
14. Kassam A, Kassam L, editors. . UK: Woodhead Publishing; 2021: 444.
15. Kassam A, Kassam L. Paradigms of agriculture. In: . UK: Elsevier; 2021: 181–218.
16. Global meat production, 1961 to 2018. [cited 2021 Dec 18]. Available from: https://ourworldindata.org/grapher/global-meat-production
17. McMichael P. Political economy of the global food and agriculture system. In: . UK: Woodhead Publishing; 2021: 53–75.
18. Ritchie H, Roser M. Environmental impacts of food production. Our World in Data. 2020 [cited 2021 Dec 18]. Available from: https://ourworldindata.org/environmental-impacts-of-food
19. IPBES. Global assessment report on biodiversity and ecosystem services of the Intergovernmental Science-Policy Platform on Biodiversity and Ecosystem Services. Bonn 2019.
20. Scheffers BR, Joppa LN, Pimm SL, Laurance WF. What we know and don't know about Earth's missing biodiversity. 2012; 27(9): 501–510. doi: 10.1016/j.tree.2012.05.008
21. Ritchie H, Roser M. Drivers of deforestation. Our World in Data 2021 [cited 2021 Dec 18]. Available from: https://ourworldindata.org/drivers-of-deforestation
22. Machovina B, Feeley KJ. Meat consumption as a key impact on tropical nature: a response to Laurance et al. . 2014; 29(8): 430–431. doi: 10.1016/j.tree.2014.05.011
23. Steinfeld H, Gerber P, Wassenaar T, Castel V, Rosales M, de Haan C. Livestock's long shadow. Rome: FAO of the UN; 2006 [cited 2021 Dec 18]. www.fao.org/3/a0701e/a0701e00.htm
24. Machovina B, Feeley KJ, Ripple WJ. Biodiversity conservation: The key is reducing meat consumption. 2015; 536: 419–431. doi: 10.1016/j.scitotenv.2015.07.022
25. Stoll-Kleemann S, O'Riordan T. The sustainability challenges of our meat and dairy diets. 2015; 57(3): 34–48. doi: 10.1080/00139157.2015.1025644
26. Poore J, Nemecek T. Reducing food's environmental impacts through producers and consumers. 2018; 360(6392): 987–992. doi: 10.1126/science.aaq0216
27. Grooten M, Almond REA, editors. Living planet report - 2018: Aiming higher. Gland: WWF; 2018 [cited 2021 Dec 18]. http://pure.iiasa.ac.at/id/eprint/15549/1/%255bEMBARGO%2030%20OCT%255d%20LPR2018_Full%20Report_12.10.2018.pdf
28. Chemnitz C, Rehmer C, Wenz K, editors. Insect Atlas: facts and figures about friends and foes in farming. 2020 [cited 2021 Dec 18]. https://friendsoftheearth.eu/publication/insect-atlas-facts-and-figures-about-friends-and-foes-in-farming/
29. What is Agrobiodiversity?. FAO [cited 2021 Dec 18]. www.fao.org/3/y5609e/y5609e02.htm
30. Bar-On YM, Phillips R, Milo R. The biomass distribution on Earth. 2018; 115(25): 6506–6511. www.pnas.org/content/115/25/6506
31. van Lexmond MB, Bonmatin JM, Goulson D, Noome DA. Worldwide integrated assessment on systemic pesticides. 2014; 22(1): 1–4. https://link.springer.com/article/10.1007/s11356-014-3220-1
32. Gerber PJ, Steinfeld H, Henderson B, Mottet A, Opio C, Dijkman J, et al. Tackling climate change through livestock: a global assessment of emissions and mitigation opportunities. Tackling climate change through livestock: a global assessment of emissions and mitigation opportunities. Rome: FAO; 2013; xxi–115.
33. Twine R. Emissions from Animal Agriculture—16.5% Is the New Minimum Figure. 2021; 13(11): 6276. www.mdpi.com/2071-1050/13/11/6276/htm
34. Poore J, Nemecek T. Erratum for the Research Article "Reducing food's environmental impacts through producers and consumers" by J. Poore and T. Nemecek. 2019; 363(6429). doi: 10.1126/science.aaw9908
35. Chai BC, van der Voort JR, Grofelnik K, Eliasdottir HG, Klöss I, Perez-Cueto FJA. Which

36. Kim BF, Santo RE, Scatterday AP, Fry JP, Synk CM, Cebron SR, et al. Country-specific dietary shifts to mitigate climate and water crises. 2020; 62: 101926. doi: 10.1016/j.gloenvcha.2019.05.010
37. Lal R. Managing Soils and Ecosystems for Mitigating Anthropogenic Carbon Emissions and Advancing Global Food Security. 2010; 60(9): 708–721. doi: 10.1525/bio.2010.60.9.8
38. Kassam A, editor. . London: Burleigh Dodds Science Publishing; 2020.
39. Kassam A, editor. London: Burleigh Dodds Science Publishing; 2020; 1(1): 575.
40. Montgomery DR. . USA: University of California Press; 2007: 285.
41. UNCCD. . Bonn; 2017.
42. Lal R. Feeding 11 billion on 0.5 billion hectare of area under cereal crops. 2016; 5(4): 239–251. doi: 10.1002/fes3.99
43. Juniper T. What has nature ever done for us? How money really does grow on trees. 2013. [link?]
44. Annual freshwater withdrawals, agriculture (% of total freshwater withdrawal). [cited 2021 Dec 18]. https://data.worldbank.org/indicator/er.h2o.fwag.zs
45. Diaz RJ, Rosenberg R. Spreading dead zones and consequences for marine ecosystems. 2008; 321(5891): 926–929. doi: 10.1126/science.1156401
46. Global Animal Slaughter Statistics And Charts – Faunalytics. [cited 2021 Dec 18]. https://faunalytics.org/global-animal-slaughter-statistics-and-charts/
47. Numbers of farmed fish slaughtered each year. fishcount.org.uk [cited 2021 Dec 18]. http://fishcount.org.uk/fish-count-estimates-2/numbers-of-farmed-fish-slaughtered-each-year
48. Numbers of fish caught from the wild each year fishcount.org.uk [cited 2021 Dec 18]. http://fishcount.org.uk/fish-count-estimates-2/numbers-of-fish-caught-from-the-wild-each-year
49. Lebreton L, Slat B, Ferrari F, Sainte-Rose B, Aitken J, Marthouse R, et al. Evidence that the Great Pacific Garbage Patch is rapidly accumulating plastic. 2018; 8(1): 1–15. doi: 10.1038/s41598-018-22939-w
50. Ritchie H, Roser M. Fish and Overfishing. Our World in Data 2021 [cited 2021 Dec 18]. https://ourworldindata.org/fish-and-overfishing#wild-fish-stocks
51. Holt-Giménez E, Shattuck A, Altieri M, Herren H, Gliessman S. We Already Grow Enough Food for 10 Billion People … and Still Can't End Hunger. 2012; 36(6): 595–598. doi: 10.1080/10440046.2012.695331
52. Hickel J. The true extent of global poverty and hunger: questioning the good news narrative of the Millennium Development Goals. 2016; 37(5): 749–767. doi: 10.1080/01436597.2015.1109439
53. Morse SS, Mazet JAK, Woolhouse M, Parrish CR, Carroll D, Karesh WB, et al. Prediction and prevention of the next pandemic zoonosis. 2012; 380(9857): 1956–1965. doi: 10.1016/S0140-6736(12)61684-5
54. Salyer SJ, Silver R, Simone K, Behravesh CB. Prioritizing Zoonoses for Global Health Capacity Building—Themes from One Health Zoonotic Disease Workshops in 7 Countries, 2014–2016. 2017; 23(Suppl 1): S55. /pmc/articles/PMC5711306/
55. WHO. Antibiotic resistance fact sheet. World Health Organization 2020 [cited 2021 Dec 18]. www.who.int/news-room/fact-sheets/detail/antibiotic-resistance
56. Ritchie H. How do we reduce antibiotic resistance from livestock?. Our World in Data 2021 [cited 2021 Dec 18]. https://ourworldindata.org/antibiotic-resistance-from-livestock
57. Bijay-Singh, Craswell E. Fertilizers and nitrate pollution of surface and ground water: an increasingly pervasive global problem. 2021; 3(4): 1–24. doi: 10.1007/s42452-021-04521-8
58. Nicolopoulou-Stamati P, Maipas S, Kotampasi C, Stamatis P, Hens L. Chemical Pesticides and Human Health: The Urgent Need for a New Concept in Agriculture. 2016; 4: 148. doi: 10.3389/fpubh.2016.00148
59. Rauh VA, Garcia WE, Whyatt RM, Horton MK, Barr DB, Louis ED. Prenatal exposure to the organophosphate pesticide chlorpyrifos and childhood tremor. 2015; 51: 80. /pmc/articles/PMC4809635/
60. Mnif W, Hassine AIH, Bouaziz A, Bartegi A, Thomas O, Roig B. Effect of Endocrine Disruptor

Pesticides: A Review. 2011; 8(6): 2265. /pmc/articles/PMC3138025/
61. IARC Monographs Volume 112: evaluation of five organophosphate insecticides and herbicides. Lyon 2015 Mar [cited 2021 Dec 18]. www.iarc.who.int/wp-content/uploads/2018/07/MonographVolume112-1.pdf
62. Pesticide Action Network (Group). United Kingdom. Pesticides on a plate: a consumer guide to pesticide issues in the food chain. Pesticide Action Network UK 2007; 36.
63. Springmann M, Clark MA, Rayner M, Scarborough P, Webb P. The global and regional costs of healthy and sustainable dietary patterns: a modelling study. 2021; 5(11): e797–807. doi: 10.1016/S2542-5196(21)00251-5
64. Nyéléni. Declaration of Nyéléni. Sélingué 2007 [cited 2021 Dec 18]. www.nyeleni.org/IMG/pdf/DeclNyeleni-en.pdf
65. Kassam A, Friedrich T, Derpsch R. Global spread of Conservation Agriculture. 2018; 76(1): 29–51. doi: 10.1080/00207233.2018.1494927
66. Briske DD, Ash AJ, Derner JD, Huntsinger L. Commentary: A critical assessment of the policy endorsement for holistic management. 2014; 125: 50–53. doi: 10.1016/j.agsy.2013.12.001
67. Carter J, Jones A, O'Brien M, Ratner J, Wuerthner G. Holistic management: misinformation on the science of grazed ecosystems. 2014; 2014. doi: 10.1155/2014/163431
68. Garnett T, Godde C, Muller A, Röös E, Smith P, de Boer I, et al. Grazed and confused?: Ruminating on cattle, grazing systems, methane, nitrous oxide, the soil carbon sequestration question-and what it all means for greenhouse emissions. Oxford 2017 [cited 2021 Dec 18]. https://web.archive.org/web/20180422094122id_/https://www.fcrn.org.uk/sites/default/files/project-files/fcrn_gnc_report.pdf
69. U.S. call to action on climate, health, and equity: A policy action agenda. 2019 [cited 2021 Dec 18]. https://climatehealthaction.org/cta/climate-health-equity-policy/
70. Wellbery CE. Climate Change Health Impacts: A Role for the Family Physician. 2019; 100(10): 602–603. www.aafp.org/afp/2019/1115/od3.htm.

Abbreviations

AA	amino acid		element binding protein	ETR	erythematotelangiectatic and
AASK	African American Study of Kidney Disease and Hypertension	CKD	chronic kidney disease		
		CNS	central nervous system	EVOO	extra virgin olive oil
		COM-B	capability, opportunity, motivation and behaviour	FDA	Food and Drug Administration (USA)
AASLD	American Association for the Study of Liver Disease			FEV	forced expiratory volume
		COPD	chronic obstructive pulmonary disorder	FFA	free fatty acid
ACC	American College of Cardiology			FGF21	fibroblast growth factor 21
		CRC	colorectal cancer	FLiO	Fatty Liver in Obesity diet
AD	atopic dermatitis	CRP	C-reactive protein	FMD	fasting mimicking diet
ADA	American Diabetes Association	CU	chronic urticaria	FODMAP	fermentable oligo-di-mono-saccharides and polyols
		CV	cardiovascular		
AGA	anti-gliadin antibody	CVD	cardiovascular disease	FV	fruit and vegetable
AGEs	advanced glycation end products	dAGE	dietary advanced glycation end product	GABA	gamma-aminobutyric acid
				GBA	gut-brain axis
AHA	American Heart Association	DAL	dietary acid load	GC	gluten-containing
		DASH	Dietary Approaches to Stop Hypertension	GFD	gluten-free diet
AHEI	Alternative Healthy Eating Index			GHG	greenhouse gas
		DHA	docosahexaenoic acid	GI	gastrointestinal
AHI	apnoea-hypopnoea index	DII	Dietary Inflammatory Index	GIANT	Genetic Investigation of Anthropometric Traits
APP	amyloid precursor protein				
ART	artificial reproductive technology	DLD	diffuse lung disease	GLP	glucagon-like peptide
		DM	diabetes mellitus	GOLD	Global Initiative for Chronic Obstructive Lung Disease
ALA	alpha-linolenic acid	DNL	de novo lipogenesis		
ALT	alanine aminotransferase	DPA	docosapentaenoic acid		
ANS	autonomic nervous system	DUB	dysfunctional uterine bleeding	GORD	gastro-oesophageal reflux disease
ApoB	apolipoprotein B				
AST	aspartate aminotransferase	EASL	European Association for the Study of the Liver	GPx	glutathione peroxidase
ATP	adenosine triphosphate			HCA	heterocyclic amines
BBB	blood-brain barrier	ED	erectile dysfunction	HCP	health care professionals
BCAA	branched-chain amino acids	EFSA	European Food Safety Authority	HDL	high density lipoprotein
				HF	heart failure
BDA	British Dietetic Association	EGCG	epigallocatechin-3-gallate	HIF-1	hypoxia inducible factor
BDNF	brain derived neurotrophic factor	EMCC	European Mentoring and Coaching Council	HLA	human leukocyte antigen
				HMB	heavy menstrual bleeding
BMD	bone mineral density	eNOS	endothelial nitric oxide synthase	HPA	hypothalamic-pituitary-adrenal
BMI	body mass index				
BMR	basal metabolic rate	ENS	enteric nervous system		
BP	blood pressure	EPA	eicosapentaenoic acid	hPDI	healthy plant-based diet index
CA	conservation agriculture	EPC	endothelial progenitor cell		
CAC	coronary artery calcium score	EPIC	European Prospective Investigation into Cancer and Nutrition study	HR	Hazard Ratio
				HRT	hormone replacement therapy
CAD	coronary artery disease				
CD	coeliac disease	ESPEN	European Society for Clinical Nutrition and Metabolism	HS	hidradenitis suppurativa
CHD	coronary heart disease			hsCRP	high sensitivity C-reactive protein
CHO	carbohydrate				
ChREBP	carbohydrate response	ESRD	end stage renal disease	IARC	International Agency for

IBD	Research on Cancer inflammatory bowel disease	NK	natural killer cell	SBP	systolic blood pressure
		NNT	number needed to treat	SACN	Scientific Advisory Commission on Nutrition
IBS	irritable bowel syndrome	NO	nitric oxide	SCFA	short chain fatty acid
IBS-C	constipation dominant	NOC	N-nitroso compound	SERM	selective (o)estrogen receptor modulator
IBS-D	diarrhoea dominant	NREM	non-rapid eye movement		
IBS-M	mixed	NSAID	non-steroidal anti-inflammatory	SFA	saturated fatty acid
IDL	intermediate density lipoprotein	OAD	obstructive airway disease	SHBG	sex hormone binding globulin
IGF-1	insulin growth factor-1	OHS	obesity hypoventilation syndrome	SIBO	small intestine bacterial overgrowth
IHD	ischaemic heart disease	OI	ovulation infertility		
IL	interleukin	OR	odds ratio	SLE	systemic lupus erythematosus
IPF	idiopathic pulmonary fibrosis	OSA	obstructive sleep apnoea		
		PAH	polycyclic aromatic hydrocarbons	SREBP	sterol regulatory element-binding protein
IVUS	intravascular ultrasound				
KDOQI	Kidney Disease Outcomes Quality Initiative	PBD	plant-based diet	SSRI	selective serotonin reuptake inhibitor
		PCOS	polycystic ovary disease		
LA	linoleic acid	PDGF	platelet-derived growth factor	T2DM	type 2 diabetes mellitus
LDL	low density lipoprotein			TC	total cholesterol
LDL-C	low-density lipoprotein cholesterol	PDI	plant-based diet index	TEE	total energy expenditure
		PENG	Parenteral and Enteral Nutrition Group	TFA	trans fatty acid
LPS	lipopolysaccharides			TG	triglyceride
LRNI	lower recommended nutrient intake	PET	positron emission tomography	Tg-Ab	thyroglobulin antibody
				TMA	trimethylamine
LTC	long term condition	PH	pulmonary hypertension	TMAO	trimethylamine N-oxide
MD	Mediterranean diet	PID	pelvic inflammatory disease	TNF	tumour necrosis factor
MHT	menopausal hormone therapy			TPO-Ab	thyroid peroxidase antibody
		PNPLA3	patatin-like phospholipase domain containing 3		
MI	Motivational Interviewing			TRP	transient receptor potential
MIND	Mediterranean-DASH Intervention for Neurodegenerative Delay diet	POP	persistent organic pollutant	tTG	tissue transglutaminase
		PPAR	peroxisome proliferative-activated receptor	TTM	Transtheoretical Model
				UC	ulcerative colitis
MMP	metalloproteinase	PR	pulmonary rehabilitation	uPDI	unhealthy plant-based diet index
MNT	medical nutrition therapy	PREDIMED	Prevention with Mediterranean Diet study		
MPO	myeloperoxidase			USDA	United States Department of Agriculture
MS	multiple sclerosis	PSA	prostate specific antigen		
mTOR	mammalian target of rapamycin complex	PUFA	polyunsaturated fatty acid	VAT	visceral adipose tissue
		RA	rheumatoid arthritis	VEGF	vascular endothelial growth factor
MUFA	monounsaturated fatty acid	RAGE	receptor for advanced glycation end products		
NAFLD	non-alcoholic fatty liver disease			VLDL	very-low density lipoprotein
		RCT	randomised controlled trial		
NASH	non-alcoholic steatohepatitis	RDA	recommended daily allowance	WCRF	World Cancer Research Fund
NCD	non-communicable disease	RDI	recommended daily intake	WFPB	whole food plant-based
NCGS	non-coeliac gluten sensitivity	REE	resting energy expenditure	WHO	World Health Organization
		RNI	reference nutrient intake		
NHANES	National Health and Nutrition Examination Survey	ROS	reactive oxygen species		
		RR	relative risk		

Index

acid load, dietary (on kidney), 141, 244
acne inversa, 262–263
acne vulgaris, 255–257
action stage (of behavioural change), 286, 298
adenosine triphosphate (ATP), 273–274
adherence/compliance, 304
    to four lifestyle habits, 302
    to PBD, 11, 13, 50, 58, 59, 105, 122
adolescents (11-18; teenagers)
    mental wellbeing, 186
    requirements/recommended intakes, 30, 35–36
advanced glycation end products, 24–25
    asthma and, 95
    cardiovascular disease and, 52–53
    fertility and, 211
    insulin resistance and, 127
    polycystic ovary syndrome and, 206
Adventist Health Studies, 8
    Alzheimer's disease, 221
    autoimmune thyroid disease, 233
    body weight, 106
    bone health, 242
    cancer, 78
        colorectal, 167
    dementia, 221
    diabetes, 121–122
    hypertension, 54
    respiratory health, 90
aerobic glycolysis, 274
affirmations in Motivational Interviewing, 297
African American Study of Kidney Disease and Hypertension (AASK), 141
African microbiomes, 232
age, 27–43, 303–304
agriculture (farming), 315–330
    chemicals (agrochemicals), 77, 318–319, 320, 321, 322, 325
    industrial, 316–318, 322, 324
airflow limitation, spirometry, 93
alcohol, 309–310
    bone health and, 250
    cancer and, 79, 310
    dementia and, 223

endometriosis and, 199
fibroids and, 201
psoriasis and, 261
alkylating signature and processed and red meat consumption and colorectal cancer, 74
alpha-gal (α-gal) allergy, 264
alpha-linolenic acid (α-linolenic acid; ALA), 32, 37, 40
    athletes, 276
    cardiovascular disease and, 57
    dementia and, 223
    elderly, 40
    pregnancy/lactation and, 37
Alternative Healthy Eating Index 2010 (AHEI2010), 50
alternative therapies see complementary therapies
Alzheimer's disease, 219–227
American Association for the Study of Liver Disease (AASLD), 157
American Association of Clinical Endocrinologists, 15, 125
American Cancer Society, 77, 80
American College of Cardiology (ACC), 15, 46
    Prevention of Cardiovascular Disease Council, 57
    Nutrition and Lifestyle Committee for, 58
American College of Endocrinology, 15
American College of Lifestyle Medicine, 15, 16, 125, 301, 303, 312, 326
American Diabetic Association (ADA), 109, 124–125
American Heart Association (AHA), 9, 46, 49, 52, 58
American Institute for Cancer Research, 79
amino acids
    in animal protein, insulin resistance and, 128
    essential, 12
    athletes, 276–277
2-amino-1-methyl-6-phenylimidazo[4,5-b]pyridine (PhIP), 76

anaemia see iron-deficiency anaemia
anaerobic glycolysis, 274
anatabine, 235–236
animal(s), farmed, 321
    grazing, 318, 319, 326
    inclusive responsibility and use of, 325–326
animal foods (incl. animal-based foods and diet)
    cancer and, 73–74
    hyperphosphataemia and, 142
    kidney health and, 140–141
    in PBD, 9
animal protein, 11, 12
    fertility and, 216
    insulin resistance and, 128
    non-alcoholic fatty liver disease, 152
    weight management and, 110–111
anisakiasis and urticaria, fish, 264
anthocyanin-rich fruit, 236
antibiotics in agriculture, 321, 322
anticancer phytonutrients, 70–71, 72
anti-inflammatory effects (of foods)
    cardiovascular disease and, 51–52
    obesity and, 114
antioxidants, 13
    cardiovascular disease and, 53
    diabetes and, 128
    respiratory health and, 92–93, 94
antipsychotic medication, 189, 190
anxiety, 181, 183, 184, 185, 189
apigenin, 71
apoprotein B, 47
appetite, 113
    overeating and, 104
arthritis, rheumatoid, 235
artificial reproductive technology, 210
assisted (artificial) reproductive technology, 210
asthma, 94–96
atherosclerosis (and atherosclerotic plaque), 46–49, 50–51
    kidney disease and, 141
    Tsimane tribe, 46
Atherosclerosis Risk in Communities study, 140, 143

*Illustrations (figures and tables) are comprehensively referred to from the text. Therefore, significant items in illustrations have only been given a page reference in the absence of their concomitant mention in the text referring to that illustration.
**Abbreviation: PBD, plant-based diet.

athletes, 271–284
Atkins diet, 106
    see also Eco-Atkins diet
atopic dermatitis (eczema), 259–261
ATP (adenosine triphosphate), 273–274
Australia, mental wellbeing study, 186
autoimmunity, 229–239
    effectiveness of PBD, 232
    environmental influences, 230
    epidemiology, 230
    latent autoimmune diabetes (type 1.5), 131
automatic motivation, 288, 293, 294

bariatric surgery, 105
basal metabolic rate, 272
BDA (British Dietetic Association), 16, 39, 169, 303
bed head elevation in gastro-oesophageal reflux disease, 165
behavioural change
    eating
        enabling, 294–296
        motivation see motivation
        patient strategies, 292
        practitioner strategies, 292–299
        theory, 285–287
    facilitating health change, 302–303
beta-glucan fibre, 183
beverages see drinks
bioactive compounds, 70–71, 223, 230, 235, 236, 236
Biobank studies (UK), 54, 173, 224
biodiversity, agricultural, 318–322
bioflavonoids (flavonoids), 13, 223
biomass, crop, 325
biosphere integrity, 315–316
bipolar disorder, 189, 190
bleeding (menstrual), heavy, 201
blood pressure, high see hypertension
Blue Zones, 3, 57, 310–311
body
    composition, bone health and, 246
    weight see weight
body mass index (BMI), 103, 104, 106
Bolivian Tsimane tribe, 45–46
bone health/status, 241–253
    factors influencing, 243
    strength assessment, 243
    vegans, 241–242
        elderly, 38–39, 245
    see also fractures
boron, 249

Bouchardat, Apollinaire, 128
bowel see colorectum; gastrointestinal tract; inflammatory bowel disease; irritable bowel syndrome; microbiome
brain, 181
    degenerative disease (neurodegeneration), 219, 220
    gut microbiome and, 182–183
branched-chain amino acids, 12
breast cancer, 82
breastfeeding and lactation, 36–38
    eczema and, 259, 260
brewer's yeast and hidradenitis suppurativa, 263
British Dietetic Association, 16, 39, 169, 303
BROAD study, 9, 109, 126
Buettner, Dan, 3
Burkina Faso, paediatric diet, 232

C-reactive protein (CRP)
    cardiovascular disease and, 45, 52
    rheumatoid arthritis, 235
caffeine, athletes, 281
calcium, 28–29
    age and, 28–29, 30–31
    elderly, 39
    athletes, 278–279
    bone health and, 248, 249, 250
    pregnancy/lactation, 36–37
calcium 'thieves', 250
calories, athlete requirements, 272
    see also low-energy (low calorie) diets/foods
Campbell, Dr T Colin, 8
Canada, 16
cancer (malignancy), 69–87
    alcohol and, 79, 310
    colorectal see colorectum
    comorbidities, 77–78
    lung, 5, 75
    meat and see meat
    pathophysiology and mechanisms of development, 69–73
    PBD following diagnosis of, 82
    prevention, 78–81
    treatment, 81–82
capability to change to PBD, 289–290
carbohydrates, 274–275
    athletes, 274–275
    fermentable, irritable bowel syndrome and, 169–170
    non-alcoholic fatty liver disease and, 152–153

see also high-carbohydrate diets; low-carbohydrate diets
carbon dioxide (CO_2) and other greenhouse gases, 316, 317, 319
carbonated fizzy drinks, 250
carcinogens (specific diet-related), 73–77
cardiometabolic diseases and severe mental illness, 189
cardiovascular disease (CVD), 45–67
    Alzheimer's disease and, 221
    depression and, 187
    erectile dysfunction and, 207
    Mediterranean diet and, 7, 15, 49, 50, 58
    national and international dietary guidelines, 15
    non-alcoholic fatty liver disease and, 157
    Portfolio diet, 8
    respiratory health and, 90
    risk factors for, 54
    trimethylamine N-oxide (TMAO) and, 14, 53
    see also microvascular complications
Cardiovascular Disease Prevention and Reversal: The Esselstyn Program, 297–298
CARDIVEG study, 56
carnitine, 74, 140–141
    supplements for athletes, 281
carotenoids, 13
    bone health and, 246
chamomile tea, menstrual period problems, 202
change talk, 295, 296, 297, 299
    see also behaviour
chemicals in agriculture (agrochemicals), 77, 318–319, 320, 321, 322, 325
chemotherapy and fasting mimicking diet, 82
children (paediatric persons), 32–35
    asthma, 95
    B12 supplements, 28
    eczema, 259, 260
    mental wellbeing, 186
    multiple sclerosis, 234
    Western vs African diet, 232
    see also infants and toddlers
China, bone health study, 245
China-Cornell-Oxford Project, 8
CHIP (Complete Health Improvement Programme), 192
cholesterol, 51, 54
    elevated (hypercholesterolaemia), 54–55
    lipid heart hypothesis and, 48

*Illustrations (figures and tables) are comprehensively referred to from the text. Therefore, significant items in illustrations have only been given a page reference in the absence of their concomitant mention in the text referring to that illustration.
**Abbreviation: PBD, plant-based diet.

reduction/lowering, 55
    foods, 7–8, 51, 56
    see also National Cholesterol Education Programme
choline, 14, 53, 128, 140–141
chromium, polycystic ovary syndrome, 207
chronic (physical) disease
    cancer risk and, 77–78
    lifestyle habits and their connection with, 302
    prevention, mechanisms, 13–15
chronic obstructive pulmonary disease (COPD), 90–94
Clean Label Project on protein powers, 281
climate change/breakdown, 315–316, 316, 319–320, 326
clinical nutritional trials, types, 3–6
clinicians see health professionals
coeliac disease, 168–169
coffee and bone health, 250
    see also caffeine
cognitive ability to change to PBD, 289
cognitive symptoms, psychosis, 190
colitis, ulcerative, 172–173
colorectum (large bowel)
    cancer, 73–74, 74, 82, 164, 166–168
        butyrate and, 164
        dairy and, 76, 77, 167–168
        fibre and, 82
        haem iron and, 75
        red meat and, 12–13, 74, 167
        whole plant foods and, 80
    diverticula, 165–166
    see also gastrointestinal tract; inflammatory bowel disease; irritable bowel syndrome; microbiome
community, interventions in, 16–17
complementary (alternative) therapies
    endometriosis, 199
    menopause, 204
Complete Health Improvement Programme (CHIP), 192
compliance see adherence
confounding variable, 4–5
conservation agriculture, 324–326
constipation
    dialysis and, 145
    in irritable bowel syndrome, 169
consultations, behavioural change, 294–299
contemplation stage (of behavioural change), 286, 298
COPD see chronic obstructive pulmonary disease
copper, 249
coronary (ischaemic) heart disease (CAD/CHD), 8, 45–46, 48–53, 197
    epigenetics and, 53

Finnish mortalities, 16–17
    primary prevention, 49
    secondary prevention, 49–50
    see also myocardial infarction
coronavirus (COVID-19), 17–18
Counterpoint Trial, 128–129, 303
country-based dietary guidelines, 15–16
COVID-19, 17–18
cow's milk allergy, 260
creatine (phosphate), 273, 281
    supplements (athletes), 281
Crohn's disease, 172–173
crops and conservation agriculture, 325
cruciferous vegetables, 71, 76
Cunningham equation, 272
curcumin, 70
cutaneous diseases, 255–269
CVD see cardiovascular disease
cysteine, 12
Czech Republic, diabetes, 125

daidzein, 199, 203, 244
dairy (milk products)
    acne and, 256, 257
    calcium in, 248
    cancer and, 76–77
        colorectal, 76, 77, 167–168
    cardiovascular disease and, 56
    eczema (children) and maternal intake of, 259
    hidradenitis suppurativa and, 263
    see also lacto-ovo vegetarian diet; lacto-vegetarian diet
Danish dietary guidelines, 16
DASH (Dietary Approaches to Stop Hypertension), 6, 9, 54, 58
    Alzheimer's disease and, 221
    diabetes and, 122
    non-alcoholic fatty liver disease and, 154, 157
deaths (from disease)
    chronic kidney disease and, 143
    low-carbohydrate diets and, 130
    weight and, 103
    WHO factsheets on leading causes of, 91, 92
deforestation, 318
dementia (incl. Alzheimer's), 219–227
Denmark (Danish) dietary guidelines, 16
depression, 181, 183, 184, 185, 186, 187–188, 192
    prevention, 187
    treatment, 187–188
dermatological conditions, 255–269
destruction, forests, 318
developed countries see high-income countries

DEXA scan, 243
DHA see docosahexaenoic acid
diabetes, 121–137
    mental wellbeing and, 186
    type 1, 131
    type 1.5 (type 3/latent autoimmune), 131
    type 2 (and unspecified or in general), 15, 121–130, 131
        alternative treatments, 128–130
        complications, 125–126
        lifestyle factors, 124, 303
        prevention, 121–123
        treatment and remission with PBD, 124–125
    see also insulin
dialysis, 140, 143, 144, 144–145
diarrhoea-predominant irritable bowel syndrome, 169
dicarbonyls, 127
diet
    age and, 27–43, 303–304
    healthy/therapeutic, 6–11
        age and planning of, 32
        core components, 2
        patterns, 6–9
        international guidelines see international dietary guidelines
        national guidelines, 15–16
        quality indices, 9–11
    see also foods and specific (types of) diets
Dietary Portfolio (Portfolio diet), 7–8, 56
differential stress resistance between healthy and cancer cells, 81
digestive system see gastrointestinal tract
DIRECT trial, 129
diseases/medical conditions (in general)
    alcohol and, 309, 310
    chronic see chronic disease
    deaths from see deaths
    exercise and its lack and, 304, 305
    foods fighting, increasing intake, 155
    foods promoting, reducing intake, 155
    infectious see infections
    PBD impact on, 1–26
    sleep and, 305, 306
    smoking and, 309
    stress and, 307
    see also health
diverticular disease, 165–166
docosahexaenoic acid (DHA), 32
    athletes, 276
    cardiovascular disease and, 57
    elderly, 40
    pregnancy/lactation and, 37
doctors see health professionals
dopamine, 183

reward system and, 113
drinks (beverages)
    fizzy, 250
    weight management and, 112
drug therapy *see* medical therapy
Dutch (Netherlands) studies, diabetes, 122, 123
dysbiosis (intestinal), 72, 164, 183, 230, 231–232, 261
dyslipidaemia (lipid dysregulation), 15
    Alzheimer's disease and, 220
    see also hypercholesterolaemia
dysmenorrhoea, 201

Eat-Lancet Commission on Food, Planet and Health, 15, 16, 316, 323
eating behaviour *see* behaviour
Eco-Atkins diet, 130
ecosystems, 315, 316, 324–325
    services, 320, 325
eczema, 259–261
eggs
    cholesterol and, 55
    diabetes and, 123
    eczema and, 259, 260
eicosapentaenoic acid (EPA), 32, 37, 40
    athletes, 276
    cardiovascular disease and, 57
    pregnancy/lactation and, 37
elderly vegans, 38–40
    bone health, 38–39, 245
ellagic acid, 71
emotional health *see* mental health
empathic connection, 294, 296
endocrinology
    endocrine disrupters
        microplastics, 77
        pesticides, 322
        soya, 204
    weight and, 113
endometriosis, 197–200
endothelium and cardiovascular disease, 46, 52, 57
energy, 271–278
    athlete requirements, 271–278
    expenditure, 271–273
    high-energy density foods/diets, infants and toddlers, 34
    low-energy density diets/foods, 109–110, 272
    protein as source of *see* protein
    reducing intake or increasing expenditure, 113

systems, 273–274
engagement in Motivational Interviewing, 295
enteric nervous system, 182
environmental factors
    autoimmune disease, 230
    behavioural change, 290–292
EPA *see* eicosapentaenoic acid
EPIC *see* European Prospective Investigation into Cancer and nutrition study
epidemiology and epidemiological studies, 4
    cardiovascular disease, 45
epigallocatechin-3-gallate, 70
epigenetics
    cancer, 70
    cardiovascular disease, 53
    eczema and, 259
    obesity, 104
erectile dysfunction, 207–209
ergogenic aids, 280–281
erythematotelangiectatic rosacea, 257
Esseltyne Program, 297–298
essential amino acids *see* amino acids
ethics with food and agriculture system, 323
European Association for the Study of the Liver (EASL), 151
European Prospective Investigation into Cancer and nutrition (EPIC) study, 90, 106, 121
    Dutch segment, 123
    EPIC-InterAct study, 123
    Greek segment, 7
    Norfolk segment, 185
    Oxford (UK) component, 54, 59, 121, 142, 167, 241, 242
evidence (medical)
    hierarchies of, 3
    in lifestyle medicine, 301–302
evoking in Motivational Interviewing, 295
exercise (physical), 304–305
    athletes, 271–284
    impact, 304–305
    in lifestyle medicine, 304–305
        exploring barriers, 305
        prescribing, 304, 305
    older people, 40
extrapulmonary/extrathoracic restriction, 98
eye, rosacea affecting (ocular rosacea), 257, 258

farming *see* agriculture
fasting during cancer treatment, 81–82
fat (dietary - in general), 275–276
    athletes and, 275–276
    bone health and, 244–245
    dementia and, 222
    fertility and, 209–210
    gastro-oesophageal reflux disease and, 165
    see also low-fat (plant-based) diet
fatty acids (and fats)
    free, non-alcoholic fatty liver disease and, 149–150
    long-chain *see* alpha-linolenic acid; docosahexaenoic acid; eicosapentaenoic acid
    omega-3 *see* omega-3 fatty acids
    omega-6 *see* omega-6 fatty acids
    saturated *see* saturated fat/fatty acids
    short-chain *see* short-chain fatty acids
    trans, 55, 222
    unsaturated *see* unsaturated fats/fatty acids
fatty liver disease, non-alcoholic, 149–161
females *see* women
fermentable oligo-di-monosaccharides and polyols (FODMAPs), diet low in, 169–170
ferritin, 29
    athletes, 279
    diabetes and, 128
fertility, 209–211
fibre (dietary), 80
    bone health and, 245–246
    cardiovascular disease and, 55–56
    colorectal cancer and, 80
    deficiency, 164, 166
    dementia and, 223
    diverticular disease and, 165–166
    elderly, 39–40
    gastro-oesophageal reflux disease, 165
    irritable bowel syndrome and, 170
    kidney disease and uraemic toxins and, 143
    non-alcoholic fatty liver disease and, 155–156
    polycystic ovary syndrome and, 206
fibroids, 200–201
Finland, 48, 56
    FINGER study (Geriatric Intervention Study to Prevent Cognitive Impairment and Disability), 224
    North Karelia Project, 16–17, 48

---

*Illustrations (figures and tables) are comprehensively referred to from the text. Therefore, significant items in illustrations have only been given a page reference in the absence of their concomitant mention in the text referring to that illustration.
**Abbreviation: PBD, plant-based diet.

fish
- anisakiasis and urticaria, 264
- colorectal cancer and, 167–168
- eczema (children) and maternal intake, 259–260
- fibroids and, 200
- polyunsaturated fatty acids (PUFAs), 262
- psoriasis and, 262
- *see also* pesco-vegetarian diet

fishing, 321
fizzy drinks, 250
flavonoids, 13
- dementia and, 223

flexitarian (casual vegetarian), 2
FLiO (Fatty Liver in Obesity) diet, 157
fluid intake
- elderly, 39
- training, 280

focusing in Motivational Interviewing, 295
FODMAPs, diet low in, 169–170
folate/folic acid
- elderly, 39
- male fertility, 210
- pregnancy, 36, 210

foods, 315–320
- allergy, 171
  - eczema and, 259, 260
  - hidradenitis suppurativa and, 264
  - urticaria and, 264
- animal *see* animal foods
- disease-fighting, increasing intake, 155
- disease-promoting, reducing intake, 155
- intolerances, 171–172
- processed *see* processed food
- sovereignty, 324
- specific/individual (and nutrients)
  - cardiovascular disease and, 56–57
  - dementia and, 222–224
  - diabetes risk and, 122–123
  - mental health/wellbeing and, 185
- systems and choices, 15, 315–330
- thermic effects, 113
- trigger, gastro-oesophageal reflux disease, 164
- ultraprocessed, 79
- *see also* diet

forests
- destruction, 318
- renewal (reforestation), 326

fortified soya foods, 249–250
fractures
- elderly vegans, 38
- osteoporotic, 242, 243

Framingham Study, 48
free fatty acids and non-alcoholic fatty liver disease, 149–150

French NutriNet Santé study, 77
fructose
- insulin resistance and, 126, 127
- non-alcoholic fatty liver disease and, 152

fruit and/or vegetable consumption
- anthocyanin-rich fruit, 236
- asthma (children) and, 95
- bioactive compounds in, 70–71, 223, 230, 235, 236, 236
- bone health and, 245
- cancer and, 80
- COPD and, 93
- dementia and, 222–223
- diabetes and, 123
- endometriosis and, 198
- erectile dysfunction and, 208
- kidney disease (chronic) and, 141, 142
- mental health and, 186
- multiple sclerosis and, 233–234
- rheumatoid arthritis and, 235

α-gal (alpha-gal) allergy, 264
gastrointestinal tract (digestive system; gut), 163–179
- disorders, 163–179
- microbiome *see* microbiome

gastro-oesophageal reflux disease (GORD), 164–165
GEICO (Government Employees Insurance Company), 109, 189
gender/sex-specific health considerations, 197–217
genetics
- obesity, 104
- osteoporosis, 242–243
- *see also* epigenetics

genistein
- bone health and, 244, 249
- cancer and, 70
- endometriosis and, 199
- menopause and, 203, 204
- psoriasis and, 262

GIANT (Genetic Investigation of Anthropometric Traits), 104
ginger, menstrual period problems, 202
gingerol, 71
Global BMI Mortality Collaboration, 103
Global Burden of Disease Project, 12
Global Burden of Disease Study (from 2019), 1
global dimensions (worldwide)
- food systems, 15, 315–330
- non-alcoholic fatty liver disease prevalence and burden, 150
- *see also* international dietary guidelines

Global Initiative for Chronic Obstructive Lung Disease, 94
Global Nutrition Report (2021), 1
GLP-1 (glucagon-like peptide), 113, 128
glucagon, 111
glucagon-like peptide (GLP-1), 113, 128
gluconeogenesis, 274
glucose *see* gluconeogenesis; glycaemic control; glycaemic index; glycolysis
gluten, 168
- intolerance (non-coeliac sensitivity), 168, 171
- psoriasis and, 261–262

gluten enteropathy (coeliac disease), 168–169
gluten-free diet/foods, 168, 262
- psoriasis, 262
- vegan, 106

glycaemic control, 123, 124, 125, 126, 129
glycaemic index (GI), 9–10
- acne and, 256
- anxiety and, 189
- hidradenitis suppurativa and, 263, 264

glycation, advanced end products *see* advanced glycation end products
glycogen and athletes, 274–275
N-glycolylneuraminic acid, 233
glycolysis, 273–274
glyphosate, 322
Government Employees Insurance Company (GEICO), 109, 189
grains, whole, cancer and, 80
Graves' disease, 233
grazing (farmed animals), 318, 319, 326
Greece
- in European Prospective Investigation into Cancer and nutrition (EPIC) study, 7
- Ikaria, 3, 57

green Mediterranean diet, 7, 157
Green Revolution, industrial, 316–317, 320, 324, 325
green tea and weight management, 112
greenhouse gases (GHGs incl. carbon dioxide/CO2), 316, 317, 319
gut, 232
- anxiety and, 189
- brain connections with, 183–184
- microbiome *see* microbiome
- profile, plant-based/vegan diet, 232
- *see also* gastrointestinal tract

gynaecological health, 197–209

habits and motivation to change to PBD, 288
haem iron, 52, 74, 75, 128, 199, 231, 232
haemodialysis, 140, 143, 144, 144–145
haemorrhagic stroke, 59

Harris–Benedict equation, 272
Hashimoto disease, 242
HDL (high-density lipoprotein), 47, 48
HeAL (Healthy Active Lives), 189
health, human (in general), 321–322
    impact on
        PBD, 1–26
        sleep, 306
        social connections, 310–311
    see also disease
health, planetary, 15, 315–330
health professionals (healthcare practitioners; clinicians; doctors; physicians) roles
    behavioural change, 292–299, 303, 304
    planetary health, 326–327
Health Professionals Follow-up study, 11, 56, 74, 78, 122, 123, 130, 166
Healthy Active Lives (HeAL), 189
Healthy Eating Index, 9
    Alternative, 9, 50
heart
    coronary disease see coronary heart disease
    healthy, 46–48
        mechanisms underpinning, 51–53
    lipid heart hypothesis, 48–49
HELFIMED (Healthy Eating for Life with a Mediterranean Diet), 188
herbal remedies, endometriosis, 199–200
herbicides (and pesticides in general), 77, 317, 318–319, 322
heterocyclic amines, 75–76, 151
hidradenitis suppurativa, 262–263
high-carbohydrate diets, athletes, 275
high-density lipoprotein (HDL), 47, 48
high-energy density foods/diets, infants and toddlers, 34
high-income (developed) countries
    behavioural change, 288, 290
    chronic disease, 302
    colorectal cancer, 166
high-protein diets
    athletes, 277
    autoimmunity and, 231
Hill Criteria, 5
hip fractures in osteoporosis, 242, 243
HOLISM study, 233–234
hydration, athletes, 280
    see also fluid intake
hypercholesterolaemia, 54–55
hyperkalaemia, 143–144
hyperphosphataemia, 142–143

hypersensitivity, food, 171–172
hypertension, 141–142
    kidney disease as cause or consequence of, 141–142
    pulmonary, 96
    systemic/arterial, 54
hypoventilation in obesity, 97–98

identity (personal) and motivation to change to PBD, 288
Ikaria, 3, 57
immune response, 229
    gut microbiome and, 17, 229
    see also autoimmunity
inclusively responsible food and agriculture system, 322–326
indole-3-carbinol, 71
    industrial agriculture, 316–318, 322, 324
industry, pollutants, 77
infants and toddlers (birth to 2 or 3 years), 32–34
    eczema, 259, 260
infections
    autoimmune disease and, 230
    zoonotic, 321–322
infertility, 209–211
inflammation (chronic), 13, 229–239
    cancer and, 72
    cardiovascular disease and, 51–52
    mental disorders and, 183–184
    obesity and, 114
inflammatory bowel disease (IBD), 172–173
inositol
    bone health and, 246
    polycystic ovary syndrome and, 207
insecticides (and pesticides in general), 77, 317, 318–319, 322
insulin, 111, 130, 131
    resistance, 113, 124, 126–128, 206
    cancer and, 73
    hidradenitis suppurativa and, 263
    prevention mechanisms (with PBDs), 126–128
    therapeutic use, 131
insulin growth factor-1 (IGF-1), 76
    acne and, 256
    cancer and, 76
    hidradenitis suppurativa and, 263
intensive care unit (ICU), 99
intermediate-density lipoprotein (IDL), 47, 48
International Agency for Research on Cancer (IARC), 73, 74, 77, 79, 167

international dietary guidelines, 15–16
    cancer prevention, 79–80
    see also global dimensions
international dimensions see global dimensions; international dietary guidelines
International Organisation for the Study of Inflammatory Bowel Diseases, 173
intestine see colorectum; gastrointestinal tract; inflammatory bowel disease; irritable bowel syndrome; microbiome
iodine, 29, 37, 210–211
    age-related recommended intakes, 30–31
    birth to 3 year-olds, 34
    athletes, 280
    fertility and, 210–211
    pregnancy/lactation and, 37
Iran, Tehran Lipid and Glucose Study (TLGS), 139
iron, 29, 37
    age-related requirements/recommended intakes, 30–31
    birth to 3 year-olds, 30, 33
    athletes, 279
    haem, 52, 74, 75, 128, 199, 231, 232
    non-haem, 29, 75
    pregnancy, 37
iron-deficiency anaemia
    athletes and, 279
    heavy periods and, 202
    pregnancy and, 37
irritable bowel syndrome, 169–171
ischaemic heart disease see coronary heart disease
ischaemic stroke, 58, 59
isoflavones
    bone health and, 249
    diffuse lung disease and, 96–97
    menopause and, 203, 204
    psoriasis and, 262

Japanese
    depression prevention, 187
    Ni-Hon San Study, 48

Kempner, Walter, 124, 126
ketogenic diet, 129–130, 231
kidney, 139–149
    chronic disease (CKD), 139–143, 143
    complications, 141–143
    incidence and progression, 139–141

---

*Illustrations (figures and tables) are comprehensively referred to from the text. Therefore, significant items in illustrations have only been given a page reference in the absence of their concomitant mention in the text referring to that illustration.
**Abbreviation: PBD, plant-based diet.

potential concerns of PBD, 143–144
dietary acid load, 141, 244
end-stage disease, 140
stones, 145

lactation *see* breastfeeding and lactation
lactic acid and lactate, 274
Lactobacilli and rheumatoid arthritis, 234
lacto-ovo vegetarian diet, 2
lacto-vegetarian diet, 2
Lancet
 Eat-Lancet Commission on Food, Planet and Health, 15, 16, 316, 323
 Lancet Commission on Obesity (2019), 316
land use change, 318
large bowel *see* colorectum
Laron syndrome, 256
latent autoimmune diabetes (type 1.5), 131
LDL *see* low-density lipoprotein
legumes and cancer, 80–81
leiomyomas, uterine, 200–201
leucine and acne, 257
lifestyle factors (and modification/intervention)
 acne, 255–256
 bone health, 242, 243, 250
 cancer, 77–78, 81
 chronic disease burden and, 302
 dementia prevention, 224
 diabetes type 2, 124, 303
 endometriosis, 200
 erectile dysfunction, 207–208
 irritable bowel syndrome, 170–171
 menstrual period problems, 202
 obesity, 105
 pillars, 303–311
 polycystic ovary syndrome, 205
lifestyle medicine (and lifestyle modification/therapeutic interventions), 16–17, 301–313
 bone health, 243
 future, 311–312
 hierarchies of evidence applied to (HEALM), 5
 meaning of, 301–302
Lifestyle Medicine Global Alliance (LMGA), 312
lignans and menopause, 203
D-limonene, 71
linoleic acid (LA), 7, 37, 140
α-linolenic acid *see* alpha-linolenic acid
lipid(s), 47–49
 dysregulation *see* dyslipidaemia; hypercholesterolaemia
 lowering, 56
lipid heart hypothesis, 48–49

lipoprotein(s), 47
 high-density (HDL), 47, 48
 intermediate-density (IDL), 47, 48
 low-density *see* low-density lipoprotein
 very-low-density, 47, 48
lipoprotein(a) (Lp(a)), 47, 48
liver disease, non-alcoholic fatty, 149–161
Loma Linda, 3
loneliness, 311
long-chain fatty acids *see* alpha-linolenic acid; docosahexaenoic acid; eicosapentaenoic acid
low-calorie diets *see* low-energy diets/foods
low-carbohydrate diets
 diabetes and, 129–130
 unhealthy, 47
low-density lipoprotein (LDL), 55
 atherosclerosis and, 46, 47, 49, 50, 51
 non-alcoholic fatty liver disease and, 155
low-energy (low calorie) diets/foods, 109–110, 272
 immune system and, 272
 very, 128–129
low-fat (plant-based) diet, 105, 113, 129
 athletes, 276
 body weight and, 109, 111
 cardiovascular disease and, 49
low-income (resource poor) countries
 leading causes of deaths, WHO factsheet, 92
 non-alcoholic fatty liver disease, 150
lung (pulmonary) disease
 cancer, 5, 75
 diffuse, 96
 obstructive *see* chronic obstructive pulmonary/airway disease
 restrictive, 98
luteolin, 71
lycopene, 71
Lyon Diet Heart Study, 7, 50, 51

macronutrients
 bone health and, 244–246
 optimal ratio, 273
 see also carbohydrate; fat; protein
magnesium and bone health, 248
maintenance stage (of behavioural change), 286, 298
males *see* men
malignancy *see* cancer
malnutrition, 321
 elderly vegans, 38
manganese, 248
marine environment and fishing, 321
maternal factors, childhood eczema, 259, 259–260

meal size and timing and gastro-oesophageal reflux disease, 164
meat, 173, 290
 chronic inflammation and autoimmune disease and, 231–232
 cooking, 128, 259
 digestive health and, 173
 eczema and maternal consumption of, 259
 endometriosis and, 199
 fibroids and, 200
 identity as eater of, 288
 red *see* red meat
medical conditions *see* diseases
medical evidence *see* evidence
medical nutrition therapy, polycystic ovary syndrome, 206
medical therapy (incl. drugs)
 gastro-oesophageal reflux disease, 164
 hidradenitis suppurativa, 262–263
 menopause, 203
 polycystic ovary syndrome, 207
 psychosis, 189, 190
Mediterranean diet, 6–7
 Alzheimer's disease and, 220–221
 cardiovascular disease and, 7, 15, 49, 50, 58
 depression treatment, 188
 diabetes and, 122
 erectile dysfunction and, 208
 green, 7, 157
 non-alcoholic fatty liver disease and, 154
men (males), 207–209
 fertility, 209–211
menopause (and postmenopausal women), 202–204
 bone health, 242, 243, 245, 246
 vitamin B6 and B12 supplements, 247
 weight, 106
menstrual problems, 201–202
mental (psychological/emotional) health, 191–196
 biological mechanisms of diet affecting, 181–185
 diabetes diagnosis impacting on, 126
 severe disorders, 189–190
metabolic acidosis, 141
metalloproteinases, 52
metformin, polycystic ovary syndrome, 207
methionine, 12
microbiome (gut/intestine), 14–15, 53, 163–164
 antipsychotics and, 190
 autoimmune disease and, 230, 231
  rheumatoid arthritis, 234
 brain and, 182–183

cancer and, 73, 75, 80, 81
cardiovascular disease and, 53
COVID-19 and, 17
diabetes and, 127, 128
digestive health and, 163–164
dysbiosis, 72, 164, 183, 230, 231–232, 261
erectile dysfunction and, 209–210
fibre and, 80
immune response and, 17, 229
inflammation (chronic) and autoimmune disease and, 231–232
kidney disease and uraemic toxins and, 143
Slovenian study, 232
weight regulation and, 112
micronutrients
    acne and, 257
    athletes, 278–280
    bone health and, 246–250
microplastics, 77
microvascular complications, diabetes, 126
milk products *see* dairy
Millennium Ecosystem Assessment, 315
Million Women study, 77
minerals and bone health, 248–249
monounsaturated fatty acids (MUFAs), 8, 49, 57, 155
mortalities *see* deaths
mothers as factor in childhood eczema, 259, 259–260
motivation (to change to PBD), 287–289
    automatic, 288, 293, 294
    intrinsic, 294, 295
    Motivational Interviewing (MI), 294–295, 296, 298, 299
    reflective, 287, 288, 293, 294
Mount Abu Open Heart Trial, 51
mTOR
    acne and, 256–257, 257
    American diet and, 151
Multiethnic Study of Atherosclerosis (MESA), 139
multiple sclerosis, 233–234
muscle strength loss (sarcopenia), 244, 246
mushrooms, vitamin D, 28
myeloperoxidases, 52
myocardial infarction (MI), Lyon Diet Heart Study, 7, 50

N-nitroso compounds (incl. nitrosamines), 74, 128
National Cancer Institute, 76

National Cholesterol Education Programme (NCEP) in USA, 9, 106
national dietary guidelines, 15–16
National Health and Nutrition Examination Survey (NHANES), 90, 95, 130
National Kidney Foundation's Kidney Disease Outcomes Quality Initiative (KDOQI), 141
negative symptoms, psychosis, 189, 190
nephrology *see* kidney
Netherlands (Dutch) studies, diabetes, 122, 123
Neu5Gc, 233
neural tube defects and folate, 36, 210
neurodegeneration, 219, 220
neuropathy, diabetic, 126
New Zealand
    BROAD study, 9, 109, 126
    mental wellbeing study, 186
NFκ-B, 72–73
NHANES (National Health and Nutrition Examination Survey), 90, 95, 130
Nicoya Peninsula, 3
Ni-Hon San Study, 48
nitrates
    athletes and, 281
    cancer and, 74
    cardiovascular disease and, 52
    erectile dysfunction and, 208
    polluting, 322
nitric oxide, 46
    erectile dysfunction and, 207–208
nitrites, 167
    cancer and, 74
    cardiovascular disease and, 52
    diabetes and, 128
nitroso compounds (incl. nitrosamines), 74, 128
non-alcoholic fatty liver disease, 149–161
non-alcoholic steatohepatitis (NASH), 149, 150, 151, 153, 155, 156, 157, 158
non-REM (NREM) sleep, 306
Norfolk, EPIC, 185
North American Research Committee on MS, 234
North Karelia Project, 16–17, 48
nuclear factor kappa-B, 72–73
Nurses' Health Study, 11, 53, 56, 74, 122–123, 165, 167, 183, 199, 221, 247
nut(s), (mixed), erectile dysfunction, 208
nutrients, plants sources of various types, 31
    see also food; macronutrients; micronutrients

nutritional studies, types, 3–6

OARS acronym in Motivational Interviewing, 295, 297
obesity and overweight, 103–120
    BMI as measure of, 103
    bone health and, 246
    cancer and, 73
    central obesity, 246, 262
    COPD and, 94
    eczema and, 260
    erectile dysfunction and, 209
    genetics, 104
    hidradenitis suppurativa and, 263
    mental health and, 184–185
    pandemic, 216
    psoriasis and, 261
obesity hypoventilation syndrome, 97–98
observational studies, 3, 5
    weight gain, 106
obstructive pulmonary/airway disease
    chronic (COPD), 90–94
    smoking-related, 92, 93
obstructive sleep apnoea, 96–97
ocular rosacea, 257, 258
oestrogens, plant (phyto-oestrogens), 199, 200, 203
older people *see* elderly
olive oil
    bone health and, 245
    cardiovascular disease and, 57
omega-3 fatty acids, 32
    athletes, 276
    bone health and, 244–245
    cardiovascular disease and, 57
    elderly, 40
    infertility and, 309
    mental disorders and, 185
    polycystic ovary syndrome and, 207
    pregnancy/lactation and, 37
    short-chain *see* short-chain fatty acids
omega-6 fatty acids, 7, 244–245
    athletes, 276
One Blue Dot campaign, 16
open-ended questions in Motivational Interviewing, 297
opportunities for behavioural change, 290–292
organic conservation agriculture, 325
organic food and cancer, 77
organic pollutants, persistent (POPs), 77
organophosphates, 322
Ornish (Lifestyle Heart) Study, 50, 51, 106

---

*Illustrations (figures and tables) are comprehensively referred to from the text. Therefore, significant items in illustrations have only been given a page reference in the absence of their concomitant mention in the text referring to that illustration.
**Abbreviation: PBD, plant-based diet.

Orthodox Christians during Lent, 109
osteoporosis, 242–243, 246, 250
ovaries, polycystic disease, 205–207
overweight *see* obesity and overweight
ovulation infertility (OI), 209–210
Oxford
    EPIC-Oxford study, 54, 59, 121, 142, 167, 241, 242
    Oxford Vegetarian Study, 78–79
oxidative stress, 13, 95, 114
    chronic inflammation and autoimmune disease and, 231
    mental disorders and, 184
oxygen
    consumption, maximal (VO2 max), 274, 276
    reactive species of (ROS), 13, 52

palmitic acid, 127
pandemics
    COVID-19, 17–18
    synergy of (obesity/undernutrition/climate change), 316
papulopustular rosacea, 257
patient factors in behavioural change, 292
PCOS *see* polycystic ovary syndrome
performance enhancers (ergogenic aids), 280–281
perimenopause, 202
period problems, 201–202
persistent organic pollutants (POPs), 77
personal identity and motivation to change to PBD, 288
pesco-vegetarian diet, 2
pesticides (incl. insecticides and herbicides), 77, 317, 318–319, 322
pharmacotherapy *see* medical therapy
PhIP (2-amino-1-methyl-6-phenylimidazo[4,5-b]pyridine), 76
phosphate (blood), elevated, 142–143
phosphocreatine energy system, 273
phosphorus and bone health, 248
physical environment and behavioural change, 290–292
physical exercise *see* exercise
physical opportunity for behavioural change, 289–290, 293
physicians *see* health professionals
phytate, 142
    zinc and, 29
phytochemicals and phytonutrients
    anticancer, 70–71, 72
    bone health, 245
phytoestrogens, 199, 200, 203
phytosterols
    autoimmune thyroid disease, 233
    cardiovascular disease and, 56

planetary health, 15, 315–330
Planetary Health Plate, 15
planning in Motivational Interviewing, 295
plant(s), sources of various nutrients, 30–31
    see also entries under phyto-
plant-based diet (basics/generalities)
    adopting, 285–300
    age and, 27–43, 303–304
    barriers, 287–292
    concept, 105
    definition, 2
    differences from other eating patterns, 109–112
    health and disease and impact of, 1–26
    as Pillar 1 of lifestyle medicine, 303–304
    unhealthy, 47
    whole *see* whole food PBD
plant-based diet index (provegetarian score), 7, 10–11
plastic, tiny particles of (microplastics), 77
Pleasure Trap, 289
pollutants from agriculture (incl. agrochemicals), 77, 318–319, 320, 321, 322, 325
polycyclic aromatic hydrocarbons, 75–76
polycystic ovarian syndrome, 205–207
polyphenols, 53, 128, 156, 223, 233
polyunsaturated fats/fatty acids (PUFAs)
    athletes and, 276
    bone health and, 244
    cardiovascular disease and, 57
    dementia and, 223
    in fish, 262
    non-alcoholic fatty liver disease and, 155
    see also omega-3 fatty acids
population-based interventions, 16–17
Portfolio diet, 7–8, 56
positive symptoms, psychosis, 189
post-exercise (post-training) period
    carbohydrate, 275
    fat, 276
    fluids, 280
    protein, 277
    pseudo-anaemia, 279
postmenopausal women *see* menopause
potassium (blood), high (hyperkalaemia), 143–144
potato consumption, 11
poultry and digestive health, 173
POUNDS LOST study, 110, 111
PPARs (peroxisome proliferator-activated receptors), 152, 155
practitioners *see* health professionals
prebiotics, 183, 231
    fibre as, 80
pre-conception health, 209, 211

pre-contemplation stage (of behavioural change), 286, 298
PREDIMED, 7, 49, 51, 59, 90, 220–221
pregnancy, 36–38
    eczema (infants) and, 259, 260
    folate/folic acid, 36, 210
    preconception health, 209, 211
preparation stage (of behavioural change), 286, 298
prescribing exercise, 304, 305
Prevotella, 232
Primary Prevention of Cardiovascular Disease, 15
Pritikin programme, 124
processed food, Alzheimer's disease and, 220
processed meat, 151–152
    cancer and, 12–13, 73–74, 74
    digestive health and, 173
    insulin resistance and, 123, 128
    non-alcoholic fatty liver disease and, 151–152
prospective cohort study, 3–5, 8, 10–11
prostate cancer, 76, 82
protein
    age-related recommended intakes, 30–31
    elderly, 39
    animal *see* animal protein
    athletes, 276–278
        supplements, 280–281
    bone health and, 244
    as energy source, 276–278
        as last resort, 274
    fertility and, 216
    kidney disease and, 144
    pregnancy/lactation AND, 37–38
    weight management and, 110–111
    see also high-protein diets
proton pump inhibitors, 164
provegetarian score, 7, 10–11
provitamin A, 28
psoriasis, 261–262
psychological capability to change to PBD, 289, 293
psychological health *see* mental health
psychosis, 189, 189–190
Public Health England
    Eatwell Guide, 32
    vitamin D supplements, 278
pulmonary disease (non-vascular) *see* lung
pulmonary hypertension (vascular), 96
pulses and weight management, 111–112

quercetin, 71

randomised controlled trials (in general), 3, 4, 5

reactive oxygen species (ROS), 13, 52
receptors for advanced glycation end products (RAGES), 95, 211
red meat, 151–152, 290
    cancer and, 12–13, 73–74, 74–75
        colorectal, 12–13, 74, 167
        prevention of, 80
    diabetes and, 122–123
    digestive health and, 173
    endometriosis and, 199
    fibroids and, 200
    non-alcoholic fatty liver disease and, 151–152
    processed, 123, 151–152, 199, 222
reflections in Motivational Interviewing, 297
reflective motivation, 287, 288, 293, 294
reforestation, 326
REM sleep, 306
renal problems *see* kidney
resource poor-countries *see* low-income countries
respiratory disorders, 89–102
restrictive lung disease, 98
resveratrol, 70
retinopathy, diabetic, 124, 126
reward system, 113
rheumatoid arthritis, 235
risky substances, 308–310
rosacea, 257–258
rosmarinic acid, 71
Rotterdam Study, diabetes, 122

St Thomas' Atheroma Regression Study (STARS), 51
salt (dietary), 250
Sao Paulo Declaration (on planetary health), 326
sarcopenia, 244, 246
Sardinia, 3, 57
satiety, 113
saturated fat/fatty acids (SFA), 5, 6, 48, 111
    bone health and, 244–245
    dementia/Alzheimer's disease and, 222
    non-alcoholic fatty liver disease and, 152
    psoriasis and, 261
    reduction, 55, 152
scarring lung diseases, 96
Scientific Advisory Committee on Nutrition, 129
Scotland, bone health study, 246
sea environment and fishing, 321

seaweed and endometriosis, 198
sedentary behaviour, 304–305
    physical activity factors to calculate energy requirements, 273
selenium, 29–32
    age-related recommended intakes, 30–31
Seven Countries Study, 48
sex/gender-specific health considerations, 197–217
sex hormone binding globulin (SHBG), 198
short-chain fatty acids (SCFAs), 14, 223, 232
    athletes and, 276
    diabetes and, 127–128
    gut microbiome and, 164, 183, 232
    mental health and, 183
silicon and bone health, 249
skeletal framework and osteoporosis, 243
skin diseases, 255–269
sleep, 305–307
    alcohol and, 310
    assessment and recommendations, 306–307
    cycles, 306
    hygiene practices, 307
    insufficient, impact of, 306
sleep apnoea, obstructive, 96–97
Slovenian study of gut microbiota, 232
SMILES trial, 184, 188
smoking, 5, 308–309
    cancer and, 5, 76
    cessation, 309
        gastro-oesophageal reflux disease and, 165
    COPD and, 90, 91, 92, 93
    heart disease and, 48
social environment and relationships
    as behavioural change opportunity, 290–292, 293
    as pillar of lifestyle medicine, 310–311
soil degradation and erosion, 320
soy(a)
    bone health and, 244
    cancer and, 81
    fibroids and, 200
    fortified soya foods, 249–250
    male hormones and, 208
    menopause and, 204
    weight management and, 110
spinal fractures in osteoporosis, 242
sportspersons, 271–284
STABILITY (Stabilization of Atherosclerotic Plaque by Initiation of Darapladib Therapy), 50
stachyose, 249
stages of change model, 285–287, 296
Stancic, Dr Saray, 301
STARS (St Thomas' Atheroma Regression Study), 51
steatohepatitis, non-alcoholic (NASH), 149, 150, 151, 153, 155, 156, 157, 158
sterols (plant) *see* phytosterols
stigma with PBDs, 288
stones, kidney, 145
stress
    differential stress resistance between healthy and cancer cells, 81
    oxidative *see* oxidative stress
    personal/psychological, and its management, 307–308
stroke, 58–59
substances, risky, 308–310
sugars (added)
    Alzheimer's disease, 222
    non-alcoholic fatty liver disease, 152–153
sulphoraphene, 71
sulphur-containing amino acids, 12
summary in Motivational Interviewing, 297
sunlight and vitamin D, 28
supplements (in general)
    athletes, 278, 279, 280–281
    birth to 3 year-olds, 33–34
    dementia prevention, 223
    polycystic ovary syndrome (PCOS), 206–207
support systems, 310–311
sweating, athletes, 280
systemic lupus erythematosus (SLE), 233

Taiwanese
    diabetes, 122
    Tzu Chi health/vegetarian studies, 8, 59, 221
taste and motivation to change to PBD, 288
teenagers *see* adolescents
Tehran Lipid and Glucose Study (TLGS), 139
telomeres, 53, 307
thermic effects of foods, 113
thymoquinone, 71
thyroid
    autoimmune disease, 233
    hormones, fertility and, 210
tick bites and urticaria, 264

---

*Illustrations (figures and tables) are comprehensively referred to from the text. Therefore, significant items in illustrations have only been given a page reference in the absence of their concomitant mention in the text referring to that illustration.
**Abbreviation: PBD, plant-based diet.

tillage agriculture, 317, 318, 319–320, 320, 325
TMAO *see* trimethylamine N-oxide
tobacco control efforts, 309
　see also smoking
tofu, 249
toxoplasmosis, 36
trans fats/fatty acids, 55, 222
transient receptor potential (TRP) channels, 257–258
transtheoretical model of change, 285–287, 296
trials (nutritional), types, 3–6
trigger foods, gastro-oesophageal reflux disease, 164
triglyceride reduction, 56
trimethylamine N-oxide (TMAO), 14, 53, 113–114
　cancer and, 74–75
　cardiovascular disease and, 74–75
　diabetes and, 127, 128
　erectile dysfunction and, 209
　hidradenitis suppurativa and, 263
　non-alcoholic fatty liver disease and, 151
　weight and, 113–114
Tsimane case study, 45–46
Tzu Chi health/vegetarian studies, 8, 59, 221

UK *see* United Kingdom
ulcerative colitis, 172–173
ultraprocessed foods and cancer, 79
undernutrition, 316, 321
underweight, 40, 103
　fasting and, 82
United Kingdom (UK)
　Biobank studies, 54, 173, 224
　COVID-19, 17
United States (USA)
　cardiovascular disease and unhealthy diet patterns in southern states, 47
　COVID-19, 17
　National Cholesterol Education Programme (NCEP), 9, 106
　non-alcoholic fatty liver disease in prevalence and burden, 150
　standard diet and, 151
　see also entries under American
unsaturated fats/fatty acids
　monounsaturated (MUFAs), 8, 49, 57, 155
　polyunsaturated *see* polyunsaturated fats/fatty acids
uraemic toxins, 143
ursolic acid, 71
urticaria, 264
USA *see* United States

uterine leiomyomas, 200–201

vagus nerve, 182, 183
vegan diet, 8–9
　bone health *see* bone health
　cancer and, 78–79
　definition, 2
　diabetes and, 121, 122, 124–125, 126, 127
　elderly, 38–40
　gluten-free, 106
　gut profile, 232
　weight changes and, 106–109
vegetables *see* cruciferous vegetables; fruit and/or vegetable consumption
vegetarian diet, 2, 8–9
　bone health and, 241–242
　cancer and, 78–79
　cardiovascular disease and, 52
　casual (flexitarian), 2
　diverticular disease and, 166
　weight changes and, 106, 109
very-low-calorie diets, 128–129
very-low-density lipoprotein (VLDL), 47, 48
Vietnam, bone health in postmenopausal women, 245
vitamin A, 28
　age-related recommended intakes, 30–31
　bone health and, 246
vitamin B12, 27–28
　acne and, 257
　age and, 27, 27–28, 30–31
　elderly, 39
　athletes, 278
　bone health and, 247
　dementia prevention and, 223
　pregnancy and, 36
　supplements, 27–28, 36
vitamin C and bone health, 245, 247
vitamin D, 28
　age and, 27, 28, 30–31
　elderly, 39
　athletes, 278
　atopic dermatitis and, 261
　bone health and, 242, 246–247, 248
　fertility and, 210
　fibroids and, 200–201
　menstrual period problems, 202
　polycystic ovary syndrome and, 206
　pregnancy/lactation and, 36–37
　urticaria and, 264
vitamin K and K2
　bone health and, 245, 247–248
　dialysis and, 144–145

water
　agricultural use, 321
　in fruit and vegetables, 112
　see also fluid intake; hydration
weight (body), 103–120
　cancer and, 73, 83
　mental health and gain in, 184–185
　severe, 190
　respiratory health and, 89–90, 95
　see also obesity; underweight
weight loss
　elderly, 40
　interventions for, 105–112
　　gastro-oesophageal reflux disease and, 165
　　limitation of current pharmaceuticals and lifestyle modification, 105
　　menopause, 203
　　non-alcoholic fatty liver disease and, 155
　　polycystic ovary syndrome, 206
　observational evidence, 106
Westernised diet, 321
　African diet and, microbiomes, 232
　autoimmune disease and, 229, 230, 231, 232
　depression and, 187
　dermatology and, 256
　endometriosis and, 198
　irritable bowel disease and, 170
　kidney disease (chronic) and, 141
Whitehall Study, 220
WHO *see* World Health Organization
whole diet interventions, mental disorders, 185
whole food PBD (whole plant foods; WFPBD), 8–9
　bone health and, 241, 243
　cancer and, 80
　definition, 2
　diabetes and, 125
　endometriosis and, 198
　erectile dysfunction and, 209
　in Esseltyne Program, 297–298
　group consultations and, 296–297
　kidney disease (chronic) and, 139
　menopause and, 203
　polycystic ovary syndrome and, 206
whole grains
　beta-glucan fibre in, 183
　cancer and, 80
Wolff's law, 243
women (females), 197–207
　fertility, 209–211
　see also menopause
Women's Health Initiative study, 4, 8, 82

WONCA (World Organization of Family Doctors), 16
World Cancer Research Fund, 15, 76, 79, 166, 167
World Health Organization (WHO), 2
  colorectal cancer and, 73
  definition of healthy diet, 6
  dementia, 222
  leading causes of death factsheets, 91, 92
World Heart Federation (2015), 46
World Organization of Family Doctors (WONCA), 16
World Vegetarian and Vegan Congress, gut profile of attendees, 232
worldwide *see* global dimensions

yeast (brewer's) and hidradenitis suppurativa, 263

zinc, 29
  age-related recommended intakes, 30–31
  athletes, 280
  bone health and, 249
  fertility, 210
Zoe COVID-19 symptom study, 17
zoonoses, 321–322

---

*Illustrations (figures and tables) are comprehensively referred to from the text. Therefore, significant items in illustrations have only been given a page reference in the absence of their concomitant mention in the text referring to that illustration.
**Abbreviation: PBD, plant-based diet.